Wilcox's Surgical Anatomy of the Heart

Wilcox's Surgical Anatomy of the Heart

Robert H. Anderson
Institute of Genetic Medicine, Newcastle University, UK

Andrew C. Cook
University College London, UK

Diane E. Spicer
Johns Hopkins All Children's Hospital, USA

Anthony M. Hlavacek
Medical University of South Carolina, USA

Carl L. Backer
Cincinnati Children's Hospital, USA

Justin T. Tretter
Cleveland Clinic, USA

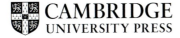

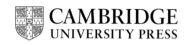

Shaftesbury Road, Cambridge CB2 8EA, United Kingdom

One Liberty Plaza, 20th Floor, New York, NY 10006, USA

477 Williamstown Road, Port Melbourne, VIC 3207, Australia

314–321, 3rd Floor, Plot 3, Splendor Forum, Jasola District Centre,
New Delhi – 110025, India

103 Penang Road, #05–06/07, Visioncrest Commercial, Singapore 238467

Cambridge University Press is part of Cambridge University Press & Assessment,
a department of the University of Cambridge.

We share the University's mission to contribute to society through the pursuit of
education, learning and research at the highest international levels of excellence.

www.cambridge.org
Information on this title: www.cambridge.org/9781009387392
DOI: 10.1017/9781009387408

© Robert H. Anderson, Andrew C. Cook, Diane E. Spicer, Anthony M. Hlavacek, Carl
L. Backer, and Justin T. Tretter 2024

This publication is in copyright. Subject to statutory exception and to the provisions
of relevant collective licensing agreements, no reproduction of any part may take
place without the written permission of Cambridge University Press & Assessment.

This fifth edition published 2024
Fourth edition first published 2013
Third edition first published 2004

Printed in the United Kingdom by TJ Books Limited, Padstow Cornwall

A catalogue record for this publication is available from the British Library

Library of Congress Cataloging-in-Publication Data
Names: Anderson, Robert H. (Robert Henry), 1942– author. | Cook, Andrew C.,
author. | Spicer, Diane E., author. | Hlavacek, Anthony M., author. | Backer, Carl L.,
author. | Tretter, Justin T., author.
Title: Wilcox's surgical anatomy of the heart / Robert H. Anderson, Andrew C. Cook,
Diane E. Spicer, Anthony M. Hlavacek, Carl L. Backer, Justin T. Tretter.
Other titles: Surgical anatomy of the heart.
Description: 5. | Cambridge, United Kingdom ; New York, NY : Cambridge
University Press, 2024. | Includes bibliographical references and index.
Identifiers: LCCN 2023042773 (print) | LCCN 2023042774 (ebook) | ISBN
9781009443913 (hardback) | ISBN 9781009387408 (ebook) | ISBN 9781009387392
(mixed media)
Subjects: MESH: Cardiac Surgical Procedures | Heart – anatomy & histology | Atlas
Classification: LCC QM181 (print) | LCC QM181 (ebook) | NLM WG 17 |
DDC 611/.12–dc23/eng/20231102
LC record available at https://lccn.loc.gov/2023042773
LC ebook record available at https://lccn.loc.gov/2023042774

ISBN 978-1-009-44391-3 Hardback
ISBN 978-1-009-38740-8 Cambridge Core
ISBN 978-1-009-38739-2 Mixed Media

Cambridge University Press & Assessment has no responsibility for the persistence
or accuracy of URLs for external or third-party internet websites referred to in this
publication and does not guarantee that any content on such websites is, or will
remain, accurate or appropriate.

Every effort has been made in preparing this book to provide accurate and up-to-date
information that is in accord with accepted standards and practice at the time of
publication. Although case histories are drawn from actual cases, every effort has been
made to disguise the identities of the individuals involved. Nevertheless, the authors,
editors, and publishers can make no warranties that the information contained herein is
totally free from error, not least because clinical standards are constantly changing through
research and regulation. The authors, editors, and publishers therefore disclaim all liability
for direct or consequential damages resulting from the use of material contained in this
book. Readers are strongly advised to pay careful attention to information provided by the
manufacturer of any drugs or equipment that they plan to use.

Contents

Preface vii
Acknowledgements viii

1 Surgical Approaches to the Heart 1
2 Development of the Heart 11
3 Anatomy of the Cardiac Chambers 41
4 Surgical Anatomy of the Valves of the Heart 77
5 Surgical Anatomy of the Coronary Circulation 113
6 Surgical Anatomy of Cardiac Conduction 133
7 Analytic Description of Congenitally Malformed Hearts 153

8 Lesions with Normal Segmental Connections

8.1 **Septal Defects** 175
8.2 **Atrioventricular Septal Defects** 191
8.3 **Ventricular Septal Defects** 215
8.4 **Malformations of the Valves of the Heart** 234
8.5 **Tetralogy of Fallot and Pulmonary Atresia with an Intact Ventricular Septum** 261
8.6 **Hypoplastic Left Heart Syndrome** 283

9 Lesions in Hearts with Abnormal Segmental Connections

9.1 **Functionally Univentricular Heart** 299
9.2 **Discordant Ventriculo-Arterial Connections** 321
9.3 **Double Outlet Ventricle** 353
9.4 **Common Arterial Trunk** 369
9.5 **Concordant Ventriculo-Arterial Connections with Parallel Arterial Trunks** 392

10 Abnormalities of the Great Vessels

10.1 **Anomalous Systemic Venous Connections** 407
10.2 **Anomalous Pulmonary Venous Connections** 418
10.3 **Obstructive Abnormalities of the Extrapericardial Systemic Pathways** 427
10.4 **Vascular Rings** 437
10.5 **Pulmonary Arterial and Ductal Anomalies** 448
10.6 **Anomalies of the Coronary Arteries and Aortoventricular Tunnels** 456

11 Positional Anomalies of the Heart 465

Index 478

This book provides access to an online version on Cambridge Core, which can be accessed via the code printed on the inside of the cover

Preface

The books and articles devoted to technique in cardiac surgery are legion. This is most appropriate, since the success of cardiac surgery is greatly dependent upon excellent operative technique. But excellence of technique can be dissipated without a firm knowledge of the underlying cardiac morphology. This is just as true for the normal heart as for those hearts with complex congenital lesions. It is the feasibility of operating on such complex malformations that has highlighted the need for a more detailed understanding of the basic anatomy in itself. Thus, in recent years surgeons have come to appreciate the necessity of avoiding damage to the coronary vessels, often invisible when working within the cardiac chambers, and particularly to avoid the vital conduction tissues, invisible at all times. Although detailed and accurate descriptions of the conduction system have been available since the time of their discovery, only rarely has its position been described with the cardiac surgeon in mind. At the time the first edition of this volume was published, to the best of our knowledge, there had been no other books that specifically displayed the anatomy of normal and abnormal hearts as perceived at the time of operation. We tried to satisfy this need in the first volume by combining the experience of a practicing cardiac surgeon with that of a professional cardiac anatomist. We added significantly to the illustrations in the second edition, whilst seeking to retain the overall concept, since feedback from those who had used the first edition was very positive. In the third edition, we sought to expand and improve still further on the changes made in the second edition. In the second edition, we had added an entirely new chapter on cardiac valvar anatomy, and greatly expanded our treatment of coronary vascular anatomy. We retained this format in the third edition, since we were gratified that, as hoped, readers were able to find a particular subject more easily. The third edition also contained still more new illustrations, retaining the approach of orienting these illustrations, where appropriate, as seen by the surgeon working in the operating room, but reverting to anatomical orientation for most of the pictures of specimens. So as to clarify the various orientations of each individual illustration, we continued to include a set of axes showing, when appropriate, the directions of superior, inferior, anterior, posterior, left, right, apex, and base. All accounts were based on the anatomy as it is observed. In the previous editions, however, except in the case of malformations involving the aortic arch and its branches, we had avoided embryological speculations. That has now changed, since as we show in our new chapter devoted to development, it is now possible to describe the changes taking place on the basis of evidence rather than speculation.

In May of 2010, just prior to the preparation of the fourth edition, our original surgical author, Benson Wilcox, sadly died. Although it was difficult to replace such a pioneer and champion of surgical education, we were gratified that Carl Backer agreed to join us, and assume the role of surgical editor. We were also pleased to add Diane Spicer to our anatomical team, along with Tony Hlavacek. Tony had been at the forefront of providing quite remarkable images obtained using computed tomography and magnetic resonance imaging, showing that the heart could be imaged with just as much accuracy during life as when the anatomists amongst us are able to hold the specimens in our hands. We are now also delighted, as we prepare the fifth edition, to be joined by Justin Tretter, who is equally skilled in the art of virtual dissection of three-dimensional computed tomographic datasets.

In seeking to recognize the huge contributions of Ben Wilcox, we had re-named the fourth edition as *Wilcox's Surgical Anatomy of the Heart*. We are proud to retain this title for our fifth edition. As with the previous editions, it is our hope that the new edition will continue to be of interest not only to the surgeon, but also to the cardiologist, anaesthesiologist, and surgical pathologist. All of these practitioners ideally should have some knowledge of cardiac structures and their exquisite intricacies, particularly those cardiologists who increasingly treat lesions that previously were the province of the surgeon. Our senior anatomist still remains active, despite his increasing years. It has been his association with Diane Spicer and Justin Tretter that has permitted him to continue to advance his knowledge of the normal and congenitally malformed heart, sharing all that information with Carl Backer and Andrew Cook, with Andrew now bringing still more advanced information from hearts imaged using synchrotron-based phase-contrast tomography. We remain confident that, in the hands of our new team, and if supply demands, the book will pass through still further editions, hopefully continuing to improve with each version.

Robert H. Anderson, Andrew C. Cook, Diane E. Spicer, Anthony M. Hlavacek, Justin T. Tretter, Carl L. Backer
London, Tampa, Charleston, Cleveland, and Lexington
April 2023

Acknowledgements

A good deal of the material displayed in these pages, and the concepts espoused, are due in no small part to the help of our friends and collaborators. Despite the alleged 'retirement' of our senior anatomist from the Institute of Child Health at Great Ormond Street Children's Hospital prior to the appearance of the previous edition, his added time has continued to permit him to establish new connections, with ongoing additions to our team of authors. More new hearts have been specifically photographed for this new edition, due to the ongoing efforts of Diane Spicer and Andrew Cook. The addition of Justin Tretter to the team has permitted us to include many more wonderful images obtained using virtual dissection of computed tomographic datasets. For this edition, however, our greatest debt is owed to those who collaborated in producing the new chapter on cardiac development. Hence, we express our deepest gratitude to Jill Hikspoors, Wout Lamers, and Tim Mohun. We have sought to improve on our illustrations as new material comes to hand, but it remains the fact that we could not have produced our book without the help of Anton Becker, long retired from the University of Amsterdam, and Bob Zuberbuhler of Pittsburgh Children's Hospital, Pennsylvania, United States of America, who sadly passed on since the appearance of the fourth edition. We also remain indebted to the initial contributions of Siew Yen Ho, still associated with the National Heart and Lung Institute and part of Imperial College in London. Yen produced many of the original drawings from which we prepared our artwork, and photographed many of the hearts in the Brompton archive. The initial photographs and surgical artwork could not have been produced without the considerable help given by the Department of Medical Illustrations and Photography, University of North Carolina. As with all the previous editions, we owe an equal debt of gratitude to Gemma Price, who has continued to improve our series of cartoons. For the previous editions, and now this one, she has worked over and above the call of duty. Finally, it is a pleasure to acknowledge the ongoing support provided by Cambridge University Press. The Press has ensured that all the good parts of the previous editions were retained and encouraged us to make the changes needed for this edition. In particular, we thank Nicholas Dunton and Jessica Papworth for all their help during the preparation of the book for publication. We are equally indebted to Beth Morel for her eagle-eyed copy-editing.

Chapter 1
Surgical Approaches to the Heart

When we describe the heart in this chapter, and in subsequent chapters, our account will be based on the organ as viewed in its anatomical position.[1] Where appropriate, the heart will be illustrated as it would be viewed by the surgeon during an operative procedure, irrespective of whether the pictures are taken in the operating room, or are photographs of autopsied hearts. When we show an illustration in non-surgical orientation, this will be clearly stated.

In the normal individual, the heart lies in the mediastinum, with two-thirds of its bulk to the left of the midline (Figure 1.1). The surgeon can approach the heart, and the great vessels, either laterally through the thoracic cavity, or directly through the mediastinum anteriorly. To make such approaches safely, knowledge is required of the salient anatomical features of the chest wall, and of the vessels and the nerves that course through the mediastinum (Figure 1.2). The approach used most frequently is a complete median sternotomy, although increasingly the trend is to use more limited incisions. The incision in the soft tissues is made in the midline between the suprasternal notch and the xiphoid process. Inferiorly, the white line, or linea alba, is incised between the two rectus sheaths, taking care to avoid entry to the peritoneal cavity, or damage to an enlarged liver, if present. Reflection of the origin of the rectus muscles in this area reveals the xiphoid process, which is then incised to provide inferior access to the anterior mediastinum. Superiorly, a vertical incision is made between the sternal insertions of the sternocleidomastoid muscles. This exposes the relatively bloodless midline raphe between the right and left sternohyoid and sternothyroid muscles. An incision through this raphe then gives access to the superior aspect of the anterior mediastinum. The anterior mediastinum immediately behind the sternum is devoid of vital structures, so that the superior and inferior incisions into the mediastinum can safely be joined by blunt dissection in the retrosternal space. Having split the sternum, retraction will reveal the pericardial sac, lying between the pleural cavities. Superiorly, the thymus

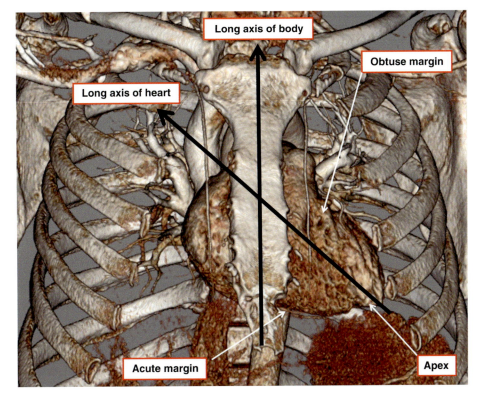

Figure 1.1 The computed tomogram, with the cardiac cavities delimited subsequent to injection of contrast material, shows well the relationships of the heart to the thoracic structures. Note the discordance between the long axis of the heart and the long axis of the body.

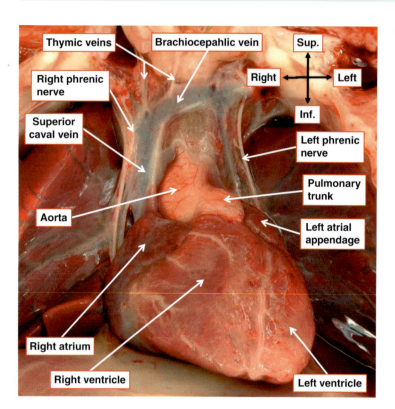

Figure 1.2 This view, taken at autopsy, demonstrates the anatomical relationships of the vessels and nerves within the mediastinum.

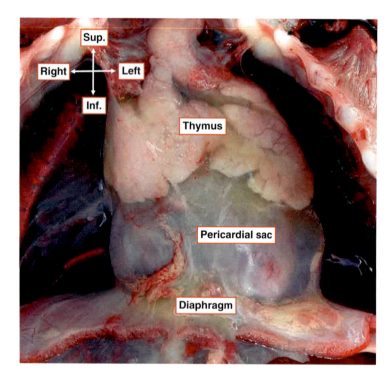

Figure 1.3 This view, taken at autopsy, demonstrates the extent of the thymus as it extends over the anterior and lateral aspects of the pericardial sac at the base of the heart.

gland wraps itself over the anterior and lateral aspects of the pericardium in the area of exit of the great arteries, the gland being a particularly prominent structure in the infant (Figures 1.3, 1.4). It has two lateral lobes, joined more or less in the midline. Sometimes this junction between the lobes must be divided, or partially excised, to provide adequate exposure. The arterial supply to the thymus is from the internal thoracic and inferior thyroid arteries. If divided, these arteries tend to retreat into the surrounding soft tissues, and can produce troublesome bleeding. The veins draining the thymus are fragile, often emptying into the left brachiocephalic, or innominate, vein via a common trunk (Figure 1.5). Undue traction on the gland can lead to damage to this major vessel.

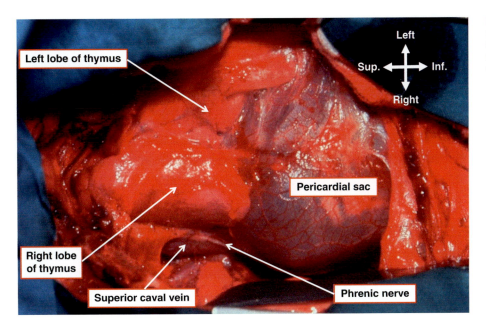

Figure 1.4 This view, taken in the operating room through a median sternotomy in an infant, shows the extent of the thymus gland. Note the right phrenic nerve adjacent to the superior caval vein.

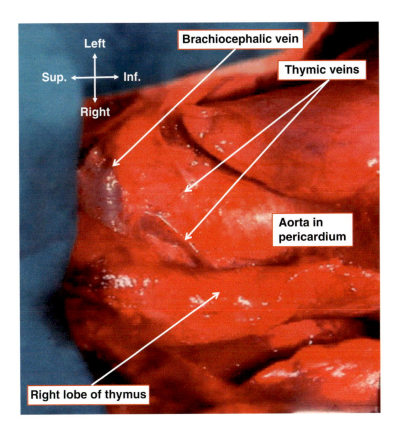

Figure 1.5 This operative view, again taken through a median sternotomy, shows the delicate veins that drain from the thymus gland to the left brachiocephalic veins.

When the pericardial sac is exposed within the mediastinum, the surgeon should have no problems in gaining access to the heart. The vagus and phrenic nerves traverse the length of the pericardium, but are well lateral (Figures 1.2, 1.6). The phrenic nerve on each side passes anteriorly, and the vagus nerve posteriorly, relative to the hilums of the lungs (Figure 1.6).

At operation, the course of the phrenic nerve is seen most readily through a lateral thoracotomy (Figure 1.7). It is when the heart is approached through a median sternotomy, therefore, with the nerve not immediately evident, that it is most liable to injury. Although it can sometimes be seen through the reflected pericardium (Figure 1.8), its proximity to the superior caval vein (Figures 1.2, 1.9, 1.10), or to a persistent left caval vein when that structure is present (Figure 1.11), is not always easily appreciated when these vessels are dissected from the anterior approach. Near the thoracic inlet, it passes close to the internal thoracic artery (Figures 1.6, 1.10),

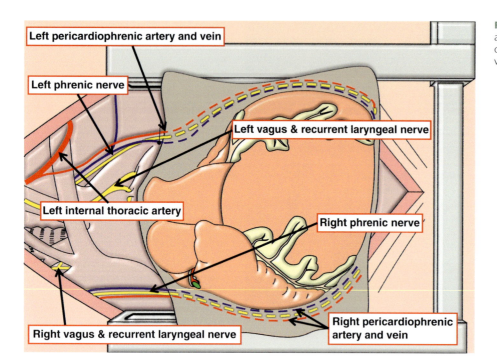

Figure 1.6 As shown in this cartoon of a median sternotomy, the pericardium can be opened in the midline so that the phrenic and vagus nerves stay well clear of the operating field.

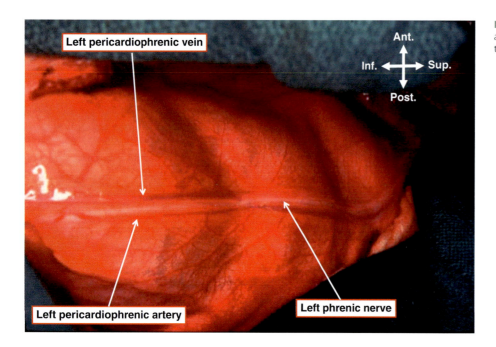

Figure 1.7 This operative view, taken through a left lateral thoracotomy, shows the course of the left phrenic nerve over the pericardium.

exposing it to injury either directly during takedown of that vessel, or by avulsing the pericardiophrenic artery with excessive traction on the chest wall. The internal thoracic arteries themselves are most vulnerable to injury during closure of the sternum. The phrenic nerve may be injured when removing the pericardium to use as a cardiac patch, or when performing a pericardiectomy. Injudicious use of cooling agents within the pericardial cavity may also lead to phrenic paralysis or paresis.

A standard lateral thoracotomy provides access to the heart and great vessels via the pleural space. Left-sided incisions provide ready access to the great arteries, left pulmonary veins, and the chambers of the left side of the heart. Most frequently, the incision is made in the fourth intercostal space. The posterior extent is through the triangular, and relatively bloodless, space between the edges of the latissimus dorsi, trapezius, and teres major muscles (Figure 1.12). The floor of this triangle is the sixth intercostal space. Division of the latissimus dorsi, and a portion of trapezius posteriorly, frees the scapula so that the fourth intercostal space can be identified. Its precise identity should be confirmed by counting down the ribs from above. The so-called

1 Surgical Approaches to the Heart

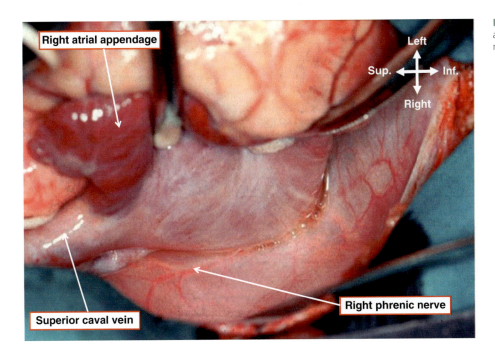

Figure 1.8 This operative view, taken through a median sternotomy, shows the right phrenic nerve as seen through the reflected pericardium.

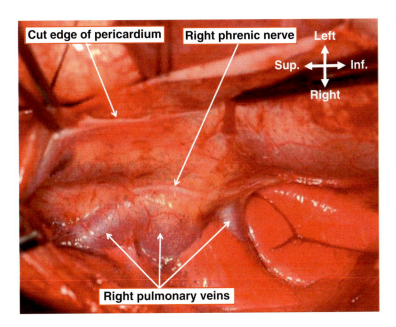

Figure 1.9 This operative view, taken through a median sternotomy having pulled back the edge of the pericardial sac, shows the right phrenic nerve in relation to the right pulmonary veins.

muscle-sparing thoracotomy is designed to preserve the latissimus dorsi and serratus anterior. In cases requiring greater degrees of exposure, the latissimus dorsi can be partially divided. It is rarely, if ever, necessary to divide the serratus anterior. The intercostal muscles are then divided equidistant between the fourth and fifth ribs. The incision is rarely carried forward beyond the midclavicular line in a submammary position, being careful to avoid damage to the nipple and the tissue of the breast. The intercostal neurovascular bundle is well protected beneath the lower margin of the fourth rib. Having divided the musculature as far as the pleura, the pleural space is entered and the lung permitted to collapse away from the chest wall. Posterior retraction of the lung reveals the middle mediastinum, in which the left lateral lobe of the thymus, with its associated nerves and vessels, is seen overlying the pericardial sac and the aortic arch. Intrapericardial access is usually gained anterior to the phrenic nerve. On occasion, the thymus gland may require elevation when the incision is extended superiorly, taking precautions to avoid unwanted damage, as discussed above. The lung is retracted anteriorly to approach the aortic isthmus and descending thoracic aorta, and the parietal pleura is divided on its mediastinal aspect. This is usually done posterior to the vagus nerve. In this area, the vagus nerve gives off its left recurrent laryngeal branch, which then passes around the inferior border of the arterial

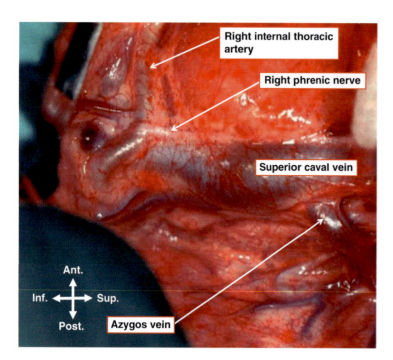

Figure 1.10 This operative view, taken through a right thoracotomy, shows the relationship of the right phrenic nerve to the right internal thoracic artery and the superior caval vein.

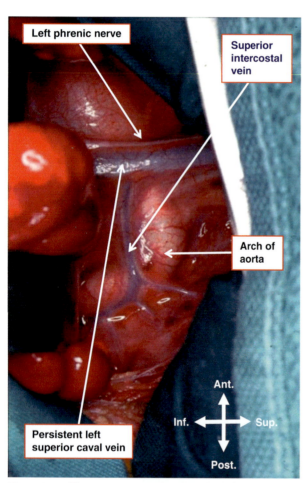

Figure 1.11 This operative view, taken through a left thoracotomy, shows the relationship of the left phrenic nerve to a persistent left superior caval vein. Note also the course of the superior intercostal vein.

ligament, or the duct if the arterial channel is still patent (Figure 1.13). The recurrent nerve then ascends towards the larynx on the medial aspect of the posterior wall of the aorta, running adjacent to the oesophagus. Excessive traction of the vagus nerve as it courses into the thorax along the left subclavian artery can cause injury to the recurrent laryngeal nerve just as readily as can direct trauma to the nerve in the environs of the ligament. The superior intercostal vein is seen crossing the aorta, then insinuating itself between the phrenic and vagus nerves (Figures 1.11, 1.14, 1.15). This structure is rarely of surgical significance, but is frequently divided to provide surgical access to the aorta. The thoracic duct (Figure 1.16) ascends through this area, draining into the junction of the left subclavian and internal jugular veins. Accessory lymph channels draining into the duct, which is usually posteriorly located, and runs along the vertebral column, can be troublesome when dissecting the origin of the left subclavian artery.

A right thoracotomy, in either the fourth or fifth interspace, is made through an incision similar to that for a left thoracotomy. The fifth interspace is used when approaching the heart, while the fourth permits access to the right-sided great vessels. Access to the pericardium is gained by incising anterior to the phrenic nerve, this approach often necessitating retraction of the right lobe of the thymus. To reach the right pulmonary artery, and its adjacent mediastinal structures, it is sometimes useful to divide the azygos vein near its junction with the superior caval vein (Figure 1.17). Extension of this incision superiorly exposes the origin of the right subclavian branch of the brachiocephalic trunk. Laterally, this artery is crossed by the right vagus nerve. The right recurrent laryngeal nerve takes origin from the vagus, and curls around the postero-inferior wall of the artery before ascending into the neck (Figure 1.18). Also encircling the

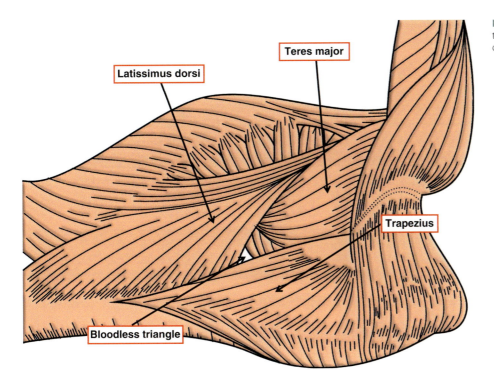

Figure 1.12 The cartoon shows the location of the bloodless area overlying the posterior extent of the sixth intercostal space.

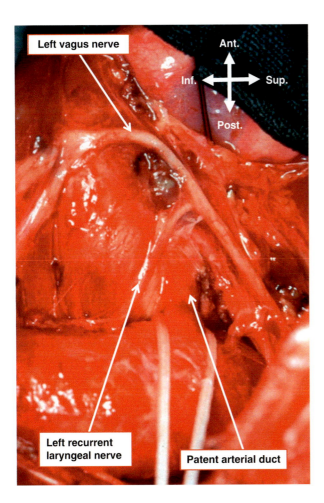

Figure 1.13 This operative view, taken through a left lateral thoracotomy in an adult, shows the left recurrent laryngeal nerve passing around the arterial duct.

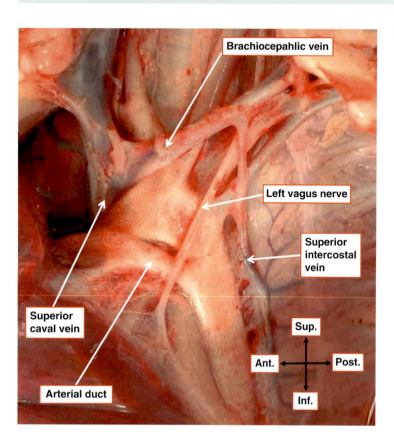

Figure 1.14 The anatomical image shows the course of the left superior intercostal vein.

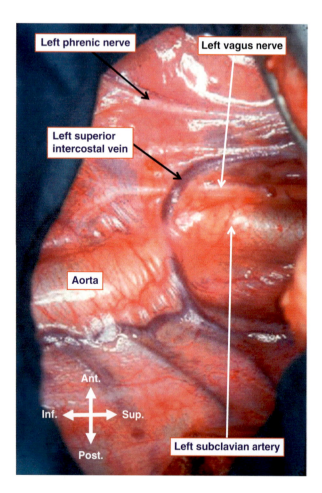

Figure 1.15 This operative view, taken through a left lateral thoracotomy, shows the course of the left superior intercostal vein. Compare with Figure 1.14.

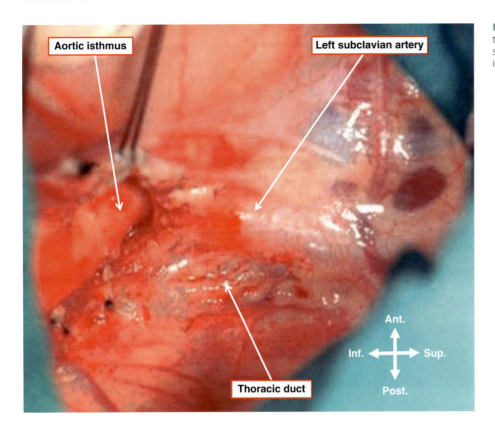

Figure 1.16 In this operative view, taken through a left thoracotomy, the thoracic duct is seen coursing below the left subclavian artery to its termination in the brachiocephalic vein.

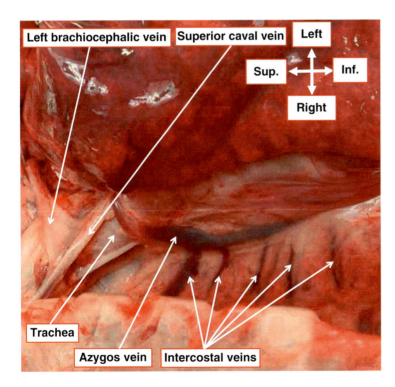

Figure 1.17 This anatomical image, taken at autopsy, shows the normal location of the azygos vein as it branches from the superior caval vein over the root of the right lung and extends along the spine.

subclavian origin on this right side is the subclavian sympathetic loop, the so-called ansa subclavia. This is a branch of the sympathetic trunk that runs up into the neck. Damage to this structure can produce Horner's syndrome.

An anterior right or left thoracotomy is occasionally used in treating congenital malformations. Once the chest is opened, the same basic anatomical rules apply as described above. Thus far, our account has presumed the presence of normal anatomy. In many instances, the disposition of the thoracic structures will be altered by a congenital malformation. These alterations will be described in the appropriate sections.

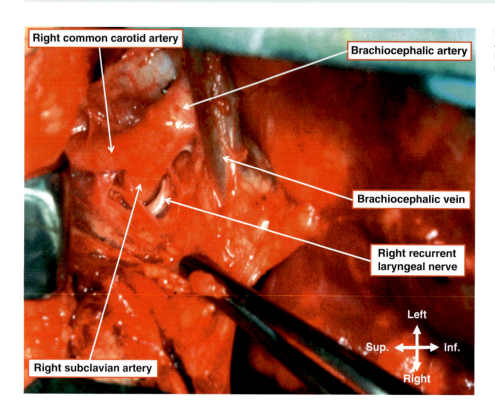

Figure 1.18 This operative view, taken through a median sternotomy, shows the course of the right recurrent laryngeal nerve relative to the right subclavian artery.

Reference Cited

1. Cook AC, Anderson RH. Attitudinally correct nomenclature. *Heart* 2002; **87**: 503–506.

Chapter 2

Development of the Heart

Robert H. Anderson,[1] Jill P.J.M Hikspoors,[2] Wouter H. Lamers,[2] and Timothy J. Mohun[3]

(1) Biosciences Institute, Newcastle University, Newcastle-upon-Tyne, UK
(2) Department of Anatomy and Embryology, Maastricht University, Maastricht, The Netherlands
(3) Francis Crick Institute, London, UK

Introduction

Cardiac surgeons, like paediatric cardiologists, consider that knowledge of cardiac development, and morphogenesis, is a major aid to the understanding of the anatomy of both the normal and the congenitally malformed heart. In previous editions of our textbook, we have eschewed the option of including a chapter on development. We had taken the stance that, until recently, accounts of the complex changes occurring during cardiac development were based on speculations, rather than evidence. Since the turn of the century, all that has changed. Evidence now exists not only to underpin accurate descriptions of the changes in morphology that occur during development, but also to reveal the lineages and molecular biology of the multiple tissues found in the definitive structures.[1] In this chapter, however, we will confine ourselves to description of the key morphological features of cardiac development.

The Linear Heart Tube

It used to be thought that all the components of the definitive organ were already present at the stage when the developing heart could be recognized as a linear tube, enclosed in a pericardial sac, and with a solitary cavity. We now know this is not the case. New material is added to the developing heart from the heart-forming regions within the embryo at both its arterial and venous poles.[2] It remains the case, nonetheless, that a solitary tube can still be recognized. It is observed in human development after about four weeks have passed subsequent to fertilization. The stages of human development are described on the basis of the system developed at the Carnegie Institute in the United States during the early part of the twentieth century.[3,4] In terms of that system, it becomes possible to recognize the linear tube at Carnegie stage 10 (Figure 2.1). The linear tube itself is formed by fusion of bilaterally symmetrical endocardial primordiums located in front of the developing foregut. Surrounded by acellular cardiac jelly, encased in myocardial walls, and initially lacking lumens, the endothelial tubes canalize as they become continuous caudally with an extensive venous plexus, made up of the vitelline vessels of the yolk sac and the umbilical veins connecting with the placenta (Figure 2.1A). At the cranial pole, the cavity of what will become the outflow tract is continuous with channels that pass around the developing pharynx. These are the ventral aortas. They provide continuity between the developing heart and the paired dorsal aortas (Figure 2.1). The cavity itself is shaped as an hourglass (Figure 2.1B), with the developing left ventricle at its caudal end, and the developing outflow tract cranially. The myocardium surrounding the developing left ventricle is known to have arisen from the so-called first heart field. The myocardium enclosing the outflow tract, in contrast, is derived from the so-called second heart field. An earlier contribution from the second field had formed the basis of the right ventricle, whilst further contributions form the atrial chambers, with still further contributions eventually producing the walls of the systemic venous sinus. The venous plexuses themselves merge outside the pericardial cavity to form hepatocardiac channels. These conduits, as they develop, provide the systemic venous inflows, which are initially bilaterally symmetrical. Within the myocardial walls, a thick layer of cardiac jelly still surrounds the solitary endocardial tube. The myocardial components are contiguous at the venous and arterial poles with the pharyngeal mesenchyme. These connections, known as mesocardium, connect the developing heart tube with the adjacent pharyngeal floor, providing portals for additional tissues to enter the heart as it develops.

Looping of the Heart Tube

By Carnegie stage 11, representing around 29 days of development, the linear tube has changed to an S-shaped configuration and has begun to beat. It is possible, at this stage, to recognize the ventricular loop. This connects at its leftward margin with the developing atrial component through a discrete atrioventricular canal. At its rightward end, it supports the outflow tract (Figure 2.2). Initially believed to reflect rapid growth of the tube within the constraining pericardial sac,[5] the process of looping is now considered an intrinsic feature of development, reflecting the known presence of Tbx2, which inhibits cellular proliferation, in the inner curvature of the developing loop. In normal development, the loop curves to the right.[6] Such rightward turning, independent of morphologically rightness or leftness within the heart, is part of the breaking of embryonic symmetry. Within the embryo itself, the neural plate by this stage has partially transformed into a tube. Although the pharynx has extended cranially and widened, as yet it has not produced any individual pharyngeal pouches. All of the endothelial cardiac tube, except for the venous inflows, is now invested in cardiac jelly and has myocardial walls (Figure 2.2A). The hepatocardiac channels continue to receive vitelline and umbilical tributaries

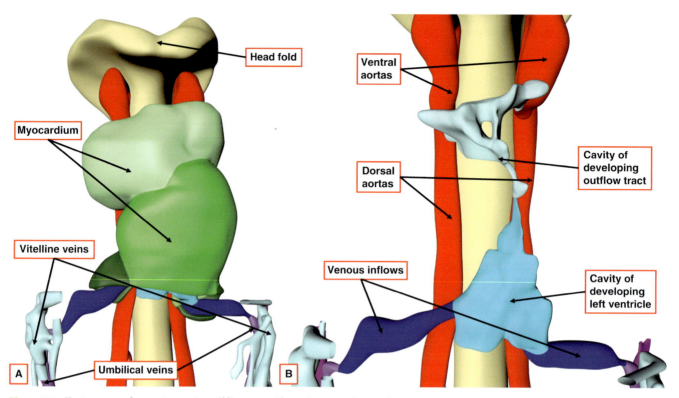

Figure 2.1 The images are from an interactive pdf file prepared from a human embryo at Carnegie stage 10. This represents around 28 days of development. The different parts of the heart were reconstructed to provide the images shown, but the segmented components can be removed to show the relationship of the various entities.[2] Panel A shows a frontal view, having removed the pericardium and the endodermal components. Panel B is an enlarged frontal view showing the cavity of the linear tube contained within the myocardial components.

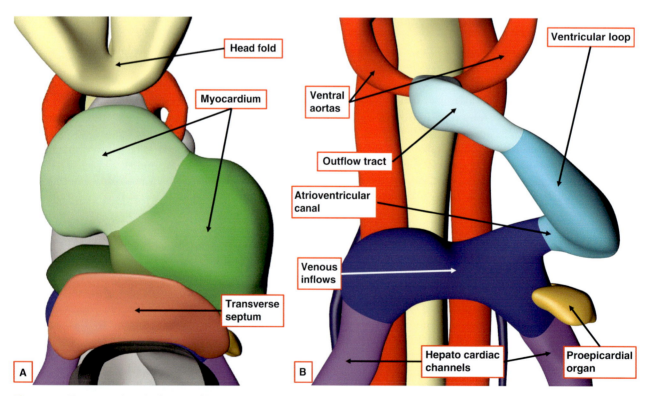

Figure 2.2 The images show the features of the developing heart at Carnegie stage 11, representing 29 days of development. The colours of the components are comparable with those shown in Figure 2.1. Panel A shows a frontal view having taken away the pericardium, with panel B showing an enlarged view of the cavities, having removed the myocardium and the cardiac jelly.

and provide the venous inflows (Figure 2.2B). Cardinal veins are beginning to form within the embryo, but without any connection, at this stage, with the venous inflows. The pro-epicardial organ can now be recognized at the junction of the left hepatocardiac channel and the developing atrial component.

Formation and Separation of the Atrial Chambers

It becomes possible to recognize the appearance of the atrial chambers, discrete from their venous inflows, when about 30 days have passed since fertilization. This is equivalent to Carnegie stage 12. By this stage, cardinal veins have developed cranially and caudally within the embryo to join the hepatocardiac channels (Figure 2.3A). The latter channels already drain the vitelline and umbilical veins in relatively symmetrical fashion, with the intrapericardial components now recognizable as the sinus horns (Figure 2.3B). Even at these early stages, the right side of the channels that will form the systemic venous sinus, or sinus venosus, is expanding more rapidly than the left side. It is also possible, by now, to identify a midline strand in the pharyngeal mesenchyme adjacent to the mesocardium still present at the venous pole. Over the next two Carnegie stages of development, in other words by the end of the fifth week of development, the strand will have canalized to form the common pulmonary vein. This opens into the left atrium dorsal to the developing left atrioventricular junction (Figure 2.4).

The opening of the pulmonary vein to the left atrium is flanked by the margins of the mesocardium, which at this stage, when viewed from the atrial aspect, are seen as obvious mounds (Figure 2.5). The growth of pharyngeal mesenchyme into the right mound of tissue produces a projection first described in the nineteenth century by Wilhelm His as the 'spina vestibuli', which we translate as the vestibular spine. As development proceeds, the spine, also known as the dorsal mesenchymal protrusion, will fuse with the mesenchymal cap carried on the leading edge of the primary atrial septum. This reinforces the closure of the primary atrial foramen, and at the same time commits the canalizing pulmonary vein to the cavity of the left atrium. Even before the pulmonary vein is committed to the left atrium, however, it is possible to recognize the beginning of formation of the trabeculations of the right and left ventricles (Figure 2.3). Although the changes in the ventricles and atriums are taking place concurrently, it is convenient to describe them separately. We will continue, therefore, to describe the changes taking place at the venous pole. It is these changes that set the scene for subsequent atrial septation. We have already described how, at Carnegie stage 12, the systemic venous tributaries join the developing atrial component in relatively symmetrical fashion via the sinus horns (Figure 2.3). The precise arrangement is better seen when assessed from the back, since at this stage each sinus horn connects directly with the atrial component (Figure 2.6). It is during these stages that the lungs have budded from the tracheobronchial rudiment, itself growing from the gut (Figure 2.4). Over the short period encompassing these stages, there has been a marked realignment of the systemic venous tributaries. The major change is the incorporation of the left sinus horn into the developing left atrioventricular groove, with retention of its own discrete walls (Figures 2.4, 2.7). Subsequent to the incorporation of the left sinus horn into the left atrioventricular groove, its orifice drains to the right side of the developing atrial component as part of the systemic venous sinus. As the systemic venous sinus itself becomes incorporated into the right atrium, so folds are formed between the venous and atrial parts. These folds are known as the venous valves (Figures 2.5, 2.7). During the initial stages of commitment of the venous sinus to the developing morphologically right atrium, the

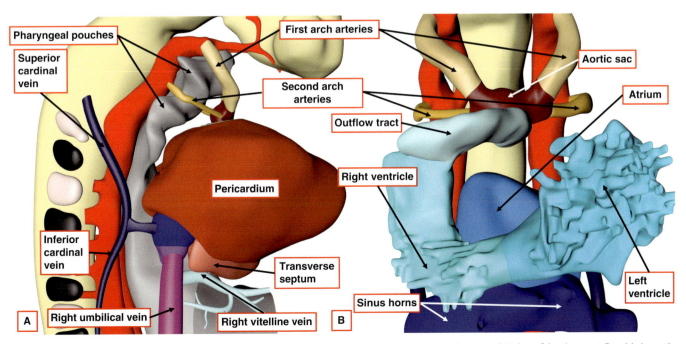

Figure 2.3 The images show the features of a reconstructed human embryo at Carnegie stage 12, representing around 30 days of development. Panel A shows the view from the right side, with panel B showing a frontal view of the cavities, having removed the pericardium, the myocardium, and the cardiac jelly.

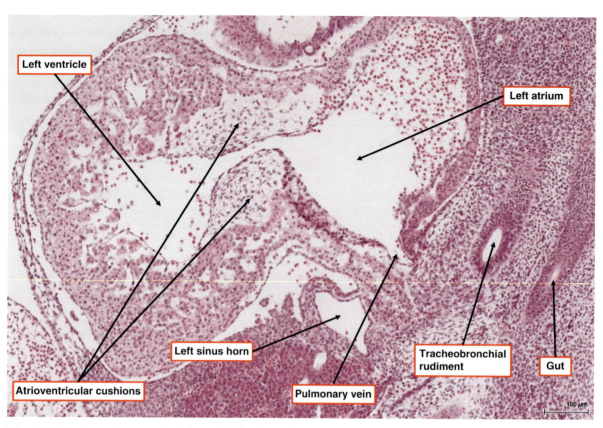

Figure 2.4 The image shows a section in the sagittal plane from a human embryo at Carnegie stage 13, The midpharyngeal strand has canalized to produce the common pulmonary vein, which now opens into the developing left atrium adjacent to the developing left atrioventricular junction. The left sinus horn, with its own discrete walls, is also part of the left atrioventricular groove.

cardinal, vitelline, and umbilical venous tributaries retain their connections bilaterally to both horns (Figure 2.8).

By the end of the fifth week of development, venous channels have also appeared within the developing lung buds, communicating with channels developing within the pharyngeal mesenchyme to join the cavity of the common pulmonary vein. During the same period, there is growth of a myocardial protrusion from the roof of the atrial part of the initial heart tube. This is the primary atrial septum, or septum primum. As soon as it appears, it carries on its leading edge a cap of mesenchyme (Figure 2.5), which is continuous ventrally and dorsally with the mesenchyme of the atrioventricular cushions (Figure 2.5). Ongoing growth of the septum takes its leading edge, and the mesenchymal cap, closer to the atrial margins of the atrioventricular cushions. The space between the cap and the cushions is the primary atrial foramen (Figure 2.9). When the heart tube was first formed, it was lined throughout by cardiac jelly. By the time of appearance of the primary atrial septum, the process of endothelial-to-mesenchymal transformation has changed the jelly within the atrioventricular canal into the superior and inferior atrioventricular cushions. As we will describe in our next section, the orifice of the canal is initially supported exclusively above the cavity of the developing left ventricle. During Carnegie stage 14, it expands rightward, with this process providing the developing right ventricle with its own inlet component. It is these changes that permit growth of the primary atrial septum to fuse with the atrial surfaces of the cushions, separating the canal into the right- and left-sided atrioventricular orifices (Figure 2.10). Before the primary septum can be closed, it is necessary to provide an alternative route for the richly oxygenated umbilical venous blood to reach the left side of the developing heart. This is achieved by the breakdown of the cranial margin of the primary septum, thus forming the secondary interatrial foramen. Creation of the secondary foramen permits the primary foramen to be closed by fusion of the mesenchymal cap carried on its leading edge with the atrioventricular endocardial cushions, which are then able also to fuse with each other. The obliteration of the primary foramen is then reinforced by the vestibular spine, which fuses both with the mesenchymal cap and the inferior atrioventricular cushion (Figure 2.11).

It is towards the end of the embryonic period of development, which extends to the end of the eighth week of gestation, that muscularization occurs in the mesenchymal tissues derived from both the vestibular spine and the mesenchymal cap. These muscularized tissues then form the antero-inferior buttress of the definitive atrial septum. This structure is the true second atrial septum. It serves to anchor the base of the primary atrial septum to the insulating tissues of the atrioventricular junctions, the latter entities derived from the fused atrioventricular cushions. By this stage, there has also been movement of the pulmonary vein from its initial location adjacent to the left atrioventricular junction. This process involves the incorporation of the right and left pulmonary veins into the cavity of the left atrium. As the veins are incorporated, so their orifices are

2 Development of the Heart

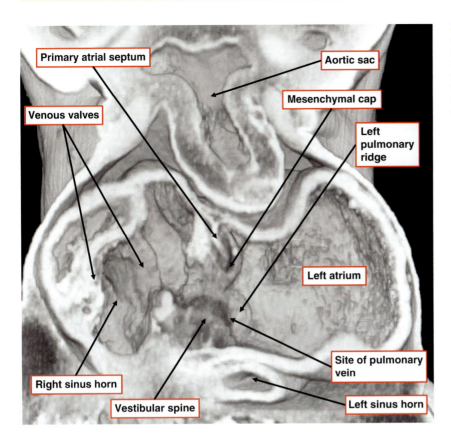

Figure 2.5 The image is taken from an episcopic dataset prepared from a human embryo at Carnegie stage 14, representing around 34 days of development. It shows the margins of the dorsal mesocardium, with the right-sided margin expanded by growth of tissues from the pharyngeal mesenchyme to form the vestibular spine. The venous valves mark the boundaries of the systemic venous sinus, which now opens to the developing right atrium.

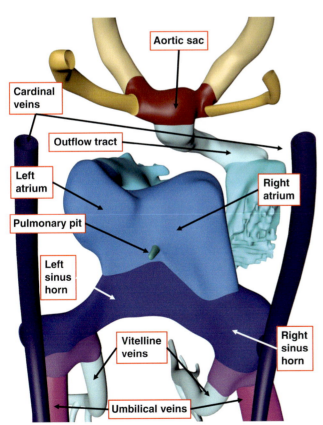

Figure 2.6 The image shows a reconstruction of the developing venous tributaries in a human embryo at Carnegie stage 12, also shown in Figure 2.3. This reconstruction shows the view from behind. At this stage, each sinus horn is connected directly and respectively to the left and right sides of the developing atrial component. Note the location of the pulmonary pit. This marks the site of the midpharyngeal strand, which canalized to form the pulmonary vein (Figure 2.4).

moved onto the dome of the atrium, at the same time producing a fold between the orifices of the right pulmonary veins and the junction of the superior caval vein with the walls of the right atrium. This fold then forms the cranial margin of the oval fossa, with the primary septum itself then forming the floor, or flap valve, of the oval foramen. The beginning of this process is evident by Carnegie stage 21, which is at the beginning of the eighth week of development (Figure 2.12). It is not until several weeks after the end of the embryonic period that the pulmonary veins achieve their definitive location at the four corners of the roof of the left atrium.[7] The fold produced superiorly between the right pulmonary veins and the superior caval vein then provides the buttress against which the flap valve, derived from the primary septum, is able to appose so as the close the oval foramen in postnatal life.[8] Fusion between the flap valve and the infolded superior rim of the foramen is found in only three-quarters to two-thirds of the overall population.[9] It is failure of this anatomical fusion that accounts for persistent patency of the oval foramen. When the foramen retains its patency, it is a tunnel rather than a simple hole, a feature of significance for those seeking to close the foramen by transcatheter insertion of devices in postnatal life. During the formation of the oval foramen, the terminal part of the left sinus horn has become transformed into the coronary sinus. Retention of the left-sided superior caval venous tributary to the horn becomes manifest as persistence of the left superior caval vein. Almost always, this venous channel drains to the right atrium through an enlarged mouth of the coronary sinus. When development proceeds normally, the cranial part of the left sinus horn regresses, persisting only as the oblique vein of the left atrium, or the vein of Marshall.

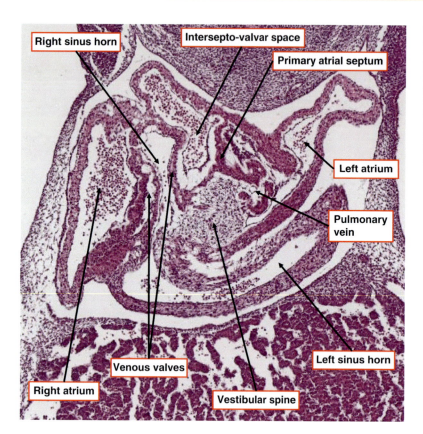

Figure 2.7 The image is a frontal section through the developing systemic venous sinus in a human embryo at Carnegie stage 15. The plane of section is comparable to the image from the episcopic dataset shown in Figure 2.5. It shows how the left sinus horn has been incorporated into the left atrioventricular groove, but with the retention of its own walls, which are separate from the walls of the left atrium. Note the space between the left venous valve and the primary atrial septum. This area, known as the intersepto-valvar space, represents the part of the initial atrial component of the primary heart tube, which is committed to the morphologically right atrium subsequent to the growth of the primary atrial septum.

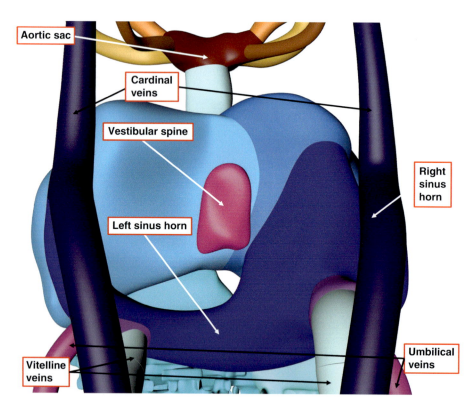

Figure 2.8 The image shows a reconstruction of the developing venous tributaries in a human embryo at Carnegie stage 13. Over the short period of time of two to three days elapsing from stage 12 (see Figure 2.6), the left sinus horn has been incorporated as part of the developing left atrioventricular junction. Its opening has shifted along with the overall systemic venous sinus, such that all the venous tributaries now drain into the cavity of the developing right atrium (see also Figure 2.7).

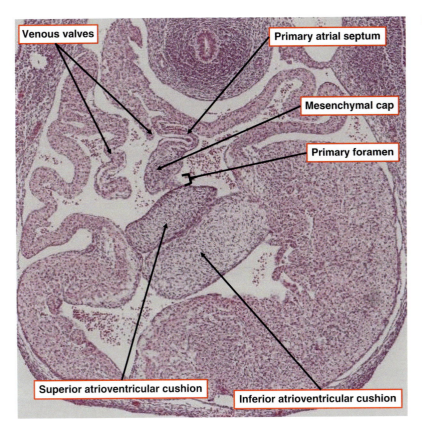

Figure 2.9 The image shows the consequence of growth of the primary atrial septum. The 'four-chamber' section is from a human embryo at Carnegie stage 16. The growth of the septum has brought the mesenchymal cap closer to the atrial surface of the superior atrioventricular cushion, and thus diminishing the size of the primary foramen.

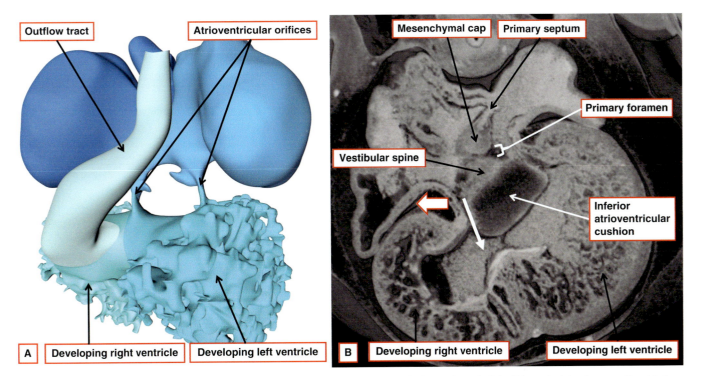

Figure 2.10 The images show the features of the developing heart at Carnegie stage 14, which is at the end of the fifth week of development. Panel A shows a reconstruction of the cavities, with panel B showing a frontal cut through an episcopic dataset. Panel B shows the rightward expansion of the atrioventricular canal (white arrow with red borders), thus providing the direct inlet from the right atrium to the right ventricle (white arrow). The atrioventricular cushions, although not yet fused, have now separated the cavity of the atrioventricular canal into the right and left atrioventricular orifices, as shown in panel A. The primary foramen has still to close (panel B).

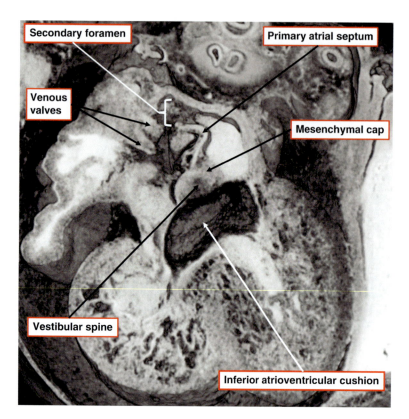

Figure 2.11 The image is a frontal section through an episcopic dataset prepared from a human embryo at Carnegie stage 17, which is almost at the end of the sixth week of development. The mesenchymal cap on the primary atrial septum has now fused with the atrioventricular cushions, with the attachment of the vestibular spine to the rightward surfaces of the atrioventricular cushions reinforcing their zone of fusion. Breakdown of the primary septum at the atrial roof has produced the secondary foramen, permitting the richly oxygenated blood arriving from the placenta to continue to reach the left side of the heart.

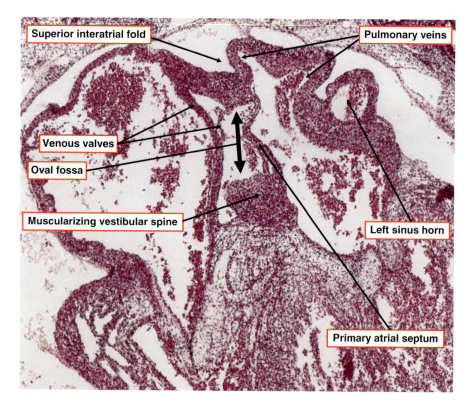

Figure 2.12 The image shows a frontal section from a human embryo at Carnegie stage 21, which is at the beginning of the eighth week of development. The vestibular spine, which reinforced the right side of fusion of the mesenchymal cap with the atrial margins of the atrioventricular cushions, is now muscularizing to form the inferior buttress of the oval fossa. The superior rim of the fossa, which is shown by the double-headed arrow, is formed by the superior interatrial fold, itself developing as the pulmonary veins migrate to reach their position on the dome of the left atrium.

Formation and Septation of the Atrioventricular Canal

Subsequent to formation of the ventricular loop, the connection between the developing atrial chambers and the loop is recognizable as the atrioventricular canal, which at this stage possesses its own discrete myocardial walls. At Carnegie stage 13, when the embryo is around 32 days old, the circumference of the canal is supported exclusively by the myocardium of the inlet part of the ventricular loop (Figure 2.13). The ventricular

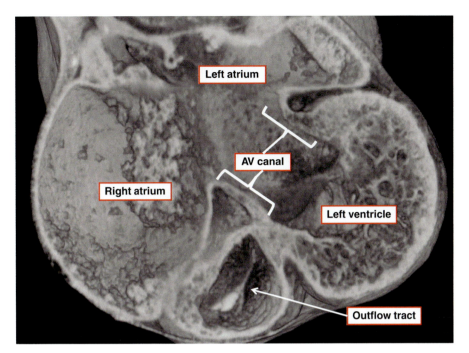

Figure 2.13 The image shows a 'four-chamber' section through an episcopic dataset prepared from a human embryo at Carnegie stage 13, which represents around 32 days of development after fertilization. The discrete walls of the atrioventricular canal are supported exclusively by the developing left ventricle.

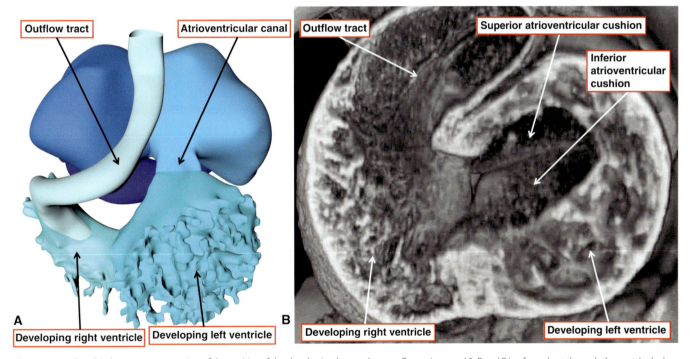

Figure 2.14 Panel A shows a reconstruction of the cavities of the developing human heart at Carnegie stage 13. Panel B is a frontal cut through the ventricular loop made from an episcopic dataset of another human embryo at Carnegie stage 13. The atrioventricular canal, as shown in Figure 2.13, is supported exclusively above the developing left ventricle, while the outflow tract arises exclusively from the developing right ventricle. In the inner curvature, although the atrioventricular canal opens only to the left ventricle, its rightward wall is in continuity between the walls of the developing right atrium and ventricle.

loop itself at this stage has obvious inner and outer curvatures (Figure 2.14). The right-sided wall of the canal, although supported above the cavity of the left ventricle, is in direct continuity, as part of the inner curvature, with the cranial wall of the developing right ventricle (Figure 2.14A). The apical components of both ventricles are themselves ballooning from the outer curvature of the loop, with the developing right ventricle supporting the outflow tract. The atrioventricular cushions formed within the canal are positioned superiorly and inferiorly. Although they have yet to fuse, they lie edge-to-edge, thus dividing the orifice of the canal into right-sided and left-sided channels. As the apical components balloon from the outer curvature, so the primordium of the muscular ventricular septum is formed between them. At this stage, the interventricular foramen is bounded caudally by the crest of the muscular septum and cranially by the inner heart curvature. All the blood passing through the atrioventricular canal, therefore, must pass through the foramen to reach the outflow tract. It follows that the primary foramen, as seen at Carnegie stage 13 (Figure 2.14), can never be closed. Instead, with ongoing development it is remodelled. The consequence of the first part of this remodelling is that the right half of the canal expands so as to provide the direct inlet to the right ventricle (Figure 2.10). As part of this process, the caudal margins of the primary interventricular foramen become the right atrioventricular junction.[10] With still further development, to be described in the next section, and as the second part of the remodelling, the ventral part of the primary foramen will become the outflow tract for the developing left ventricle. Prior to any remodelling, however, the right-sided atrioventricular groove interposes between the cavities of the developing right atrium and right ventricle (Figure 2.15).

The walls of the developing right-sided chambers, nonetheless, are already in continuity, as part of the inner curvature, in the cranial margin of the primary interventricular foramen. And, by Carnegie 14, the atrioventricular canal has expanded rightward, thus providing the direct inlet to the right ventricle (Figure 2.10). The proof of the expansion of the canal was provided by tracking the fate of a ring of cells serendipitously marked in the human heart by an antibody to the nodose ganglion of the chick.[10] The dorsal part of the ring, which initially surrounded the primary interventricular foramen, was found surrounding the right atrioventricular junction subsequent to expansion of the canal. As the canal expands, so is the developing muscular ventricular septum brought beneath the ventricular surfaces of the atrioventricular cushions. With still further development, the rightward margins of the cushions will drape themselves across the crest of the septum, leaving the bulk of the fused cushion mass positioned above the cavity of the left ventricle. As part of the same process of remodelling, the myocardium of the atrioventricular canal is eventually sequestrated on the atrial aspect of the atrioventricular junctions, forming the vestibules of the developing atrial chambers (Figure 2.16). Over the period of expansion of the canal, additional cushions have been formed in the lateral margins of the newly separated ventricular inlets. These lateral cushions, along with the fused major cushions, then provide the primordiums for development of the leaflets of the atrioventricular valves (Figure 2.17). The lateral cushion in the left atrioventricular junction provides the primordium for the mural leaflet of the mitral valve. In the right atrioventricular junction, the lateral cushion will eventually remodel to produce both the antero-superior and antero-inferior, or mural, leaflets of the tricuspid valve. The rightward margins of the conjoined atrioventricular cushions, subsequent to draping themselves across the crest of the muscular ventricular septum, provide the substance for formation of the septal leaflet of the tricuspid valve. Delamination of this leaflet, however, does not take place until the fetal period of development.

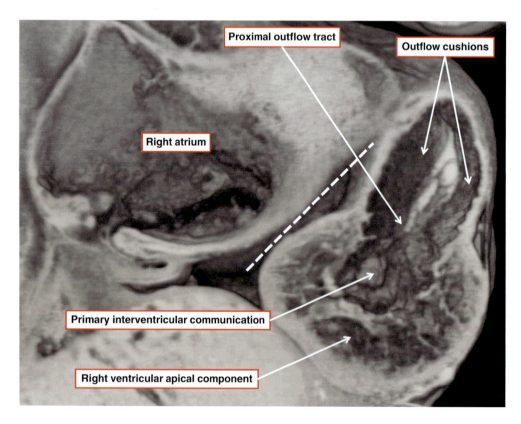

Figure 2.15 The image is taken from another episcopic dataset prepared from a human embryo at Carnegie stage 13. It shows the right atrioventricular groove (white dashed line) interposed, at this stage, between the cavities of the developing right atrium and right ventricle.

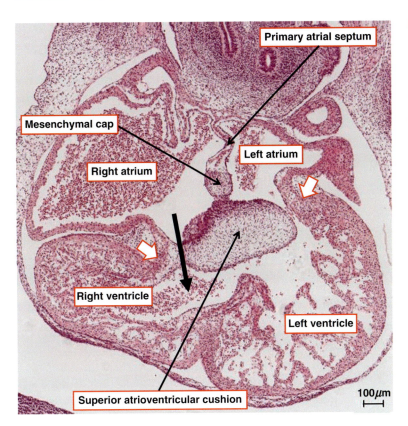

Figure 2.16 The image is a four-chamber histological section from a human embryo at Carnegie stage 16, representing around 38 days of development. The atrioventricular canal has expanded rightward, providing the right ventricle with its own inlet (large black arrow). The canal myocardium, with ongoing development, will be sequestrated to produce the atrial vestibules of the atrioventricular junctions, with the eventual plane of insulation shown by the white arrows with red borders. The atrioventricular cushions are straddling the crest of the developing muscular ventricular septum.

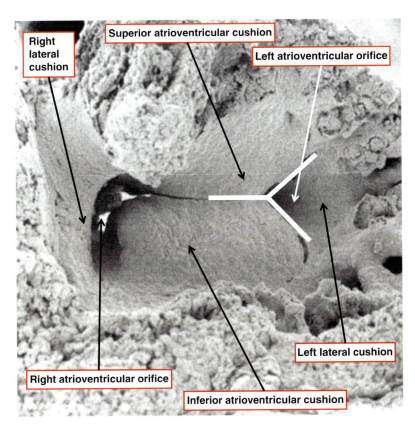

Figure 2.17 The image is a scanning electron micrograph showing a dissected heart from a human embryo at Carnegie stage 17. The developing atrioventricular junctions are seen from their ventricular aspect. The major atrioventricular cushions lie edge-to-edge in supero-inferior relationship, with the formation of lateral cushions in both atrioventricular junctions producing the primordiums of the atrioventricular valves. The developing mitral valve has a trifoliate configuration at this stage of development (white Y configuration).

In addition, tubercles from these rightward margins of the cushions serve to close the tertiary interventricular foramen. These tubercles then provide the basis for formation of the membranous septum. On the left side, furthermore, the developing mitral valve initially has a trifoliate configuration (Figure 2.17). It is only subsequent to much later expansion of the left atrioventricular junction that the lateral cushion becomes the mural leaflet of the mitral valve. The bulk of the mass formed by fusion of the major cushions then becomes the aortic leaflet of the mitral valve. A significant component of these left-ventricular parts of the fused cushions also produces the fibrous roof of the infero-septal recess of the left ventricular outflow tract (Figure 2.18). The processes are not completed until after the end of the embryonic period of development. In both ventricles, it is coalescence of the initial trabecular layers of the ventricular walls that forms the papillary muscles, which initially extend to the margins of the cushions (Figure 2.18B). Delamination of the cushions from the parietal ventricular walls and the muscular septum then produces the inferior and septal leaflets of the tricuspid valve, with comparable delamination from the parietal wall producing the mural leaflet of the mitral valve. The junctions between the cushions and the papillary muscles then remodel to produce the tendinous cords, with leaflets and cords both having an endocardial rather than a myocardial lineage. The transformation into tendinous cords does not take place until the tenth and eleventh weeks of development.

Formation of the Ventricles

Ballooning of the apical components from the outer curvature of the ventricular loop heralds the formation of the right and left ventricles.[11] By Carnegie stage 13, the apical part of the left ventricle is already ballooning from the inlet component of the loop, with the apical part of the right ventricle beginning its formation from the outlet component (Figure 2.14). The ballooning of the two apical components produces the primordium of the muscular ventricular septum between them, with the septum initially formed by coalescence of apical trabeculations. It is then the rightward expansion of the atrioventricular canal, as already described, which brings the cavity of the right atrium into direct continuity with the cavity of the developing right ventricle (Figures 2.10, 2.16). And, as also explained, the process of endothelial-to-mesenchymal transformation has by now produced the atrioventricular endocardial cushions, A similar process of endothelial-to-mesenchymal transformation, but with the added involvement of cells derived from the neural crest, then converts the cardiac jelly within the outflow tract into paired cushions. These cushions also lie edge-to-edge, initially spiralling throughout the outflow tract. They eventually fuse to separate the solitary cavity into aortic and pulmonary channels. We will discuss the fate of the distal outflow cushions when considering development of the outflow tract. At the stage described thus far, subsequent to expansion of the atrioventricular canal, the right ventricle will have acquired its own inlet, but still supports both outlets. The

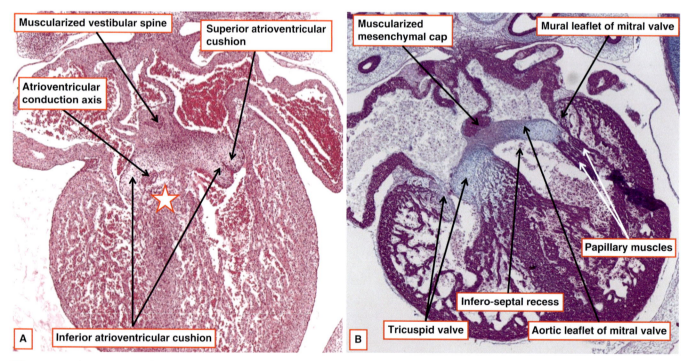

Figure 2.18 The images show 'four-chamber' histological sections through developing human hearts at Carnegie stages 18 (panel A) and 19 (panel B). This is at the end of the seventh week of development. The heart shown in panel A is stained with haematoxylin and eosin, whereas the heart in panel B was processed using the periodic acid Schiff stain. The images show how the bulk of the fused major cushions remain above the roof of the left ventricle, where they become the aortic leaflet of the mitral valve. The rightward margins eventually form the septal leaflet of the tricuspid valve, but have yet to delaminate from the septum at this stage. The mural leaflets of the valves have not yet developed to any great extent. The images also show how the trabeculations forming the larger parts of the ventricular walls at these stages are beginning to coalesce to form the papillary muscles, which extend to the margins of the cushions at this stage, with no formation yet of tendinous cords. The fused cushions also form the roof of the infero-septal recess of the left ventricle (panel B), supporting the muscularized vestibular spine, which becomes the antero-inferior buttress of the atrial septum.

formation of the definitive ventricles is completed by transfer of the ventral part of the initial interventricular foramen to the developing left ventricle as the subaortic outflow tract (Figure 2.19A).

When the shelf is built in the roof of the right ventricle, the aortic root remains supported above the cavity of the right, rather than the left, ventricle (Figure 2.19B). At this stage, furthermore, an additional communication is still present dorsal to the fusing cushions between the cavities of the aortic root and the apical part of the right ventricle. This space, which can be considered as the tertiary interventricular foramen, in reality is an aorto–right ventricular foramen (Figure 2.20). Irrespective of the name, the foramen is closed by expansions from the rightward margins of the atrioventricular cushions, which are known as the tubercles (Figure 2.20B). Subsequent to closure by the tubercles, the secondary interventricular foramen has become the entrance to the left ventricular outflow tract. At the initial stage of this remodelling, the roof of the outflow tract, made up by the inner heart curvature, is myocardial. Even at the end of the embryonic period, eight weeks subsequent to fertilization, by which time the tertiary foramen has closed, and the aortic root is in exclusive communication with the cavity of the left ventricle, the aortic root remains aligned with the cavity of the right ventricle. It is during the early part of the fetal period that the inner curvature becomes converted to fibrous tissue, with the aortic root becoming positioned between the aortic leaflet of the mitral valve and the ventricular septum. The tubercles that closed the persisting tertiary part of the initial interventricular foramen then become the fibrous, or membranous, part of the ventricular septum. This process occurs prior to delamination of the septal leaflet of the tricuspid valve. When initially formed, therefore, the fibrous partition is exclusively an atrioventricular septum. It is only with subsequent delamination of the septal leaflet, in the weeks following completion of the ventricular septation, that the membranous septum is separated into its interventricular and atrioventricular components.[12]

During the early stages of ventricular formation, the compact parts of the ventricular walls themselves are very thin, but an extensive layer of trabeculations fills the larger part of the ventricular cavities. The trabeculations subsequently coalesce to form the papillary muscles of the atrioventricular valves (Figure 2.18B). They also coalesce to form the muscular ventricular septum. The superficial components then persist as the subendocardial ventricular conduction pathways. There is no evidence, however, to substantiate the notion that the trabeculations coalesce to form the compact ventricular walls. Instead, the growth of the initially thin compact wall, as seen at Carnegie stage 12, outstrips that of the trabecular layer, which hence becomes increasingly insignificant. Should the growth of the trabeculations match that of the compact layer, then the picture that emerges is one of excessive trabeculation, this being the term that should be used to describe so-called ventricular non-compaction.[13]

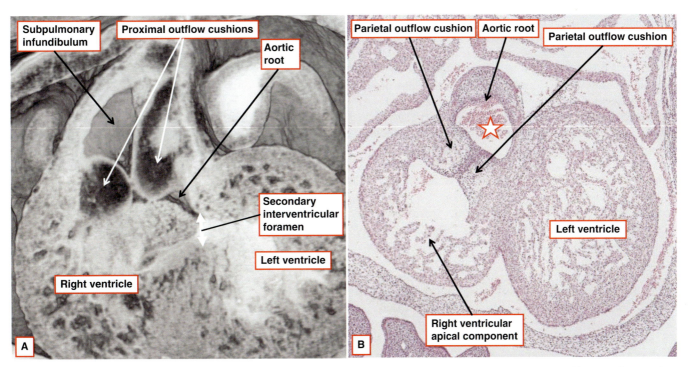

Figure 2.19 Panel A shows an image from an episcopic dataset prepared from an embryo at Carnegie stage 17. The persisting channel between the ventricles is the secondary interventricular foramen. It provides the outlet from the left ventricle to the aortic root. At stage 17, the proximal cushions have still to fuse. Panel B shows a histological section at stage 18. As the cushions fuse, they build a shelf in the roof of the right ventricle, which then sequestrates part of the right ventricular cavity as the aortic root (star with red borders).

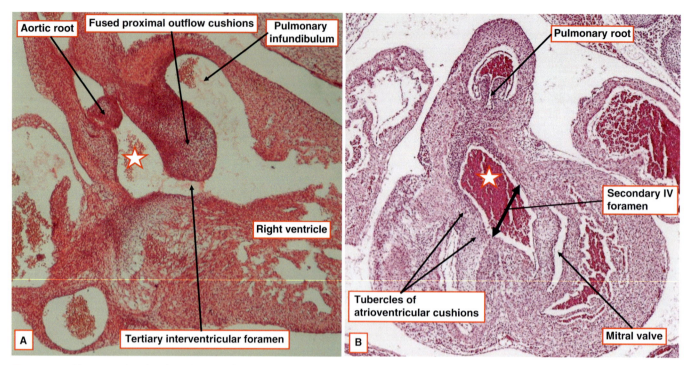

Figure 2.20 The images show histological sections from human embryos at Carnegie stages 19 (panel A) and 20 (panel B). Panel A shows how, subsequent to the formation of the shelf in the roof of the right ventricle, cut obliquely in this section, the aortic root remains in communication with the right ventricle via the tertiary interventricular foramen. As shown in Figure 2.19B, however, the space supporting the aortic root initially belonged to the right ventricle. The area undergoing closure, therefore, is an aorto–right ventricular foramen. When closed by the tubercles of the atrioventricular cushions, as shown in panel B, the space becomes part of the left ventricle. The secondary interventricular (IV) foramen then becomes the entrance to the left ventricular outflow tract. The stars show the subaortic outflow tract, which in panel A remains part of the cavity of the right ventricle, but which, in panel B, has become part of the cavity of the left ventricle.

Formation, Septation, and Separation of the Aortic and Pulmonary Pathways

Subsequent to formation of the ventricular loop, the outflow tract is supported exclusively above the cavity of the developing right ventricle (Figure 2.14). At this early stage of development, the walls of the outflow tract, from its origin from the developing right ventricle to its termination at the margins of the pericardial cavity, are exclusively myocardial (Figure 2.21). At the margins of the pericardial cavity, its lumen is continuous with the cavity of the aortic sac. The latter entity is the manifold within the pharyngeal mesenchyme, which gives rise to the bilaterally symmetrical arteries of the developing pharyngeal arches (Figure 2.22). At the earlier Carnegie stage 12, when around 30 days have elapsed since fertilization, it is possible to recognize the formation of the first two pharyngeal pouches. The pouches, which bud from the pharynx, meet two ectodermal clefts to delimit the arches. Two sets of arteries extend through the pharyngeal mesenchyme, uniting dorsally with the bilateral aortas (Figure 2.23). The arteries are formed cranially relative to the position of the corresponding pharyngeal pouches. With two additional days of development, at Carnegie stage 13, the first set of arteries has disappeared, but two additional arches have formed, containing the third and fourth sets of arch arteries. Only three pouches, however, can be recognized at this stage (Figure 2.24). With the passage of two further days of development, at Carnegie stage 14, the second set of arteries has also disappeared, but it is now possible to

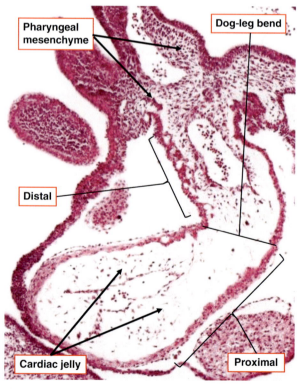

Figure 2.21 The image shows a histological section, in frontal plane, from a human embryo at Carnegie stage 13, representing around 32 days of development. The outflow tract has exclusively myocardial walls, with cardiac jelly surrounding its solitary cavity. It has an obvious dog-leg bend, delimiting its proximal and distal parts.

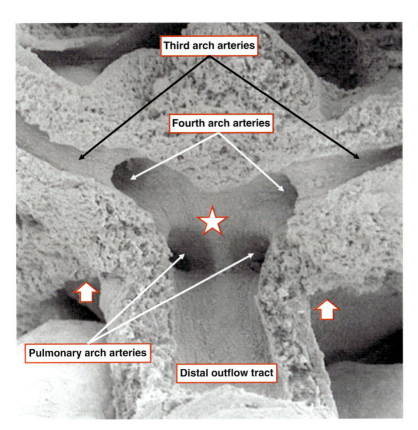

Figure 2.22 The image is a scanning electron micrograph showing a dissection of a human heart at Carnegie stage 13. It shows how the cavity of the outflow tract, at the margins of the pericardial cavity (white arrows with red borders), becomes confluent with the aortic sac, the manifold within the pharyngeal mesenchyme which gives rise to the arteries that run within the pharyngeal arches. At this stage, it is possible only to recognize the arteries of the third, fourth, and ultimate arches. The ultimate arch arteries will become the pulmonary arteries. The dorsal wall of the sac (white star with red borders), with ongoing development, will protrude into the distal outflow tract as the aortopulmonary septum.

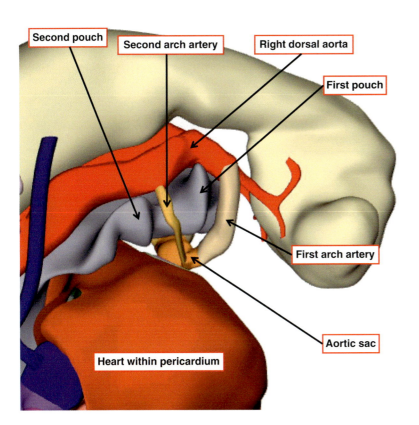

Figure 2.23 The image shows a reconstruction of the right side of a developing human embryo at Carnegie stage 12, representing around 30 days of development. By this time, two pharyngeal pouches have delimited two pharyngeal arches, with the arteries of these arches extending through the pharyngeal mesenchyme, having taken origin from the aortic sac, to join the dorsal aortas in symmetrical fashion.

recognize the fourth pharyngeal pouch. An ultimate set of arteries then develops in the pharyngeal mesenchyme caudal to the fourth pouch. There is never formation of any additional pouches. The arteries appearing caudal to the fourth pouch, therefore, are the fifth set of pharyngeal arch arteries (Figure 2.25).

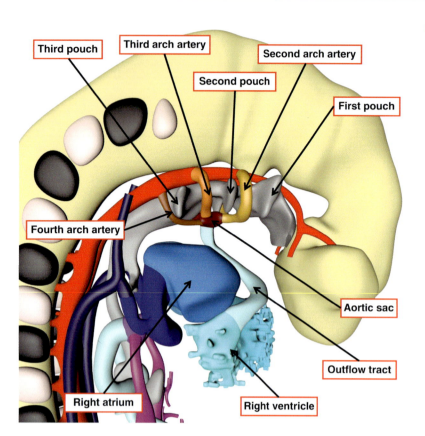

Figure 2.24 The image shows a comparable reconstruction to the one shown in Figure 2.23, but this time for the human embryo at Carnegie stage 13, the stage shown also in Figures 2.21 and 2.22. There are now three pharyngeal pouches, and three arch arteries, but the arteries initially present in the first arch have disappeared.

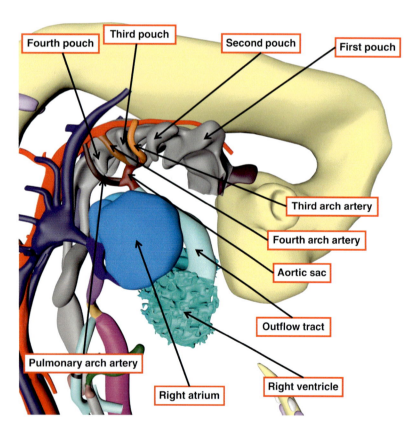

Figure 2.25 The image shows reconstructions of a human embryo at Carnegie stage 14, which is at the end of the fifth week of development. The view is from the right side, and is comparable to the images shown in Figures 2.23 and 2.24. The artery of the second arch has by now attenuated. This permits recognition of three sets of arteries. The ultimate set of arteries has conventionally been called the sixth set. They are, however, only the fifth set of arteries ever to be formed. To label them as 'fifth arch arteries' would be confusing, since such presumed arteries are often implicated to explain anomalous arrangements. For this reason, and since they eventually supply the pulmonary circulation, we have chosen to designate them as the pulmonary arch arteries.

The pharyngeal mesenchyme surrounding this ultimate set of arteries is different from that forming the first four arches. All of the cranial four arches contain endodermal, bony, and neural components. It is arguable, therefore, that the pharyngeal mesenchyme surrounding the ultimate set of arteries is not a pharyngeal arch at all. The arteries themselves, with ongoing development, will give rise to the right and left pulmonary arteries. It is unfortunate that, by tradition, these arteries have been labelled as representing the sixth set. Six segments of pharyngeal mesenchyme, with contained arteries, have never been found, neither in human nor other mammalian embryos.[14] The arteries, logically, should now be described as the fifth set. It would be confusing, however, to label them in this fashion. This is because so-called fifth arch arteries, presumed to represent the 'missing' set in the system based on six arches, have been implicated as the basis for anomalous arrangements, such as the double-barrelled aorta. It is now established that better explanations can be offered for these anomalous patterns, such as the presence of collateral channels, or remodelling of the aortic sac.[15] For all of these reasons, it is better to describe the ultimate set as the arteries of the pulmonary arches.[16] By the time that it has become possible to recognize the arteries of the pulmonary arches, at the end of the fifth week of development, remodelling of the aortic sac has already begun. Its cranial component has now separated into right and left horns. Each of these horns feeds the arteries of the fourth and third arches. The caudal component now supplies the arteries of the pulmonary arches, with an extensive dorsal wall interposing between the cranial and caudal parts. This wall, with ongoing development, will protrude into the distal part of the outflow tract to become the aortopulmonary septum (Figure 2.26). At the end of the fifth week of development, the arteries arising from the aortic sac are symmetrical, joining dorsally with the paired dorsal aortas (Figure 2.27). We will return to describe the features of remodelling of the extrapericardial arterial pathways. This involves attenuation of several of the right-sided components of the initially symmetrical arrangement. During the changes taking place in the extrapericardial pathways, equally significant changes are to be found in the outflow tract itself. The result is its separation into the intrapericardial arterial trunks, the arterial roots, and the ventricular outflow tracts. At the end of the fifth week of development, the walls of the outflow tract are exclusively myocardial. It has a solitary lumen enclosed within a thick layer of cardiac jelly. Due to the presence of the dog-leg bend, it also has obvious proximal and dorsal components (Figure 2.28).

The boundaries of the pericardial cavity serve to underscore the description of the ongoing remodelling of the distal component. At this stage of development, the aortic sac has also begun to remodel. Its cranial part now gives rise to the arteries of the third and fourth pharyngeal arches, leaving the arteries of the pulmonary arches arising from the caudal part (Figure 2.26). Subsequent to this remodelling, the dorsal wall of the sac is extensive and elongated. As development proceeds, its dorsal wall between the third and fourth, and pulmonary arch, arteries will protrude anteriorly, entering the cavity of the distal part of the outflow tract as the aortopulmonary septum. Additional significant changes then involve the most distal parts of the walls. Tissues continue to enter these walls from the heart-forming areas. Unlike the previous populations entering the arterial pole, however, the new tissues are non-myocardial. The intrusion of the non-myocardial tissues, furthermore, is far from uniform. The first signs of the intercalations of non-myocardial components becomes apparent

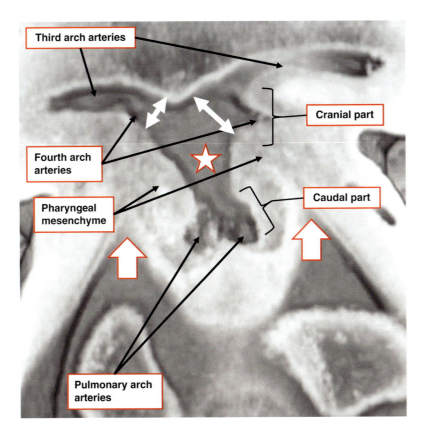

Figure 2.26 The image shows a frontal section through an episcopic dataset prepared from a human embryo at Carnegie stage 14, which represents around 34 days of development. At the margins of the pericardial cavity (white arrows with red borders), the cavity of the outflow tract becomes confluent with that of the aortic sac. The aortic sac has been remodelled into cranial and caudal parts, with the cranial part itself now having right and left horns (double-headed white arrows). The dorsal wall of the sac (white star with red borders) will itself protrude with ongoing development to become the aortopulmonary septum.

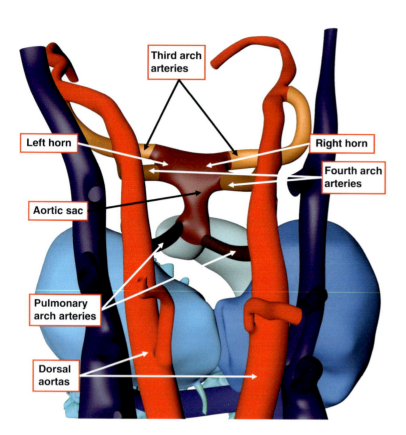

Figure 2.27 The image shows the posterior view of a reconstructed human embryo at Carnegie stage 14, representing around 34 days of development. The arteries arising from the aortic sac are bilaterally symmetrical, opening dorsally into the paired aortas.

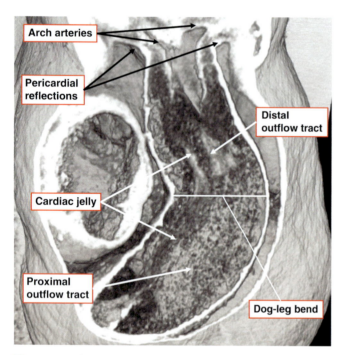

Figure 2.28 The image shows a frontal section through an episcopic dataset prepared from a human embryo at Carnegie stage 14. The outflow tract takes an obvious bend, permitting distinction of its proximal and distal parts. As was shown in Figure 2.21, the walls of both parts are myocardial at this stage of development, with the lumen lined by a thick layer of cardiac jelly.

with the appearance of buttons of non-myocardial cells at the cranial and caudal attachments of the myocardial walls of the distal outflow tract with the non-myocardial pharyngeal mesenchyme. As these non-myocardial tissues infiltrate the distal walls, they rotate. During Carnegie stage 14, the cranial button becomes a right-sided rod, with the caudal button producing a more elongated left-sided counterpart (Figure 2.29A). As the non-myocardial tissues come to occupy the distal walls of the outflow tract during Carnegie stages 15 and 16, so there is a concomitant retreat of the myocardial walls away from the pericardial boundaries (Figure 2.29B,C). At the same time, the process of endothelial-to-mesenchymal transformation results in the cardiac jelly lining the cavity of the outflow tract becoming opposing and spiralling cushions. When first formed, the cushions, initially described by some investigators as ridges, are located cranially and caudally at their pericardial boundaries. When traced proximally, the cushions spiral around each other. In consequence, the cranial cushion occupies a parietal proximal position, while the caudal distal cushion is aligned proximally with the muscular ventricular septum. Throughout the parts of the outflow tract that have retained their myocardial wall, the cushions lie edge-to-edge, thus separating the initially solitary cavity into aortic and pulmonary channels. Although lying edge-to-edge, the cushions are not initially fused. Fusion, when it occurs, takes place in a distal-to-proximal direction. The initial fusion distally also coincides with fusion of the distal margins of the cushions with the aortopulmonary septum, which by now has grown obliquely into the cavity of the distal outflow tract from the dorsal wall of the aortic sac. The protrusion is now functioning as an aortopulmonary septum because, subsequent to the initial remodelling of the aortic sac, it has come to separate the cranial aortic and the caudal pulmonary components (Figure 2.26). Its growth into the distal outflow tract also coincides with the effective retreat of the distal myocardial border away from the pericardial boundary. By using 'retreat', we do not imply that there is active movement of the distal myocardial border. On the contrary, the change is likely the consequence of the growth of the non-myocardial distal walls. As the protrusion approaches the distal margins of the fusing cushions, there is a transient aortopulmonary foramen between their edges (Figure 2.30).

At the beginning of the sixth week of development, the leading edge of the protrusion fuses with the distal margins of the outflow cushions, thus obliterating the aortopulmonary foramen. This serves to connect the cranial part of the aortic sac with the aortic channel formed within the outflow tract by fusion of the cushions themselves, leaving the caudal part of the sac in continuity with the pulmonary channel. The changes are accompanied by further effective retreat of the distal myocardial border away from the margins of the pericardial cavity. During the initial appearance of the non-myocardial walls, the persisting distal myocardial border had an obvious fishmouth arrangement (Figure 2.29). By the time the aortopulmonary foramen has been closed, the ongoing retreat of the myocardial walls has provided the distal myocardial boundary with a relatively planar margin, with the overall outflow tract itself losing its dog-leg bend. The formation of the swellings from the distal margins of the initial non-myocardial rods now permits the recognition of a middle part of the outflow tract, which has retained its myocardial walls (Figure 2.31).

By the time of closure of the aortopulmonary foramen, therefore, the walls of the distal outflow tract have become exclusively non-myocardial. Significant changes by this stage are also taking place within the middle and proximal parts of the outflow tract, which have retained their myocardial walls. As the aortopulmonary septum grew to separate the distal outflow tract, it was populated by cells migrating from the neural crest. These cells derived from the neural crest also enter the distal ends of the major cushions. And, by this time, the non-myocardial tissues infiltrating to form the walls between the jaws of the myocardial fishmouth have seeded parts of the cardiac jelly to produce swellings discrete from the major cushions. As the swellings form within the middle part of the outflow tract, they interpose between the unfused parietal margins of the major cushions, thus creating the primordiums of the arterial roots (Figures 2.32).

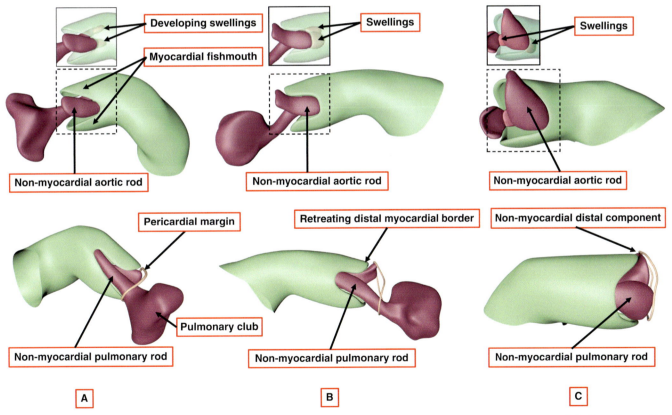

Figure 2.29 The images are reconstructions from human embryos at Carnegie stages 14 (panel A), 15 (panel B), and 16 (panel C). They illustrate the changes that take place at the border between the distal outflow tract and the pharyngeal mesenchyme of the aortic sac. The mesenchymal cells initially intercalate into the walls of the distal outflow tract to form non-myocardial rods. By Carnegie stage 16, the rods have rotated and broadened at their bases to become more triangular. The rods then interact with the cardiac jelly in the distal part of the outflow tract that has retained its myocardial walls to produce swellings. These swellings, subsequently, will give rise to the non-adjacent leaflets of the arterial valves. The cells making up the pulmonary rod can be traced into continuity with a peritracheal club within the pharyngeal mesenchyme. As the rods extend further proximally, so they produce a distal collar of non-myocardial tissues. This results in a gradual retreat of the distal myocardial border away from the pericardial margins, producing an outflow tract with myocardial proximal and middle portions, and a distal part with non-myocardial walls.

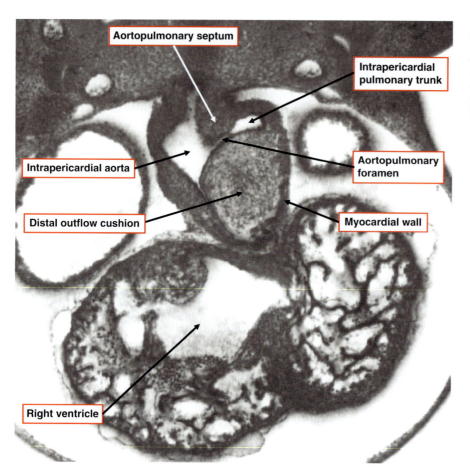

Figure 2.30 The image shows a two-dimensional cut through an episcopic dataset made from a human embryo at Carnegie stage 15. The dorsal wall of the aortic sac has protruded obliquely into the cavity of the distal outflow tract as the aortopulmonary septum. At the stage shown, there is a transient aortopulmonary foramen between the protrusion and the distal margins of the cushions.

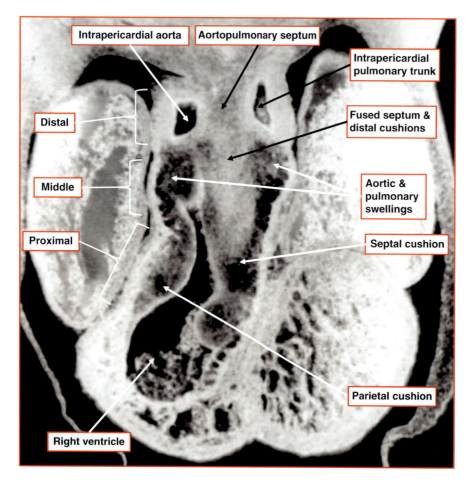

Figure 2.31 The image is a long-axis section through an episcopic dataset prepared from a human embryo late during Carnegie stage 15, which is at the end of the fifth week of development. Due to the ingrowth of the non-myocardial tissues, it has become possible to recognize three parts within the outflow tract. The distal part has non-myocardial walls, while the middle and proximal parts retain their myocardial walls. The aortopulmonary septum by this stage has fused with the cushions in the middle part, which have also fused with each other. The cushions in the proximal part, in contrast, have still to fuse.

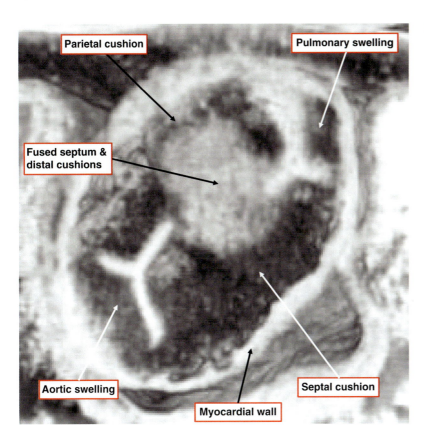

Figure 2.32 The image is prepared from the same episcopic dataset used to produce Figure 2.31. The cut is taken across the short axis of the middle part of the outflow tract, through the area of fusion between the aortopulmonary septum and the fused distal cushions. It shows how the swellings occupying the middle part of the outflow tract interpose between the parietal unfused ends of the major cushions to produce the primordiums for the arterial roots. The area of fusion is condensed mesenchyme. It is made up of the cells derived from the neural crest.

The swellings, and their role in forming the scaffolds for the future arterial roots, were first recognized by Kramer.[17] On the basis of his observations, Kramer had proposed that the outflow tract could be described in terms of the 'truncus' and the 'conus'. These terms remain contentious. This, in part, reflects the fact that Kramer neglected to specify to which part of the developing outflow tract the arterial roots belonged. The 'conus' as defined by Kramer is the proximal part of the muscular outflow tract. When fusion has taken place between the aortopulmonary septum and the margins of the distal cushions, the cushions within the proximal part have still to fuse. It is open to debate as to which part of the outflow tract Kramer considered to represent the 'truncus'. That is why it is now better to approach development in tripartite fashion. There is no question but that it is the middle part of the outflow tract, initially retaining its myocardial walls, which subsequently remodels to produce the arterial roots.[2,18] Kramer, however, had described the major entities spiralling through the myocardial part of the outflow tract as ridges rather than cushions, as had de Vries and Saunders when reviewing earlier accounts.[19] There is some justification for continuing to consider these entities as ridges. Unlike the cushions that separate the atrioventricular canal, the entities spiralling through the muscular outflow tract are populated by cells derived from the neural crest. It is the influence of the neural crest cells that induces the structures to fuse with each other, and also with the aortopulmonary septum. Nowadays, nonetheless, it is more usual to find the entities described as 'cushions', largely because they look more like cushions than ridges.

With ongoing development, the cushions within the proximal part of the outflow tract also fuse. At the time of their fusion, the entirety of the proximal component of the outflow tract remains supported above the cavity of the developing right ventricle. As we have already shown, therefore, the fusion of the proximal cushions serves to create a shelf in the roof of the ventricle, thus committing the aortic root to the cavity of the left ventricle (Figure 2.17). And then, by virtue of the fusion of the tubercles derived from the atrioventricular cushions, ventricular septation is completed. These processes are taking place during the seventh and eighth weeks of development (Figure 2.18). The tubercles of the atrioventricular cushions then form the membranous part of the ventricular septum.[20] Significant remodelling then involves the distal ends of the cushions and swellings, converting them into the leaflets of the developing arterial valves (Figure 2.33). The leaflets, which have become recognizable by Carnegie stage 20, remain supported as they remodel by the myocardial walls of the middle part of the outflow tract. The remodelling process involves further addition of non-myocardial tissues to form the arterial walls of the developing valvar sinuses. This results in an ongoing effective retreat of the distal myocardial border (Figure 2.34). As the additional non-myocardial tissues form the arterial walls of the valvar sinuses, the arterial roots themselves continue to separate one from the other. During this process, the core of the fused proximal cushions remodels to become an area of fibro-adipose tissue that separates the aortic root from the developing subpulmonary infundibulum (Figure 2.35). The wall of the pulmonary infundibulum

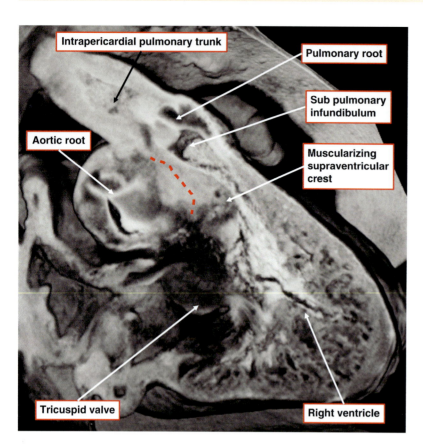

Figure 2.33 The image is an oblique section taken from an episcopic dataset prepared from a human embryo at Carnegie stage 20, which is in the seventh week of development. By this stage, the distal ends of the cushions and swellings in the middle part of the outflow tract are beginning to remodel to form the semilunar leaflets of the arterial valves. The proximal part of the outflow tract has now separated into the free-standing subpulmonary infundibulum and the aortic vestibule, with the cushion mass muscularizing to form the supraventricular crest. An area of fibro-adipose tissue is developing within the core of the fused proximal cushions (red dashed line).

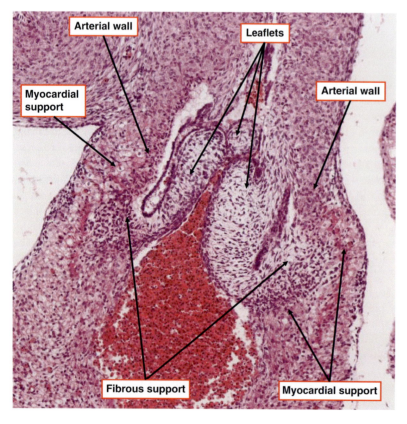

Figure 2.34 The image is a histological section through the developing pulmonary root of a human embryo at Carnegie stage 21, which is reached during the seventh week of development. The cushions and swellings are remodelling to form the valvar leaflets, which retain their myocardial support from the wall of the middle part of the outflow tract. There is ongoing appearance of non-myocardial tissues to form the arterial walls of the sinuses.

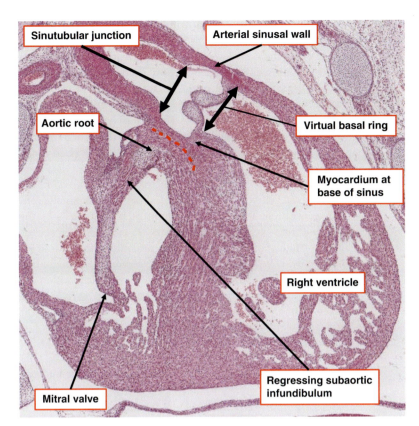

Figure 2.35 The image is a histological section cut in the plane simulating the oblique subcostal echocardiographic projection from a human embryo at Carnegie stage 23, which is the end of the embryonic period of development. The pulmonary root now extends from the virtual basal ring to the sinutubular junction. The free-standing infundibular sleeve now separates the right ventricular outflow tract from the aortic root (red dashed line).

adjacent to the aortic root has been formed by muscularization of the shell of the proximal cushions. The core of the cushion mass also contains the columns of condensed mesenchyme formed from the cells that migrated into the heart from the neural crest. These cells become the so-called tendon of the conus, which eventually extends through the fibrous adipose tissue between the walls of the aortic and pulmonary roots.

The myocardium of the subpulmonary infundibulum adjacent to the aortic root, therefore, is new tissue formed by muscularization of the shell of the fused proximal outflow cushions. As was the case initially for the aortopulmonary septum, and for the distal parts of the outflow cushions, the fused proximal outflow cushions functioned transiently as a septal structure.[21] As occurred with the separation of the intrapericardial arterial trunks, and the arterial roots one from the other, the tissues forming the transient muscular outlet septum lose their septal position as the subpulmonary infundibulum becomes separated from the aortic root by the development of the extracavitary tissues from the core of the tissue mass (Figures 2.33, 2.35). The overall arrangement has frequently been described in terms of an 'aortopulmonary septal complex'. During the initial stages of development, when the protrusion and cushions, in combination, produce a partition between the aortic and pulmonary channels, there is justification for this terminology. The structures, however, fulfil a septal role for only a short time. With the formation of the discrete walls of the intrapericardial arterial trunks, the arterial roots, and the subpulmonary infundibulum, so do the intervening structures cease to be septal. By Carnegie stage 23, therefore, which represents the end of the embryonic period of development, there are no septal components remaining in the outflow tracts. In the setting of deficient ventricular septation, nonetheless, the proximal cushions are able to persist as either a muscular or a fibrous outlet septum.[21]

Development of the Extrapericardial Arterial Pathways

Whilst all the remodelling of the outflow tract has been taking place during the latter part of the embryonic period of development, the heart itself has been moving caudally within the embryo. Accompanying this change, there has also been major and rapid remodelling of the arteries arising from the aortic sac. At Carnegie stage 14, the arrangement was one of symmetry, with the third, fourth, and pulmonary arch arteries extending through the pharyngeal mesenchyme on each side of the gut to join the dorsal aortas (Figure 2.27). It is not only the arch arteries that are involved in the remodelling. Also involved are the seventh cervical intersegmental arteries. These vessels take their origin from the dorsal aortas, but initially at a site markedly caudal to the location of the heart. During the sixth week of development, the caudal movement of the heart brings the seventh segmental arteries closer to the arteries of the fourth arch, with the dorsal aorta on each side providing the arterial continuity (Figure 2.36). With ongoing remodelling, the arteries of the third arches are becoming the carotid arteries. The right horn of the aortic sac, along with the right fourth arch artery, have become the brachiocephalic artery, with the artery of the right fourth arch now

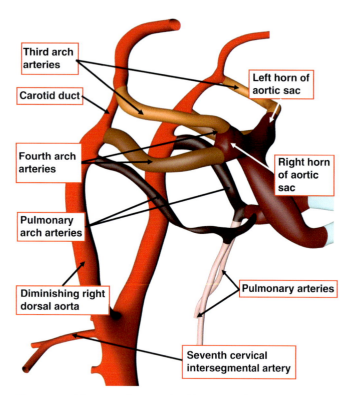

Figure 2.36 The image shows a right oblique view of the reconstructed extrapericardial arterial pathways from a human embryo at Carnegie stage 17, representing around 40 days of development. The caudal movement of the heart has brought the seventh cervical intersegmental arteries, which will become the subclavian arteries, closer to the arteries of the fourth arch arches. It is possible now to recognize the beginnings of diminution in size of the right dorsal aorta and the artery of the right pulmonary arch.

providing the continuity between the right horn of the sac and the seventh cervical segmental artery (Figure 2.37). The left horn of the aortic sac is then transformed into the first part of the transverse aortic arch. The part of the transverse arch between the origins of the left common carotid artery, which is derived from the artery of the left third arch, and the left seventh cervical intersegmental artery, is then the artery of the left fourth arch. As on the right side, the segmental artery will eventually become the subclavian artery. On the left side, however, during the process of remodelling, the artery must cross the junction between the pulmonary arch artery and the left dorsal aorta. With attenuation of the artery of the right pulmonary arch, so has the left artery become the arterial duct. The transfer of the left seventh cervical intersegmental artery across the junction between the duct and the descending aorta then produces the aortic isthmus. This point has been reached at Carnegie stage 20, during the seventh week of development, by which time the arterial pathways are essentially in their definitive situations (Figure 2.38).

Development of the Cardiac Conduction System

In the postnatal heart, it is the sinus node that creates the sinus impulse. The impulse, having spread through the atrial myocardium, is then slowed by the atrioventricular node, thus permitting atrial contraction to fill the ventricles prior to ventricular systole. The working ventricular myocardium is then activated by the ramifications of the atrioventricular conduction axis. The atrioventricular node, responsible for producing the atrioventricular delay, forms the atrial component of the axis. It is only the atrioventricular conduction axis, in the normal heart, which penetrates the insulating tissues formed at the atrioventricular junctions. These elements responsible for generation and transmission of the cardiac impulse are usually described as the conduction system. All the working cardiomyocytes, however, are also able to conduct. It is arguable that the make-up of the working cardiomyocytes is more specialized than that of the cells that generate and transmit the impulse. It is the cells of the transmitting system, nonetheless, that are labelled as representing the conduction system. All of the cardiomyocytes are coupled electrically. It is those with the highest pacemaking activity that generate the impulse. Almost always, this takes place within the sinus node. The developing sinus node can be recognized at the junction of the superior caval vein with the developing right atrium as early as Carnegie stage 15, when the embryo is just beginning its sixth week of development (Figure 2.39). During the early stages of development, all the cardiomyocytes making up the initial heart tube are poorly coupled and display intrinsic automaticity. When the heart begins to beat, the depolarizing impulse is conducted slowly along the cardiac tube, with peristaltic waves of contraction serving to propel the blood from the venous to the arterial pole. As the atrial appendages balloon from the atrial component of the primary tube, and the ventricular apical components from the ventricular loop, so the heart begins to generate an adult type of electrocardiogram. This is characterized by rapid atrial depolarization, a period of atrioventricular delay, and subsequent rapid ventricular depolarization. By the stage of closure of the primary atrial foramen, it has become possible to recognize the appearance of the sinus node (Figure 2.39). Over the period of the following week, by Carnegie stage 19, the node has established its definitive position within the terminal groove, with an obvious body and a well-formed tail (Figure 2.40).

It is the working cardiomyocytes that depolarize rapidly. They express atrial natriuretic factor, with their linking gap junctions containing the proteins connexin 40 and 43, which permit fast conduction. At the initial stages, when the atrioventricular canal is supported by the developing left ventricle, and the outflow tract is positioned above the developing right ventricle, the areas permitting rapid conduction are separated by the cardiomyocytes of the atrioventricular canal itself. This is part of the primary heart tube, and its contained cardiomyocytes all conduct slowly. This slowly conducting myocardium of the atrioventricular canal, with ongoing development, becomes sequestered on the atrial sides of the developing atrioventricular junctions as the atrial vestibules. Prior to expansion of the atrioventricular canal, its right side is also part of the initial margins of the primary interventricular foramen (Figure 2.14). And, at this early stage, the cells surrounding the foramen can be recognized on the basis of their response to an epitope prepared from the nodose ganglion of the chick heart[22] as being part of the so-called primary ring (Figure 2.41).

2 Development of the Heart

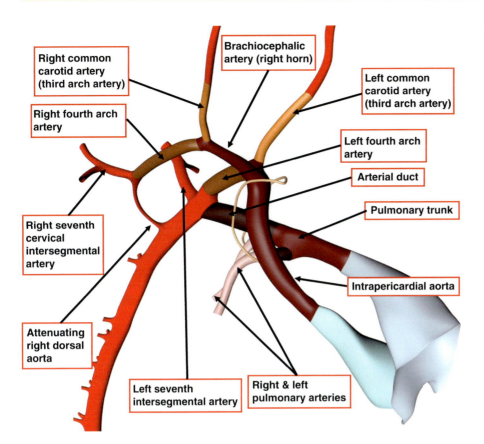

Figure 2.37 The image shows the state of the developing extrapericardial arterial pathways at Carnegie stage 18, when the embryo is around 43 days after fertilization. With ongoing attenuation of the dorsal part of the right dorsal aorta, the right seventh cervical intersegmental artery has continued to move cranially to join the base of the right fourth arch artery, with the right horn of the aortic sac transforming into the brachiocephalic artery.

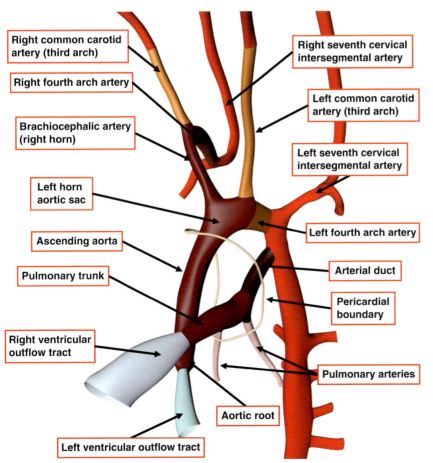

Figure 2.38 The image shows a view of the reconstructed arterial pathways from the left side and anterior in a human embryo at Carnegie stage 20, representing the situation towards the end of the seventh week of development. By this stage, the pathways are essentially in their postnatal arrangement, albeit that the arterial duct will close after birth.

It is rightward expansion of the atrioventricular canal that gives the right atrium its inlet component (Figures 2.10, 2.14). The process of expansion also serves to incorporate the cranial part of the primary ring within the vestibule of the developing right atrioventricular junction (Figure 2.42).

Subsequent to the formation of the insulating tissues of the atrioventricular junctions, there are two potential transitions created by the primary ring with the atrial myocardium. It is the inferior transition that will become the atrioventricular node. Extensions from the primary ring into the vestibules of the tricuspid and mitral valves form the right and left inferior extensions of the node. It is muscularization of the vestibular spine that then provides the inputs to the node from the atrial septum (Figure 2.43). It is components of the trabecular meshwork that initially filled the larger part of both ventricular apical components that then remodel to produce the ventricular bundle branches and their apical ramifications. Parts of the initial primary ring also persist in the vestibule of the tricuspid valve as the so-called atrioventricular ring tissues (Figure 2.42). The part directly adjacent to the inferior transition becomes the inferior right extension of the atrioventricular node. The inferior left extension is part of the atrioventricular canal myocardium, but does not contain any component of the primary ring. Initially, the ring also encircled the secondary interventricular foramen, which remodels to become the entrance to the aortic root. Most of these ventral parts of the primary ring attenuate and disappear, although some parts can extend into the aortic root on the crest of the muscular ventricular septum as the so-called dead-end tract.[23] The atrial component of the superior transition can still be identified in many postnatal hearts as the retro-aortic node.[24] The locations of these remnants of the primary ring, as we will describe in the appropriate chapters of our book, provide the

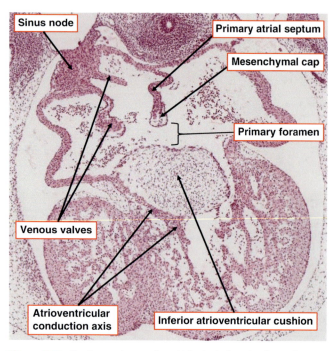

Figure 2.39 The image shows a frontal histological section from a human embryo at Carnegie stage 15, when around 36 days have passed after fertilization. The sinus node can be recognized at the superior cavoatrial junction. It is also possible to recognize the beginning of the atrioventricular conduction axis, which is extending between the left ventricular trabeculations and the atrioventricular canal myocardium.

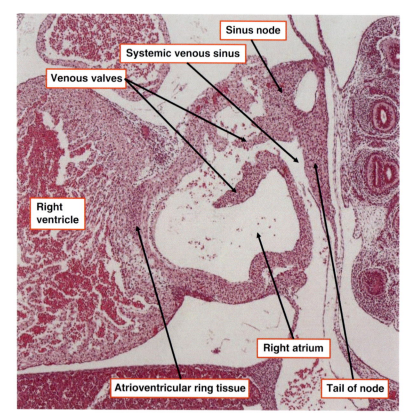

Figure 2.40 The image is a sagittal histological section from a human embryo at Carnegie stage 19, at the beginning of the seventh week of development. It shows the sinus node now occupying the junction between the systemic venous sinus, which receives the superior and inferior caval veins at its poles, and the remainder of the right atrium. By this stage, the node has an obvious body and an elongated tail. There is also an obvious aggregation of cardiomyocytes in the vestibule of the tricuspid valve. These cardiomyocytes are part of the ring that initially encircled the primary interventricular foramen, and which forms the basis of the atrioventricular conduction axis.

2 Development of the Heart

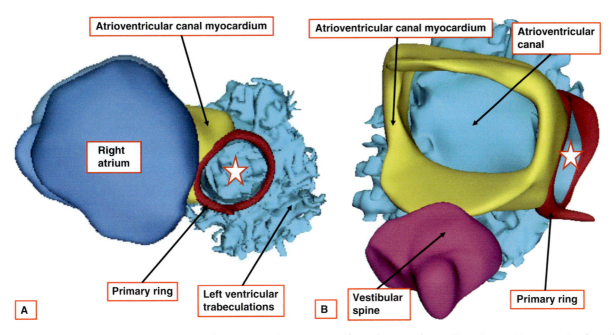

Figure 2.41 The images show reconstructions from the same dataset, prepared from a human embryo at Carnegie stage 14, representing the end of the fifth week of development. The primary ring is shown encircling the primary embryonic interventricular foramen (white stars with red borders). The image in panel A is shown from the right side, having removed the developing right ventricle. Panel B shows the same reconstruction, but viewed from above with the addition of the vestibular spine. The cranial part of the primary ring is part of the right wall of the atrioventricular canal.

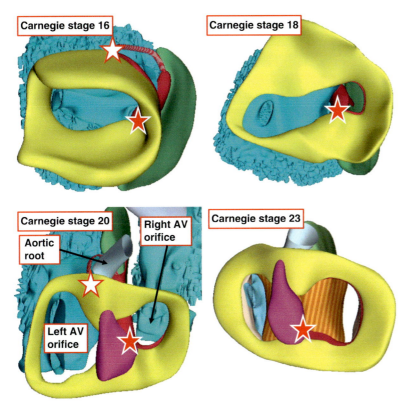

Figure 2.42 The reconstructions show the influence of expansion of the atrioventricular canal on the fate of the primary ring. With the cranial part of the ring becoming incorporated into the vestibule of the tricuspid valve, there are two transitions across the developing insulating tissues of the atrioventricular junctions. The inferior transition becomes the penetrating atrioventricular bundle (red stars with white borders). The superior transition attenuates, but the atrial component becomes the retro-aortic node (white stars with red borders). At the end of the embryonic period, however, at Carnegie stage 23, the point of penetration is at the crux of the heart.

basis for interpreting the atypical disposition of the conducting system in congenital malformations such as straddling tricuspid valves, double inlet left ventricles, and congenitally corrected transposition. As we will also describe, they can also explain the variant of ventricular pre-excitation known as Mahaim conduction.[25]

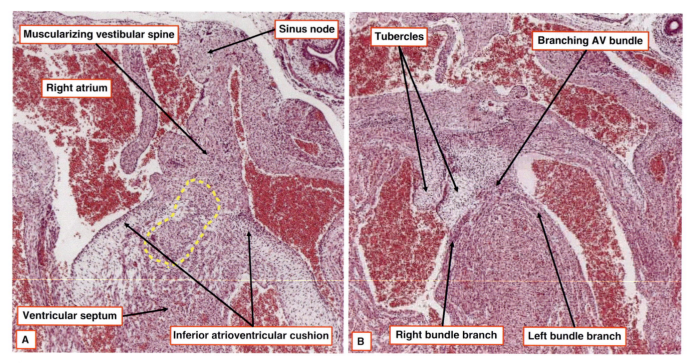

Figure 2.43 The images show two serial histological sections, in the frontal plane, from a human embryo at Carnegie stage 22, which represents around eight weeks of development. Panel A shows the inferior transition of the primary ring (yellow dashed line), which is forming the atrioventricular node as it makes contact with the atrial cardiomyocytes in the muscularizing vestibular spine. Panel B shows the continuation of the primary ring through the trabecular cardiomyocytes of the ventricles, which are remodelling to form the right and left bundle branches. Note also the tubercles of the atrioventricular cushions, which have closed the tertiary interventricular communication.

Development of the Coronary Circulation

The coronary arteries are derived from the epicardium, which in turn is derived from the pro-epicardial organ. Cells derived from this organ subsequently expand over the epicardial surface of the heart, reaching as far as the distal outflow tract. The cells then penetrate the developing myocardial walls, providing not only the fibrous matrix of the compact myocardium, but also the muscular walls of the coronary arteries and veins.[26] It had been suggested long since that the developing epicardial coronary arteries were connected to the aortic root by virtue of stems budding out from the aortic valvar sinuses. Indeed, such buds were intimated to develop not only from the aortic valvar sinuses, but also the sinuses of the pulmonary trunk.[27] It then became fashionable to argue that the proximal epicardial coronary arteries grew into the aortic root.[28] The evidence from both histological sections and episcopic datasets now shows that stems do grow out from the proximal margins of distal non-myocardial outflow tract as the walls become converted into the arterial valvar sinuses (Figure 2.44). Even in hearts that are congenitally malformed, it is almost always the case that the major epicardial coronary arteries take their origin from the aortic sinuses adjacent to the pulmonary trunk. There is no obvious pattern of sinusal origin, however, when the middle part of the outflow tract fails to separate in the setting of common arterial trunk. These facts suggest that fusion of the distal outflow cushions plays a role in guiding the epicardial coronary arteries to their appropriate aortic origin. Further support for this notion is provided by the frequent finding of anomalous origin of a major coronary artery from the pulmonary trunk in the setting of aortopulmonary window.

Development during the Fetal and Neonatal Periods

The end of the embryonic period of development, coinciding with around eight weeks of development subsequent to conception, is represented by Carnegie stage 23. The anatomical arrangements we have demonstrated at that stage indicate that additional marked changes are needed during ongoing fetal development so as to produce the definitive anatomy of the four-chambered organ. At the end of the embryonic period, for example, the pulmonary venous tributaries have only just begun their migration to the roof of the left atrium. The septal leaflet of the tricuspid valve has still to delaminate from the ventricular septum. Both atrioventricular junctions have still to expand to form the inferior pyramidal space, and the aortic root remains relatively distant from the left atrioventricular junction, with the myocardial subaortic infundibulum only just beginning to attenuate. It is with the ongoing commitment of the pulmonary veins to the roof of the left atrium that the superior interatrial fold becomes much deeper. All these changes begin at the end of the third month of gestation, and continue through the fourth and fifth months. In the ongoing months of fetal life, therefore, major differences remain when compared with the definitive situations. The long axis of the heart, for example, is horizontal, but points anteriorly rather than to the left. The absence of air in the lungs does mean that it is much easier for the fetal echocardiographer to display the intracardiac structures, and hence to identify congenital malformations throughout gestation.

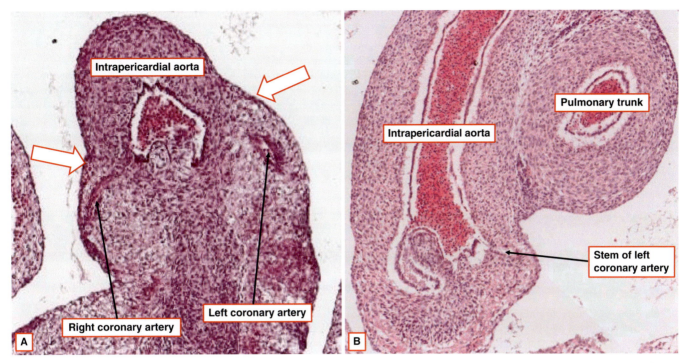

Figure 2.44 The images are from frontal histological sections prepared from human embryos at Carnegie stages 18 (panel A) and 21 (panel B). Panel A shows the major epicardial coronary arteries within the myocardial collar that continues to enclose the middle part of the outflow tract at this stage. Now, the arteries within the myocardial collar have no obvious connection with the developing aortic valvar sinuses. The white arrows with red borders are showing the distal extent of the myocardial wall of the outflow tract. Panel B shows that, by the later stage of development, the stem of the left coronary artery has developed from the non-myocardial tissues that are becoming incorporated into the aortic root to form the arterial valvar sinuses.

With birth, and with the equalization of atrial pressures, the flap valve of the atrial septum, derived from the primary atrial septum, is pushed firmly against the left atrial rims of the oval fossa, thus promoting subsequent anatomical fusion. The foramen remains probe patent, nonetheless, in up to one-third of all normal individuals.[4] At birth, since the right ventricle has been working against systemic pressures during fetal life, its thickness is comparable to that of the left ventricle. By the end of the third postnatal month, the left ventricle has become thicker than the right. This growth continues, with the left ventricular walls being twice as thick by the second year, and three times as thick at puberty. Conversion of the fetal to the postnatal circulation also requires closure of the arterial and venous ducts. Physiological closure takes place on the first day of life, with the muscular walls of the ducts becoming converted into arterial ligaments over the ensuing weeks.

References Cited

1. Meilhac SM, Buckingham ME. The deployment of cell lineages that form the mammalian heart. *Nat Rev Cardiol* 2018; **15**: 705–724.

2. Hikspoors JP, Kruepunga N, Mommen G, et al. A pictorial account of the human embryonic heart between 3.5 and 8 weeks of development. *Commun Biol* 2022; **5**: 1–22.

3. Davis CL. Development of the human heart from its first appearance to the stage found in embryos of twenty paired somites. *Contributions Embryol, Carnegie Inst* 1927; **107**: 247–284.

4. O'Rahilly R, Müller F. Developmental stages in human embryos: revised and new measurements. *Cells Tissues Organs* 2010; **192**: 73–84.

5. Manner J. On the form problem of embryonic heart loops, its geometrical solutions, and a new biophysical concept of cardiac looping. *Ann Anat* 2013; **195**: 312–323.

6. Rodgers LS, Lalani S, Runyan RB, Camenisch TD. Differential growth and multicellular villi direct proepicardial translocation to the developing mouse heart. *Dev Dyn* 2008; **237**: 145–152.

7. Webb S, Kanani M, Anderson RH, Richardson MK, Brown NA. Development of the human pulmonary vein and its incorporation in the morphologically left atrium. *Cardiol Young* 2001; **11**: 632–642.

8. Jensen B, Spicer DE, Sheppard MN, Anderson RH. Development of the atrial septum in relation to postnatal anatomy and interatrial communications. *Heart* 2017; **103**: 456–462.

9. Hagen PT, Scholz DG, Edwards WD. Incidence and size of patent foramen ovale during the first 10 decades of life: an autopsy study of 965 normal hearts. *Mayo Clin Proc* 1984; **59**: 17–20.

10. Lamers WH, Wessels A, Verbeek FJ, et al. New findings concerning ventricular septation in the human heart. Implications for maldevelopment. *Circulation* 1992; **86**: 1194–1205.

11. Christoffels VM, Habets PE, Franco D, et al. Chamber formation and morphogenesis in the developing mammalian heart. *Dev Biol* 2000; **223**: 266–278.

12. Allwork SP, Anderson RH. Developmental anatomy of the membranous part of the ventricular septum in the human heart. *Heart* 1979; **41**: 275–280.

13. Anderson RH, Jensen B, Mohun TJ, et al. Key questions relating to left ventricular noncompaction cardiomyopathy: is the emperor still wearing any clothes? *Can J Cardiol* 2017; **33**: 747–757.
14. Graham A, Poopalasundaram S, Shone V, Kiecker C. A reappraisal and revision of the numbering of the pharyngeal arches. *J Anat* 2019; **235**: 1019–1023.
15. Anderson RH, Bamforth SD, Gupta SK. How best to describe the pharyngeal arch arteries when the fifth arch does not exist? *Cardiol Young* 2020; **30**: 1708–1710.
16. Anderson RH, Bamforth SD. Morphogenesis of the mammalian aortic arch arteries. *Front Cell Dev Biol* 2022; **10**: 892900.
17. Kramer TC. The partitioning of the truncus and conus and the formation of the membranous portion of the interventricular septum in the human heart. *Am J Anat* 1942; **71**: 343–370.
18. Anderson RH, Chaudhry B, Mohun TJ, et al. Normal and abnormal development of the intrapericardial arterial trunks in humans and mice. *Cardiovasc Res* 2012; **95**: 108–115.
19. De Vries PA, Saunders JB. Development of the ventricles and spiral outflow tract in the human heart: a contribution to the development of the human heart from age group IX to age group XV. *Cont Embryol* 1962; **37**: 87–114.
20. Odgers PN. The development of the pars membranacea septi in the human heart. *J Anat* 1938; **72**: 247–259.
21. Anderson RH, Tretter JT, Spicer DE, Mori S. The fate of the outflow tract septal complex in relation to the classification of ventricular septal defects. *J Cardiovasc Dev Dis* 2019; **6**:9.
22. Wessels A, Vermeulen JL, Verbeek FJ, et al. Spatial distribution of 'tissue-specific' antigens in the developing human heart and skeletal muscle. III. An immunohistochemical analysis of the distribution of the neural tissue antigen GlN2 in the embryonic heart; implications for the development of the atrioventricular conduction system. *Anat Rec* 1992; **232**: 97–111.
23. Anderson RH, Spicer DE, Mori S. Of tracts, rings, nodes, cusps, sinuses, and arrhythmias – a comment on Szili-Torok et al.'s paper entitled 'The "Dead-End Tract" and Its Role in Arrhythmogenesis'. *J Cardiovasc Dev Dis* 2016; **3**: 17.
24. Hikspoors JP, Macías Y, Tretter JT, et al. Miniseries 1 – part I: the development of the atrioventricular conduction axis. *EP Europace* 2022; **24**: 432–442.
25. Sternick EB, Sanchez-Quintana D, Wellens HJ, Anderson RH. Mahaim revisited. *Arrhythm Electrophysiol Rev* 2022; **11**: e14.
26. Anderson RH, Turner JE, Henderson DJ. The morphogenesis of abnormal coronary arteries in the congenitally malformed heart. *J Thorac Cardiovasc Surg* 2022; **164**: 344–349.
27. Hackensellner HA. Akzessorische Kranzgefäßanlagen der Arteria pulmonalis unter 63 menschlichen Embryonen-Serien mit einer größten Länge von 12 bis 36 mm. *Z Mikrosk Anat Forsch* 1956; **62**: 153–164.
28. Bogers AJ, Gittenberger-de Groot AC, Poelmann RE, Peault BM, Huysmans HA. Development of the origin of the coronary arteries, a matter of ingrowth or outgrowth? *Anat Embryol* 1989; **180**: 437–441.

Chapter 3

Anatomy of the Cardiac Chambers

Regardless of the surgical approach, once having entered the mediastinum, the surgeon will be confronted by the heart enclosed in its pericardial sac. In the strict anatomical sense, this sac has two layers, one fibrous and the other serous. From a practical point of view, the pericardium is essentially the tough fibrous layer, since the serous component forms the lining of the fibrous sac, and is reflected back onto the surface of the heart as the epicardium. It is the fibrous sac, therefore, which encloses the mass of the heart. By virtue of its own attachments to the diaphragm, it helps support the heart within the mediastinum. Free-standing around the atrial chambers and the ventricles, the sac becomes adherent to the adventitial coverings of the great arteries and veins at their entrances to and exits from it, these attachments closing the pericardial cavity.[1] The cavity of the pericardium is limited by the two layers of serous pericardium, which are folded on one another to produce a double-layered arrangement. The outer, or parietal, layer is densely adherent to the fibrous pericardium, while the inner layer is firmly attached to the myocardium, and is the epicardium (Figure 3.1). The pericardial cavity, therefore, is the space between the inner parietal serous lining of the fibrous pericardium and the surface of the heart (Figure 3.2). There are two recesses within the cavity that are lined by serous pericardium. The first is the transverse sinus, which occupies the inner curvature of the heart (Figure 3.3). It is bounded anteriorly by the posterior surface of the great arteries. Posteriorly, it is limited by the right pulmonary artery and the roof of the left atrium. There is a further recess from the transverse sinus that extends between the superior caval and the right upper pulmonary veins, with its right lateral border being a pericardial fold between these vessels (Figure 3.4). When exposing the mitral valve through a left atriotomy, incisions through this fold, along with mobilization of the superior caval vein, provide excellent access to the superior aspect of the left atrium and the right pulmonary artery. This fold is also incised when a snare is placed around the superior caval vein. On each side, the ends of the transverse sinus are in free communication with the remainder of the pericardial cavity.

The second pericardial recess is the oblique sinus. This is a blind-ending cavity behind the left atrium (Figure 3.5). Its upper boundary is formed by the reflection of serous pericardium between the upper pulmonary veins. The right border is the reflection of pericardium around the right pulmonary veins and the inferior caval vein, while the left border is the reflection of pericardium around the left pulmonary veins (Figure 3.6).

With the usual surgical approach through a median sternotomy, the fibrous pericardium is opened more-or-less in the midline and retracted laterally, exposing the anterior sternocostal surface of the heart and great vessels. The pulmonary trunk and aorta are then seen leaving the base of the heart. They extend in a superior direction, with the aortic root in posterior and rightward position (Figure 3.2). Should the aortic root not be in this expected relationship, then almost always the ventriculo-arterial connections will be abnormal (see Chapter 9.2). The atrial appendages are usually seen one to either side of the prominent arterial pedicle.

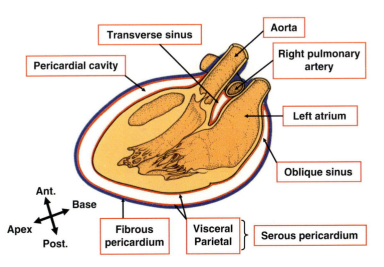

Figure 3.1 The cartoon shows the arrangement of the pericardial cavity as seen in parasternal long-axis view.

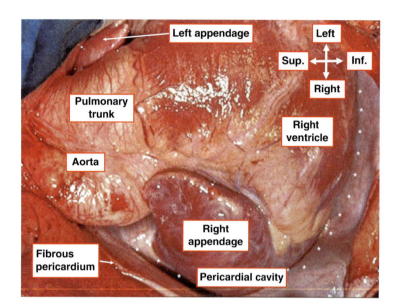

Figure 3.2 The operative view, through a median sternotomy, shows the anterior surface of the heart following a pericardial incision. The white asterisks show the extent of the pericardial cavity.

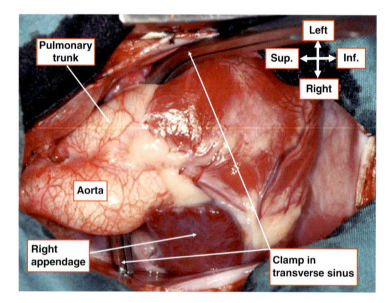

Figure 3.3 Operative view through a median sternotomy. The clamp has been passed through the transverse sinus.

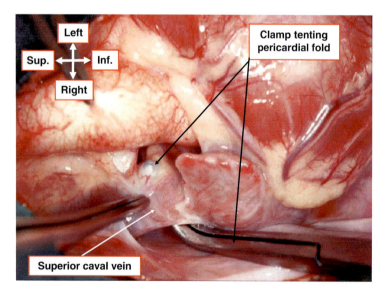

Figure 3.4 Operative view through a median sternotomy showing the posterior recess of the transverse sinus limited by a pericardial fold around the superior caval vein. In this picture, the fold is being tented by a right-angled clamp passed behind the superior caval vein.

3 Anatomy of the Cardiac Chambers

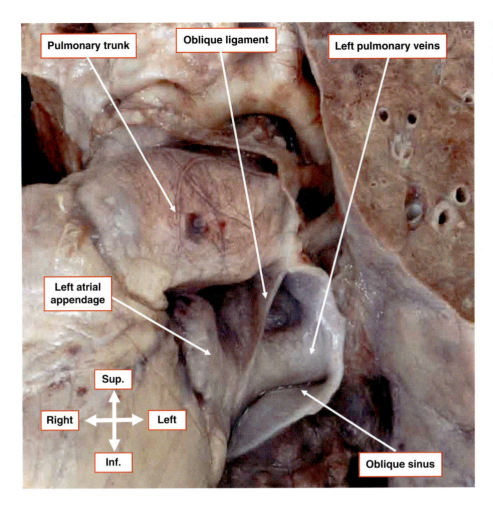

Figure 3.5 Anatomical view showing the oblique sinus of the pericardial cavity, which lies behind the left atrium. Note the oblique ligament, which occupies the site during development of the left superior caval vein.

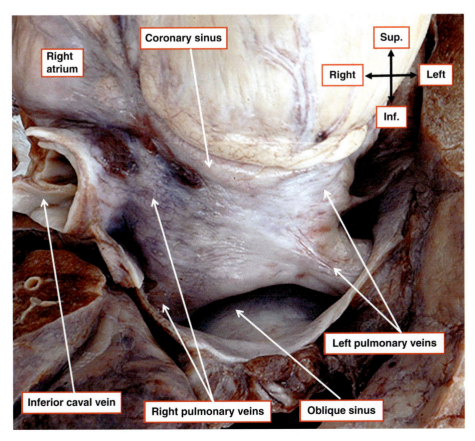

Figure 3.6 The heart has been reflected superiorly from its pericardial cradle to show the location of the oblique sinus.

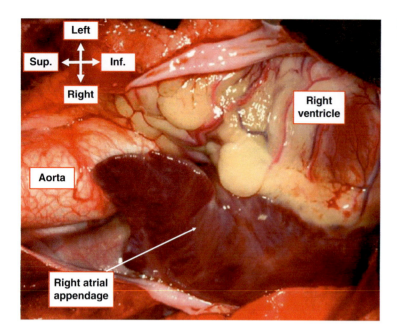

Figure 3.7 Operative view through a median sternotomy showing the typical triangular shape of the morphologically right atrial appendage.

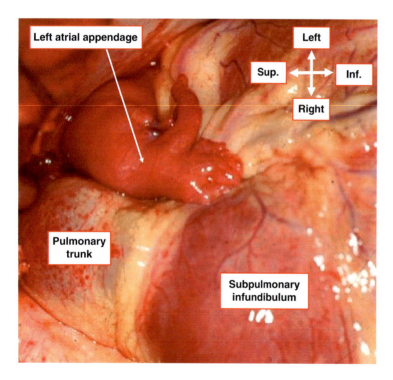

Figure 3.8 Operative view through a median sternotomy showing the tubular morphologically left atrial appendage.

The morphologically right appendage is more prominent. It has a blunt triangular shape, and possesses a broad junction with the atrial vestibule and the systemic venous sinus (Figure 3.7). The morphologically left appendage may not be seen immediately. When found at the left border of the pulmonary trunk, it is a tubular structure, having a narrow junction with the rest of the atrium (Figure 3.8). Presence of the two appendages on the same side of the arterial pedicle is an anomaly in itself, which is called juxtaposition. This arrangement is almost always associated with additional malformations within the heart (see Chapter 11). Inspection of the left border of the heart should always include a search for persistence of the left superior caval vein. When present, the venous channel will be found by following the course of the left pulmonary artery. The vein crosses anterior to the left pulmonary artery. It is seen superiorly within the pericardial cavity, with the left atrial appendage located anteriorly and laterally (Figure 3.9). Within the pericardial cavity, it then extends down the posterior aspect of the left atrium, passing through the inferior left atrioventricular groove to reach the right atrial orifice of the coronary sinus (Figure 3.10).

The ventricular mass extends from the atrioventricular grooves to the apex, and usually extends into the left hemithorax. An anomalous position of the ventricular mass, or its

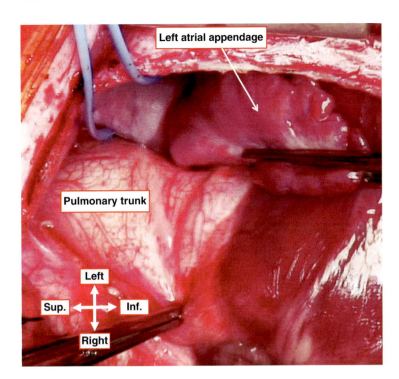

Figure 3.9 The operative view through a median sternotomy shows the location of a persistent left superior caval vein, snared by the surgeon in this image.

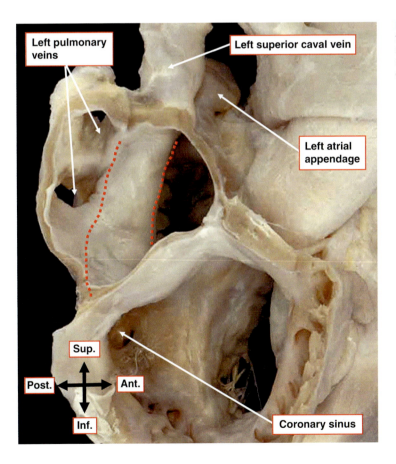

Figure 3.10 The base of the heart has been dissected by removing the atrial walls. The dissection now shows the course of a persistent left superior caval vein as it passes through the left atrioventricular groove (red dotted lines), emptying into the right atrium through the enlarged orifice of the coronary sinus.

apex, is again highly suggestive of the presence of congenital cardiac malformations (see Chapter 11). In shape, the ventricular mass is a three-sided pyramid, with inferior diaphragmatic, anterior sternocostal, and posterior pulmonary surfaces (Figure 3.11). The margin between the first two surfaces is sharp. Because of this, it is described as the acute margin. The angulations of the margins between the pulmonary and the sternocostal surfaces anteriorly, and the pulmonary and diaphragmatic surfaces posteriorly, are much more obtuse. The surgeon encounters these obtuse marginal areas

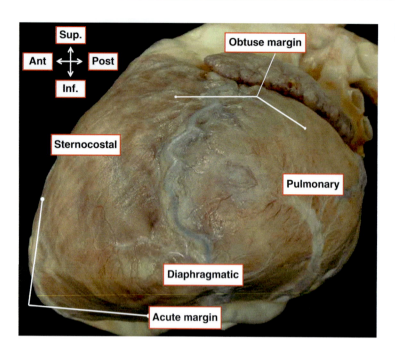

Figure 3.11 The heart has been removed from the chest and is viewed from its apex, showing the surfaces of the ventricular cone.

when the apex of the heart is tipped out of the pericardium. They are supplied by the obtuse marginal branches of the circumflex coronary artery. The greater part of the anterior surface of the ventricular mass is occupied by the morphologically right ventricle, with its left border marked by the anterior interventricular, or descending, branch of the left coronary artery. This artery curves onto the ventricular surface between the left atrial appendage and the basal origin of the pulmonary trunk. The right border of the morphologically right ventricle is marked by the right coronary artery, which runs obliquely in the atrioventricular groove. Unusually prominent coronary arteries coursing on the ventricular surface should always raise the suspicion of significant cardiac malformations.

The surface anatomy of the heart is helpful in determining the most appropriate site for an incision to gain access to a given cardiac chamber. For example, the relatively bloodless outlet portion of the right ventricle just beneath the origin of the pulmonary trunk affords ready access to the cavity of the subpulmonary infundibulum (Figure 3.8). The important landmark for the right atrium is the terminal groove, or sulcus terminalis. This marks the junction between the appendage and the systemic venous component of the right atrium (Figure 3.12). The sinus node is located within this groove. It is usually positioned laterally and inferiorly relative to the superior cavoatrial junction (Figures 3.13). On occasion, it extends over the crest of the appendage (Figure 3.14). The clinically significant artery to the sinus node can also be seen on occasion, either as it crosses the crest of the right appendage, or as it courses behind the superior caval vein to enter the terminal groove between the orifices of the caval veins. Posterior to, and parallel with, the terminal groove is a second, deeper, groove. This second groove interposes between the cavity of the right atrium and the right pulmonary veins. Known as Waterston's or Sondergaard's groove, it can be used to gain access to the left atrium (Figure 3.15). Such access can be gained either by making an incision in the floor of the groove, or directly through the left atrial roof. The roof is seen behind the aorta, to the left of the superior cavoatrial junction (Figure 3.12).

Morphologically Right Atrium

The right atrium, and, as we will see, its left atrial counterpart, has four basic parts. These are the body, the appendage, the venous component, receiving the systemic venous return, and the vestibule of the tricuspid valve. The atrial septum then interposes between the atrial cavities. The body is the remnant of the initial atrial component of the heart tube (see Chapter 2). The majority of the body, in the postnatal heart, is committed to the left atrium, but a small part is found in the right atrium between the left venous valve, when present, and the atrial septum. The space is larger during development, when it is known as the intersepto-valvar space (see Figure 2.7). When it is possible to recognize the left venous valve, which is not always the case, the body of the right atrium can then be identified (Figure 3.16). The venous valves form the boundaries between the systemic venous sinus and, to the right, the appendage, and, to the left, when present, the small part of the body. The right venous valves persist to some extent as the Eustachian and Thebesian valves (Figure 3.17). It is less frequent to find a remnant of the left valve to provide an anatomical boundary between the systemic venous sinus and the septum (Figure 3.17). The venous sinus is much smaller when viewed externally, with only that part extending between the terminal and Waterston's grooves being visible to the surgeon (Figures 3.12, 3.15). It receives the superior and inferior caval veins at its extremities. The coronary sinus also opens into the venous sinus, with its orifice found on the septal aspect of the opening of the inferior caval vein (Figure 3.17). The junction of the systemic venous sinus with the appendage is much more obvious. It is identified externally by the prominent terminal groove (Figure 3.12). Internally, the groove corresponds with the terminal crest. This

3 Anatomy of the Cardiac Chambers

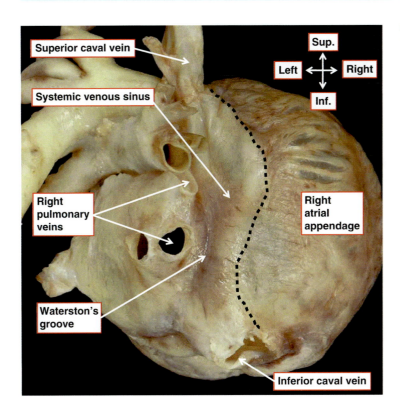

Figure 3.12 The heart is photographed from the right side to show the location of the terminal groove (black dots) between the appendage and the systemic venous sinus.

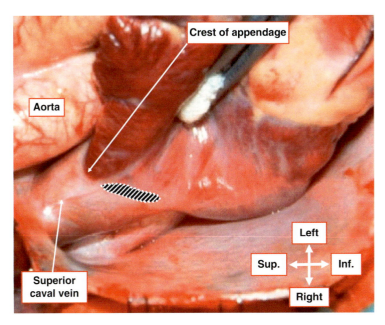

Figure 3.13 Operative view through a median sternotomy demonstrating the usual site of the sinus node. The node can often be seen as a pale cigar-shaped area located antero-laterally in the terminal groove. This anticipated site is highlighted in the photograph by the black and white cross-hatched area.

prominent muscular strap gives origin to the pectinate muscles of the appendage (Figures 3.17, 3.18). In shape, the appendage is blunt and triangular, having a wide junction to the venous sinus across the terminal groove. Superiorly and anteriorly, the appendage has a particularly important relation with the superior caval vein. Here, the appendage terminates in a prominent crest (Figure 3.13). This forms the summit of the terminal groove. It can be traced as it extends into the transverse sinus behind the aorta to become contiguous with the interatrial groove (Figure 3.14). Absence of such a right-sided crest should alert the surgeon to the presence of isomerism of the left atrial appendages (see Chapter 7). As already discussed, almost always

the sinus node lies immediately subepicardially within the terminal groove. Spindle-shaped, it usually lies to the right of the crest as seen by the surgeon, in other words, lateral and inferior to the superior cavoatrial junction (Figure 3.13). In about one-tenth of cases, the node extends across the crest into the interatrial groove. It is then draped across the cavoatrial junction in horseshoe fashion[2] (Figure 3.14).

Also of significance is the course of the artery to the sinus node (Figure 3.19). This artery is a branch of the right coronary artery in just over half the population, and a branch of the circumflex artery in the remainder.[3] Irrespective of its origin, it usually courses through the anterior interatrial groove towards

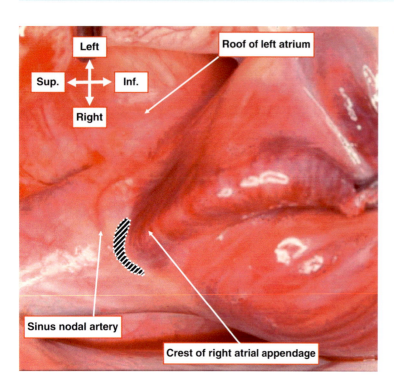

Figure 3.14 Operative view through a median sternotomy showing a sinus node arranged in horseshoe fashion across the crest of the right atrial appendage, with one limb in the terminal groove and the other extending towards the interatrial groove. The nodal location is again highlighted by the black cross-hatched area. Note the course of the artery to the node.

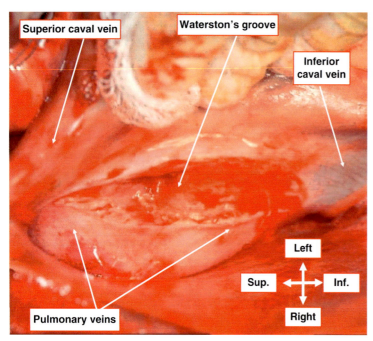

Figure 3.15 Waterston's groove seen through a median sternotomy. The tissue plane between the atrial chambers has been partially dissected.

the superior cavoatrial junction (Figure 3.20), frequently running within the atrial myocardium. It usually takes its origin from the proximal segment of its parent coronary artery (Figure 3.21). A significant variant is found when the artery originates from either coronary artery some distance from the aorta. If taking origin from the right coronary artery, it then courses over the lateral surface of the appendage to reach the terminal groove (Figure 3.22). If originating from the circumflex artery, it crosses the roof of the left atrium (Figure 3.23). Such lateral origin is rare in normal hearts,[4,5] but more frequent in association with congenital malformations.[6] Irrespective of its origin, as it enters the sinus node, the artery may cross the crest of the appendage,

course retrocavally (Figure 3.24), or even divide to form an arterial circle round the junction (Figure 3.25). All these variations should be taken into account when planning the safest right atrial incision, particularly when the nodal artery crosses the lateral margin of the right appendage, or courses over the roof of the left atrium. Although it might seem obvious, care should be taken to ensure that the incision cuts across neither the terminal crest nor the right coronary artery.

Opening the atrium through the most appropriate incision shows that the terminal groove (Figure 3.26) is the external counterpart of the prominent internal muscle bundle, the terminal crest. This separates the pectinate muscles of the

3 Anatomy of the Cardiac Chambers

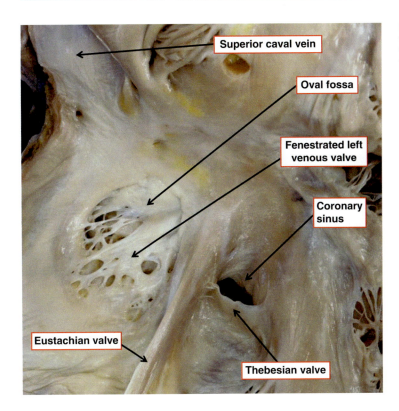

Figure 3.16 The right atrium has been opened to show a heart in which it is possible to recognize the remnants of the left venous valve, which is fenestrated. The body of the atrium is the small space between the venous remnant and the floor of the oval fossa, which is itself patent.

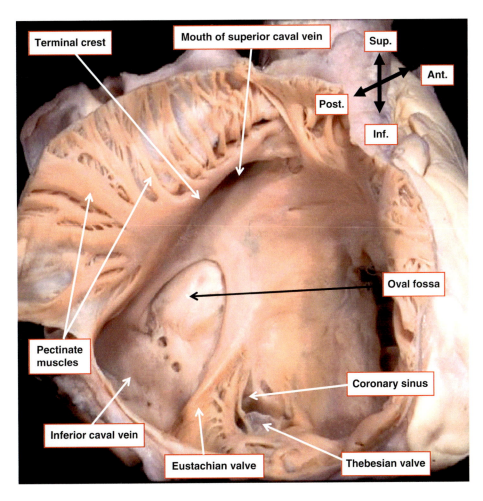

Figure 3.17 The heart has been opened by reflecting the wall of the right atrial appendage, showing the more usual arrangement when it is not possible to recognize any remnant of the left venous valve. The systemic venous sinus now abuts the septal structures. Note the location of the terminal crest and the pectinate muscles in the appendage.

49

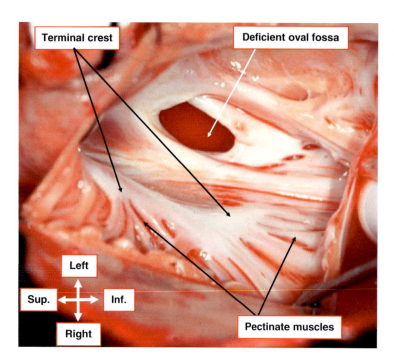

Figure 3.18 Operative view through a median sternotomy having opened the right atrium. The terminal crest is seen giving rise to the pectinate muscles of the right atrial appendage. Note that, in this patient, the floor of the oval fossa is deficient, producing an atrial septal defect.

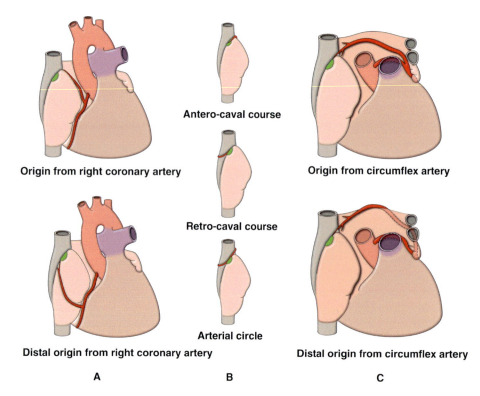

Figure 3.19 The cartoon, drawn in anatomical orientation, shows the variations in the origin of the artery to the sinus node, and the variability relative to the cavoatrial junction. Panel A shows the usual arrangement with origin from the right coronary artery, found in 55% of the population, with the rare variant of distal origin with coursing across the appendage (lower panel A). Panel C show proximal origin from the circumflex artery, found in around 45% of the population, with the rare variant of distal origin with coursing across the dome of the left atrium. Panel B shows the variation relative to the superior cavoatrial junction. The sinus node is shown in green.

appendage from the smooth walls of the systemic venous sinus (Figures 3.17, 3.18). The cardiomyocytes are aligned along the long axis of the crest, thus providing one of the major routes for conduction from the sinus node towards the atrioventricular node.[7] Anteriorly, the crest curves in front of the orifice of the superior caval vein, with its medial extension forming the border between the appendage and the superior rim of the oval fossa. The crest then continues through the superior interatrial groove as Bachmann's bundle. This is the major route for conduction into the left atrium.[7]

On first sight, when inspecting the right atrium through this incision, there appears to be an extensive septal surface between the openings of the caval veins and the orifice of the tricuspid valve (Figure 3.27). The apparent extent of this septum is spurious.[8] The true septum[9] is confined to the floor of the oval fossa, which is formed by the flap valve, and its antero-inferior buttress (Figures 3.28, 3.29). The extensive superior rim of the fossa is produced by the superior interatrial groove. This fold separates the mouth of the superior caval vein from the entrances of the pulmonary veins to the left atrium

3 Anatomy of the Cardiac Chambers

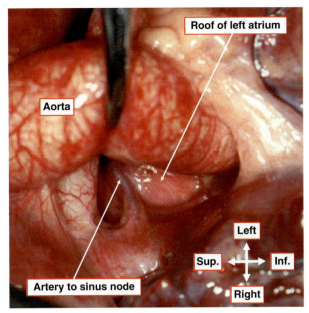

Figure 3.20 Operative view through a median sternotomy showing the artery to the sinus node, which in this case originates from the circumflex coronary artery and extends across the dome of the left atrium.

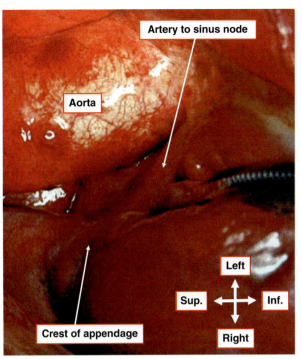

Figure 3.21 Operative view through a median sternotomy showing the artery to the sinus node originating proximally from the right coronary artery.

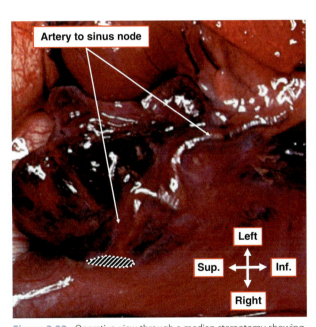

Figure 3.22 Operative view through a median sternotomy showing the artery to the sinus node originating distally from the right coronary artery and coursing over the lateral surface of the right atrial appendage. The site of the sinus node is shown by the black and white cross-hatched area.

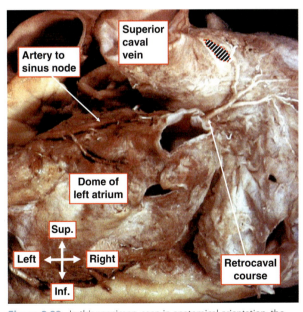

Figure 3.23 In this specimen, seen in anatomical orientation, the artery to the sinus node originates laterally from the circumflex coronary artery and courses over the dome of the left atrium. The site of the sinus node is shown by the black and white cross-hatched area.

(Figure 3.29). The postero-inferior rim is another fold, this time formed by reflection of the musculatures forming the mouth of the coronary sinus and the orifice of the inferior caval vein (Figure 3.30). These muscular structures continue anteriorly within the atrium as the Eustachian ridge. This is seen to advantage when the floor of the oval fossa, or the flap valve, is itself deficient (Figure 3.31). Because of the limited extent of these septal components, it is an easy matter for the surgeon to pass outside the heart when attempting to gain access to the left atrium through a right atrial approach.

In addition to the position of the sinus node, and the extent of the atrial septum, the other major area of surgical significance within the right atrium is the site of the atrioventricular node. This vital structure is contained within the triangle of Koch.[10] The triangle is bounded by the tendon of Todaro, the attachment of the septal leaflet of the tricuspid valve, and the orifice of the coronary sinus (Figure 3.32). The tendon of Todaro is a fibrous structure formed by the junction of the Eustachian valve, the valve of the inferior caval vein, and the Thebesian valve, the valve of the coronary sinus. The fibrous continuation of these two valvar structures buries itself in the anterior continuation of the Eustachian ridge. It then runs medially as the tendon of Todaro before inserting into the atrioventricular part of the membranous septum (Figure 3.33). The entire atrial component of the axis of atrioventricular conduction tissues is contained within the confines of the triangle of Koch. If, in hearts with normal segmental connections, this area is scrupulously avoided during surgical procedures, the atrioventricular conduction tissues will not be damaged. Should the node need to be identified more precisely, it should be remembered that the attachment of the tricuspid valve is some way down the surface of the septum relative to that of the mitral valve (Figure 3.34).

The relationship between the atrial and ventricular muscular walls within the triangle of Koch is complex.[10] At first sight, because of the off-setting of the attachments of the mitral and tricuspid valves, the entire muscular area seems to interpose between the cavities of the right atrium and the left ventricle. Indeed, in earliest editions of the book, we described this area as representing an atrioventricular muscular septum. In the floor of the triangle, however, the atrial musculature is separated from the underlying ventricular myocardium by a superior extension of the inferior atrioventricular groove. The fibrofatty tissue in this area serves to insulate the atrial from the ventricular muscular layers.[10] The extent of this insulating layer can be demonstrated by dissecting away the superficial atrial musculature, revealing at the same time the location of the artery supplying the atrioventricular node (Figure 3.35). It follows that the larger part of Koch's triangle, as seen by the surgeon, is formed by the atrial layer of an atrioventricular muscular sandwich, rather than representing a true muscular atrioventricular septum.

Much was written in the latter part of the twentieth century concerning the role of allegedly specialized pathways of myocardium in conducting the sinus impulse to the atrioventricular node.[11] All of the atrial myocardium, apart from the nodal components, is made up of working, rather than specialized, cardiomyocytes.[7] There is no anatomical evidence to support

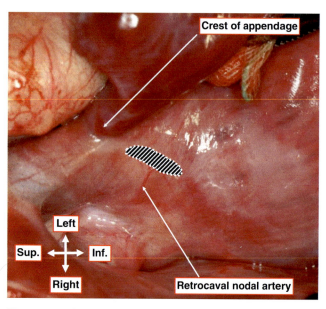

Figure 3.24 Operative view through a median sternotomy showing a retrocaval course of the artery to the sinus node, the site of the node itself being emphasized by the black cross-hatching.

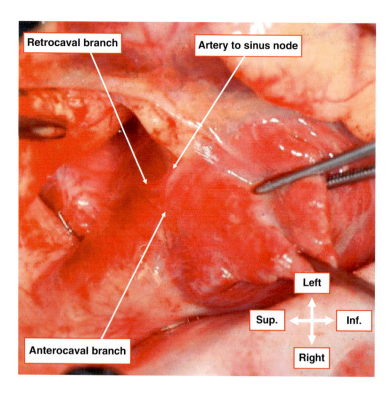

Figure 3.25 Operative view through a median sternotomy showing the artery to the sinus node dividing to form an arterial circle around the cavoatrial junction.

3 Anatomy of the Cardiac Chambers

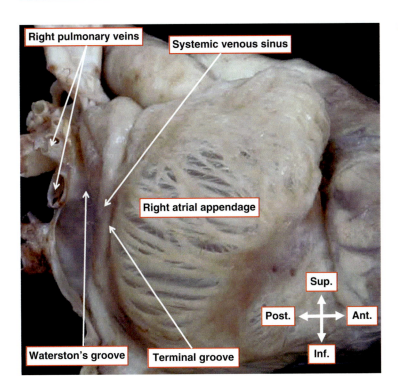

Figure 3.26 The heart is shown from the right side. The terminal groove and Waterston's groove form the boundaries of the systemic venous sinus.

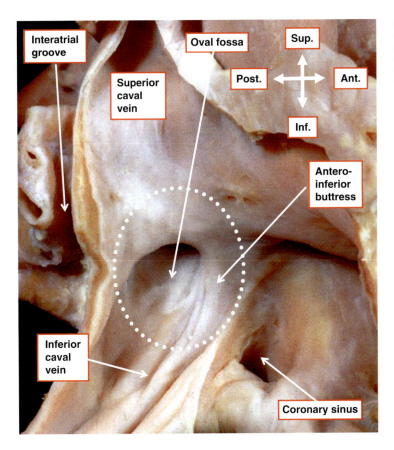

Figure 3.27 The right atrium has been opened to show its posterior surface, which is dominated by the oval fossa. At first sight, there is an extensive septal area interposing between the cavities of the atrial chambers (white dotted oval). This is deceptive, since as is shown by taking sections, almost all of the rims of the fossa, with the exception of the antero-inferior buttress, and infoldings of the atrial walls.

suggestions that surgical operations should be specially modified to avoid presumed specialized internodal tracts. The anatomical paradigm for tracts of myocardium modified for conduction in the heart is provided by the ventricular conduction system, which is insulated by fibrous sheaths from the adjacent working ventricular myocardium.[12] There are no such insulated and isolated tracts within the atrial walls.[11,13,14] The major muscle bundles of the atrial chambers, nonetheless, serve as preferential pathways of conduction. Their location is dictated by the overall geometry of the chambers. Ideally,

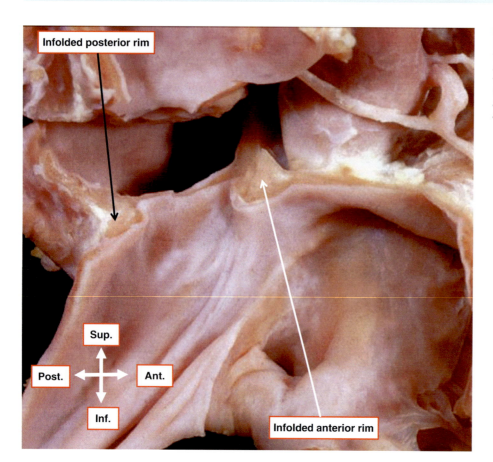

Figure 3.28 The specimen shown in Figure 3.27 has been transected through the oval fossa, showing that the rims are infoldings of the atrial walls. The floor of the fossa is the flap valve derived from the primary atrial septum. Note the relationship of the anterior fold to the aortic root, the right coronary artery, and the artery to the sinus node.

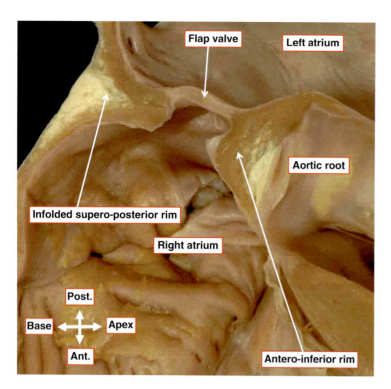

Figure 3.29 This heart has been sectioned in a four-chamber plane, showing that the supero-posterior rim of the oval fossa is also a deep infolding between the systemic venous sinus of the right atrium and the entry of the pulmonary veins into the left atrium. the section again shows how the so-called flap valve forms the floor of the fossa.

therefore, prominent muscle bundles, such as the terminal crest, the superior rim of the oval fossa, the myocardium of the Eustachian ridge, and the superior interatrial fold, should be preserved during atrial surgery. Even if they cannot be preserved, the surgeon can rest assured that internodal conduction will continue as long as viable atrial myocardium interposes between the nodes, providing that the arterial supply to the nodes, or the nodes themselves, are not traumatized.

3 Anatomy of the Cardiac Chambers

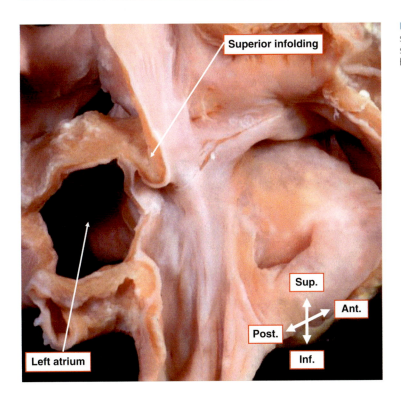

Figure 3.30 The heart shown in Figures 3.27 and 3.28 has been sectioned in the long axis of the venous sinus, again showing that the superior rim of the oval fossa is an infolding of the interatrial groove. The heart is viewed in anatomical orientation from the back.

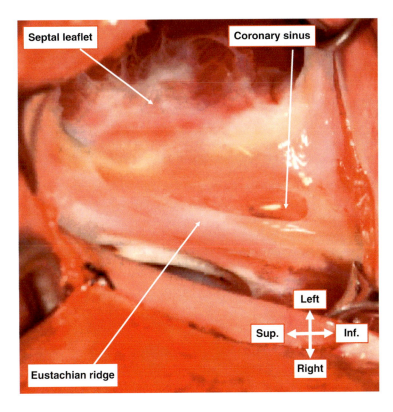

Figure 3.31 The heart has been opened through an atriotomy, and the interior surface of the right atrium is shown in surgical orientation. Note the Eustachian ridge separating the mouth of the coronary sinus from the orifice of the inferior caval vein. The floor of the oval fossa is deficient, producing an atrial septal defect.

The key to avoiding postoperative atrial arrhythmias is the fastidious preservation of the sinus and atrioventricular nodes, along with their arteries, rather than concern about non-existent tracts of purportedly specialized atrial myocardium.

Much is also written about the fibrous skeleton of the heart. The strongest part of this skeleton is the central fibrous body. This area of fibrous tissue touches on three of the four cardiac chambers, but is seen most clearly by the surgeon when working from the right atrium (Figure 3.36). The morphologist appreciates the area best when viewing it through the subaortic outflow tract of the left ventricle (Figure 3.37). This shows that, rather than being considered as a specific body, it is better conceptualized as the area within the heart where the

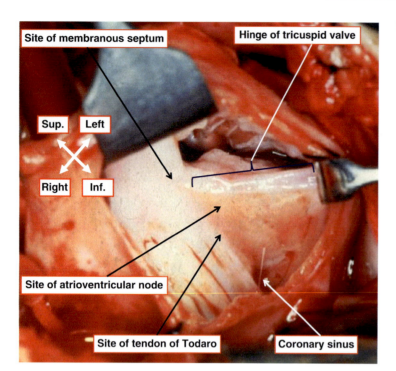

Figure 3.32 This operative view through a right atriotomy shows the location of the triangle of Koch.

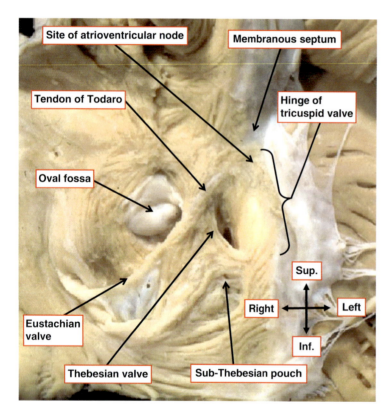

Figure 3.33 The endocardium has been removed from this heart, viewed in anatomical orientation, to demonstrate the boundaries of the triangle of Koch. Note the non-uniform anisotropic arrangement of the aggregated cardiomyocytes.

membranous septum, the hinges of the leaflets of the atrioventricular valves, and the fibrous components of the aortic root join in fibrous continuity. The membranous septum, usually divided by the hinge of the septal leaflet of the tricuspid valve into atrioventricular and interventricular components, forms the part of the fibrous area interposed between the left ventricle and the right-sided chambers (Figure 3.38). An area of fibrous continuity between the leaflets of the tricuspid valve in the right ventricle, and the mitral valve in the left ventricle, then forms the part of the body that provides the fibrous support for the antero-inferior buttress of the atrial septum (Figure 3.39). This area also forms the roof of the infero-septal recess of the subaortic outflow tract.[10] It is continuous to the left with the much larger area of fibrous continuity between the leaflets of

3 Anatomy of the Cardiac Chambers

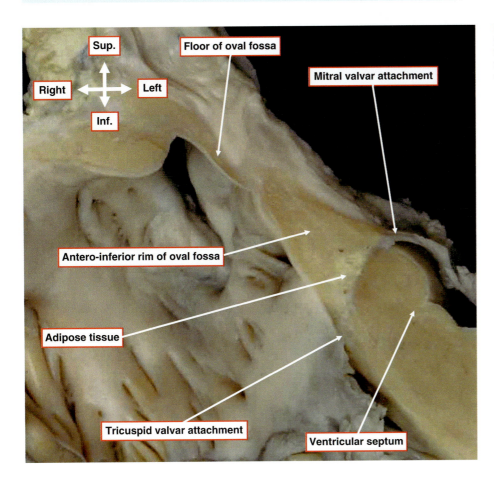

Figure 3.34 The heart has been sectioned in four-chamber plane to show the off-setting of the hinges of the tricuspid and mitral valves. Note the adipose tissue separating the atrial and ventricular musculatures in the area of off-setting.

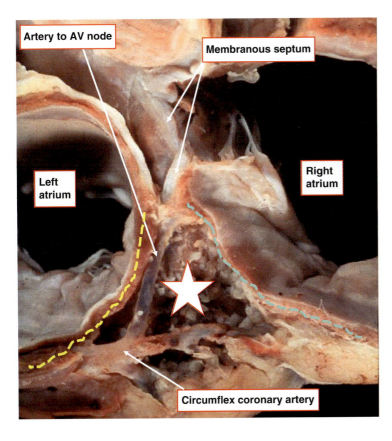

Figure 3.35 This dissection, in anatomical orientation having removed the non-coronary sinus of the aortic valve, shows the fibrofatty tissue (white star with red borders) interposed between the atrial and ventricular muscular layers of the atrioventricular muscular sandwich. The remnant of the left atrial vestibule is shown by the dashed yellow line, with the dashed green line showing the remnant of the right atrial vestibule. Note the artery to the atrioventricular node.

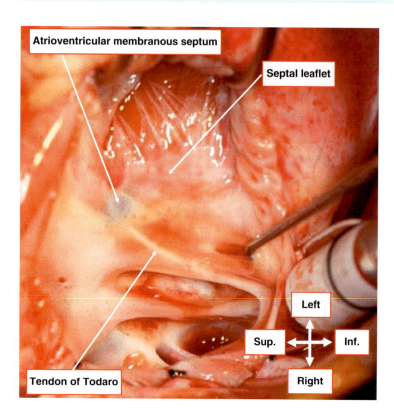

Figure 3.36 Operative view through a right atriotomy, showing the tendon of Todaro inserting into the atrioventricular component of the membranous septum, which forms the rightward component of the central fibrous body.

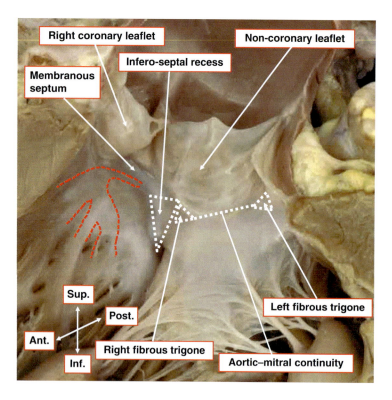

Figure 3.37 This specimen, viewed in anatomical orientation, is opened to show the origin of the aorta from the left ventricle, with the membranous septum in fibrous continuity with the leaflets of the aortic and mitral valves. The site of the fascicles of the left bundle branch is marked by the red dots. The white-dotted areas show the components of the so-called central fibrous body.

the mitral and aortic valves. This more extensive area forms the roof of the left ventricle itself. It is thickened at both its ends to form the so-called right and left fibrous trigones (Figure 3.37). By convention, the right fibrous trigone is also usually considered to be an integral part of the central fibrous body. Indeed, many consider the roof of the infero-septal recess to be part of the right fibrous trigone.

The central fibrous body, however it is defined, serves as an anatomical focal point for the cardiac surgeon. Operations involving valvar replacement or repair, closure of septal defects, and control of arrhythmias require the surgeon to understand implicitly its anatomical relationships from both the obvious right (Figure 3.36) and also the usually invisible left (Figure 3.37) sides. Knowledge of the location of the atrioventricular component of

3 Anatomy of the Cardiac Chambers

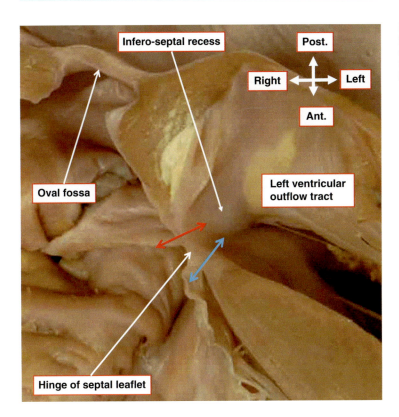

Figure 3.38 The heart is sectioned to replicate the echocardiographic four-chamber plane. The section passes through the membranous part of the septum, which is divided by the hinge of the septal leaflet of the tricuspid valve into atrioventricular (red double-headed arrow) and interventricular (blue double-headed arrow) components.

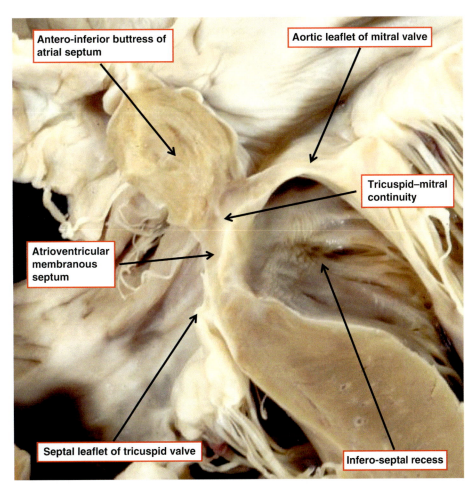

Figure 3.39 The close-up of a heart sectioned in four-chamber plane shows how the roof of the infero-septal recess, formed by an area of fibrous continuity between the leaflets of the tricuspid and mitral valves, supports the muscular antero-inferior buttress of the atrial septum.

59

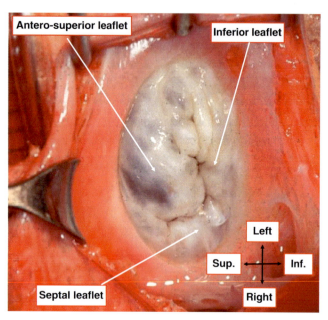

Figure 3.40 This operative view through a right atriotomy, seen in surgical orientation, shows the vestibule of the right atrium and the three leaflets of the tricuspid valve.

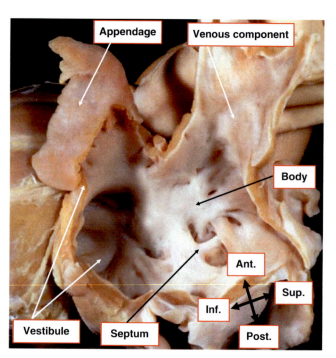

Figure 3.41 In this heart, shown in anatomical orientation, the left atrium is opened to show its components. Note the extensive body.

the membranous septum (Figure 3.38) is then the key to understanding the occurrence of the so-called Gerbode septal defect.[15] Septal deficiency at this site produces a direct shunt from the left ventricular outflow tract to the right atrium (see Figure 4.37).

The final atrial component, the vestibule to the right ventricle, surrounds the orifice of the tricuspid valve. This smooth-walled atrial component is contiguous with both the systemic venous component and the appendage of the right atrium. The anterior junction of these two parts of the atrium overlies the peripheral attachment of the antero-septal commissure of the tricuspid valve and the supraventricular crest of the right ventricle (Figure 3.40). The posterior junction is at the orifice of the coronary sinus, where there is usually an extensive inferior trabeculated diverticulum. Although usually called the post-Eustachian sinus, it is sub-Thebesian when the heart is viewed relative to the anatomical position (Figure 3.33).

Morphologically Left Atrium

As with the right atrium, the left atrium possesses a body, an appendage, an extensive venous component, and a vestibule. The left atrial body, representing the initial atrial component of the linear heart tube, is much more extensive than its right atrial counterpart (Figure 3.41). The chamber, of course, is also separated from its neighbour by the septum. The body of the atrium is confluent with all the other components. Unlike in the right atrium, the narrow junction between the body and the appendage is unmarked by either a terminal groove or crest (Figure 3.41). Because of the posterior position of the left atrium, and its firm anchorage by the four pulmonary veins, it can be difficult for the surgeon to gain direct access to the left atrium. Knowledge of the salient anatomy can help best exposure of the cavity. Probably the most popular route is provided by an incision made just posterior to the right lateral aspect of the interatrial groove (Figure 3.42). As we have explained, this groove, the extensive infolding between the right pulmonary veins and the venous sinus of the right atrium, produces the superior rim of the oval fossa (Figure 3.29). A posteriorly directed incision within this groove takes the surgeon directly into the left atrium. If necessary, the incision can be extended to the superior aspect of the left atrium by incising the pericardial fold between the superior caval vein and the right pulmonary artery (Figure 3.4). Because the infolding of the interatrial groove also forms the superior border of the oval fossa, much the same access can be gained by approaching through the right atrium, and incising just superiorly within the fossa. It must then be remembered that an extensive incision may take the surgeon out of the confines of the atrial chambers and into the pericardial space. Perhaps more importantly, it should be noted that such an incision may damage the artery to the sinus node, either in the interatrial groove or on the roof of the left atrium. The left atrium can also be entered superiorly by incising directly through its roof. If the aorta is pulled anteriorly, and to the left, an extensive trough is seen between the two atrial appendages (Figure 3.43). An incision through the floor of this trough enters the left atrium directly. When making such an incision, it must again be remembered that the artery to the sinus node may be coursing through this area when it takes origin from the circumflex artery (Figure 3.23). In other instances, this artery may pass through the infolding of the interatrial groove to reach the terminal groove.

Once access is gained to the left atrium, the small size of the opening of the appendage is apparent (Figure 3.44). The mouth of the appendage lies to the left of the mitral orifice as viewed by the surgeon. It is positioned above the superior end of the

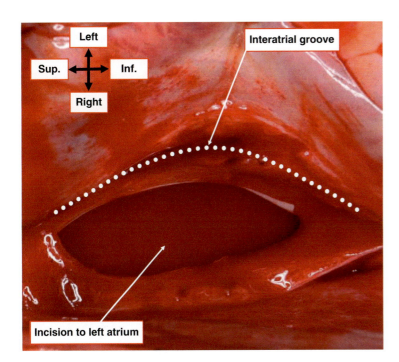

Figure 3.42 This operative view, through a median sternotomy, shows how an incision through the bottom of Waterston's groove (white dotted line) takes the surgeon into the left atrium.

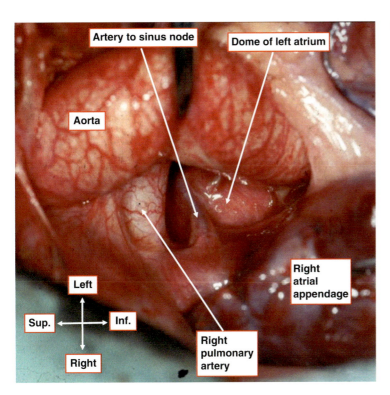

Figure 3.43 This operative view, through a median sternotomy, shows how retraction of the aorta to the left reveals the deep trough inferior to the right pulmonary artery and between the atrial appendages. Note that, in this heart, the artery to the sinus node courses through this trough.

zone of apposition between the leaflets of the mitral valve. The greater part of the pulmonary venous sinus, confluent with the smooth-walled atrial body, will usually be located inferiorly, away from the operative field. It is the vestibule of the mitral orifice that dominates the picture (Figure 3.45). The septal aspect will be anterior, exhibiting the typically roughened flap valve aspect of its left side (Figure 3.46). The large sweep of tissue between the flap valve of the septum and the opening of the appendage is the internal aspect of the deep anterior interatrial groove.

Morphologically Right Ventricle

The musculature of the right ventricle extends from the atrioventricular to the myocardial–arterial junctions. Its cavity, however, extends to the sinutubular junction. Understanding of ventricular morphology in general is greatly aided by considering the ventricles in terms of three components. These are the inlet, apical trabecular, and outlet parts, respectively (Figure 3.47). The inlet portion of the right ventricle contains, and is limited by, the tricuspid valve and its tension apparatus.

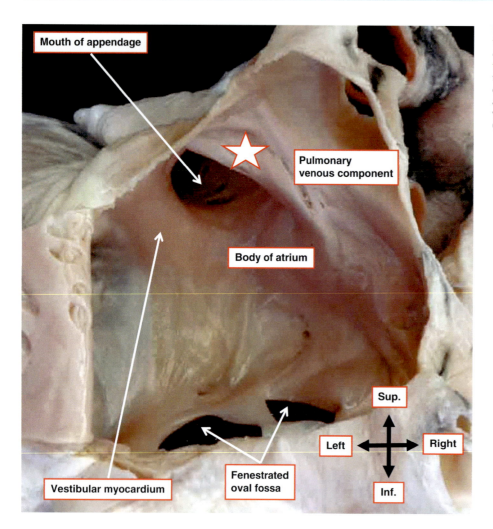

Figure 3.44 The left atrium is photographed from behind to show the relations of the mouth of the left atrial appendage. All components of the atrial chamber can be seen. Note the isthmus formed by the vestibular myocardium, and the extensive fold between the mouth of the appendage and the origin of the left pulmonary veins from the pulmonary venous component (star).

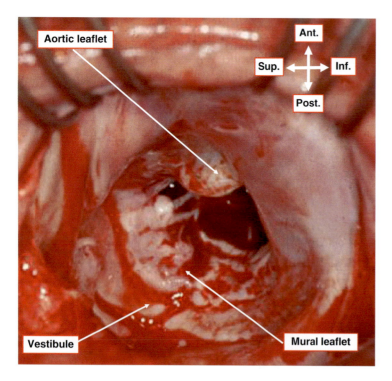

Figure 3.45 On gaining access through a right-sided left atriotomy, the vestibule of the mitral orifice dominates the surgical picture. Note the location of the leaflets of the mitral valve.

3 Anatomy of the Cardiac Chambers

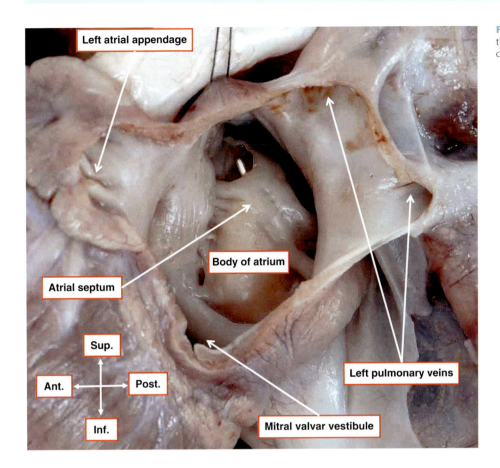

Figure 3.46 The left atrium is windowed from the left and posterior aspect, showing its component parts.

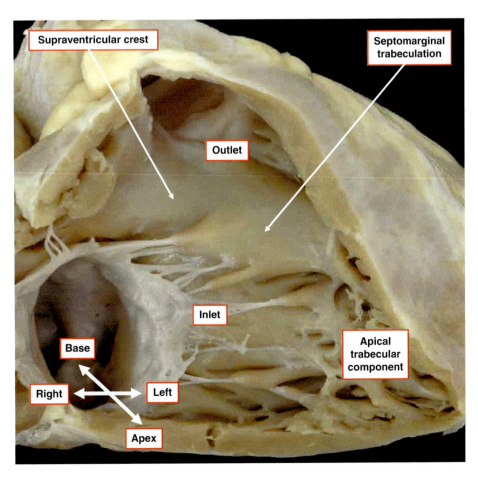

Figure 3.47 This specimen, viewed in anatomical orientation, shows the three components of the morphologically right ventricle.

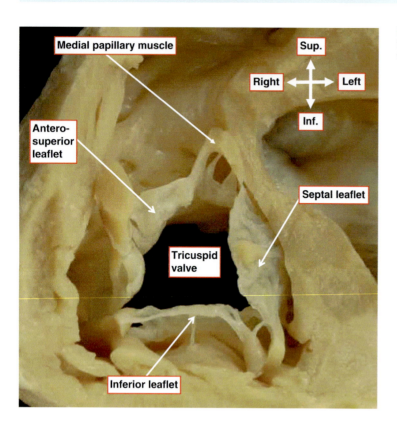

Figure 3.48 The right atrioventricular junction is photographed from the ventricular apex, showing the location of the leaflets of the tricuspid valve.

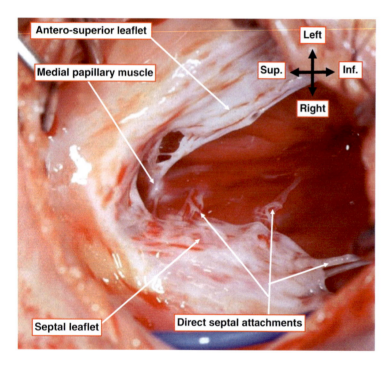

Figure 3.49 Operative view through a right atriotomy showing the direct cordal attachments to the septum of the septal leaflet of the tricuspid valve.

Although there is anatomical variability, it is often in most instances to distinguish three leaflets in the valvar orifice. They guard the antero-superior, -septal, and -inferior or mural zones of the atrioventricular junction (Figures 3.48, 3.49). When seen in closed position, their boundaries are clearly marked by their zones of apposition, which extend to the centre of the valvar orifice. The entirety of the zones of apposition could, logically, be defined as the commissures. It is the peripheral parts of the zones of apposition that are usually described as the commissures. In the atrioventricular valves, these areas do not abut directly on the so-called valvar annulus. The zones of apposition between the leaflets in these commissural areas are usually tethered by fan-shaped cords arising atop prominent papillary muscles. We discuss the details of this valvar and commissural anatomy in our next chapter. In anatomical terms, the most constant distinguishing morphological feature of the tricuspid valve is the direct attachments to the septum of the cords tethering its septal leaflet (Figure 3.49).

The apical component of the right ventricle, as the name suggests, extends to the ventricular apex, where its wall is particularly thin. It is then especially vulnerable to perforation by cardiac catheters and pacemaker electrodes. Its trabeculations, when compared with those of the left ventricle, are uniformly coarse. The outlet component of the right ventricle is a complete muscular sleeve (Figure 3.50), the infundibulum. This extends from the ventricular base to support the leaflets of the pulmonary valve. The leaflets of the valve are attached to the infundibular musculature in semilunar fashion. These hinges cross the circular anatomical myocardial–arterial junction so as to incorporate triangles of arterial wall within the ventricle, and crescents of ventricular muscle in the bases of the pulmonary valvar sinuses (Figure 3.51). Another distinguishing morphological feature of the right ventricle is the prominent muscular shelf that interposes between the tricuspid and pulmonary valvar orifices. This is the supraventricular crest. At first sight, it has the appearance of a thick muscle bundle. In reality, its larger part is no more than the infolded inner heart curve (Figure 3.52). Incisions, or deep sutures, through this part run into the transverse sinus and right atrioventricular groove. They can jeopardize the right coronary artery.[16] We used to think that a small part of the most medial area of the crest could be removed so as to create a hole between the subpulmonary and subaortic outflow tracts, suggesting that the musculature might represent an 'outlet septum'. We now know this not to be the case. The entirety of the crest is separated by extracavitary tissues from the right coronary aortic valvar sinus (Figure 3.53). The crest includes, as its most distal component, the free-standing infundibular muscular sleeve (Figure 3.50). It is the presence of this sleeve that permits the valve itself to be removed as an autograft for use in the Ross procedure (Figures 3.54). Considered as a whole, the supraventricular crest inserts between the limbs of an equally prominent and important right ventricular septal

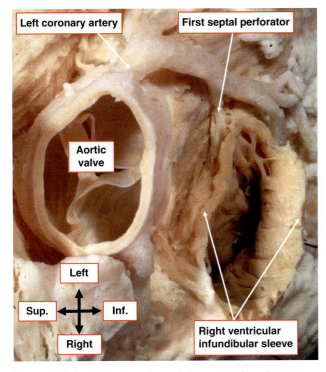

Figure 3.50 In this heart, also shown in Figure 3.54, the pulmonary infundibulum has been removed from the base of the heart, revealing the free-standing myocardial sleeve that 'lifts' the valvar leaflets away from the left ventricle. Note the site of the first septal perforating artery.

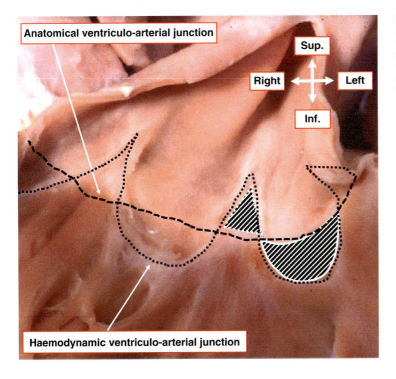

Figure 3.51 In this heart, shown in anatomical orientation, the leaflets of the pulmonary valve have been removed. Note how the semilunar attachment of the pulmonary valvar leaflets crosses the myocardial–arterial junction (dashed line), the dotted lines and cross-hatchings emphasizing the crescents of ventricular muscle incorporated in the valvar sinus and the triangles of arterial wall within the ventricle.

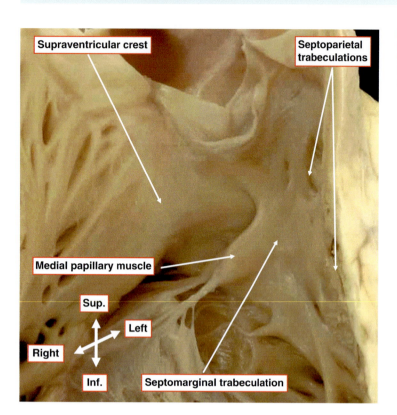

Figure 3.52 Opening the outflow tract of the right ventricle reveals the supraventricular crest, which interposes between the hinges of the leaflets of the tricuspid and pulmonary valves. It is the inner heart curvature, or ventriculo-infundibular fold, and inserts to the septal surface between the limbs of the septomarginal trabeculation.

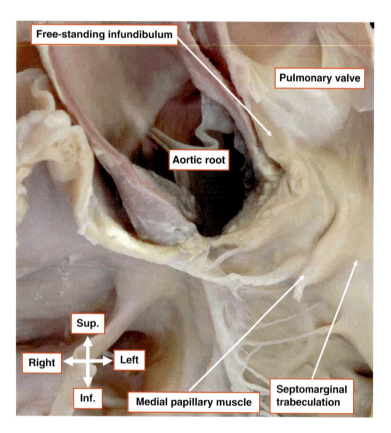

Figure 3.53 Dissection of the right ventricular outflow tract reveals the inner heart curvature that separates the cavity of the right ventricle from the aortic root. It continues as the free-standing sleeve of infundibular muscle that supports the leaflets of the pulmonary valve.

trabeculation. This structure, described by us as the septomarginal trabeculation, but also known as the septal band, has antero-superior and postero-inferior limbs that clasp the septal attachment of the crest (Figure 3.55). The antero-superior limb runs up to the attachment of the leaflets of the pulmonary valve. The postero-inferior limb extends backwards, extending inferior to the interventricular component of the membranous septum. It reinforces the crest of the muscular septum. It was the part of the crest reinforcing the muscular septum that we removed previously, considering it to

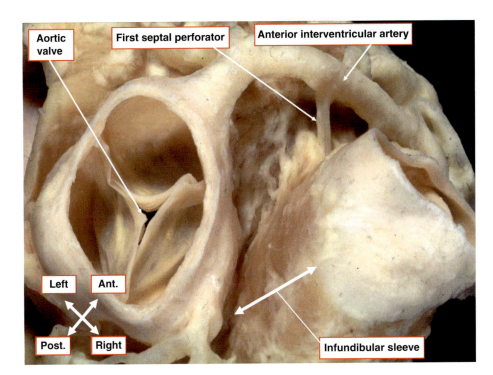

Figure 3.54 This heart, shown also in Figure 3.50, was photographed prior to removal of the sleeve of free-standing infundibular musculature. It is the presence of the sleeve that makes possible the Ross procedure.

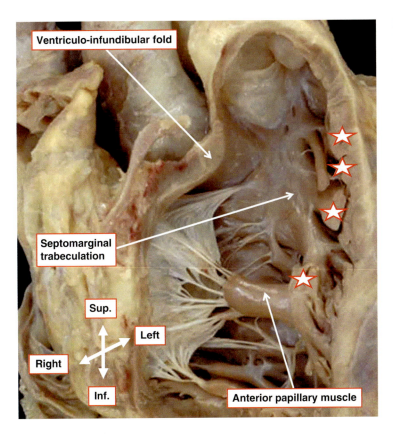

Figure 3.55 The right ventricle has been opened from the front, with the heart oriented anatomically, to show the septoparietal trabeculations (stars). The most inferior of the trabeculations is the moderator band.

represent an 'outlet septum'. The medial papillary muscle usually arises from this postero-inferior limb. The body of the septomarginal trabeculation itself extends towards the apex of the ventricle, breaking up into a sheath of smaller trabeculations. Some of these mingle into the apical trabecular portion, and some support the tension apparatus of the tricuspid valve. Several of these trabeculations are often particularly prominent. One becomes the anterior papillary muscle, while another extends from the septomarginal trabeculation to the papillary muscle, being termed the moderator band. Additional significant right ventricular trabeculations arise from the anterior margin of the septomarginal trabeculation. Variable in number, these are the septoparietal trabeculations (Figure 3.55).

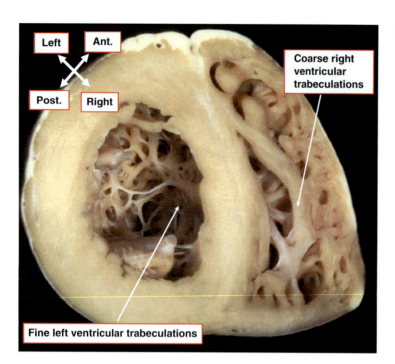

Figure 3.56 The apical component of the ventricular mass has been transected, and is photographed from above to show the different patterns of the apical trabeculations of the two ventricles.

It is the uniformly coarse apical trabeculations that, for the morphologist, serve as the most constant anatomical feature of the morphologically right ventricle. Additional morphological differences between the ventricles also permit their distinction. These include the arrangement of the leaflets of the atrioventricular valves and their tension apparatus, the ventricular shape, the thickness of the ventricular walls, and the configuration of the outflow tracts. These features, however, can be altered or lacking in the congenitally abnormal heart. In final arbitration of ventricular morphology, therefore, the morphologist relies on the contrast, in the same heart, between the coarse and broad trabeculations of the right ventricle, and the much finer trabeculations seen in the apical part of the left ventricle (Figure 3.56).

Morphologically Left Ventricle

As with the right ventricle, the musculature of the left ventricle extends from the atrioventricular to the myocardial–arterial junctions. And again, extensions of the ventricular cavity reach to the sinutubular junction. Taken overall, the ventricle is again conveniently considered in terms of inlet, apical trabecular, and outlet components (Figure 3.57). In the left ventricle, there is marked overlapping of the inlet and outlet components. The inlet component surrounds, and is limited by, the mitral valve and its tension apparatus. Its two leaflets, supported by two prominent papillary muscle groups and their tendinous cords, have widely differing appearances (Figure 3.58). The antero-superior leaflet is squat and relatively square. It guards only one-third of the circumference of the valvar orifice. Being in fibrous continuity with the leaflets of the aortic valve, it is best termed the aortic leaflet.[17] The other leaflet is narrower, guarding two-thirds of the valvar circumference. It is supported by the parietal part of the left atrioventricular junction. Reflecting this support, and being positioned postero-inferiorly, it is accurately termed the mural leaflet.[17] Because the aortic leaflet of the mitral valve forms part of the outlet of the left ventricle, the boundary between the inlet and outlet is somewhat blurred. The papillary muscles of the valve, located in supero-lateral and infero-medial positions, are close to each other at their origin (Figure 3.59). It is incorrect to describe the muscles as being antero-lateral and postero-medial, these terms reflecting the bad habit of morphologists of removing the heart from the body and describing it as positioned on its apex.[18] Unlike the tricuspid valve, the leaflets of the mitral valve have no direct septal attachments. This is because the deep infero-septal recess of the subaortic outflow tract displaces the aortic leaflet of the valve away from the muscular ventricular septum (Figure 3.60). The apical component of the left ventricle extends to the ventricular apex. It has characteristically fine trabeculations (Figure 3.57). As in the right ventricle, the myocardium is surprisingly thin at the apex. This feature is important to the cardiac surgeon, who may have reason to place catheters and electrodes in the right ventricle, or drainage tubes in the left side. Immediate perforation, or delayed rupture, may occur. This may be a particular problem should catheters stiffened by hypothermia be pushed against the apical endocardium by surgeons manipulating the heart during coronary arterial surgery.[19]

The outlet component of the left ventricle supports the aortic valve. Unlike its right ventricular counterpart, it is not a complete muscular structure. The septal wall is largely composed of muscle, but in this area is found the membranous septum, forming part of the central fibrous body in the sub-aortic outflow tract (Figure 3.37). The postero-lateral portion of the outflow tract is composed exclusively by fibrous tissue. Its larger part is the fibrous curtain joining the leaflets of the aortic valve to the aortic leaflet of the mitral valve. The left lateral quadrant, continuing around to the septum, is

3 Anatomy of the Cardiac Chambers

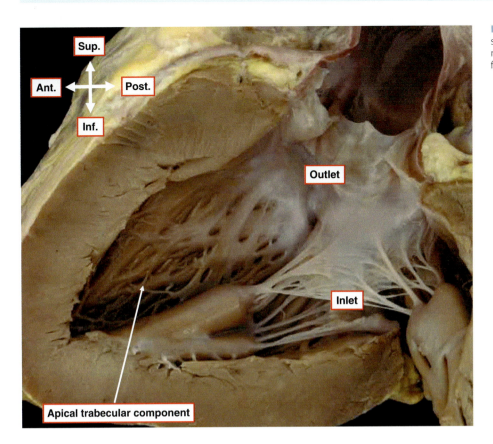

Figure 3.57 In this specimen, viewed from the side in anatomical orientation, the morphologically left ventricle is opened in clam fashion to show its three components.

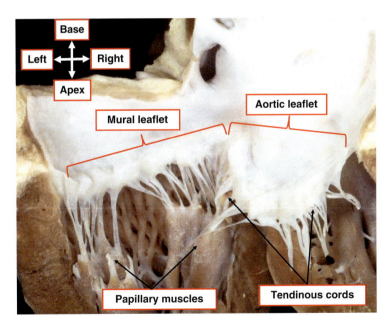

Figure 3.58 This specimen, viewed from behind, and opened through a cut in the left atrioventricular junction adjacent to the septum, demonstrates the marked differences in the arrangement of the aortic and mural leaflets of the mitral valve.

a muscular structure representing the lateral margin of the inner heart curvature, and separating the cavity of the left ventricle from the transverse sinus. The muscular septal surface of the outflow tract is characteristically smooth, with the fan-like left bundle branch cascading down from the septal crest. The landmark of its descent is the inferior margin of the membranous septum immediately beneath the zone of apposition between right coronary and non-coronary leaflets of the aortic valve (Figure 3.61). The bundle descends, initially, as a relatively narrow, solitary fascicle, but soon divides into three interconnected fascicles that radiate into superior, septal, and inferior divisions. The interconnecting radiations do not fan out to any degree until the bundle itself has descended to between one-third and one-half the length of the septum. Importantly, the superior fascicle continues to encircle the septal component of the outflow tract. It is typically the part of the axis most closely related to the aortic valve, specifically its right coronary leaflet. The fascicle can be found within one millimetre of the nadir of the hinge of the leaflet.[20] As with the pulmonary valve, the leaflets of the aortic valve are

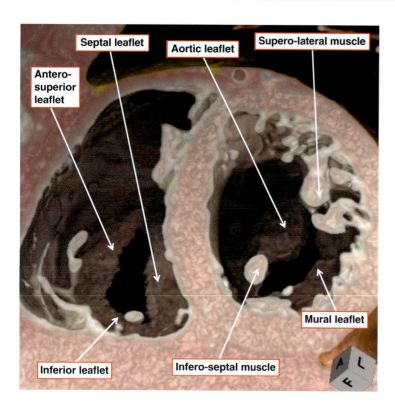

Figure 3.59 The image shows a virtual dissection from a computed tomographic dataset prepared from an individual with a normal heart. The cube in the lower right-hand corner shows the orientation of the section relative to the bodily coordinates. The papillary muscles of the mitral valve are positioned infero-septally and supero-laterally, rather than being 'postero-medial' and 'antero-lateral', as they are usually described. It can also be seen that the mural leaflet of the mitral valve wraps around the aortic leaflet. The section also shows that the leaflets of the tricuspid valve are located antero-superiorly, septally, and inferiorly.

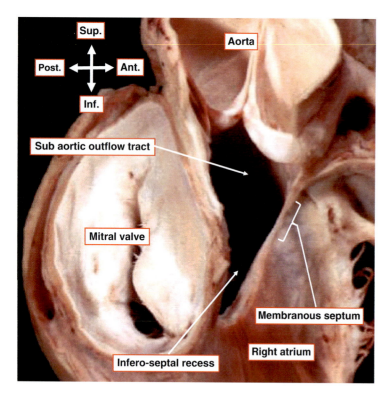

Figure 3.60 This heart, seen from above and from the right in anatomical orientation, has been prepared by removing the base of the atrial septum and the non-coronary sinus of the aortic valve to illustrate the infero-septal recess of the subaortic outflow tract separating the mitral valve from the septum.

not attached in circular fashion to a supporting ring of fibro-collagenous tissue. Instead, the leaflets are attached in semilunar fashion, but with only the hinges of the two coronary aortic leaflets crossing the myocardial-arterial junction (Figure 3.62). This arrangement again means that crescents of ventricular muscle are incorporated into the bases of two of the aortic sinuses.[21] The three triangles of fibrous tissue separating the valvar sinuses then line the extensions of the cavity that reach to the sinutubular junction.[22]

The Aorta

The ascending aorta begins at the distal extremity of the three aortic sinuses, the sinutubular junction, which forms the distal extent of the left ventricular cavity (Figure 3.63).

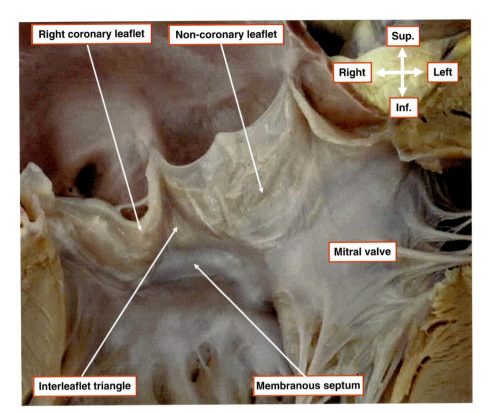

Figure 3.61 This specimen, oriented in anatomical position, demonstrates the relationship of the zone of apposition between the right and non-coronary leaflets to the membranous septum and the interleaflet triangle between the right coronary and non-coronary leaflets of the aortic valve.

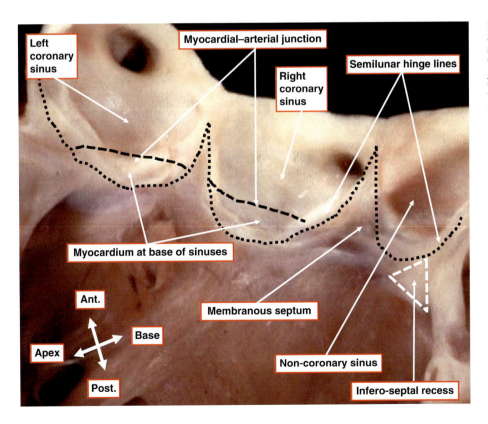

Figure 3.62 This dissection demonstrates that, as in the pulmonary valve (see Figure 3.51), the attachments of the coronary leaflets of the aortic valve (dotted line) cross the myocardial–arterial junction (dashed line), incorporating crescents of ventricular tissue into the arterial valvar sinuses. Triangles of arterial tissue are also incorporated into the ventricular base.

The ascending aortic trunk then runs its short course, passing superiorly, and obliquely to the right, and slightly forward, towards the sternum. It is contained within the fibrous pericardial sac, so its surface is covered with serous pericardium. Its anterior surface abuts directly on the pulmonary trunk, which is also covered with serous pericardium. The two vessels together make up the vascular pedicle of the heart (Figure 3.64). The ascending aorta is related antero-medially to the right atrial appendage, and postero-laterally to the right ventricular outflow tract and the pulmonary trunk.

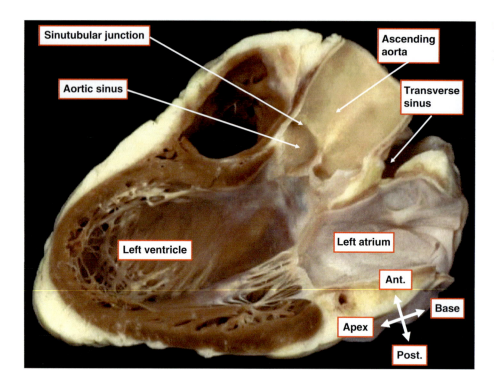

Figure 3.63 This long-axis section shows the sinutubular junction at the line of peripheral attachment of the zones of apposition between the leaflets of the aortic valve.

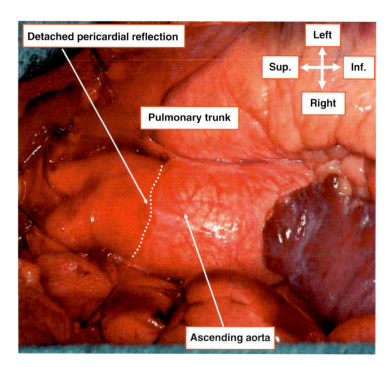

Figure 3.64 This operative view through a median sternotomy shows the vascular pedicle leading to the beginning of the aortic arch, which gives rise to the brachiocephalic and left common carotid arteries just distal to the detached pericardial reflection (white dotted line). The origin of the left subclavian artery is not seen.

Extrapericardially, the thymus gland lies between it and the sternum. The medial wall of the right atrium, the superior caval vein, and the right pleura relate to its right side. On the left, its principal relationship is with the pulmonary trunk. Posterior to the ascending aorta lies the transverse sinus of the pericardium (Figure 3.3), which separates it from the roof of the left atrium and the right pulmonary artery. The arch of the aorta begins at the superior attachment of the pericardial reflection. This is usually just proximal to the origin of the brachiocephalic artery. It continues superiorly for a short distance, before coursing posteriorly and to the left, crossing the lateral aspect of the distal trachea. It terminates on the lateral aspect of the vertebral column. Here, it is tethered by the parietal pleura and the arterial ligament. During its course, it gives off the brachiocephalic trunk, and then the left common carotid and left subclavian arteries (Figure 3.65). Bronchial arteries arise from the underside of the arch (Figure 3.66). They can be particularly troublesome if

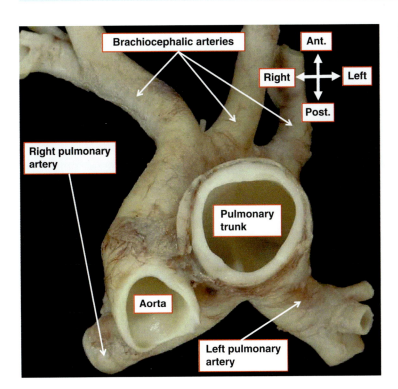

Figure 3.65 The arterial trunks have been removed from the base of the heart, and photographed from the apical aspect, showing their patterns of branching.

not carefully identified in the presence of aortic coarctation. The left phrenic and vagus nerves run over the antero-lateral aspect of the arch just beneath the mediastinal pleura. The left recurrent laryngeal nerve takes origin from the vagus. It curls superiorly around the arterial ligament before passing on to the postero-medial side of the arch. Here, the arch relates to the tracheal bifurcation and esophagus on its medial border, but also to the left main bronchus and the left pulmonary artery inferiorly.

The descending, or thoracic, aorta continues from the arch, running an initial course lateral to the vertebral bodies, and reaching an anterior position at its termination. It gives off many branches to the organs of the thorax throughout its course, as well as the prominent lower nine pairs of intercostal arteries. These latter vessels are of critical concern for the cardiac surgeon (see Chapter 10.3). In coarctation of the aorta, they serve as primary collateral vessels to bypass the obstructed aorta, accounting for the rib notching seen in older children with this lesion. These vessels, and their branches to the chest wall, can be a source of troublesome bleeding if not properly secured when operating on such patients. The surgeon must also remember that the dorsal branches of the intercostal vessels contribute a spinal branch that is important in supplying blood to the spinal cord. Because it is difficult to predict exactly the site of origin of these vital branches, the surgeon must make every attempt to protect their origin from permanent occlusion. The important bronchial arteries (Figure 3.66) also arise from the descending segment of the thoracic aorta. These vessels can become dilated in the presence of pulmonary atresia, when they serve as a source of pulmonary vascular supply.

The Pulmonary Arteries

The pulmonary trunk is a short vessel, usually less than five centimetres in length in the adult (Figure 3.67). It is completely contained within the pericardium (Figure 3.68). As with its running mate, the ascending aorta, it is covered with a layer of serous pericardium except where the two vessels abut each other in the vascular pedicle. It takes origin from the most anterior aspect of the heart, lying just behind the lateral edge of the sternum and the second left intercostal space. Initially, the pulmonary trunk overlies the aorta and left coronary artery. It soon moves to a side-by-side relationship with the ascending aorta. The left coronary artery turns abruptly anteriorly to lie between the left atrial appendage and the pulmonary trunk. The arterial ligament extends from the aorta to the very end of the pulmonary trunk as the latter divides into left and right pulmonary arteries. The left pulmonary artery then courses laterally in front of the descending aorta and the left main stem bronchus before it sends branches to the hilum of the lung. Postero-inferiorly, the left pulmonary artery is connected to the left superior pulmonary vein by a fold of serous pericardium that contains a ligamentous remnant of the left superior caval vein, the ligament of Marshall (Figure 3.68). The right pulmonary artery is somewhat longer than the left, having to traverse the mediastinum beneath the aortic arch, and then behind the superior caval vein, to reach the hilum of the lung (Figure 3.69). It lies in a postero-inferior position relative to the azygos vein, and is anterior to the left main bronchus. The right pulmonary artery often branches before reaching the lateral wall of the superior caval vein posterior to the transverse sinus of the pericardium. In this situation, a large upper lobar branch may be mistaken for the right pulmonary artery itself.

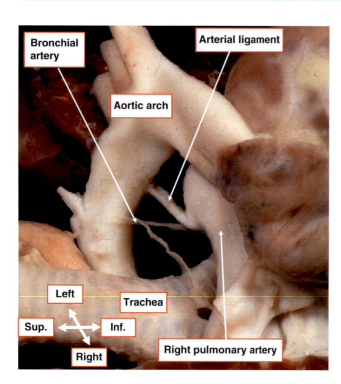

Figure 3.66 This dissection, viewed from the right side in surgical orientation, shows a bronchial artery arising from the aorta in the midline and dividing to supply both bronchuses.

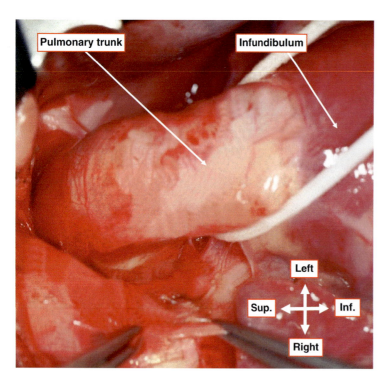

Figure 3.67 This operative view, taken through a median sternotomy, shows the short course of the pulmonary trunk prior to its bifurcation.

References Cited

1. Mori S, Bradfield JS, Peacock WJ, Anderson RH, Shivkumar K. Living anatomy of the pericardial space: a guide for imaging and interventions. *Clin Electrophysiol* 2021; 7: 1628–1644.

2. Anderson KR, Ho SY, Anderson RH. The location and vascular supply of the sinus node in the human heart. *Br Heart J* 1979; **41**: 28–32.

3. James TN. *Anatomy of the Coronary Arteries*. New York: Hoeber; 1961: pp. 103–106.

4. McAlpine WA. *Heart and Coronary Arteries. An Anatomical Atlas for Clinical Diagnosis, Radiological Investigation and Surgical Treatment*. New York: Springer-Verlag; 1975: p. 152.

5. Busquet J, Fontan F, Anderson RH, Ho SY, Davies MJ. The surgical significance of the atrial branches of the coronary arteries. *Int J Cardiol* 1984; **6**: 223–234.

6. Barra Rossi M, Ho SY, Anderson RH, Rossi Filho RI,

3 Anatomy of the Cardiac Chambers

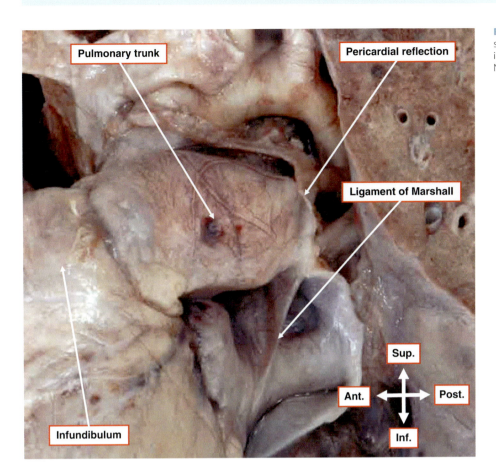

Figure 3.68 The anatomical specimen is shown from the left side, illustrating the short intrapericardial course of the pulmonary trunk. Note the location of the ligament of Marshall.

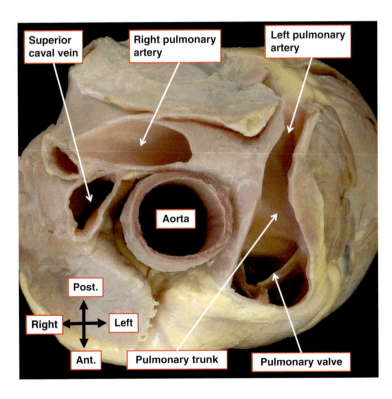

Figure 3.69 The heart has been sectioned in the short axis, and photographed from above, showing the branching pattern of the pulmonary trunk.

75

Lincoln C. Coronary arteries in complete transposition: the significance of the sinus node artery. *Ann Thorac Surg* 1986; **42**: 573–577.

7. Anderson RH, Sánchez-Quintana D, Spicer DE, Farré J, Sternick EB. How does the cardiac impulse pass from the sinus to the atrioventricular node? *Heart Rhythm* 2022; **19**: 1738–1746.

8. Anderson RH, Webb S, Brown NA. Clinical anatomy of the atrial septum with reference to its developmental components. *Clin Anat* 1999; **12**: 362–374.

9. Jensen B, Spicer DE, Sheppard MN, Anderson RH. Development of the atrial septum in relation to postnatal anatomy and interatrial communications. *Heart.* 2017; **103**: 456–462.

10. Tretter JT, Spicer DE, Sánchez-Quintana D, et al. Miniseries 1 – part III: 'behind the scenes' in the triangle of Koch. *EP Europace* 2022; **24**: 455–463.

11. James TN. The connecting pathways between the sinus node and the A-V node and between the right and the left atrium in the human heart. *Am Heart J* 1963; **66**: 498–508.

12. Anderson RH, Ho SY. Anatomic criteria for identifying the components of the axis responsible for atrioventricular conduction. *J Cardiovasc Electrophysiol* 2001; **12**: 1265–1268.

13. Janse MJ, Anderson RH. Internodal atrial specialised pathways – fact or fiction? *Eur J Cardiol* 1974; **2**: 117–137.

14. Anderson RH, Ho SY, Smith A, Becker AE. The internodal atrial myocardium. *Anat Rec* 1981; **201**: 75–82.

15. Gerbode F, Hultgren H, Melrose D, Osborn J. Syndrome of left ventricular-right atrial shunt. *Ann Surg* 1958; **148**: 433–446.

16. McFadden PM, Culpepper WS, Ochsner JL. Iatrogenic right ventricular failure in tetralogy of Fallot repairs: reappraisal of a distressing problem. *Ann Thor Surg* 1982; **33**: 400–402.

17. Anderson RH, Garbi M, Zugwitz D, Petersen SE, Nijveldt R. Anatomy of the mitral valve relative to controversies concerning the so-called annular disjunction. *Heart* 2023; **109**: 734–739.

18. Anderson RH, Frater RWM. Editorial. How can we best describe the components of the mitral valve? *J Heart Valve Dis* 2006; **15**: 736–739.

19. Breyer RH, Lavender S, Cordell AR. Delayed left ventricular rupture secondary to transatrial left ventricular vent. *Ann Thorac Surg* 1982; **3**: 189–191.

20. Macías Y, Tretter JT, Sánchez-Quintana D, et al. The atrioventricular conduction axis and the aortic root – inferences for transcatheter replacement of the aortic valve. *Clin Anat* 2022; **35**: 143–154.

21. Toh H, Mori S, Tretter JT, et al. Living anatomy of the ventricular myocardial crescents supporting the coronary aortic sinuses. *Sem Thorac Cardiovasc Surg* 2020; **32**: 230–241.

22. Sutton JPIII, Ho SY, Anderson RH. The forgotten interleaflet triangles: a review of the surgical anatomy of the aortic valve. *Ann Thorac Surg* 1995; **59**: 419–427.

Chapter 4

Surgical Anatomy of the Valves of the Heart

It is axiomatic that a thorough knowledge of valvar anatomy is a prerequisite for successful surgery, be it valvar replacement or reconstruction. The surgeon will also require a firm understanding of the arrangement of other aspects of cardiac anatomy to ensure safe access to a diseased valve or valves. These features were described in the previous chapter. Knowledge of the surgical anatomy of the valves themselves, however, must be founded on appreciation of their component parts, the relationships of the individual valves to each other, and their relationships to the chambers and arterial trunks within which they reside. This requires understanding of, first, the basic orientation of the cardiac valves, emphasizing the intrinsic features that make each valve distinct from the others. Such information must then be supplemented by attention to their relationships with other structures that the surgeon must avoid, notably the conduction tissues and the major channels of the coronary circulation. For this chapter, throughout our narrative, we will presume the presence of a normally structured heart, lying in its usual position, and without any co-existing congenital cardiac malformations.

The Valvar Complexes

When considering the valves, we distinguish between the atrioventricular valves, which guard the atrioventricular junctions, and the arterial valves, which guard the ventriculo-arterial junctions (Figure 4.1). Both sets of valves are best analysed in terms of the valvar complex, which for the atrioventricular valves is made up of the annulus, the leaflets, the tendinous cords, the papillary muscles, and the supporting ventricular musculature (Figure 4.2). All of these components must work in harmony so as to achieve valvar competence.[1] The leaflets of the atrioventricular valves are supplied with a complex tension apparatus, since they must withstand the full force of ventricular systole so as to retain their competence when in their closed position. The arterial valves are also a combination of complex anatomical parts. Often named the semilunar valves, it is the leaflets that are semilunar, being hinged within the overall valvar complex, which extends from the proximal ventriculo-arterial orifice, a virtual ring constructed at the nadir of the hinges of the leaflets, to the sinutubular junction (Figure 4.3). The components of the arterial valvar complex are the leaflets, their supporting arterial sinuses, and the fibrous interleaflet triangles. In the right ventricle, each of the arterial sinuses is supported at the ventricular base exclusively by infundibular myocardium. For the right ventricle, the myocardial–arterial junction thus formed is one of the two true anatomical rings to be found within the pulmonary root (Figure 4.4). The other obvious anatomical ring is the sinutubular junction. In the left ventricle, only the two sinuses of the aortic root giving rise the

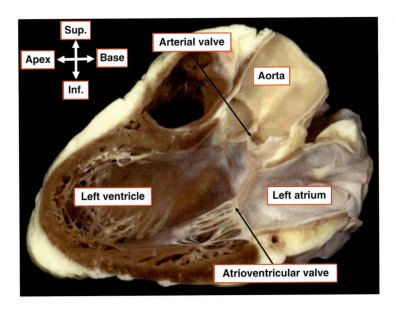

Figure 4.1 The heart has been sectioned in the long-axis plane, and oriented so as to replicate the long-axis parasternal section as obtained by echocardiographers. The cut shows well how, in the left heart, the mitral valve guards the atrioventricular junction, and the aortic valve the ventriculo-arterial junction.

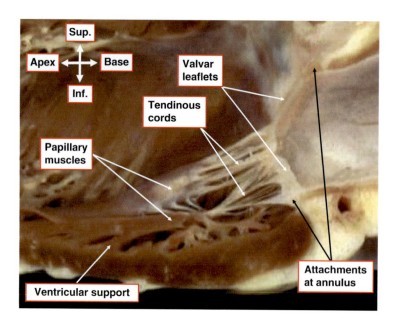

Figure 4.2 The close-up view of the mitral valve, taken from the long-axis section illustrated in Figure 4.1, shows the components of the atrioventricular valvar complex.

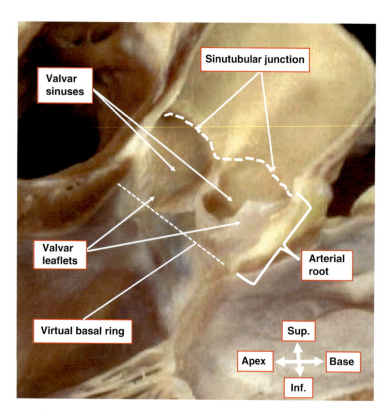

Figure 4.3 A comparable close-up of the aortic valve from Figure 4.1 shows the components of the arterial valvar complex, which extends from the virtual plane at the nadir of the attachments of the leaflets (white dotted line) to the sinutubular junction (dashed line).

coronary arteries are supported by ventricular musculature, with the sinus and leaflet of the non-coronary aortic sinus being contiguous with one of the leaflets of the mitral valve (Figure 4.5). It is still possible, nonetheless, to recognize the myocardial–arterial junction formed at the base of the coronary aortic sinuses, and to note the myocardium incorporated within these sinuses. In both arterial roots, it is also possible to recognize the fibrous interleaflet triangles extending distally to the level of the sinutubular junction. In the aortic root, as was the case for the pulmonary root, the sinutubular junction is the other obvious anatomical ring (Figures 4.4, 4.5). In both of the roots, furthermore, the distal margins of the semilunar hinges of the leaflets are attached at the sinutubular junctions, forming the peripheral extent of their zones of apposition (Figures 4.4, 4.5).

When comparisons are made between the overall arrangement of the atrioventricular and arterial valvar complexes, one fundamental difference is that the leaflets of the atrioventricular valves are suspended in relatively annular fashion at the atrioventricular junctions, although the orifices formed are far from circular. In the arterial roots, in contrast, the leaflets are hinged in semilunar fashion, with the semilunar attachments

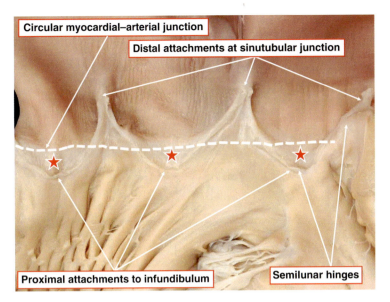

Figure 4.4 The ventriculo-arterial junction of the right ventricle has been cut anteriorly, and opened out. The valvar leaflets have been removed, their remnants revealing their initial semilunar attachments. Note how these hinges cross the junction between the muscular infundibulum and the walls of the pulmonary valvar sinuses (white dashed line). All the leaflets are supported by muscle, which therefore forms the basal part of each of the sinuses of Valsalva (red stars with white borders). The distal attachments, however, are at the sinutubular junction.

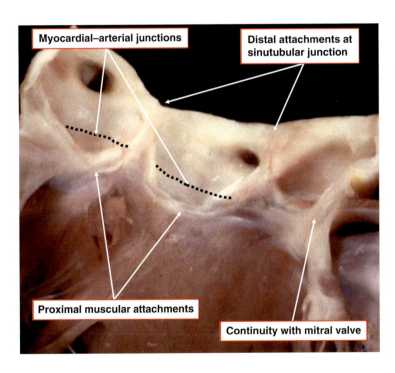

Figure 4.5 The ventriculo-arterial junction of the left ventricle has been opened and splayed in comparable fashion to Figure 4.4, and again, the leaflets of the aortic valve have been removed, revealing the semilunar attachments. In the left ventricle, however, because of the fibrous continuity with the aortic leaflet of the mitral valve, only two of the aortic valvar leaflets have muscular support. It is only within these sinuses, which give rise to the coronary arteries, that the semilunar hinges cross the myocardial–arterial junction (dotted lines).

crossing the myocardial–arterial junctions (Figures 4.4, 4.5). This difference underscores the problems currently existing in the use of 'annulus' when describing the morphology of the cardiac valves.[2] The fashion in which the same words are used in different ways to describe the components of the valves has led to much of the confusion surrounding their specific anatomy. This was exemplified by the answers to a questionnaire circulated amongst cardiac surgeons working in worldwide centres.[3] Thus, some consider that, while the atrioventricular valves possess leaflets, the moving components of the arterial valves should be considered as cusps. Our preference is to achieve uniformity by describing these working parts in both the atrioventricular and arterial valves as the leaflets.[2] This is the more so since, over the past decade, electrophysiologists and interventionists have used the word 'cusp' also to account for the arterial valvar sinuses.[4] As we have already discussed, it is the individual leaflets of the arterial valves that are semilunar, rather than the roots themselves. The overall anatomical complexes guarding the ventriculo-arterial junctions, therefore, are best considered as being arterial rather than semilunar. When considering the leaflets, it then follows that, because of their semilunar shape, they are supported in crown-like fashion within the arterial roots. There is often a degree of fibrous thickening that reinforces these attachments. The fibrous thickenings are more obvious in the aortic than the pulmonary valve (compare Figures 4.4 and 4.5), but become more marked in the pulmonary valve with ageing. When considered as a unit, the semilunar attachments are not strictly circular, and hence not annular. The remnants of the leaflets are often described during surgical procedures as representing

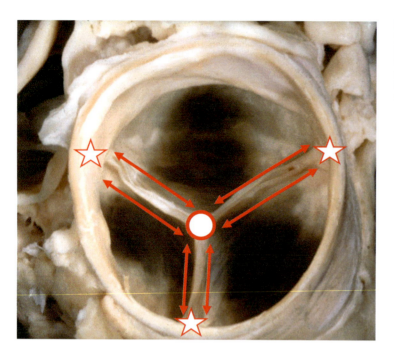

Figure 4.6 The aortic valve has been photographed from above, with the leaflets in their closed positions. As can be seen, the zones of apposition between the leaflets (double-headed red arrows) extend from the peripheral sinutubular junction to the valvar centroid. In anatomical terms, these zones are the commissures between the leaflets. Conventionally, however, it is the peripheral attachments (stars) that are usually defined as the commissures.

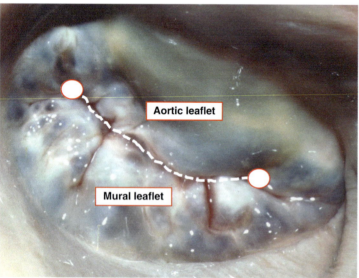

Figure 4.7 The mitral valve has been photographed in its closed position, showing the view obtained from the left atrium. There is but a solitary zone of apposition between the aortic and mural leaflets (dashed line), but conventionally it is the ends of this zone of apposition (white circles) that are defined as the valvar commissures. The photograph was taken by Dr Van S. Galstyan, from Armenia, and we thank him for permitting us to use it in our book.

the valvar 'annulus'.[3] Echocardiographers, in contrast, measure the virtual ring marking the entrance to the valvar complex as the 'annulus', and report this dimension to the surgeon.[2] This discrepancy must harbour the potential for confusion.[5] Consensus is now growing, therefore, that surgeons should also consider this virtual ring as representing the valvar annulus.[2,3,5] It would be optimal if the entrance to the roots was simply described as the valvar diameter, but might this be too much to hope for?

Further potential difficulties arise with the use of 'commissure'. When used anatomically, a commissure describes a line of junction between adjacent structures, as in the eyelids or lips. These structures, with two moving parts, have a solitary commissure, which has two ends. An alternative definition for 'commissure' is the end-point of a zone of apposition.[2] It is in this fashion in which 'commissure' has traditionally been used when describing the cardiac valves. Such usage is unlikely to change.[3] In addition to taking note of the ends of the zones of apposition, therefore, it is also important to acknowledge the structure of the zones of apposition themselves. They extend from the commissures as traditionally defined to the valvar centroid.[5] There are three such zones of apposition to be found in the arterial valves (Figure 4.6), and also in the tricuspid valve. The leaflets of the mitral valve, in contrast, have but a solitary zone of apposition (Figure 4.7).[6]

Position and Support of the Valves within the Heart

In the left heart, the leaflets of the atrioventricular and arterial valves are in proximity to each other within the atrioventricular and ventriculo-arterial junctions (Figure 4.1). Their

4 Surgical Anatomy of the Valves of the Heart

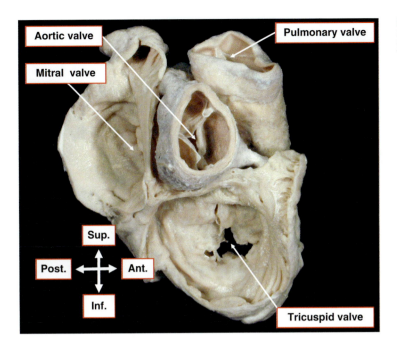

Figure 4.8 This superior view of a cylindrical section of the base of the heart taken at the level of the atrioventricular and ventriculo-arterial junctions shows the relationship of all four cardiac valves.

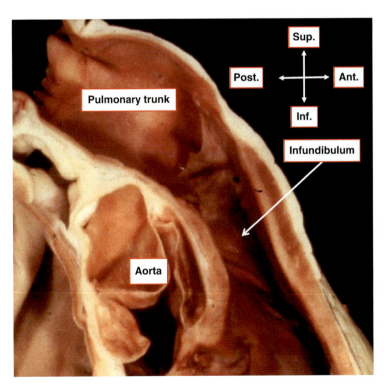

Figure 4.9 The cut across the heart to replicate the oblique subcostal echocardiographic section shows the muscular infundibular sleeve of the right ventricle supporting the leaflets and sinuses of the pulmonary valve. See also Figure 4.3.

hinges are well separated within the right heart. These differences, and the overall arrangement of the four cardiac valves, are best appreciated by examining the short-axis cylindrical section of the heart (Figure 4.8). Within this cylinder, the leaflets of three of the valves can be seen to be in fibrous continuity with one another. Descriptions of a fibrous skeleton providing support for the leaflets within the atrioventricular junctions, however, are grossly exaggerated. The arterial sinuses of the pulmonary valve are supported exclusively by ventricular muscle, specifically by the free-standing right ventricular infundibulum (Figures 4.3, 4.9). More distally, the valvar leaflets are hinged from the arterial wall rather than the infundibular muscle. The distal attachments are at the sinutubular junction, where they form the commissures. A similar arrangement then pertains for the aortic valve (Figure 4.10). When considered in attitudinally appropriate fashion, the pulmonary valve is the most anterior and superior valve, the tricuspid valve is the most inferior, with the mitral valve being the most posterior of the four (Figure 4.11). The aortic valve is centrally located relative to its neighbours, and is rightward and posterior to the pulmonary valve, even though it guards the exit of the left ventricle.

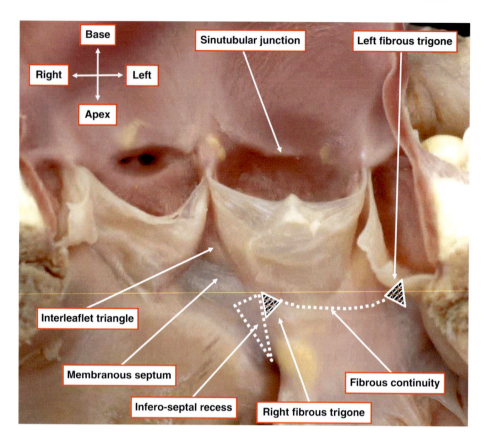

Figure 4.10 The aortic root has been opened to show the combination of fibrous tissues making up the so-called central fibrous body, with this image showing the view as seen from the left ventricle in anatomical orientation. The body is made up of the membranous septum, the area of fibrous continuity forming the roof of the infero-septal recess (white dashed triangle), and the right fibrous trigone, the latter being the rightward end of the continuity between the leaflets of the aortic and mitral valves (cross-hatched triangle seen to the left hand). The left fibrous trigone is shown by the right-hand cross-hatched triangle. The membranous septum is continuous with the fibrous triangle between the superior parts of the semilunar attachments of the right coronary and non-coronary leaflets of the aortic valve.

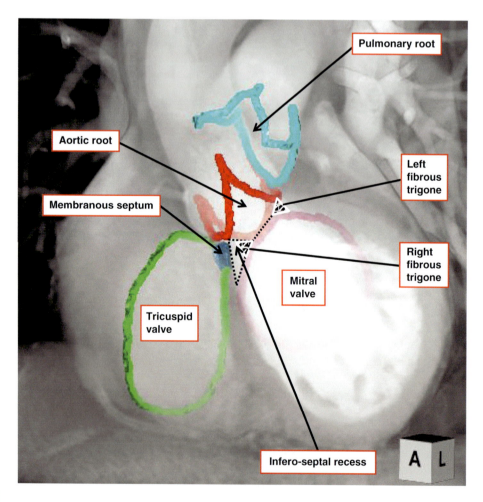

Figure 4.11 The virtual dissection of a computed tomographic dataset, shown in modified frontal projection as indicated by the compass cube in the lower-right corner, reveals the locations in space of the four cardiac valves as seen in attitudinally appropriate orientation. The semilunar hinges of the arterial valves have been reconstructed, showing the separate nature of the pulmonary root (light blue semilunar lines) and the continuity between the hinges of the aortic (red semilunar lines) and mitral valves (faint purple oval). The location of the fibrous trigones and the infero-septal recess have been superimposed on the image, using comparable markers as shown in Figure 4.10.

4 Surgical Anatomy of the Valves of the Heart

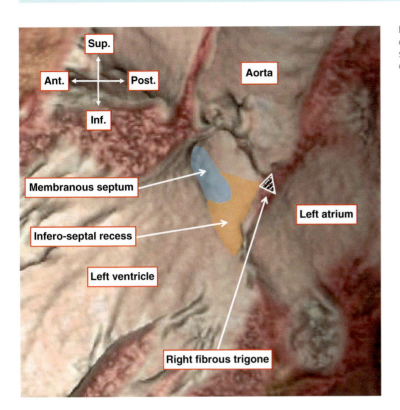

Figure 4.12 Another virtual dissection of a computed tomographic dataset has been segmented to show the contributions made to the so-called central fibrous trigone by the membranous septum, the roof of the infero-septal recess, and the right fibrous trigone.

The concept of an extensive fibrous skeleton supporting the leaflets of all four valves within the muscular cylinder forming the base of the ventricular mass, appealing as it may be, is far from reality. The pulmonary valvar leaflets have no direct relationship to the leaflets of the other valves (Figures 4.8, 4.11). The leaflets of the two atrioventricular valves have limited fibrous support within the atrioventricular junctions. It is the relationships of the aortic leaflet of the mitral valve that underscore the presence of the greatest fibrous support within the cardiac base. This leaflet of the mitral valve is in direct fibrous continuity with two of the leaflets of the aortic valve. The area of continuity produces the aortic–mitral curtain, which forms the roof of the left ventricle. The area is thickened at both its ends, serving to anchor the aortic–mitral valvar unit to the ventricular musculature across the short axis of the left ventricle (Figure 4.10). These thickenings are called the right and left fibrous trigones, respectively. The right fibrous trigone is itself continuous with the fibrous components that form the strongest part of the fibrous support. The conjoined structure is called the central fibrous body. It has three parts, the right fibrous trigone, the roof of the infero-septal recess, and the membranous septum (Figures 4.11, 4.12). The fibrous area formed by the membranous septum does not extend distally to reach the level of the sinutubular junction. The most distal parts of the walls of the aortic root, interposing between the valvar sinuses, are the interleaflet fibrous triangles (Figure 4.10).

The location of the fibrous triangle interposing between the right coronary and non-coronary aortic sinuses is best perceived from the right side, having removed the fibrous tissue forming its floor (Figure 4.13). The triangle is then seen to extend superiorly to the level of the aortic sinutubular junction, thus separating the most distal part of the left ventricular cavity from the right side of the transverse sinus. Similar small triangles of fibrous tissue form the most distal parts of the spaces between the other leaflets of the aortic valve.[7] The triangle between the non-coronary and the left coronary leaflets is itself confluent with the area of fibrous continuity between the aortic and mitral valves (Figure 4.14). When the triangle is removed, and the heart photographed from behind, the fibrous tissue can be seen to separate the left ventricular outflow tract from the middle part of the transverse sinus (Figure 4.15). The much smaller triangle separating the two coronary leaflets of the aortic valve separates the left ventricular outflow tract from the area of extracavitary tissue running between the aortic root and the free-standing right ventricular infundibulum (Figure 4.16). Taken overall, therefore, the fibrous components of the aortic root form a three-pronged crown extending to the level of the sinutubular junction (Figure 4.17). Extensions from the fibrous tissue forming the crown-like aortic root continue to a limited extent into both atrioventricular junctions. These extensions have been described as the 'coronary files' ('fila coronaria'). They are usually believed to support the hinges of the atrioventricular valves, providing the valvar 'annulus'. The extent of such fibrous support, however, varies markedly from heart to heart.[8] It is questionable whether it is ever the case that a complete ring of fibrous tissue supports the leaflets of the mitral valve. In some places, the hinge of the leaflet can be supported by a fibrous shelf (Figure 4.18A). In many more sites in the same heart, however, the leaflet is supported only by the fibrofatty tissues of the left atrioventricular groove (Figure 4.18B). It is the fibro-adipose tissues, furthermore, which serve to insulate the atrial from the ventricular myocardium. This arrangement, in which the fibrofatty tissues

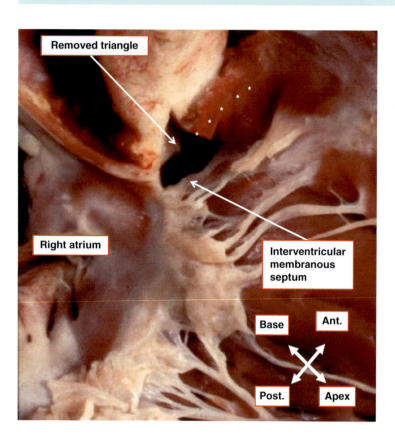

Figure 4.13 This image was produced by removing the interleaflet triangle between the right and non-coronary aortic leaflets, with the heart then photographed from the right side. The base of the triangle is formed by the interventricular component of the membranous septum. The white asterisks show the cut edge of the ventriculo-infundibular fold, which forms the greater part of the supraventricular crest. The most apical part of the removed triangle encroaches on the transverse sinus.

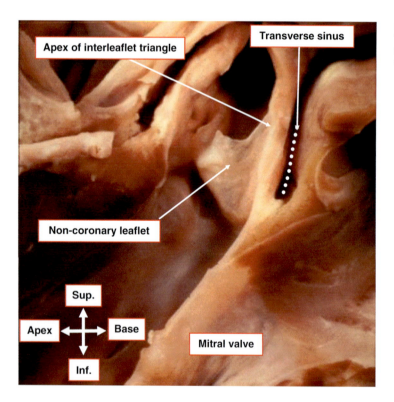

Figure 4.14 The heart has been sectioned through the interleaflet triangle between the non-coronary and left coronary aortic leaflets, showing how the fibrous wall interposes between the left ventricular outflow tract and the transverse sinus (white dotted line).

insulate the atrial from the ventricular muscles masses (Figure 4.19), is the rule around the orifice of the tricuspid valve. It is again questionable as to whether the leaflets of the tricuspid valve are ever supported by a true fibrous 'annulus'. Paradoxically, the solitary area of atrioventricular muscular continuity to be found in the normal heart, namely the site of penetration of the atrioventricular conduction axis, is within perhaps the strongest part of the fibrous skeleton, specifically the atrioventricular component of the membranous septum. This point is conveniently marked for the surgeon by the

4 Surgical Anatomy of the Valves of the Heart

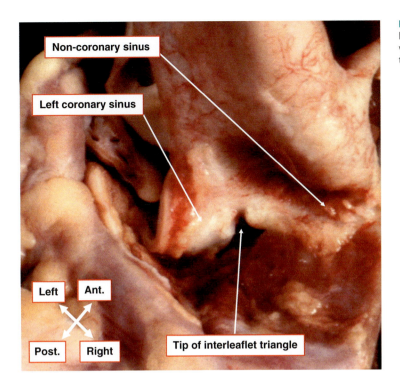

Figure 4.15 In this heart, the tip of the fibrous triangle between the left coronary and non-coronary aortic valvar leaflets has been removed, with the heart then photographed from the transverse sinus to show the location of the apex of the triangle.

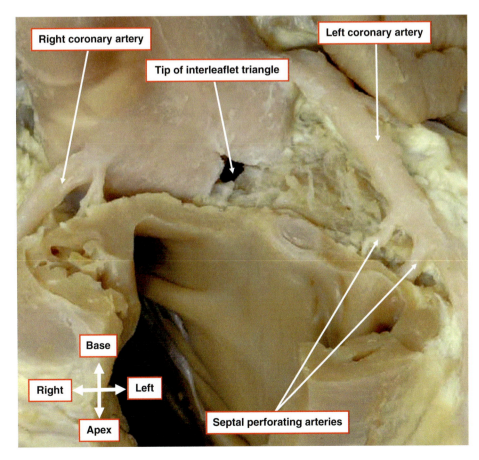

Figure 4.16 This dissection shows the location of the interleaflet fibrous triangle between the two sinuses of the aortic valve that give rise to the coronary arteries. The triangle itself has been removed, as has the free-standing sleeve of subpulmonary infundibulum. The heart is photographed from the right ventricular aspect. Note the position of the septal perforating arteries.

attachment to the central fibrous body of another fibrous structure, the tendon of Todaro. This fibrous cord extends through the myocardium of the right atrial wall, attaching to the right-sided aspect of the membranous septum. It forms the atrial boundary of the triangle of Koch (Figure 4.20).

The issue of fibrous shelves supporting the leaflets has become controversial over recent years. The feature has been identified as so-called disjunction, with the finding of disjunction allegedly associated with prolapse of the leaflets of the mitral valve, and potentially lethal arrhythmias.[8] As already

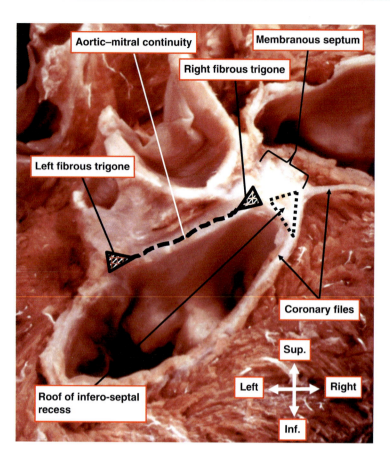

Figure 4.17 This heart has been dissected by removing the entirety of the atrial myocardium, and is photographed from behind. The walls of the aortic sinuses have been removed to the level of the semilunar hinge points of the valvar leaflets, showing the overall crown-like arrangement of the fibrous part of the root supporting the leaflets. Note how the membranous septum, the roof of the infero-septal recess (black dashed triangle), and the right fibrous trigone (right-hand cross-hatched triangle) together produce the central fibrous body. Note also the fibrous extensions extending from the fibrous tissue of the aortic root into the orifices of the mitral and tricuspid valves. These are the so-called coronary files (fila coronaria).

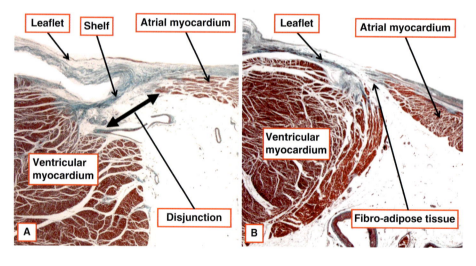

Figure 4.18 These histological sections are taken across the left atrioventricular junction of the same heart. In panel A, there is a fibrous shelf supporting the hinge of the valvar leaflet, and producing so-called disjunction between the crest of the ventricular myocardium and the leading edge of the left atrial vestibule. In panel B, the areas of myocardium are separated only by the fibro-adipose tissue of the atrioventricular junction, with no 'disjunction'. This type of variability is ubiquitous in normal hearts. The sections were prepared by Professor Damian Sanchez-Quintana, and are reproduced with his kind permission.

indicated, such a feature is to be found at certain points of the left atrioventricular junction in all hearts.[9] Indeed, McAlpine, when producing his *Atlas*, went as far as to suggest that such a left ventricular 'membrane' supported the entirety of the mural leaflet of the mitral valve.[10] This is an exaggeration. Studies using either computed tomography or magnetic resonance imaging,[11,12] nonetheless, confirm the fact that such 'disjunction' is an almost ubiquitous finding within some part of the normal left atrioventricular junction.[6]

Returning to the arrangement of the arterial roots, it is incorrect to speak of either an aortic or a pulmonary valvar 'ring' in the sense of a collagenous structure supporting the valvar leaflets. Rather than being hinged in uniplanar circular fashion, the leaflets of the arterial valves have semilunar attachments within the arterial roots (Figures 4.4, 4.5). Uniplanar rings are to be found within the structure of each arterial root, but not confluent with the semilunar attachments of the leaflets. Paradoxically, the rings that do exist are not taken by surgeons to represent a valvar annulus. The most obvious anatomical ring, albeit found only in the pulmonary root, becomes evident only when the valvar leaflets themselves have been removed (Figure 4.4). It is the myocardial–arterial junction. The semilunar hinges of the valvar leaflets cross this ring, incorporating myocardium at the bases of all three sinuses of the pulmonary

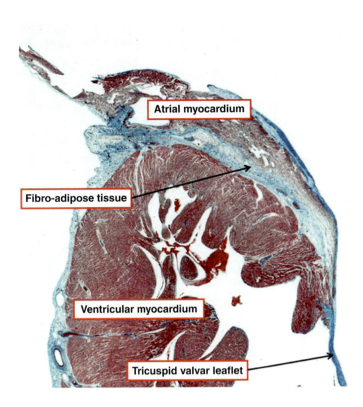

Figure 4.19 The histological section across the right atrioventricular junction shows that it is the fibrofatty tissue of the atrioventricular groove that, at all points except the penetration of the bundle of His, insulates the right atrial from the right ventricular myocardium. There is no fibrous 'annulus' supporting the hinge of the tricuspid valve.

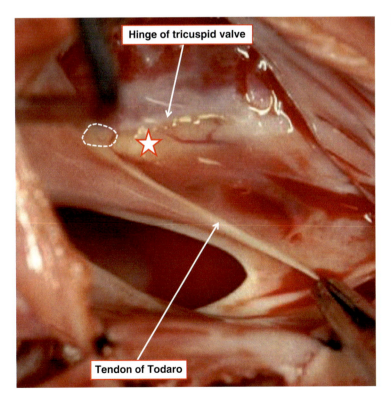

Figure 4.20 This picture, taken in the operating room, shows how the continuation of the Eustachian valve, inserting as the tendon of Todaro into the membranous septum (white dotted circle) demarcates the atrial border of the triangle of Koch. The star marks the site of the atrioventricular node, located at the apex of the triangle.

root (Figure 4.4). Such myocardial–arterial junctions in the aortic root are found only in the sinuses that give rise to the coronary arteries (Figure 4.5). The distal extremities of all the leaflets in both arterial roots, nonetheless, are then attached to another obvious anatomical ring, namely the sinutubular junction (Figure 4.3). There is then a third 'ring' within the arterial roots, but this one is a virtual, rather than an anatomical, structure. It is formed by joining together the most proximal parts of the valvar hinges (Figure 4.3). The virtual ring has particular clinical significance, since this is the ring identified by echocardiographers as the valvar annulus.[2] As was suggested by the German Working Group concerned with surgical treatment of the aortic valve,[3] the overall situation would become much clearer if surgeons also accepted this virtual ring as representing the valvar annulus.

Basic Morphology of the Atrioventricular Valves

The mitral and tricuspid valves, as we have seen, have several important features in common. These features permit their collective description in terms of a valvar complex (Figure 4.2).[1] The first feature is the attachments of the valvar leaflets within the atrioventricular junctions. As has been discussed above, this arrangement is usually described as the annulus of the atrioventricular valves. It is questionable if the leaflets are ever uniformly supported by a firm and continuous collagenous cord. A second feature is the arrangement of the leaflets. Histologically, these structures have a spongy atrial, and a fibrous ventricular, layer. The atrial myocardium inserts for varying distances between the endocardium and the spongy layer. On rare occasions, fronds of ventricular musculature may extend into the fibrous layer. In normal valves, blood vessels are found only within the segment of leaflet containing muscular fronds. The leaflets are then supported by the tendinous cords, which themselves insert into the papillary muscles, or else directly into the ventricular myocardium. These cordal attachments are the third feature common to both tricuspid and mitral valves, although there are fundamental differences in the way each of the cordal units is arranged. This is also the case with the fourth feature, namely the papillary muscles. The differences in these various features readily permit the morphological differentiation of the valves. Indeed, the morphological differences are sufficient to distinguish between the morphologically right and left ventricles. This is important, since the valves always go with their morphological ventricle. Before describing these differences, however, emphasis must be placed on the features of the leaflets and their tension apparatus which are common to both valves.

Considered as a whole, the leaflets form a continuous skirt that hangs from the atrioventricular junction. The skirt itself is divided into discrete components, with these individual sections representing the individual leaflets. There is no current consensus as to how many leaflets there are in each valve, nor as to what constitutes the point of separation of one leaflet from the other. Traditionally, the tricuspid valve, as indicated by its name, has been considered to have three leaflets. Some have argued that the valve has only two leaflets,[13,14] albeit that our studies lend no support to this concept.[15,16] The alternative name for the mitral valve is the bicuspid valve. Yet it has been suggested that this valve is best considered as having four,[17] or even six, leaflets.[18] These ongoing arguments illustrate the difficulties that exist in defining individual leaflets. Some have sought to achieve such definition by identifying the so-called commissures between them. This then necessitates defining a commissure. Surgeons usually take the commissures as the peripheral attachments of a breach in the skirt of valvar tissue. For the atrioventricular valves, these breaches are supported by fan-shaped commissural cords, such cords then inserting into a major papillary muscle or papillary muscle group (Figure 4.21). The concept of identifying the commissure on the basis of the cords supporting it amounts to defining one variable structure in terms of another that is itself variable. As we will discuss in Chapter 7, when addressed in terms of philosophy, this is a poor principle. In order to define commissures in this fashion, furthermore, the valve must be assessed in opened position. Yet, as all surgeons know, in

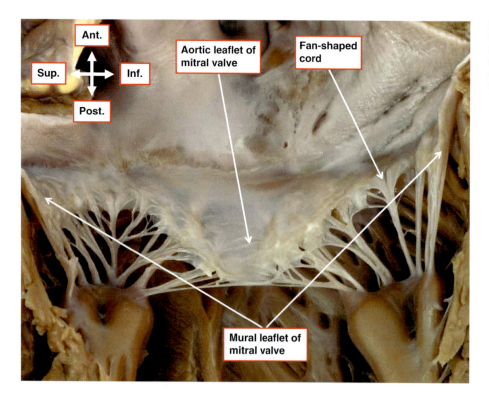

Figure 4.21 The anatomical specimen has been opened through the mural leaflet of the mitral valve, with the valvar orifice then spread open and photographed from behind. The image shows the free-edge and fan-shaped cords supporting both leaflets of the valve.

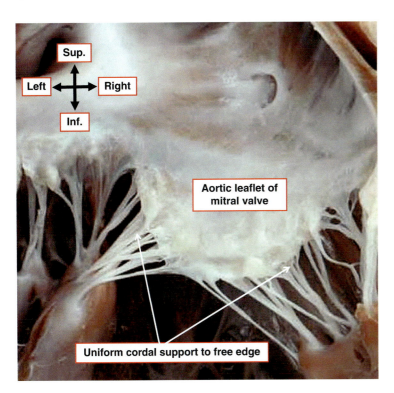

Figure 4.22 This anatomical specimen, prepared as for Figure 4.21, and viewed from the inlet aspect, shows the tendinous cords supporting the entirety of the free edge of the aortic leaflet of the mitral valve.

order to function properly, the leaflets of the valve must fit together snugly when closed. Because of this, we prefer to define the extent of the leaflets according to the location of the zones of apposition between them. It is then the peripheral extents of these zones of apposition that become the commissures. The areas of the skirt separated by the peripheral commissures then represent the leaflets.

The leaflets themselves are supported by tendinous cords. The ends of the zones of apposition between the adjacent leaflets are usually supported by fan-shaped cords. These can then be defined as commissural cords (Figure 4.21). In addition to the fan-shaped cord, the entire free edges of the leaflets are normally uniformly supported by cords (Figure 4.22). As was indicated by Frater[19] when discussing the exquisitely complex categorization of cords proposed by the group from Toronto,[20] if any of these cords supporting the free edge are cut, the valve may become regurgitant. We agree with Frater[19] that, for the purposes of categorization, it is sufficient simply to distinguish those cords supporting the free edge (Figure 4.22) from those supporting the rough zone (Figure 4.23). The detailed classification proposed by the Toronto group[20] has little, if any, surgical utility.

The cords from the rough zone are prominent structures. They extend from the papillary muscles to the ventricular aspect of the leaflets. Some of these cords are particularly prominent in the mitral valve, and are called strut cords (Figure 4.23). There is then a third type of cord that extends from the ventricular wall close to the atrioventricular junction, and again inserts into the ventricular aspect of the leaflet. These are the basal cords (Figure 4.24). There is little point in further characterizing the pattern of branching and the generations of these cords. The significant point is that, normally, all parts of the leaflets receive good cordal support. Lack of uniform cordal support is very likely a mechanism leading to prolapse of a leaflet.[21,22]

The different components of the atrioventricular valve making up the overall valve complex (Figure 4.1) must function in concert so as to produce a competent valvar mechanism. The reason that the atrioventricular valves have such a complex tension apparatus is that, while in their closed position, they must withstand the full brunt of systolic ventricular pressure. A lesion of any of the valvar components can result in regurgitation. Thus, it is essential that the atrioventricular junction be of normal size and not overly dilated. The leaflets must coapt snugly. This demands an area of overlap. Often, particularly in aged valves, this point of closure is marked by a series of nodules. The point of closure away from the free edge gives a margin of safety for dilation of the valvar orifice. Equally significant to competent closure is the support of the leaflet provided by cords attached to the free edge. As discussed above, this feature is highly significant to the mechanism of prolapse of the valve leaflets. It has been suggested[23] that prolapse of the leaflets of the mitral valve is one of the most common congenital lesions. As yet, there is no consensus as to the aetiology of such prolapse. Morphological observations[21,22] certainly suggest that lack of cordal support to the free edge of the leaflets can contribute to prolapse, along with lengthening of the persisting cords. And uniform support of the free edges of the leaflets is an integral part of a normal valve. Also important in the maintenance of competence is the correct action of the papillary muscles and the ventricular myocardium. Not only must the papillary muscles be viable, but they must also be in their appropriate position of mechanical advantage relative to the axis of the valve. Taken together, all parts of the valvar unit are significant in the normal function of the valve.[1]

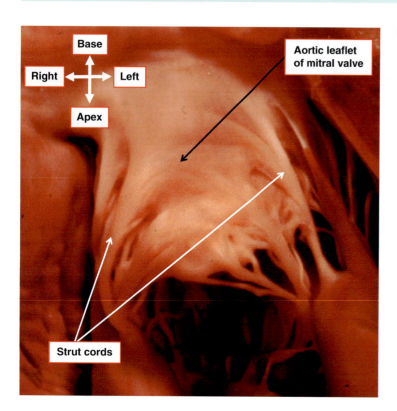

Figure 4.23 Some cords to the rough zone of the ventricular aspect of the aortic leaflet of the mitral valve are particularly prominent, and are defined as strut cords.

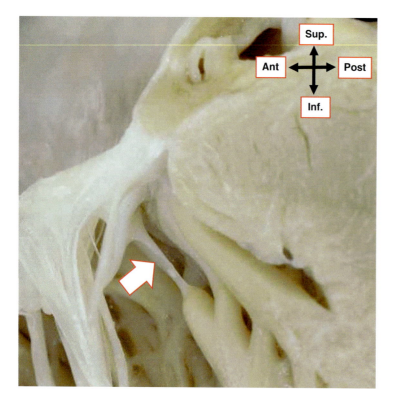

Figure 4.24 The mural leaflet of the mitral valve has been reflected upwards, showing a basal cord (white arrow with red borders), supported by its own muscular belly.

The Mitral Valve

The mitral valve has two major leaflets, which are supported by paired papillary muscles. The two leaflets have widely dissimilar circumferential lengths (Figure 4.25). The ends of the solitary zone of apposition between them, traditionally labelled the commissures, together with the papillary muscles, are positioned infero-septally and supero-laterally. They are usually described, incorrectly, as being postero-septal and antero-lateral.[6] The advent of computed tomographic imaging, which relates the location of the heart to the coordinates of the body, serves to emphasize the inappropriate nature of the conventional description (Figure 4.26). The tomographic images also

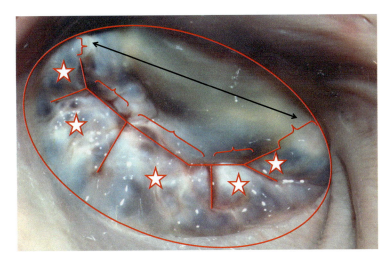

Figure 4.25 The mitral valve, photographed in Figure 4.6, is shown again here from above in closed position, as it might be seen by the surgeon. There is a solitary zone of apposition between its two major leaflets, with slits in the mural leaflet producing a number of potential subcomponents in the mural leaflet (stars). Note that the ends of the zone of apposition do not extend to the atrioventricular junction (brackets). The black double-headed arrow shows the extent of the aortic leaflet. The original photograph was kindly sent to us by Dr Van S. Galstyan, from Armenia, and we thank him for permitting us to use it in our book.

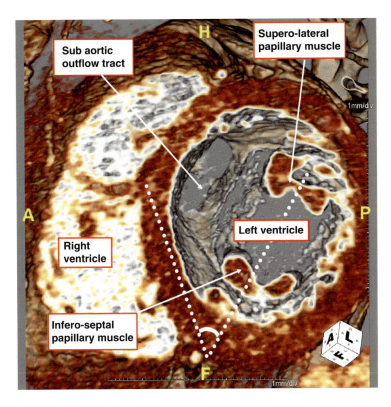

Figure 4.26 The computed tomographic image shows the orientation of the short axis of the ventricular mass relative to the bodily coordinates, indicated both by the cube seen at the bottom right-hand corner of the image, and the abbreviations showing the coordinates of the head (H), feet (F), anterior (A), and posterior (P). The tomographic section shows the angle between the line of the zone of apposition between the leaflets of the mitral valve and the plane of the inferior part of the muscular ventricular septum (dotted lines). The papillary muscles are positioned infero-septally and supero-laterally when considered in attitudinally correct orientation (see orientation cube).

show well the angle existing between the axis of opening of the valve and the plane of the inferior component of the muscular ventricular septum (Figure 4.26). The infero-septal recess occupies this angle. This arrangement is key to the disposition of the axis of atrioventricular conduction tissue (see Chapter 6). The two leaflets of the mitral valve themselves are usually described as being 'anterior' and 'posterior'. Strictly speaking, they are supero-anterior and infero-posterior, again because of the oblique axis of opening of the valve relative to the anatomical axes of the body (Figure 4.26). We prefer to describe the leaflets as being aortic and mural, this description accounting well both for their morphology and their usual location within the body.[6]

The aortic leaflet is supported by only one-third of the circumference of the left atrioventricular junction. It is trapezoidal or more semicircular in shape than the mural leaflet (Figure 4.27). The mural leaflet, supported by two-thirds of the circumferences, is long and rectangular, although its middle component can also be somewhat semicircular. It is the segments of the mural leaflet adjacent to the ends of the zone of apposition with the aortic leaflet that show the most variation in morphology. Often these segments are almost completely separate from the central component, producing the so-called scallops of the mural leaflet. Carpentier and his colleagues[24] have coded these scallops in alphanumeric fashion, along with the facing segments of the aortic leaflet. This convention has widespread surgical use (Figure 4.28). Yacoub[17] has gone so far as to nominate the scallops as separate leaflets of a quadrifoliate valve. Others[18] point out that the parts of the leaflet adjacent to the ends of the

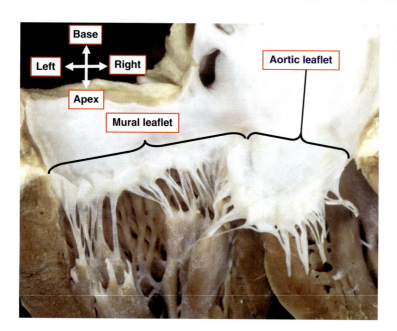

Figure 4.27 Opening the mitral valve through the end of the zone of apposition between the leaflets closest to the septum, and spreading the valve, illustrates the widely dissimilar lengths of the two leaflets at their hinge points from the atrioventricular junction.

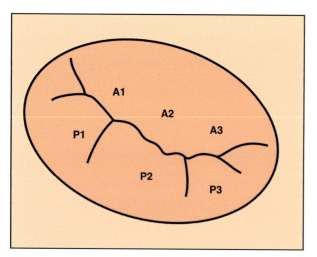

Figure 4.28 The classification of Carpentier and his colleagues[24] recognizes three major scallops in the mural leaflet (P1 through P3), and also names the facing segments of the aortic leaflet in alphanumeric fashion (A1 through A3). This classification, however, ignores the potential subcomponents of the leaflet at the ends of the solitary zone of apposition (see Figure 4.25).

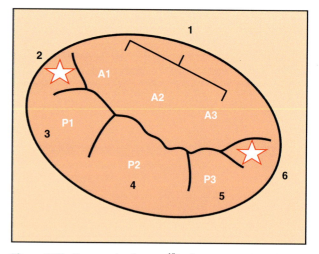

Figure 4.29 Kumar and colleagues,[18] in their suggested classification, did take into account the components of the mural leaflet adjacent to the ends of the solitary zone of apposition between the two major leaflets (stars), giving six rather than four potential subcomponents for the entire valvar skirt (compare with Figure 4.28).

zone of apposition can also take a 'scallop-like' appearance (Figure 4.29). All these categorizations are artificial. Because of the marked variability that occurs normally in the valve, the mural leaflet can be composed of four, five, or even more components. It is better to recognize that there are a variable number of slits in the mural leaflet, and that these slits act as pleats so that the normal valve can close snugly.[25] In the setting of prolapse, nonetheless, individual components of the divided mural leaflet may be deformed in isolation, and must then be recognized as such.

The supporting cords attach the leaflets either to the papillary muscles, in the form of the cords to the free edge and rough zone, or else directly to the wall of the ventricle, as with the basal cords. The cords at the ends of the zone of apposition attach adjacent sides of both the leaflets to the heads of each of the papillary muscles. Supplementary heads of both papillary muscles then support other cords running to the free edge, which usually attach uniformly along the leading edge of the leaflets. As we have discussed, the degree of support can be quite variable. The cords supporting the divisions between the scallops of the mural leaflet also often have a fan-shaped appearance. When attached to a prominent supplementary head of a papillary muscle, they can be markedly similar to the cords supporting the ends of the zone of apposition. The cords to the rough zone run from the papillary muscles to the ventricular aspect of the leaflets. Several of these cords, running from each papillary muscle to the undersurface of the aortic leaflet, are particularly prominent, and are called strut cords (Figure 4.23). The basal cords attach to the ventricular aspect of the mural leaflet, running directly

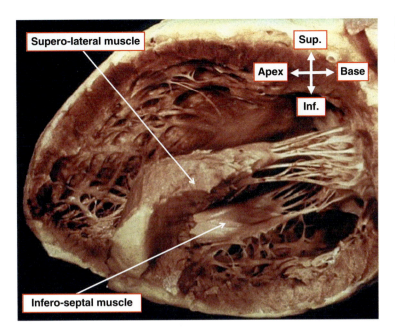

Figure 4.30 This dissection was made by removing the parietal wall of the left ventricle, and photographing the heart from behind and beneath. The papillary muscles, located infero-septally and supero-laterally, are directly adjacent at their ventricular origins.

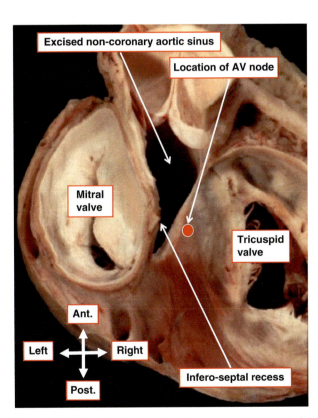

Figure 4.31 The atrial chambers have been removed, along with the non-adjacent sinus and leaflet of the aortic valve, revealing the deep infero-septal recess of the left ventricular outflow tract. Note the position of the atrioventricular (AV) node (red circle) relative to the mitral valve.

from miniature muscle heads on the parietal wall of the ventricle (Figure 4.24).

The papillary muscles of the mitral valve are almost always prominent paired structures, located on the infero-septal and supero-lateral aspects of the parietal ventricular wall (Figure 4.26). Although there can be considerable variation in the precise morphology of either muscle, neither arises from the septum. This is in contrast to the attachments of the tricuspid valve within the right ventricle. When the valve is dissected in its natural position within the left ventricle (Figure 4.30), the muscles are seen to be adjacent to each other at the junction of the apical and middle thirds of the parietal ventricular wall.

It is the area of the valvar orifice related to the rightward end of the zone of apposition between the leaflets that is most vulnerable in terms of the conduction tissues. The atrioventricular node and the penetrating atrioventricular bundle are adjacent to these areas (Figures 4.31, 4.32). The area of fibrous continuity between the aortic and mitral valves is variably related to the zone of apposition between the non-coronary and left coronary leaflets of the aortic valve. At this point, the aortic root is tented up, and an incision apparently through the atrial wall will extend into the subaortic outflow tract. If the incision is continued superiorly, it will pass into the transverse sinus of the pericardial cavity, which overlies the aortic–mitral curtain (Figure 4.15). The deep inner curvature of the heart overlies and runs to either side of the curtain, and is lined by the transverse sinus. Encircling the mural leaflet of the valve are the circumflex coronary artery from below and to the left, and the coronary sinus from below and to the right (Figure 4.32). The atrioventricular nodal artery also runs in proximity to the right side of the mitral orifice, particularly when arising from a dominant circumflex artery. Indeed, the extent of the margin directly related to the circumflex artery depends on coronary arterial dominance. When the left coronary artery is dominant, an arrangement found in one-tenth of the population, the entire attachment of the mural leaflet is intimately related to the coronary artery, including its branch supplying the atrioventricular node (Figure 4.33).

The Tricuspid Valve

When judged on its pattern of closure,[15,16] the tricuspid valve has three major leaflets (Figures 4.34, 4.35). They are positioned septally, antero-superiorly, and inferiorly (Figure 4.36). The

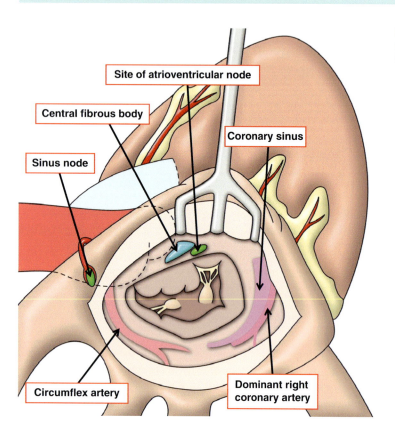

Figure 4.32 The cartoon shows the components of the mitral valve relative to the structures of surgical significance when the right coronary artery is dominant, this being the situation in 90% of individuals.

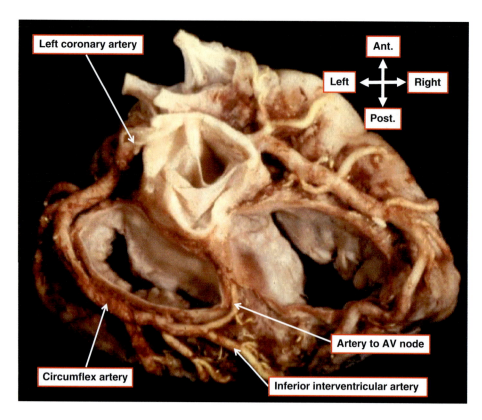

Figure 4.33 The dissection, photographed from above and behind, with the heart in anatomical position, shows the relationship of the circumflex artery to the mural leaflet of the mitral valve when the left coronary artery is dominant. Note that the inferior interventricular artery and the artery to the atrioventricular (AV) node take their origin from the circumflex artery.

inferior, or mural, leaflet is conventionally described as being posterior. This is yet another example of the description of cardiac structures as seen in the autopsy or dissecting room after the heart has been removed, rather than using the bodily coordinates for reference. The septal leaflet is supported between the relatively inconstant inferior papillary muscle, and the much more constant medial papillary muscle. Also known as the muscle of Lancisi, or the papillary muscle of the

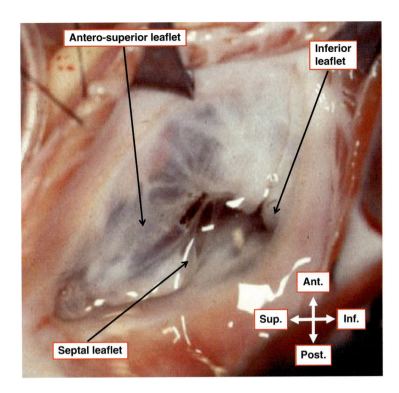

Figure 4.34 This picture, taken in the operating room, shows the arrangement of the three leaflets of the tricuspid valve, which are positioned septally, antero-superiorly, and inferiorly or murally. The latter leaflet is usually described, incorrectly, as being positioned posteriorly.

conus, it arises from the caudal limb of the septomarginal trabeculation (Figure 4.37). The attachment of the septal leaflet crosses the membranous septum, dividing it into atrioventricular and interventricular components (Figure 4.38). The distal extent of the leaflet is attached by multiple cords running from the free edge directly to the septum (Figure 4.39). It is this feature that serves to distinguish the tendinous support of the tricuspid valve from that of the mitral valve. The mitral valvar leaflets lack any septal attachments. In the area where the septal leaflet of the tricuspid valve extends across the membranous septum, the leaflet may be divided, resulting in a discrete cleft which extends towards the membranous part of the septum.

The antero-superior leaflet is hinged from the underside of the ventriculo-infundibular fold, hanging like an extensive curtain between the inlet and outlet parts of the ventricle. Its medial and superior end is supported by cords from the medial papillary muscle (Figure 4.37). There is more variability in the arrangement of its lateral and inferior component. Its zone of apposition with the inferior leaflet is usually supported by the prominent anterior papillary muscle, which takes origin from the apical portion of the septomarginal trabeculation.[16] The anterior papillary muscle can also support the midportion of the antero-superior leaflet itself.[16] The leaflet is well supported not only by cords to its free edge, but also by rough-zone and strut cords, in a fashion comparable with that seen in the aortic leaflet of the mitral valve. When the anterior papillary muscle supports the midpoint of the antero-superior leaflet, the muscle supporting its zone of apposition with the inferior leaflet is relatively indistinct. Frequently, there are extensions of muscle from either the papillary muscles or the ventriculo-infundibular fold directly into the antero-superior leaflet. The third leaflet of the tricuspid valve is the inferior, or mural, one. It is less constant than the other two, since the inferior papillary muscles are less distinct, and are variable in number. The leaflet is attached to the parietal part of the atrioventricular junction, being supported distally by several cords to the free edge, attached either to small heads of muscle or directly into the ventricular wall. There are usually also basal cords supporting the inferior leaflet (Figure 4.40). The entire parietal attachments of the leaflets of the tricuspid valve are encircled by the right coronary artery running in the atrioventricular groove (Figure 4.41). It is rare to find a well-formed collagenous tricuspid 'annulus'. Instead, the atrial and ventricular myocardial masses are separated almost exclusively by the adipose tissue within the groove, with the leaflets of the valve hinged from the endocardial surface of the ventricular wall (Figure 4.19).

Basic Arrangement of the Arterial Valves

The arterial valves are much simpler structures than the atrioventricular valves. They do not need an intricate arrangement of tension apparatus to ensure their competence. They are, nonetheless, still best analysed in terms of a valvar complex (Figure 4.3). Their design is simplicity itself. The three semilunar leaflets open into the supporting arterial sinuses during ventricular systole. They then collapse together during diastole, being held in their closed position by the hydrostatic pressure of the column of blood they then support (Figure 4.42). In terms of histological structure, the leaflets have a fibrous core with an endothelial lining (Figure 4.43). The fibrous core is thickened at the free edge, particularly at its central portion short of the edge. With age, a distinct fibrous thickening becomes evident at this site, namely the nodule of Arantius. The zone of apposition of the leaflets of

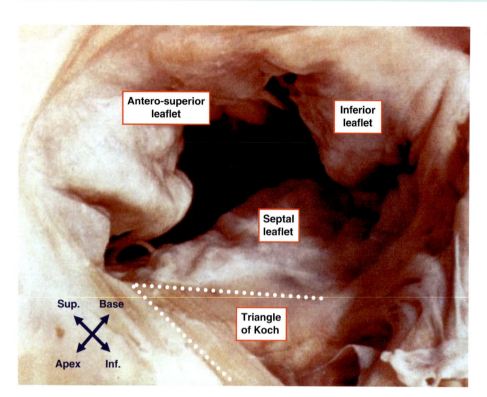

Figure 4.35 The anatomical specimen has been photographed to replicate the arrangement as seen in the operating room, as shown in Figure 4.34, confirming that the leaflets are located septally, antero-superiorly, and inferiorly. Note the relationship of the septal leaflet to the landmarks of the triangle of Koch (dotted lines).

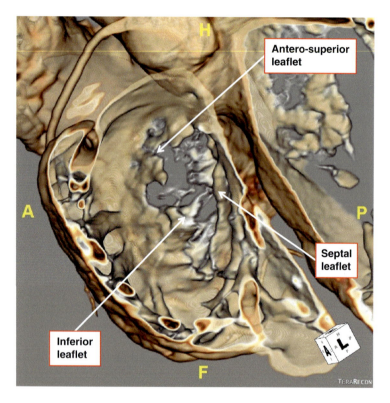

Figure 4.36 The computed tomographic image, showing the three leaflets of the tricuspid valve, confirms that they are positioned septally, antero-superiorly, and inferiorly when the heart is viewed in attitudinally appropriate fashion. Note the markers produced by the computed tomographic software. In addition to the orientation cube in the lower right-hand corner, with 'A' representing the abbreviation for anterior, and 'L' showing left, the additional abbreviations provide more attitudinal information, with 'F' representing 'feet', or inferior, and 'H' head, or superior. 'P' is the abbreviation for posterior.

the valve extends from near the midportion of the leaflet proximally to their free edge distally. It is central coaptation of the nodules of Arantius, and coaptation of the adjacent lunules on either side, which forms the surface areas of the zones of apposition. Not infrequently, the leaflets may contain an abnormal aperture or communication with the lunules of the leaflet, referred to as a fenestration. Such fenestrations are common findings. They are covered by the lunule of the opposing leaflet, and do not affect valvar function. Alternatively, larger tears or holes in the leaflet may be present, referred to as perforations. These often extend outside the components involved in the zone of apposition. These perforations are pathological, and result in valvar incompetence.

4 Surgical Anatomy of the Valves of the Heart

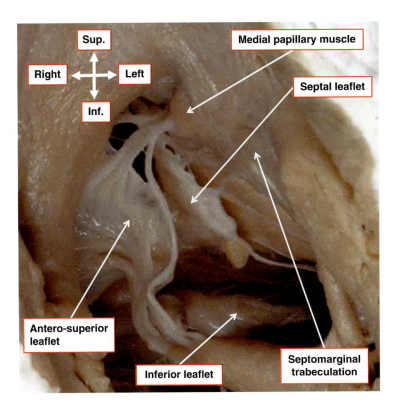

Figure 4.37 The right ventricle is photographed from the infundibular aspect in anatomical orientation, showing the medial papillary muscle, also known as the muscle of Lancisi, supporting the zone of apposition between the septal and the antero-superior leaflets.

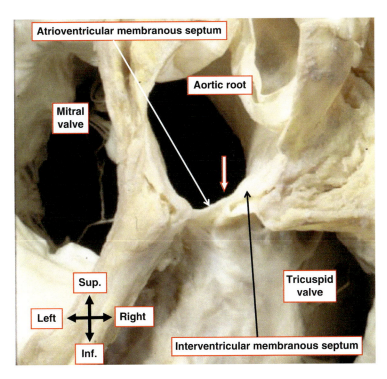

Figure 4.38 The base of the heart is shown from the atrial aspect, the atrial myocardium and the non-coronary sinus of the aortic valve having been removed. The attachment of the septal leaflet of the tricuspid valve (white arrow with red borders) divides the membranous septum into its atrioventricular and interventricular components.

It is the hinge line of the individual leaflets which is of half-moon, or semilunar, shape (Figures 4.4, 4.5). When the three semilunar hinges are considered in terms of their overall structure, the seating of the leaflets takes the form of a coronet (Figure 4.44). The attachments of the leaflets at the apex of their zones of apposition are then significantly higher than the attachments at their midportion (Figure 4.45). In the light of these arrangements, it is less than ideal to describe the hinges of the valvar leaflets in terms of the annulus. Many, if not most, surgeons still consider this to be an appropriate term.[3] As we have already shown, there are two potential anatomical rings within the extent of the arterial roots, with one being incomplete in the aortic root. Perhaps paradoxically, neither has attracted attention from surgeons for description as the valvar annulus. The most obvious anatomical ring is the sinutubular junction, this being the plane of

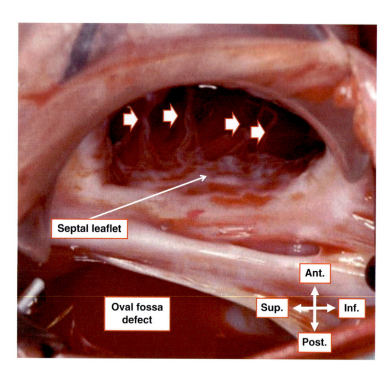

Figure 4.39 This operative view through a right atriotomy shows the cordal attachments to the septum of the septal leaflet of the tricuspid valve (white arrows with red borders). The patient also has a defect in the oval fossa.

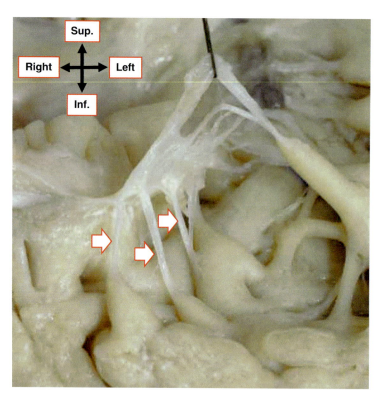

Figure 4.40 In this anatomical specimen, the inferior leaflet of the tricuspid valve has been reflected away from the ventricular wall to show the basal cords (arrows).

attachment of the valvar commissures (Figure 4.3). The other obvious anatomical ring, but seen only in the pulmonary root, is the locus over which the fibrous walls of the arterial trunks are attached to the supporting infundibulum, thus constituting the myocardial–arterial junction (Figure 4.4). Myocardial–arterial junctions in the aortic root are to be found only in the sinuses which give rise to the coronary arteries. It follows that the myocardial–arterial junction is an anatomical ventriculo-arterial junction. It is markedly different from the haemodynamic junction, which is marked in the periphery by the semilunar attachment of the leaflets, and centrally by the ventricular surface of the bellies of the leaflets. By virtue of this arrangement, parts of the arterial wall, the interleaflet triangles, haemodynamically are ventricular structures. Part of the ventricular myocardium, in contrast, when incorporated at the base of a valvar sinus is within the arterial trunk. Thus, despite the seemingly simple nature of the valvar structure, the overall arterial roots are

4 Surgical Anatomy of the Valves of the Heart

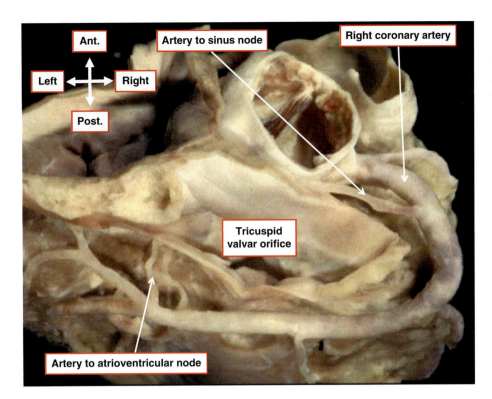

Figure 4.41 This view of the heart, also shown in Figure 4.64, with a dominant right coronary artery, is photographed in anatomical orientation from above and behind, showing the intimate relationship of the artery to the orifice of the tricuspid valve. The fibro-adipose tissue within the atrioventricular groove has been removed.

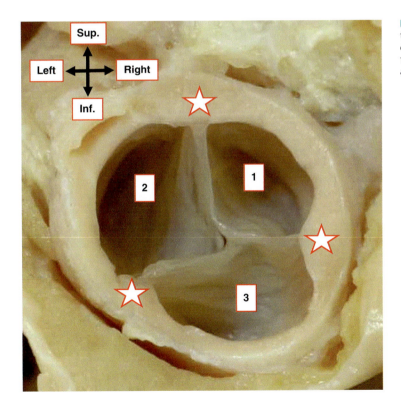

Figure 4.42 This image of the closed aortic valve from above shows the three valvar leaflets (1, 2, 3) coapting snugly, held together by the diastolic pressure of the column of blood they support. The stars mark the commissures, which are the peripheral attachments of the zones of apposition to the sinutubular junction.

complex structures. The sinuses themselves are arranged in clover-like fashion, permitting the valvar leaflets to close in the fashion of a Mercedes-Benz sign (Figure 4.42). It is the virtual basal ring, constructed by joining the nadirs of attachment of the valvar leaflets, that is taken as the point of measurement of the echocardiographic valvar annulus (Figure 4.46). This plane, therefore, does not correspond to any anatomical structure. Consensus amongst surgeons is now moving towards accepting it, nonetheless, as representing the valvar annulus.[3] In reality, it is no more than the diameter of the entrance to the arterial roots, although far from circular in either arterial root.

99

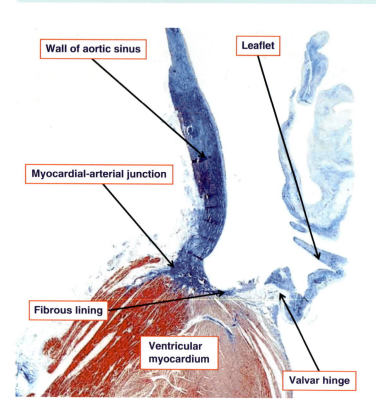

Figure 4.43 The histological section shows the fibrous core of one leaflet of the aortic valves, with its endothelial linings on the arterial and ventricular aspects. Note that the valvar hinge is well below the myocardial–arterial junction. There is a fibrous layer on the myocardium incorporated into the base of the valvar sinus.

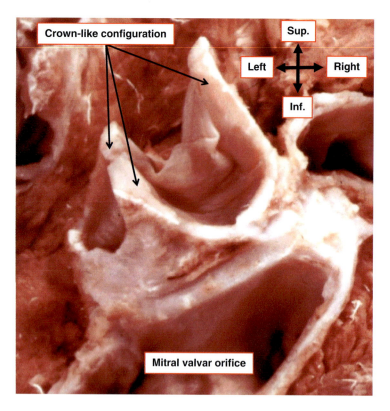

Figure 4.44 The aortic root in this specimen has been dissected by removing the valvar sinuses, leaving behind the semilunar attachments of the leaflets. It shows how the overall arrangement is crown-like.

The Aortic Valve

The semilunar leaflets of the aortic valve are attached in part to the area of fibrous continuity with the aortic leaflet of the mitral valve, and in part to the crest of the muscular ventricular septum (Figure 4.47). When naming the leaflets of the valve, advantage can be taken of the fact that, almost without exception, the major coronary arteries take origin from two of the aortic sinuses, but not the third. Thus, the aortic leaflets can accurately be described as being right coronary, left coronary, and non-coronary (Figure 4.48). Since the so-called non-coronary sinus can, rarely, give rise to one of the coronary arteries, it can more accurately be described as the

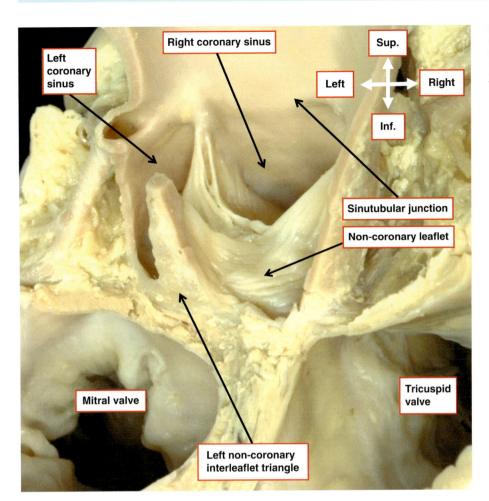

Figure 4.45 The dissection of the crown-like configuration of the aortic root shows the level of apposition of the leaflets in their closed position, which is well below the level of the sinutubular junction.

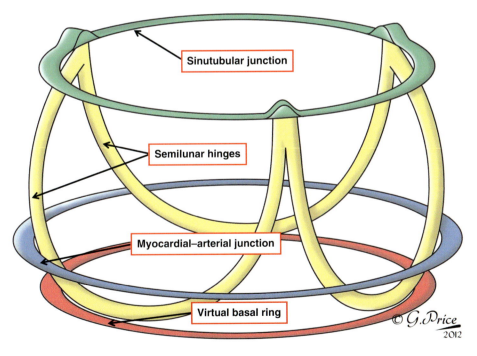

Figure 4.46 The cartoon shows the relationship of the semilunar hinges of the aortic valvar leaflets (yellow) relative to the rings to be found within the pulmonary root. The superiorly located green ring is the sinutubular junction. The blue ring shows the myocardial–arterial junction, while the red ring is the virtual basal plane, formed by joining together the nadirs of attachment of the valvar hinges.

non-adjacent sinus, referring to its position relative to the pulmonary root. It is the right and left coronary aortic leaflets that have a predominantly myocardial origin, with the supporting myocardium being incorporated within the aortic sinuses (Figure 4.49). These are the leaflets that are adjacent to the pulmonary trunk. Their more distal adjacent parts take origin from the free aortic wall. The small interleaflet fibrous triangle between them separates the cavity of the outflow tract

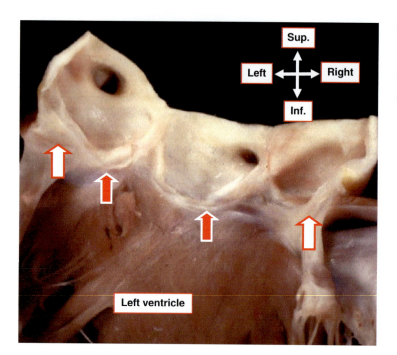

Figure 4.47 The aortic root has been displayed by removing the leaflets of the aortic valve, having opened the outflow tract between the left coronary and the non-adjacent aortic leaflets. The two sinuses giving rise to the coronary arteries have septal musculature at their base (red arrows with white borders), while part of the left coronary sinus, along with the non-coronary sinus, are supported by fibrous continuity with the aortic leaflet of the mitral valve (white arrows with red borders).

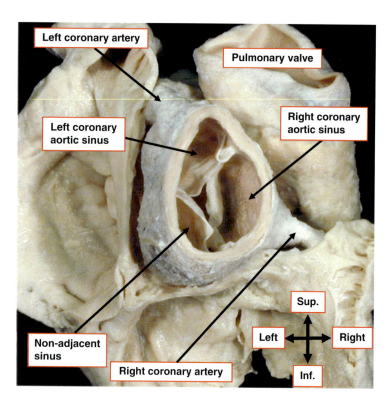

Figure 4.48 The heart has been photographed from above, the tubular aorta having been removed to reveal the valvar sinuses. The origins of the coronary arteries permit two sinuses to be named as right and left coronary aortic sinuses. The third sinus is non-adjacent relative to the pulmonary trunk. In almost all instances, it does not give rise to a coronary artery. In those circumstances, it can also be called the non-coronary sinus.

from the tissue plane between the aortic root and the subpulmonary infundibulum (Figure 4.16).

As the semilunar attachment of the right coronary leaflet is traced from its zone of apposition with the left coronary leaflet, it drops towards the crest of the muscular part of the septum in the area of the membranous septum. It then rises again to the apex of the zone of apposition with the non-adjacent leaflet (Figure 4.50). The attachment of this posterior part of the right coronary leaflet is an integral part of the fibrous skeleton. All of the non-adjacent leaflet has a fibrous origin, with the fibrous support again being part of the so-called skeleton. Half of it, extending from the zone of apposition with the right coronary leaflet, is attached to the area of the membranous septum (Figure 4.50). The triangle between these leaflets has important relationships to both right atrium and right ventricle (Figure 4.13). The extensive infero-septal recess, the continuation inferiorly of the left ventricular outflow tract, lies beneath the non-adjacent leaflet, limited anterolaterally by the atrioventricular component of the membranous septum. Usually reaching its nadir in the region of the right fibrous trigone, the

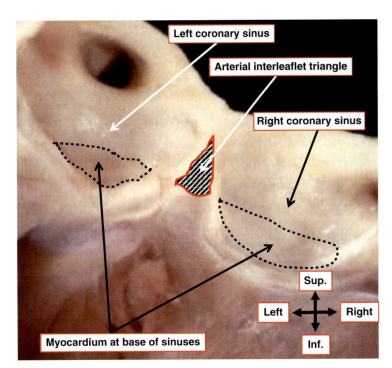

Figure 4.49 The image is an enlargement of the heart shown in Figure 4.47. It shows how the sinuses giving rise to the coronary arteries are supported by the musculature of the ventricular septum, with myocardium incorporated at the bases of both sinuses (dotted black areas). The cross-hatched red-bordered triangle shows the area of aortic wall that forms the distal extent of the outflow tract between the coronary aortic leaflets, running to the level of the sinutubular junction.

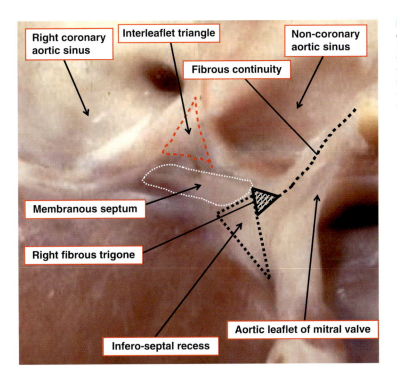

Figure 4.50 The photograph shows a close-up of the base of the zone of apposition between the right coronary and non-coronary aortic leaflets. The interleaflet red-dotted triangle is continuous at its base with the membranous septum (white dots), which in turn is continuous with the roof of the infero-septal recess (black-dotted triangle) and the right fibrous trigone (cross-hatched triangle). The black dashed line shows the area of continuity between the leaflets of the aortic and mitral valves.

non-adjacent leaflet then rises to the apex of its zone of apposition with the left coronary leaflet. The adjacent parts of both leaflets in this area are attached to the free aortic wall distally. Proximally, they are continuous with the aortic leaflet of the mitral valve. In this way, they form the aortic–mitral curtain. This separates the left ventricular outflow tract not from the left atrium, but from the transverse sinus of the pericardium (Figure 4.51). Beyond this area, the left coronary leaflet then adjoins a short segment of parietal myocardium before extending anteriorly to reach the zone of apposition with the right coronary leaflet. The precise attachments of the aortic leaflets vary from heart to heart.[26] This is particularly the case with regard to that portion of the zone of apposition between the non-coronary and left coronary leaflets, which is related to the aortic–mitral curtain. The length of the subaortic fibrous curtain also varies from heart to heart. In a very small percentage of normal hearts, the aortic valve in this area can be supported by a complete muscular infundibulum or sleeve.[27] These individual variations do not distort the basic anatomical relationships as described above.

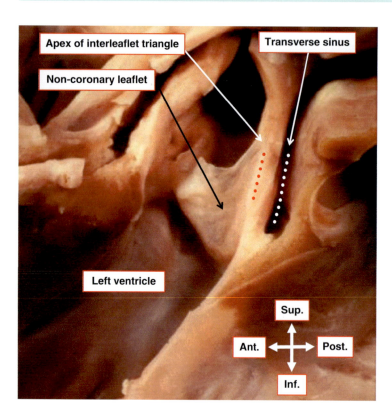

Figure 4.51 The left ventricular outflow tract in this heart is bisected through the fibrous triangle between the non-adjacent and left coronary aortic leaflets. The fibrous wall (red dotted line) separates the outflow tract from the transverse sinus (white dotted line).

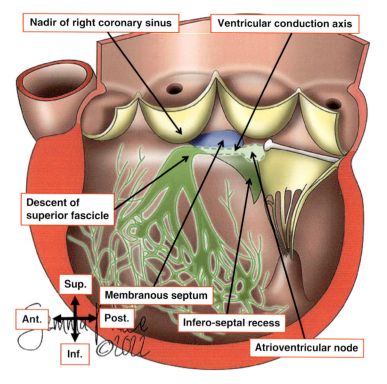

Figure 4.52 The drawing shows the location of the atrioventricular conduction axis relative to the components of the left ventricle.

Appreciation of the anatomy of the valvar hinges brings into focus the important surgical danger areas related to the aortic valve. The ascending part of the non-coronary aortic leaflet is positioned directly above the part of the atrial wall containing the atrioventricular node, while the zone of apposition with the right coronary aortic leaflet is above the penetrating atrioventricular bundle and the membranous septum (Figures 4.52, 4.53). The zone of apposition between the right coronary and left coronary leaflets is usually positioned opposite the corresponding zone of apposition between the facing leaflets of the pulmonary valve. The adjacent parts of the two aortic coronary leaflets, therefore, are directly related to the infundibulum of the right ventricle, albeit that a discrete extracavitary tissue plane interposes between them. Incisions through the right ventricular

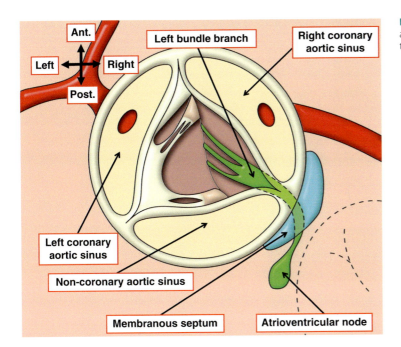

Figure 4.53 The drawing shows the relationships of the atrioventricular node and penetrating bundle as they would be seen by the surgeon working through the aortic valve.

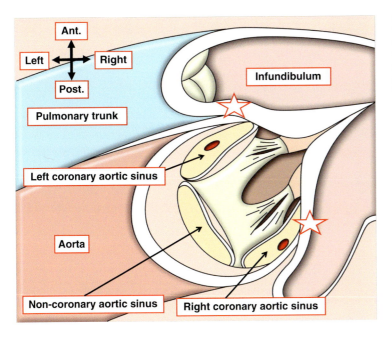

Figure 4.54 The drawing shows how, in the Konno procedure, an incision through the posterior wall of the subpulmonary infundibulum takes the surgeon into the subaortic outflow tract, the incision in the infundibular wall being carried into the muscular ventricular septum, and entering the left ventricular outflow tract between the two aortic sinuses giving origin to the coronary arteries. The two stars show how the wall has been folded open.

outflow tract at this site lead directly into the subaortic region (Figure 4.54). This is the basis of the right ventricular approach for relief of subaortic obstruction, as in the Konno, or modified Konno, procedure. Beyond this point, the lateral part of the left coronary leaflet is the only part of the aortic valve that is not intimately related to another cardiac chamber. This is the part of the valve that takes origin from the lateral margin of the inner heart curvature. It is in relationship externally with the free pericardial space.

The Pulmonary Valve

The pulmonary valve in the normal heart has exclusively muscular attachments to the infundibulum of the right ventricle (Figure 4.55). Because of its oblique position, there is difficulty in naming the pulmonary leaflets according to the body coordinates. It is better to describe them according to their relationship to the aortic valve, reflecting the location of their component parts as seen during development (Figure 4.56). The two leaflets of the aortic valve that are attached to the septum are always adjacent to two leaflets of the pulmonary valve. These two leaflets of the pulmonary valve, therefore, can simply be called the right and left adjacent leaflets. The third leaflet is then described appropriately as the non-adjacent leaflet. When assessed from the stance of the observer positioned within the non-adjacent sinus, the two adjacent sinuses are to his or her right and left hands.[28] The right-handed leaflet as seen from the pulmonary trunk, however, is positioned leftward and posteriorly in space, while the left-handed leaflet

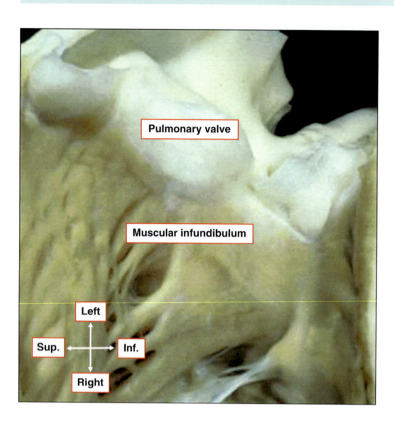

Figure 4.55 This heart, shown in anatomical orientation, is opened along the parietal wall of the right ventricle. It shows how all leaflets of the pulmonary valve are supported by infundibular musculature.

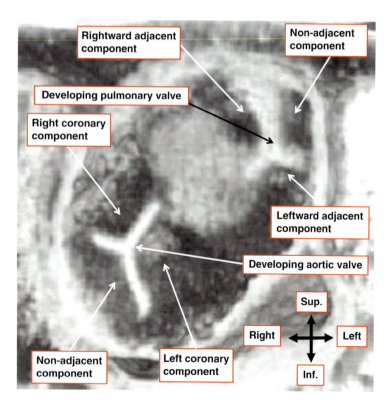

Figure 4.56 The image shows the components of the developing aortic and pulmonary roots as seen in the human heart at Carnegie stage 15, which is at the end of the fifth week of development. As we explained in Chapter 2, the cushions will excavate so as to give rise to the valvar leaflets and their supporting sinuses. The components retain their relationships, so that two of the sinuses of the pulmonary valve are always adjacent to the sinuses of the aortic valve that, eventually, will give rise to the coronary arteries. The other sinus is non-adjacent. This provides a logical means of describing the valvar sinuses and leaflets, as shown by the labels to this figure.

is adjacent to the right coronary artery. Our preference, therefore, is to account for their anatomical location. The zone of apposition between the two adjacent leaflets has traditionally been considered to be attached to the muscular outlet septum immediately above the anterior limb of the septomarginal trabeculation. In reality, it is attached to the free-standing sleeve of infundibular musculature (Figures 4.57, 4.58). As the right adjacent leaflet drops down from the apex of its zone of apposition with the other adjacent leaflet, it is supported by the inner heart curve, which separates it from the tricuspid valve. This muscular mass is the supraventricular crest of the right ventricle. The particular part separating the

4 Surgical Anatomy of the Valves of the Heart

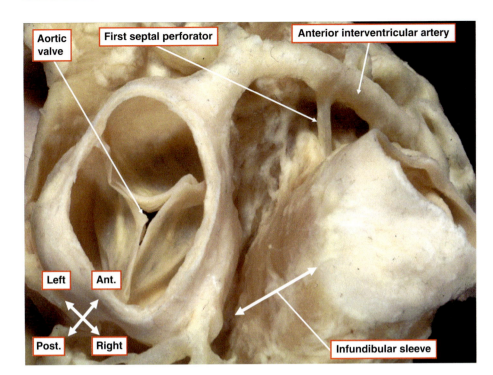

Figure 4.57 The pulmonary trunk has been tilted forward in this heart, showing the sleeve of infundibular musculature that lifts the leaflets of the pulmonary valve away from the ventricular base. Note the origin of the first septal perforating artery.

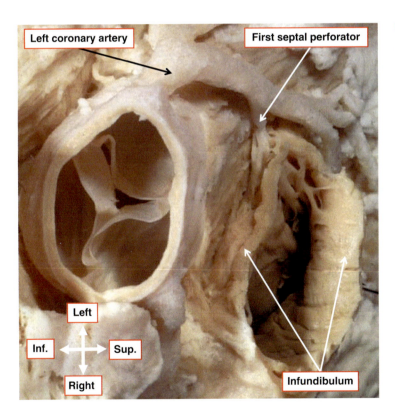

Figure 4.58 The subpulmonary infundibulum has now been removed completely from the heart shown in Figure 4.57, revealing how this can be achieved without transgressing on the left ventricle. Note again the location of the first septal perforating artery.

hinges of the atrioventricular and arterial valves is the ventriculo-infundibular fold. The zone of apposition between the right and non-adjacent leaflets is then towards the parietal extent of this fold, with the non-adjacent leaflet being supported by the anterior parietal wall of the infundibulum. The zone of apposition between the non-adjacent and left adjacent leaflets extends from the parietal attachment back towards the septum. The left adjacent leaflet, therefore, runs from the parietal wall to the area of the septum. When considered as a whole, the valve can be liberated from the right ventricle, together with its infundibular sleeve (Figure 4.57). This can be achieved without damaging any vital structures, although the left adjacent leaflet is commonly closely related to the first septal perforating artery (Figure 4.58). Preservation of this artery is one of the features that underscores the success of the Ross procedure.[29]

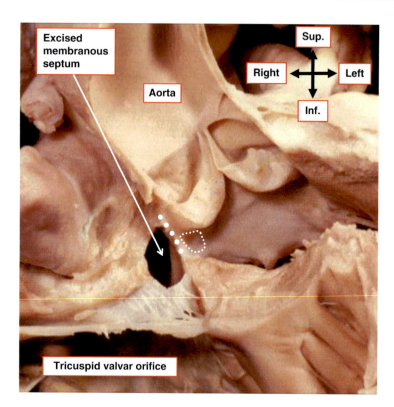

Figure 4.59 This dissection is through the membranous septum (large dotted line). The atrioventricular conduction axis penetrates through this septum to reach the crest of the muscular ventricular septum. As can be seen, the point of penetration is directly adjacent to the right end of the area of continuity between the tricuspid and mitral valves, which form the roof of the infero-septal recess of the subaortic outflow tract (dotted area).

Relationships of the Valves to Other Vital Cardiac Structures

Positioned as they are within the ventricular base, the tricuspid, mitral, and aortic valves are intimately related to two vital cardiac subsystems, namely the atrioventricular conduction system and the coronary circulation. It is mandatory to avoid damage to these structures during surgery. It is important, therefore, to know their precise locations. This must be learned relative to landmarks within the valves themselves, since the conduction tissues are largely invisible, while the course of the coronary vessels is likely to be hidden as the surgeon approaches the valves. Although we have mentioned these landmarks when discussing the individual valves, their importance is such that they justify a collective review.

The Specialized Muscular Axis for Atrioventricular Conduction

In the normal heart, the penetrating atrioventricular bundle is the only muscular communication between the atrial and ventricular muscle masses. The bundle penetrates through the membranous septal component of the central fibrous body at its junction with the fibrous roof of the infero-septal recess. It is intimately related to the leaflets of the mitral, tricuspid, and aortic valves. The axis takes its origin from the atrioventricular node and its atrial zones of transitional cells. These atrial components of the conduction axis are contained exclusively within the triangle of Koch. The inferior extent of the triangle is the junctional attachment of the septal leaflet of the tricuspid valve. As the axis penetrates the septum, it immediately enters the subaortic region of the left ventricle (Figure 4.59). The point of penetration is related to the antero-inferior end of the zone of apposition between the leaflets of the mitral valve. In this area, the atrioventricular node lies within five to ten millimetres of the atrial attachment of the medial part of the mural leaflet. Having reached the left ventricular outflow tract, the conduction axis begins to branch, either on the crest of the muscular ventricular septum, sandwiched between it and the interventricular membranous septum (Figure 4.52), or on the left ventricular aspect of the septum. This area is immediately beneath the zone of apposition between the non-adjacent and right coronary leaflets of the aortic valve (Figure 4.53). The height of the interleaflet fibrous triangle serves to separate the valvar attachments from the conduction axis. When seen from the left ventricle, the left bundle branch fans out as a continuous sheet on the smooth left septal surface beneath the zone of apposition, splitting into its three divisions as it descends the ventricular septum. The nadir of the right coronary leaflet is the closest part of the aortic valvar complex to the conduction axis (Figure 4.52). The right bundle branch takes origin from the axis beyond the take-off of the left bundle branches. It courses back across the septum as a thin, insulated cord, which emerges on the right ventricular aspect in the area of the medial papillary muscle. It then runs, usually intramyocardially, within the structure of the septomarginal trabeculation, to ramify at the ventricular apex. When considered from the right side, the site of the branching segment of the conduction axis can be imagined as a line joining the apex of the triangle of Koch to the medial papillary muscle (Figure 4.60). Care must be taken when placing sutures in this area, since the overall axis is within five millimetres of the right ventricular septal surface.

4 Surgical Anatomy of the Valves of the Heart

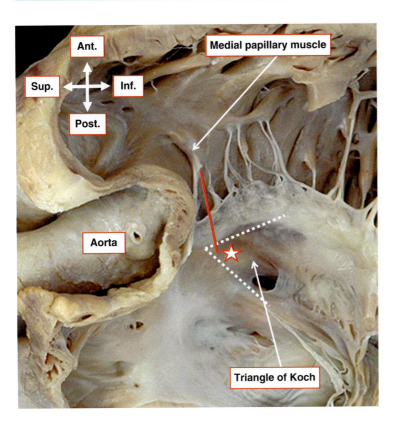

Figure 4.60 The heart is shown in surgical orientation, the parietal walls of the right atrium and ventricle having been removed. The red line shows the course of the atrioventricular conduction axis as it penetrates from the atrioventricular node (star) to reach the left ventricular outflow tract. The right bundle branch then re-emerges on the right side beneath the medial papillary muscle. The white dashed lines show two of the boundaries of the triangle of Koch.

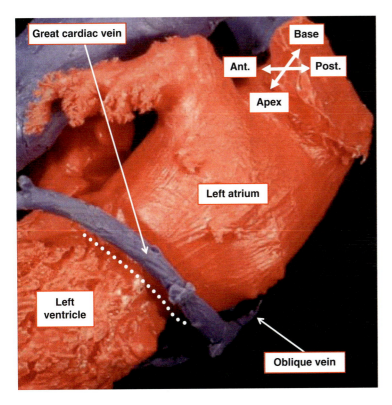

Figure 4.61 This cast shows the location of the great cardiac vein in the left atrioventricular groove (white dotted line). The vein does not become the coronary sinus until it receives the oblique vein of the left atrium.

The Vulnerable Coronary Circulation

On the venous side of the circulation, the coronary sinus is the only noteworthy structure related to the valves. The great cardiac vein runs within the left atrioventricular groove, receiving the oblique vein as it turns into the inferior part of the groove (Figures 4.61, 4.62). This confluence marks the beginning of the coronary sinus, which proceeds in the fatty tissue of the inferior atrioventricular groove to empty into the right atrium (Figure 4.63). In its course in an adult, it may approach to within five to fifteen millimetres of the medial attachment of the mural leaflet of the mitral valve. Deeply

109

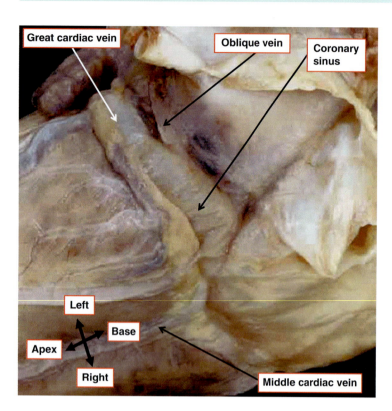

Figure 4.62 The heart has been removed from the body, and the diaphragmatic surface is photographed to show the course of the coronary sinus within the inferior left atrioventricular groove. The great cardiac vein becomes the cardiac sinus at the point where it receives the oblique vein of the left atrium.

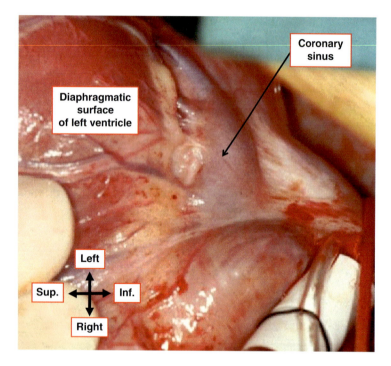

Figure 4.63 This operative view, taken through a median sternotomy, with the surgeon having reflected the heart, shows the position of the coronary sinus in the inferior atrioventricular groove. The sinus then opens to the right atrium. The cannula is in the inferior caval vein.

placed sutures in this area during replacement of the mitral valve may lead to damage to the coronary sinus. This can cause extremely troublesome bleeding. Also, when removing a previously placed mitral valvar prosthesis, care must be taken not to enter the sinus with scalpel or suture. The normal anatomy may well have been distorted by the earlier operation.

The coronary arteries are intimately related to both the mitral and tricuspid valves, since much of their course follows the atrioventricular grooves, albeit that the fibro-adipose tissue within the grooves can separate them from the epicardial surface. The main stem of the left coronary artery branches in the angle of the margin of the left-sided ventriculo-infundibular fold immediately above the left fibrous trigone. The anterior interventricular artery moves away from the valves, although its septal perforating branches commonly extend into the septum immediately beneath the left-facing leaflet of the pulmonary valve. This important artery could be damaged by extensive dissection in this area. It is the

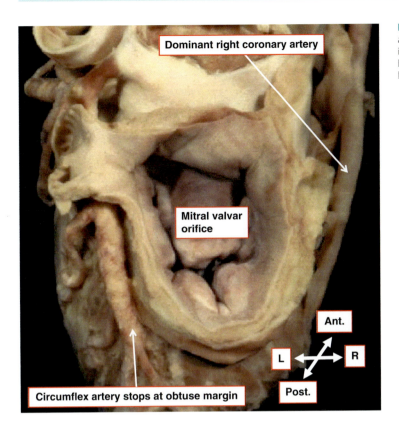

Figure 4.64 The heart in this image, also shown in Figure 4.41, has a dominant right coronary artery, which gives rise to the inferior interventricular artery, and the artery to the atrioventricular node. As can be seen, the circumflex artery is only marginally related to the mural leaflet of the mitral valve in this setting.

circumflex branch of the left coronary artery that is most intimately related to the mitral valve, particularly when the left coronary artery is dominant. When the right coronary artery is dominant, giving rise to the inferior interventricular artery as it does in about 90 per cent of cases, the circumflex artery is related only to the area around the lateral scallop of the mural leaflet of the mitral valve (Figure 4.64). When the circumflex branch becomes the inferior interventricular artery, its entire course is intimately related to the entirety of the mural leaflet (Figure 4.33).

The right coronary artery always runs a circumferential course around the mural attachments of the tricuspid valve. The initial course of the artery is through the right atrioventricular groove (Figure 4.41), where it lies on the epicardial aspect of the ventriculo-infundibular fold. It can be damaged by deeply placed sutures in this area.[30] The artery then encircles the attachment of the mural leaflet of the tricuspid valve before, in the majority of cases, turning to become the inferior interventricular artery. Just prior to its descent, the right coronary artery, when dominant, takes a prominent U-loop beneath the floor of the coronary sinus, giving off the artery to the atrioventricular node at the apex of the loop. In cases where the circumflex artery gives rise to the inferior interventricular artery, then the atrioventricular nodal artery originates from the circumflex artery (Figure 4.33). Whether arising from a dominant left or right coronary artery, this small but important vessel courses within the inferior pyramidal space towards its apex, and is related to the inferior aspect of the annular attachment of the septal leaflet of the tricuspid valve.

References Cited

1. Perloff JK, Roberts WC. The mitral apparatus. Functional anatomy of mitral regurgitation. *Circulation* 1972; **46**: 227–239.
2. Frater RWM, Anderson RH. How can we logically describe the components of the arterial valves? *J Heart Valve Dis* 2010; **19**: 438–440.
3. Sievers HH, Hemmer G, Beyersdorf F, et al. The everyday used nomenclature of the aortic root components: the Tower of Babel? *Eur J Cardiothoracic Surg* 2012; **41**: 478–482.
4. Anderson RH, Spicer DE, Quintessenza JA, Najm HK, Tretter JT. Words and how we use them – which is to be the master? *J Card Surg* 2022; **37**: 2481–2485.
5. Anderson RH. Demolishing the Tower of Babel. *Eur J Cardiothoracic Surg* 2012; **41**: 483–484.
6. Anderson RH, Garbi M, Zugwitz D, et al. Anatomy of the mitral valve relative to controversies concerning the so-called annular disjunction. *Heart* 2023; **109**: 734–739.
7. Sutton JPIII, Ho SY, Anderson RH. The forgotten interleaflet triangles: A review of the surgical anatomy of the aortic valve. *Ann Thor Surg* 1995; **59**: 419–427.
8. Garbi M, Garweg C. Arrhythmia in mitral valve prolapse: all roads lead to Rome. *J Am Coll Cardiol* 2020; **76**: 650–652.
9. Angelini A, Ho SY, Anderson RH, Davies MJ, Becker AE. A histological study of the atrioventricular junction in hearts with normal and prolapsed leaflets of the mitral valve. *Br Heart J* 1988; **59**: 712–716.
10. McAlpine WA. *Heart and Coronary Arteries: An Anatomical Atlas for Clinical Diagnosis, Radiological*

Investigation, and Surgical Treatment. New York: Springer-Verlag; 1975: Chapter 2.

11. Toh H, Mori S, Izawa Y, et al. Prevalence and extent of mitral annular disjunction in structurally normal hearts: comprehensive three-dimensional analysis using cardiac computed tomography. *Eur Heart J Cardiovasc Imag* 2021; **22**: 614–622.

12. Zugwitz D, Fung K, Aung N, et al. Mitral annular disjunction assessed by cardiovascular magnetic resonance imaging: insights from UK Biobank Population Study. *J Am Coll Cardiol Card Img* 2022; **15**: 1856–1866.

13. Victor S, Nayak VM. The tricuspid valve is bicuspid. *J Heart Valve Dis* 1994; **3**: 27–36.

14. Hołda MK, Zhingre Sanchez JD, Bateman MG, Iaizzo PA. Right atrioventricular valve leaflet morphology redefined: implications for transcatheter repair procedures. *JACC Cardiovasc Interv* 2019; **12**: 169–178.

15. Sutton JP III, Ho Sy, Vogel M, Anderson RH. Is the morphologically right atrioventricular valve tricuspid? *J Heart Valve Dis* 1995; **4**: 571–575.

16. Tretter JT, Sarwark AS, Anderson RH, Spicer DE. Assessment of the anatomical variation to be found in the normal tricuspid valve. *Clin Anat* 2016; **29**: 399–407

17. Yacoub M. Anatomy of the mitral valve chordae and cusps. In D Kalmason, ed., *The Mitral Valve. A Pluridisciplinary Approach.* London: Edward Arnold; 1976: pp. 15–20.

18. Kumar N, Kumar M, Duran CM. A revised terminology for recording surgical findings of the mitral valve. *J Heart Valve Dis* 1995; **4**: 76–77.

19. Frater R. Anatomy and physiology of the normal mitral valve. (Discussion) In D Kalmanson, ed., *The Mitral Valve.* London: Edward Arnold; 1976: p. 41.

20. Lam JHC, Ranganathan N, Wigle ED, Silver MD. Morphology of the human mitral valve. I. Chordae tendineae: a new classification. *Circulation* 1970; **41**: 449–458.

21. Becker AE, de Wit APM. Mitral valve apparatus. A spectrum of normality relevant to mitral valve prolapse. *Br Heart J* 1979; **42**: 680–689.

22. Van der Bel-Kahn J, Duren DR, Becker AE. Isolated mitral valve prolapse: chordal architecture as an anatomic basis in older patients. *J Am Coll Cardiol* 1985; **5**: 1335–1340.

23. Roberts WC. The 2 most common congenital heart diseases. (Editorial) *Am J Cardiol* 1984; **53**: 1198.

24. Carpentier A, Branchini B, Cour JC, et al. Congenital malformations of the mitral valve in children. Pathology and surgical treatment. *J Thorac Cardiovasc Surg* 1976; **72**: 854–866.

25. Victor S, Nayak VM. Definition and function of commissures, slits and scallops of the mitral valve: analysis in 100 hearts. *AustralAs J Cardiac Thorac Surg* 1994; **3**: 8–16.

26. Amofa D, Mori S, Toh H, et al. The rotational position of the aortic root related to its underlying ventricular support. *Clin Anat* 2019; **32**: 1107–1117.

27. Rosenquist GC, Clark EB, Sweeny LJ, McAllister HA. The normal spectrum of mitral and aortic valve discontinuity. *Circulation* 1976; **54**: 298–301.

28. Dodge-Khatami A, Mavroudis C, Backer CL. Congenital heart surgery nomenclature and database project: anomalies of the coronary arteries. *Ann Thorac Surg* 2000; **69**: S270–279.

29. Merrick AF, Yacoub MH, Ho SY, Anderson RH. Anatomy of the muscular subpulmonary infundibulum with regard to the Ross procedure. *Ann Thorac Surg* 2000; **69**: 556–561.

30. McFadden PM, Culpepper WS III, Ochsner JL. Iatrogenic right ventricular failure in tetralogy of Fallot repairs: reappraisal of a distressing problem. *Ann Thorac Surg* 1982; **33**: 400–402.

Chapter 5

Surgical Anatomy of the Coronary Circulation

The coronary circulation consists of the coronary arteries and veins, together with the lymphatics of the heart. Since the lymphatics, apart from the thoracic duct, are of very limited significance to operative anatomy, they will not be discussed at any length in this chapter. The veins, relatively speaking, are similarly of less interest. In this chapter, therefore, we concentrate on those anatomical aspects of arterial distribution that are pertinent to the surgeon, limiting ourselves to brief discussions of the cardiac venous drainage and the cardiac lymphatics.

The Coronary Arteries

The coronary arteries are the first branches of the ascending portion of the aorta. They take their origin from the sinuses within the aortic root, immediately above its attachment to the heart (Figure 5.1). There are three sinuses within the aortic root, but only two coronary arteries. The sinuses can be named, therefore, according to whether or not they give rise to an artery, the normal arrangement being a right coronary, left coronary, and non-coronary aortic sinus (Figure 5.2). When described in this fashion, the terms 'right' and 'left' refer to the aortic sinuses giving rise to the right and left coronary arteries, rather than to the position of the sinuses relative to the right–left coordinates of the body (Figure 5.3). It is also the case that, increasingly, examples are found of an artery arising from the sinus most distant from the pulmonary root. In these circumstances, of course, the sinus itself cannot be described as being 'non-coronary'. It is best then described as being non-adjacent, or non-facing. In the circumstance of origin of an artery from the non-adjacent sinus, it is similarly best to describe the artery involved, taking note of its course relative to the vascular pedicle.

In the normal heart, the aortic root is obliquely situated, while, in malformed hearts, the root is frequently abnormally positioned. Whatever the position of the aortic root, however, almost always the two coronary arteries, when two are present, take origin from those aortic sinuses that are adjacent to the sinuses of the pulmonary trunk. Because of this, it is more convenient, and more accurate, to consider these sinuses as being to the left hand and the right hand of the observer standing, figuratively speaking, within the non-adjacent sinus

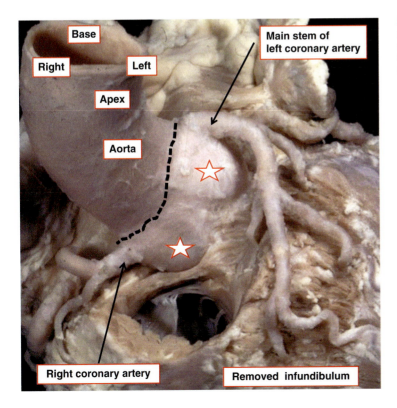

Figure 5.1 The heart has been dissected by removing the subpulmonary infundibulum. It is photographed in anatomical orientation to show the origin of the coronary arteries from the sinuses of the aortic root that lie adjacent to the pulmonary root (stars). The dashed line shows the sinutubular junction.

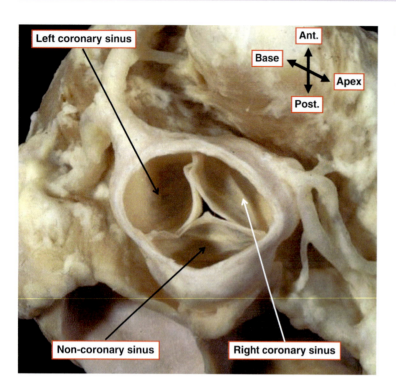

Figure 5.2 The heart is photographed from above in anatomical orientation after removal of the atrial myocardium and the arterial trunks. Two sinuses of the aortic valve give rise to coronary arteries, permitting them to be named as the right and left aortic coronary sinuses. The other sinus is usually described as the non-coronary sinus. Very rarely, it can give rise to a coronary artery. In such circumstances, it is best described as the non-adjacent, or non-facing, sinus.

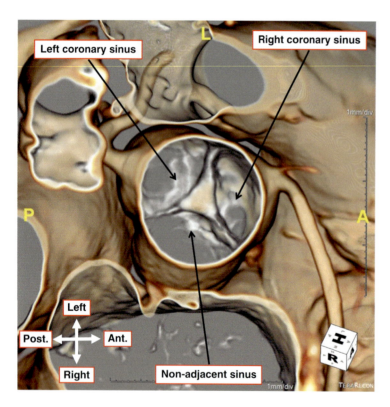

Figure 5.3 The software providing computed tomographic images also produces markers that show the orientation of the demonstrated structures relative to the anatomical position. These markers show that the so-called right and left aortic sinuses are not strictly right-sided and left-sided. The orientation cube in the lower right-hand corner shows the attitudinal coordinates, with 'H' representing 'head', or superior, and 'R' right.

and looking towards the pulmonary trunk (Figure 5.4). This approach to distinguishing the aortic sinuses that give rise to the coronary arteries, introduced by the group from Leiden,[1] holds true irrespective of the relationships of the arterial trunks. It has now become conventional to describe the right-hand sinus as '#1', and to distinguish the left-hand sinus as '#2'. The convention becomes particularly valuable when considering coronary arterial origins in malformed hearts (see Chapter 9.2).

Irrespective of the specific sinus from which they arise, the coronary arteries usually take their origin within the appropriate valvar sinus, in other words proximal to the sinutubular junction (Figure 5.5). The junction is the discrete transition between the aortic root and the tubular component of the

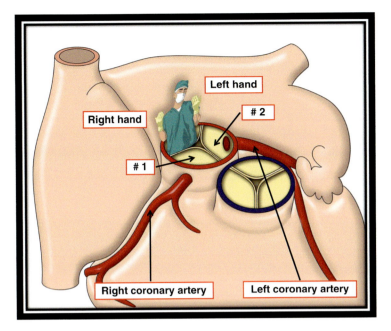

Figure 5.4 The cartoon demonstrates the basis of the so-called Leiden convention. The surgeon stands, figuratively speaking, in the non-adjacent sinus, and looks towards the pulmonary trunk. Of the sinuses adjacent to the pulmonary trunk, one is then to the left hand. This is sinus #2. The other sinus, to the right hand, is sinus #1. Almost without exception, the coronary arteries take origin from one, or both, of these sinuses. In the usual arrangement, the right coronary artery arises from sinus #1, and the main stem of the left coronary artery from sinus #2.

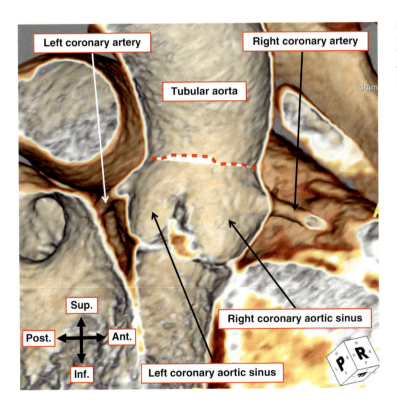

Figure 5.5 The computed tomogram shows the right and left aortic sinuses as viewed from behind. It shows the usual situation in which the coronary arteries arise within the sinuses, proximal to the sinutubular junction (red dashed line). The orientation cube again shows the attitudinal coordinates, this time with 'P' representing posterior, but 'R' still showing the surface that is to the right.

ascending aorta. It is the most obvious 'annular' structure within the aortic root. Deviations of origin of the coronary arteries relative to the junction are not uncommon.[2] The origins are considered abnormal, in adults, when arising more than one centimetre distal to the sinutubular junction, a feature said to occur in almost one-twentieth of normal hearts.[3] The arterial opening can also be deviated either towards the ventricle, so that the artery arises deep within the aortic sinus. It is more usual, nonetheless, for the origin to be deviated distally, so that it is outside the sinus (Figure 5.6). The displacement is of greater significance when combined with the artery taking an oblique course through the aortic wall and originating above or within an inappropriate aortic sinus. This arrangement, now known as anomalous aortic origin of a coronary artery,[4] is typically associated with the proximal part of the artery crossing the attachment of the zone of apposition between adjacent leaflets. It is the commonest variant of the intramural arrangement (Figure 5.7). Most usually, the right coronary artery arises from the left coronary aortic valvar sinus (Figures 5.7, 5.8), an arrangement said to occur in

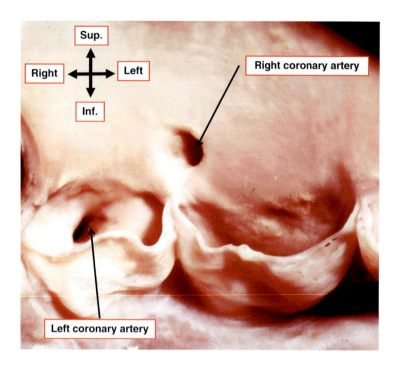

Figure 5.6 In this heart, the aortic valve has been opened and the aortic root photographed from behind to show the right and left aortic sinuses. The right coronary artery arises well above the sinutubular junction. Reproduced by kind permission of Professor Anton Becker, University of Amsterdam.

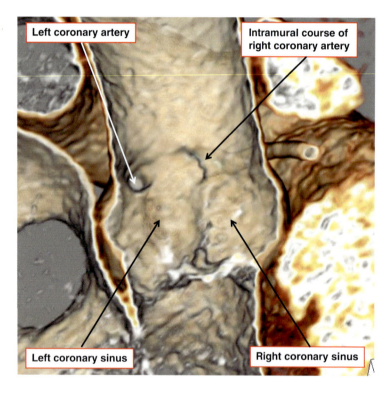

Figure 5.7 The computed tomogram, in the same orientation as Figure 5.5, shows an intramural course of the right coronary artery. The artery crosses the peripheral attachment of the zone of apposition between the valvar leaflets guarding the right and left aortic sinuses, and takes its origin, along with the left coronary artery, from the left aortic sinus (#2).

one of every 500 individuals.[5] Origin of the left coronary artery from the right coronary aortic sinus is much less frequent, found in only 0.03 per cent of cases.[5] Both variants introduce the potential for luminal narrowing, and may provoke disturbances in myocardial perfusion.[6]

The left coronary artery almost always takes origin from a single orifice within the left-hand-facing sinus. In contrast, in about half of all hearts, there are two orifices within the right coronary aortic sinus (Figure 5.9). In such instances, the orifices are unequal in size, the larger giving rise to the main trunk of the right coronary artery, while the considerably smaller second orifice usually gives rise to an infundibular artery, or rarely to the artery supplying the sinus node. In one large series,[7] two orifices were found in the right-hand-facing sinus in almost half the cases, three orifices in 7 per cent, and four orifices in 2 per cent. In contrast, multiple orifices in the left coronary aortic sinus (Figure 5.10) are considerably rarer.[7] If unrecognized, they may create problems in the

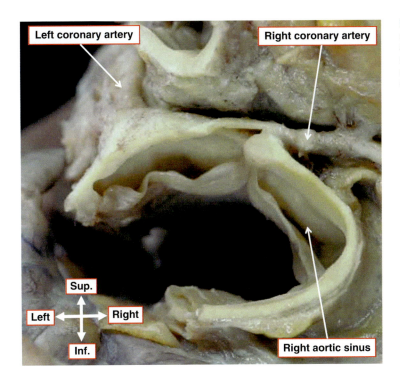

Figure 5.8 The tubular aorta has been removed at the level of the sinutubular junction to show anomalous origin of the right coronary artery from the left aortic valvar sinus, which also gives rise to the left coronary artery. Note that the right coronary artery crosses the points of attachment of the valvar leaflets to the sinutubular junction. This is the essence of the intramural arrangement.

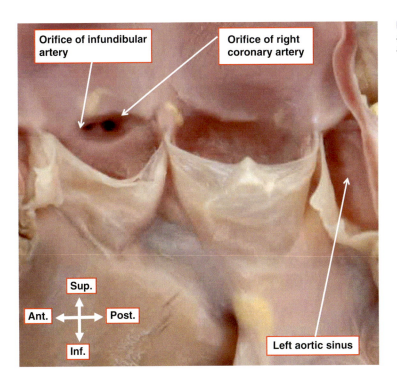

Figure 5.9 In this heart, separate orifices within the right coronary aortic sinus give rise to the right coronary artery and the infundibular artery.

interpretation of coronary angiograms. Presence of dual orifices in the same sinus, of course, is of far greater significance in the setting of anomalous aortic origin of a coronary artery, when one of the orifices gives rise to an artery taking an intraarterial and intramural course, as shown in Figures 5.7 and 5.8.

Although rare, all the coronary arteries, on occasion, can arise from a solitary orifice in the aortic root. This is usually within the right coronary aortic sinus. The artery originating from the solitary orifice can take one of two patterns. It can divide immediately into right and left coronary arteries. The left artery then passes either in front of the pulmonary trunk (Figure 5.11), between it and the aorta, or behind the arterial pedicle, before dividing into anterior interventricular and circumflex branches. The solitary artery can also arise from the left coronary aortic sinus, then branching such that the right coronary artery passes in front of the pulmonary trunk (Figure 5.12), runs between the arterial trunks, or extends

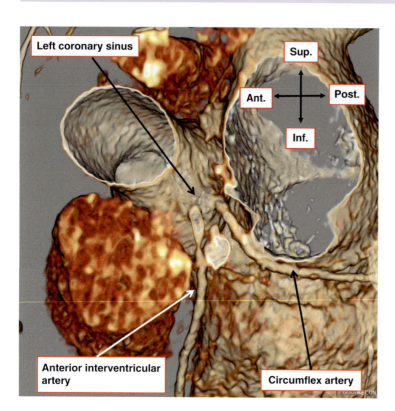

Figure 5.10 The computed tomogram shows separate origin of the interventricular and circumflex arteries from the left coronary aortic sinus.

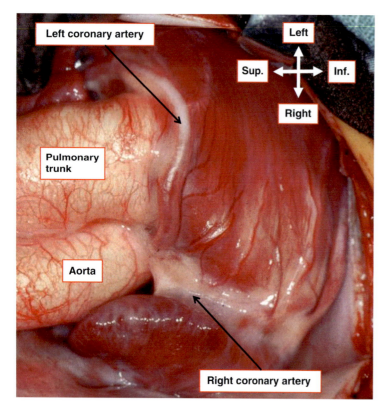

Figure 5.11 This operative view, seen through a median sternotomy, shows a solitary coronary artery taking origin from the right coronary aortic sinus. It divides immediately into right and left branches, with the main stem of the left coronary artery crossing the subpulmonary infundibulum. The left coronary artery then divides into the circumflex and anterior interventricular arteries.

behind the arterial pedicle, running through the transverse sinus. It is the variants involving a course between the great arterial trunks that are of most significance, since they can be harbingers of sudden cardiac death.[6,8] There are then subtle variations in the course taken by the artery as it passes between the trunks.[9] There are three possibilities (Figure 5.13). In the first, the artery runs between the aorta and the pulmonary trunk at the level of the aortic sinutubular junction, as shown in Figures 5.7 and 5.8. The second possibility is for the artery to extend deeply within the musculature

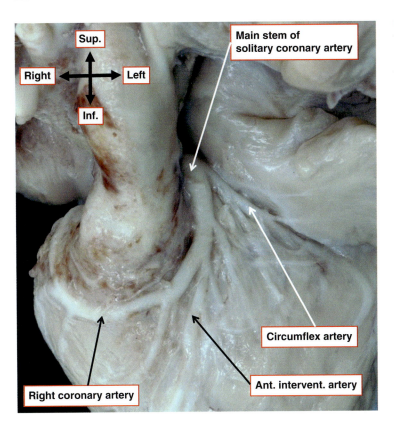

Figure 5.12 In this heart, there is a solitary coronary artery arising from the left aortic valvar sinus. It divides into circumflex and anterior interventricular (ant. intervent.) arteries, but also gives rise to the right coronary artery, which courses across the subpulmonary infundibulum to reach the right atrioventricular groove.

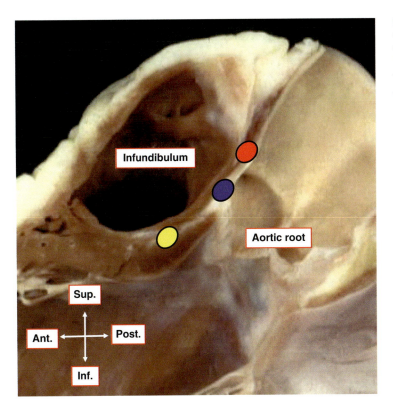

Figure 5.13 The long-axis section replicating the parasternal echocardiographic cut shows the tissue plane that exists between the aortic root and the subpulmonary infundibulum. Arteries can potentially run anomalously between the trunks at the level of the sintubular junction (red oval), within the tissue plane between the subpulmonary infundibulum and the aortic root (blue oval), or within the substance of the ventricular septum (yellow oval).

of the ventricular septum (Figure 5.14). The third possibility is for the artery to track within the tissue plane between the pulmonary infundibular sleeve and the aortic root (Figure 5.15). This course is below the level of the hinges of the pulmonary valvar leaflets, yet not buried within the muscular ventricle septum. The fact that the artery is not within the septum may not readily be appreciated when seen from the lateral aspect (Figure 5.16). It is intuitive to suggest that compression on the arterial lumen will be increased when the artery is buried within the musculature

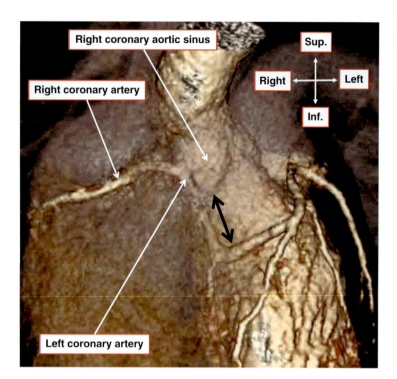

Figure 5.14 The computed tomogram shows the main stem of the left coronary artery arising from a solitary coronary artery, which itself arises from the right coronary aortic sinus. The left coronary artery extends deeply within the crest of the ventricular septum (double-headed arrow) before dividing into its anterior interventricular and circumflex branches.

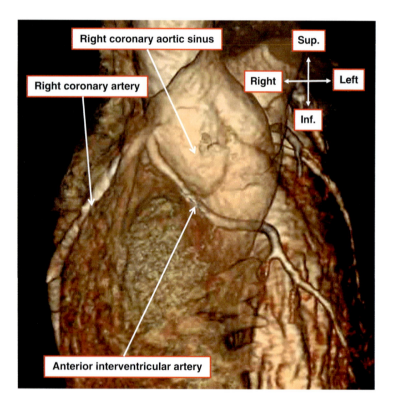

Figure 5.15 This reconstructed computed tomogram shows the anterior interventricular artery arising from the right coronary aortic sinus, and extending between the aortic root and the subpulmonary infundibulum. Unlike the situation shown in Figure 5.14, however, the artery does not burrow within the crest of the muscular septum, but runs in the tissue plane separating the aortic root from the free-standing infundibular musculature.

of the septum, but as yet there is no evidence to prove that passage through the septum adds to the risk. Indeed, it is possible that the passage through the septum is benign. Intramural course across the commissure at the level of the sinutubular junction, in contrast, is accepted as a significant risk factor. A still further alternative course for a solitary coronary artery, although less frequent, is when the single artery initially follows the path of the normal right coronary artery. It then continues beyond the crux, encircling the left atrioventricular junction through the territory usually supplied by the circumflex artery, before terminating as the anterior interventricular coronary artery.

5 Surgical Anatomy of the Coronary Circulation

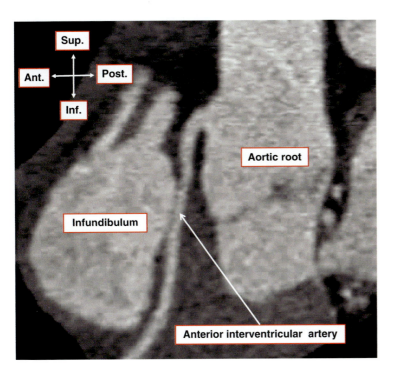

Figure 5.16 The computed tomogram shows the course of the anterior interventricular artery between the infundibulum and the aortic root previously shown in the reconstruction as Figure 5.15. It is difficult from the lateral projection to appreciate that the artery runs within the adipose tissue plane between the infundibulum and the aortic root, rather than within the musculature of the ventricular septum (see Figure 5.14).

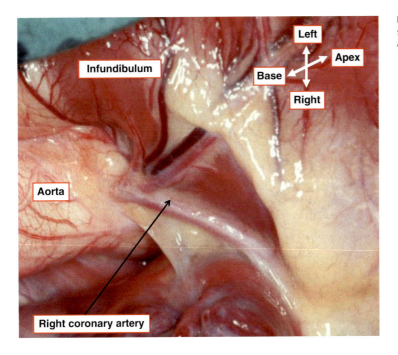

Figure 5.17 The operative view, seen through a median sternotomy, shows the right coronary artery as it emerges from its sinus into the right atrioventricular groove.

When the coronary arterial circulation is normal, the right and left coronary arteries, having taken their anticipated origin from the aortic root, extend subepicardially within the atrioventricular and interventricular grooves, with the left-sided artery giving rise to two major branches. The right coronary artery emerges from the right aortic sinus and immediately enters the right atrioventricular groove (Figure 5.17). It then encircles the tricuspid orifice, running in the right atrioventricular groove (Figure 5.18). In approximately nine-tenths of cases, the right coronary artery gives rise to an inferior interventricular artery at the crux, albeit that the artery is usually said to be posterior. Computed tomographic images now leave no doubt that the artery is inferior and interventricular (Figure 5.19). In a good proportion of these cases, the artery then continues beyond the crux, where it supplies down-going branches to the diaphragmatic surface of the left ventricle (Figure 5.20). This is right coronary arterial dominance. As the artery encircles the tricuspid orifice, it is most closely related to the origin of the leaflets of the tricuspid valve near the take-off of its acute marginal

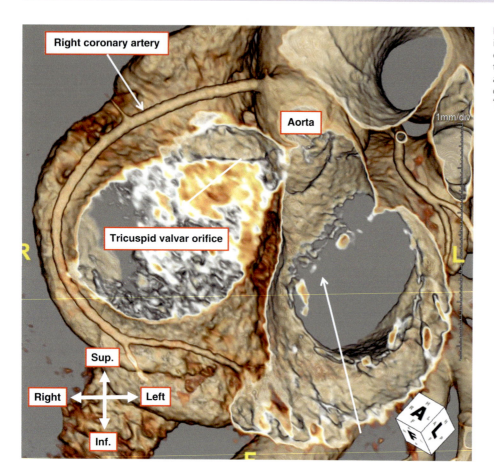

Figure 5.18 The computed tomographic image shows the right coronary artery, having emerged from its aortic valvar sinus, encircling the tricuspid valvar orifice. The orientation cube again shows the attitudinal coordinates. On this occasion, 'A' is showing the anterior surface, and 'L' the left surface.

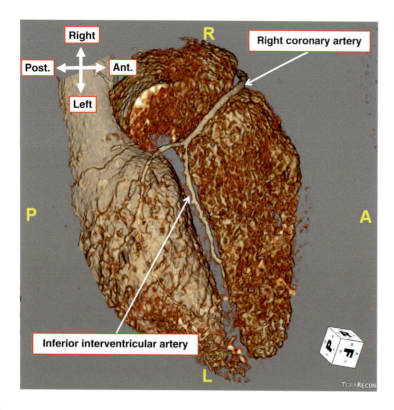

Figure 5.19 The computed tomographic image leaves no doubt that the artery supplying the diaphragmatic surface of the heart is inferior and interventricular (note the orientation marker in the lower right corner, with 'F' being the abbreviation for foot, but showing the inferior surface. The other abbreviations are 'P' for posterior, 'R' and 'L' for right and left, and 'A' for anterior).

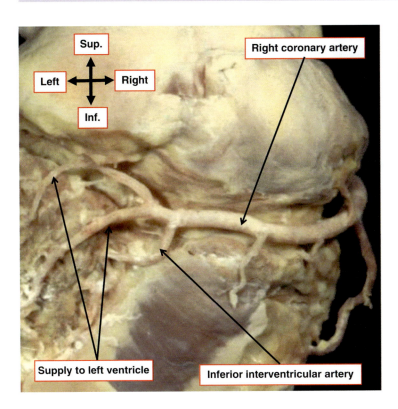

Figure 5.20 The diaphragmatic surface of the heart has been photographed from beneath, with the heart positioned on its apex. The right coronary artery, having supplied the inferior interventricular artery, continues to give branches to the diaphragmatic surface of the left ventricle. This is right coronary arterial dominance.

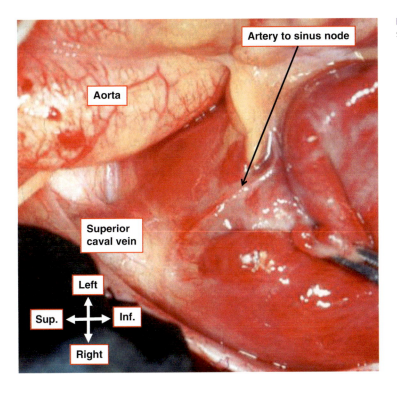

Figure 5.21 This operative view, taken through a median sternotomy, shows the artery to the sinus node arising from the right coronary artery.

branch. Other important branches also take origin from this encircling segment of the artery. Immediately after its origin, the artery lies within the rightward extent of the transverse sinus, with the adjacent muscular wall representing the ventriculo-infundibular fold of the supraventricular crest. In this course, the right coronary artery gives rise to down-going infundibular branches, which may also arise by separate orifices within the right aortic sinus. In just over half the cases, the right coronary artery gives rise to the artery supplying the sinus node (Figure 5.21). This artery typically arises from the proximal part of the right coronary artery, but on occasion the nodal artery can arise more distally, coursing over the

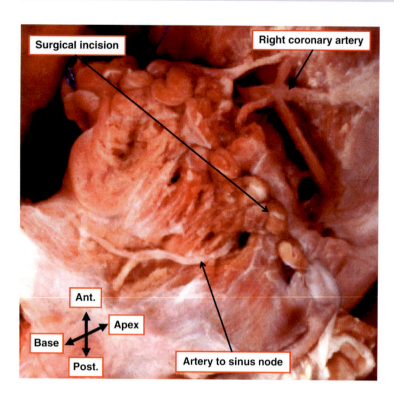

Figure 5.22 In this specimen, photographed to replicate the view seen by the surgeon working through a median sternotomy, the artery to the sinus node takes a lateral origin from the right coronary artery. It then courses over the lateral margin of the right atrial appendage to reach the terminal groove. It has been divided by the standard atriotomy.

lateral margin of the appendage to reach the terminal groove. If unnoticed, this finding is of major surgical significance (Figure 5.22).[10] As we showed in Chapter 3, however, once the surgeon is aware of the possibility, it is an easy matter to recognize the anomalous course across the right atrial appendage (see Figure 3.22).

The left coronary artery has a short confluent stem, usually called the left main artery by the surgeon. It emerges from the left coronary aortic sinus, and enters the left margin of the transverse sinus, being positioned behind the pulmonary trunk and beneath the left atrial appendage. It is a very short structure, rarely extending beyond one centimetre in length before bifurcating into its anterior interventricular and circumflex branches (Figure 5.23). In some hearts, the left main artery trifurcates, with an intermediate branch present between the two major branches (Figure 5.24). The intermediate branch supplies the pulmonary surface and obtuse margins of the left ventricle. The anterior interventricular, or descending, artery runs inferiorly within the antero-superior interventricular groove, giving off diagonal branches to the pulmonary surface of the left ventricle (Figure 5.25), and the important perforating branches which pass inferiorly into the septum (Figures 5.26, 5.27). The first septal perforating branch (Figure 5.26) is particularly important, since it is at major risk when the pulmonary valve is removed for use as a homograft. The interventricular artery then continues towards the apex, frequently curving under the apex onto the diaphragmatic surface of the ventricles.

The circumflex branch of the left coronary artery passes backwards to run in relationship with the mitral orifice. Its relationship to the orifice is most extensive when it gives rise to the inferior interventricular artery at the crux. In this circumstance, the left coronary artery is said to be dominant (Figures 5.28, 5.29). A dominant left coronary artery, however, is found in only about one-tenth of cases. When the left coronary is not dominant, the circumflex artery usually terminates by supplying branches to the obtuse margin of the left ventricle (see Figure 4.64). In almost half of normal individuals, the circumflex artery also gives rise to the artery that supplies the sinus node.

Throughout much of their epicardial course, the arteries and their accompanying veins are encased in epicardial adipose tissue. In some hearts, the myocardium itself may form a bridge over segments of the artery (Figure 5.30). The role of these myocardial bridges in the development of coronary arterial disease is not clear. They certainly can be an impediment to the surgeon in efforts to isolate the artery.

We have already emphasized the significance of the origin of the important artery supplying the sinus node. This, the largest of the atrial arteries, originates from the right coronary artery in just over half of individuals, and from the circumflex artery in the remainder (Figure 5.31). There are, however, rare variants that must also be recognized when present.[10] Lateral origin from the right coronary artery, with a course across the appendage, is an obvious potential danger for the standard atriotomy (see Figures 3.22, 5.22). The artery to the sinus node may also, rarely, take a lateral or terminal origin from the circumflex artery (Figure 5.31). Although rare in normal individuals, our experience suggests that these variants are more frequent in congenitally malformed hearts.[11] The artery

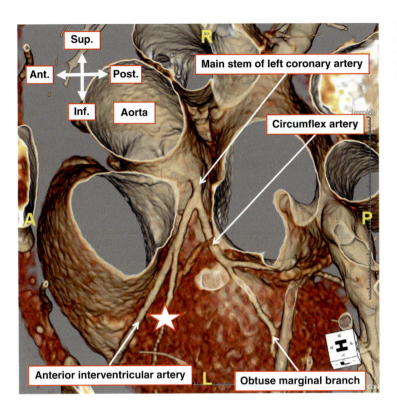

Figure 5.23 The computed tomographic image shows the left coronary artery branching into its anterior interventricular and circumflex branches. Note the diagonal branch (star) arising from the anterior interventricular artery. The attitudinal abbreviations are as for the previous images.

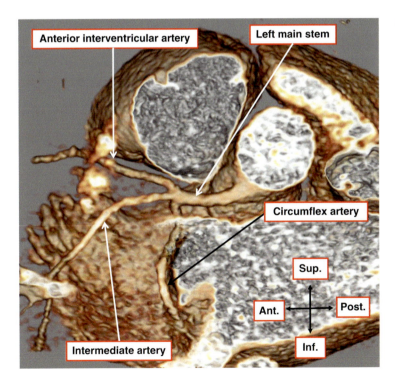

Figure 5.24 The computed tomographic image shows the left coronary artery giving rise to three, rather than two, branches. The intermediate branch supplies the obtuse margin of the left ventricle.

to the sinus node also takes a variable course relative to the cavoatrial junction. There are three possibilities (Figure 5.31). Usually, the artery courses anterocavally across the crest of the appendage to reach the node. Alternatively, it runs deeply within Waterston's groove, and passes retrocavally. It is then intimately related to the superior rim of the oval fossa. The third possibility is for the artery to branch, forming a circle around the cavoatrial junction.

The arterial supply to the ventricular conduction tissues is also of surgical significance. The atrioventricular nodal artery arises from the dominant coronary artery at

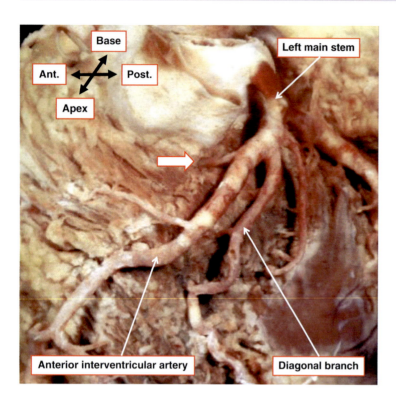

Figure 5.25 This dissection, photographed from the front in anatomical orientation, shows the course and branches of the anterior interventricular artery. Note the location of the first septal perforating branch (arrow).

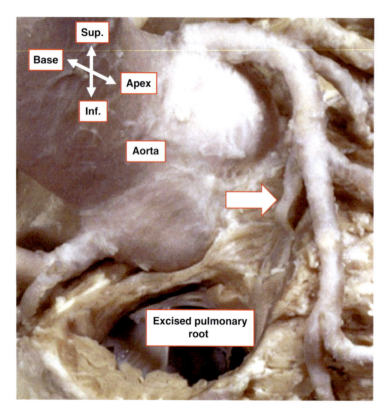

Figure 5.26 This close-up view of a specimen, in anatomical orientation subsequent to excision of the pulmonary valve, shows the origin of the first septal perforating artery (white arrow with red borders). Note its proximity to the subpulmonary infundibular area, putting it at risk when the pulmonary valve is removed for use as an autograft.

the crux, usually from a U-turn of this artery beneath the floor of the coronary sinus. The nodal artery then passes towards the central fibrous body, running within the fibrofatty plane forming the meat in the atrioventricular muscular sandwich. Having traversed the node in some hearts, it then perforates the fibrous atrioventricular junction to supply a good part of the branching atrioventricular bundle. The septal perforating arteries from the anterior interventricular artery (Figures 5.26, 5.27) always supply the anterior parts of the ventricular bundle branches. Occasionally, they also supply the greater part of the inferior ventricular conduction tissues.

5 Surgical Anatomy of the Coronary Circulation

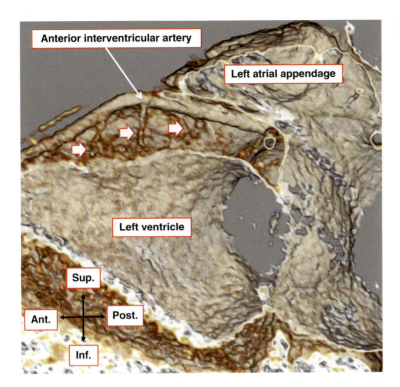

Figure 5.27 The computed tomographic reconstruction shows the course of the septal perforating arteries (white arrows with red borders).

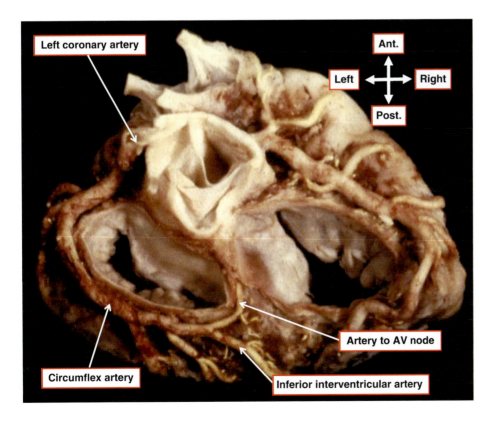

Figure 5.28 This specimen, dissected and photographed to show the base of the heart in anatomical orientation, has a dominant circumflex branch passing behind the mitral orifice and giving rise to the inferior interventricular artery at the crux.

The Coronary Veins

The coronary veins drain blood from the myocardium to the right atrium. The smaller anterior and the smallest cardiac veins drain directly to the cavity of the atrium. They are not of surgical significance. The larger veins accompany the major arteries, and drain into the coronary sinus (Figure 5.32). The great cardiac vein runs alongside the anterior interventricular artery. It becomes the coronary sinus as it encircles the mitral orifice to enter the

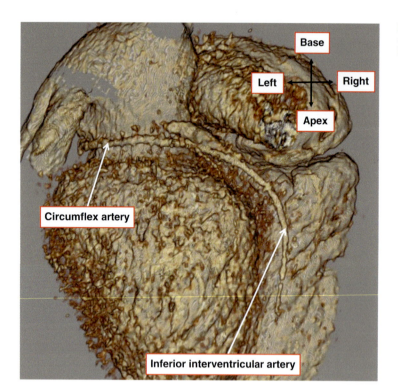

Figure 5.29 The computed tomographic reconstruction shows a dominant circumflex artery, which gives rise to the inferior interventricular artery.

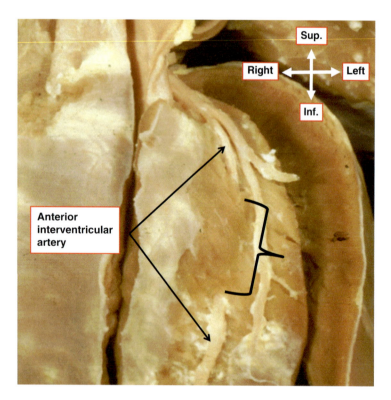

Figure 5.30 In this specimen, photographed with the heart positioned on its apex, there is extensive myocardial bridging across the anterior interventricular artery (bracket).

inferior and leftward margin of the atrioventricular groove. The coronary sinus then runs within the groove (Figure 5.33), lying between the left atrial wall and the ventricular myocardium (Figure 5.34), before draining into the right atrium between the sinus septum and the sub-Eustachian sinus. At the crux, the sinus receives the middle cardiac vein, which has ascended with the inferior interventricular artery, and the small cardiac vein, which has encircled the tricuspid orifice in company with the right coronary artery. Occasionally, these latter two veins drain directly to the right atrium. The orifice of the coronary sinus is guarded by the Thebesian valve (Figure 5.35),

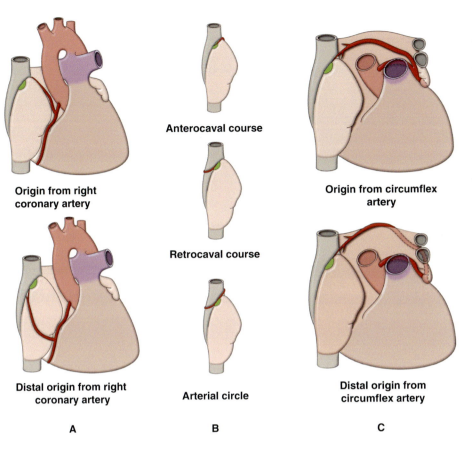

Figure 5.31 The cartoon, drawn in anatomical orientation, shows the variations in the origin of the artery to the sinus node, and the variability relative to the cavoatrial junction. Panel A shows the usual arrangement with origin from the right coronary artery, found in 55% of the population, with the rare variant of distal origin with coursing across the appendage (lower left). Panel C shows proximal origin from the circumflex artery, found in around 45% of the population, with the rare variant of distal origin with coursing across the dome of the left atrium. Panel B shows the variation relative to the superior cavoatrial junction. The sinus node is shown in green.

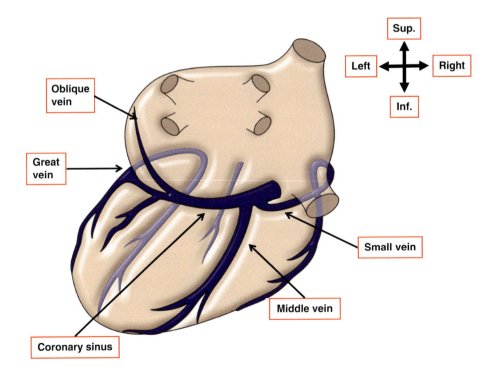

Figure 5.32 The cartoon shows the diaphragmatic surface of the heart seen from behind in anatomical orientation. It illustrates the arrangement of the coronary veins that drain into the coronary sinus.

which, on very rare occasions, may be imperforate. A prominent valve is also found in the great cardiac vein where it turns around the obtuse margin of the left ventricle. This is the valve of Vieussens.[12] Some consider that the valve marks the transition from the great cardiac vein to the coronary sinus. An alternative view is that the coronary sinus commences at the site of drainage of the oblique vein of the left atrium (Figure 5.36).

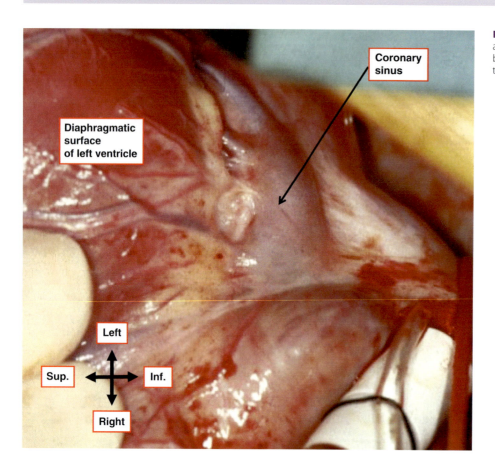

Figure 5.33 This operative view, taken through a median sternotomy, with the apex of the heart being lifted, shows the coronary sinus running through the left atrioventricular groove.

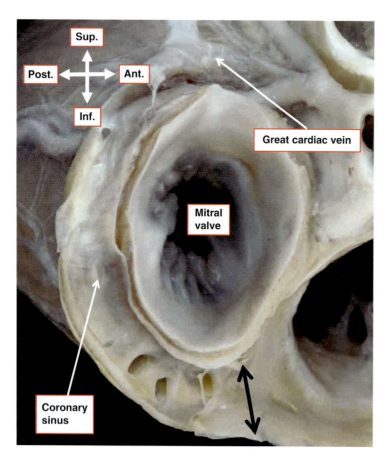

Figure 5.34 In this heart, the musculature of the atrial walls has been removed to show the course of the coronary sinus within the left atrioventricular groove. It opens to the right atrium at the base of the triangle of Koch (double-headed arrow).

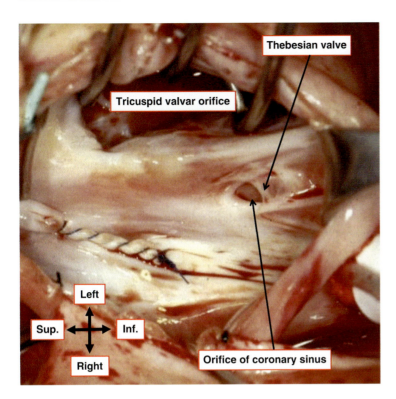

Figure 5.35 This operative view, through a right atriotomy, shows the Thebesian valve guarding the orifice of the coronary sinus.

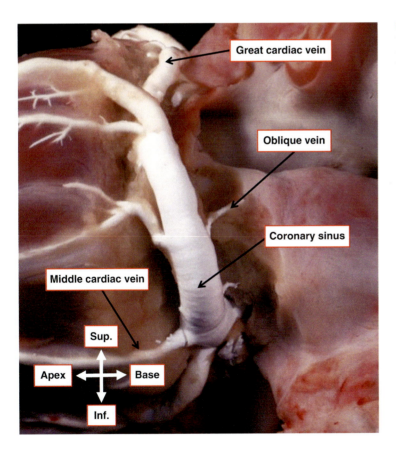

Figure 5.36 This preparation was made by casting the coronary sinus with silastic, the heart then being photographed from behind in anatomical orientation. The great cardiac vein is seen entering the coronary sinus. The location of the site of drainage of the oblique vein marks the point at which the great vein becomes the coronary sinus.

The Cardiac Lymphatics

Little is known about the surgical implications of the lymphatic drainage of the heart itself, although lymphatic structures exist as superficial, myocardial, and subendocardial networks.[13] The most important lymphatic channel within the thorax, however, is both well recognized and of particular importance. This is

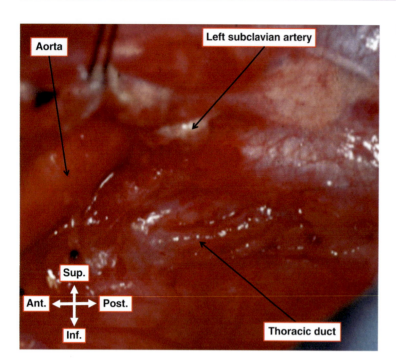

Figure 5.37 This operative view, taken through a left thoracotomy, shows the location of the thoracic duct in the vicinity of the left subclavian artery and descending thoracic aorta.

because, on occasion, the surgeon may need to ligate this vessel, the thoracic duct, in patients suffering with problems in lymphatic drainage subsequent to their conversion to the Fontan circulation. The thoracic duct originates within the abdomen in the confluence of lymphatic channels known as the chylous cistern, or cysterna chyli, this structure lying on the second lumbar vertebra. It enters the right paravertebral gutter of the thorax through the aortic opening of the diaphragm, running within the gutter to the level of the fourth thoracic vertebra. Within the lower part of the thorax, it lies on the vertebral column between the descending thoracic aorta and the azygos vein. Crossing the midline obliquely at the level of the fourth thoracic vertebra, it enters the left paravertebral gutter, running beneath the arch of the aorta (Figure 5.37). Continuing superiorly and anteriorly, and curving over the aortic arch between the left common carotid and subclavian arteries, it terminates in either the left subclavian or internal jugular vein as these structures join together to form the left brachiocephalic vein. The duct has a fibromuscular coat, and contains several valves along its course, with a bifoliate valve characteristically present at its termination in the brachiocephalic vein.

References Cited

1. Gittenberger-de Groot AC, Sauer U, Oppenheimer-Dekker A, Quaegebeur J. Coronary arterial anatomy in transposition of the great arteries: a morphologic study. *Pediatr Cardiol* 1983; 4 (Suppl.1): 15–24.
2. Neufeld HN, Schneeweiss A. *Coronary Artery Disease in Infants and Children.* Philadelphia: Lea & Febiger; 1983: pp. 73–75.
3. Bader G. Beitrag zur Systematic und Haufigkeit der Anomalien der Coronararterien des Menschen. *Virch Arch Path Anat* 1963; **337**: 88–96.
4. Kaushal S, Backer CL, Popescu AR, et al. Intramural coronary length correlates with symptoms in patients with anomalous aortic origin of the coronary artery. *Ann Thorac Surg* 2011; **92**: 986–992.
5. Cheezum MK, Liberthson RR, Shah NR, et al. Anomalous aortic origin of a coronary artery from the inappropriate sinus of valsalva. *J Am Coll Cardiol* 2017; **69**: 1592–1608.
6. Taylor AJ, Rogan KM, Virmani R. Sudden cardiac death associated with isolated congenital coronary artery disease. *J Am Coll Cardiol* 1992; **20**: 640–647.
7. Engel HJ, Torres C, Page HL Jr. Major variations in anatomical origin of the coronary arteries: angiographic observations in 4,250 patients without associated congenital heart disease. *Cathet Cardiovasc Diagn* 1975; **1**: 157–169.
8. Sharbaugh AH, White RS. Single coronary artery. Analysis of the anatomic variation, clinical importance, and report of five cases. *JAMA* 1974; **230**: 242–246.
9. Torres FS, Nguyen ET, Dennie CJ, et al. Role of MDCT coronary angiography in the evaluation of septal vs interarterial course of anomalous left coronary arteries. *J Card Comp Tomog* 2010; **4**: 246–254.
10. Busquet J, Fontan F, Anderson RH, Ho SY, Davies MJ. The surgical significance of the atrial branches of the coronary arteries. *Int J Cardiol* 1984; **6**: 223–234.
11. Barra Rossi M, Ho SY, Anderson RH, Rossi Filho RI, Lincoln C. Coronary arteries in complete transposition: the significance of the sinus node artery. *Ann Thorac Surg* 1986; **42**: 573–577.
12. Zawadzki M, Pietrasik A, Pietrasik K, Marchel M, Ciszek B. Endoscopic study of the morphology of Vieussen's valve. *Clin Anat* 2004; **17**: 318–321.
13. Walmsley T. The heart. In E Sharpey-Schafer, J Symington, TH Bryce, eds., *Quain's Elements of Anatomy.* 11th ed., vol. IV, part III. London: Longmans, Green and Co.; 1929: p. 110.

Chapter 6

Surgical Anatomy of Cardiac Conduction

The disposition of the conduction system in the normal heart has already been emphasized (see Chapter 2). In that earlier chapter, we pointed to the importance, during surgical procedures, of avoiding the cardiac nodes and ventricular bundle branches, and scrupulously protecting the vascular supply to these structures. In this chapter, we will consider the anatomy of these tissues relative to the treatment of intractable problems of cardiac rhythm, specifically the normal and abnormal atrioventricular conduction axis. The abnormal dispositions of the conduction tissues to be found in congenitally malformed hearts, features of obvious significance to the congenital cardiac surgeon, will be discussed in the sections devoted to those lesions in the chapters that follow. In this chapter, nonetheless, we will also discuss surgical procedures performed to treat arrhythmias that develop in the setting of the Fontan circulation.

Landmarks to the Atrioventricular Conduction Axis

In patients with intractable tachycardia, it may be necessary to ablate the atrioventricular bundle. Although this sometimes occurs inadvertently, it can be surprisingly difficult to divide this structure intentionally. The landmark to penetration of the atrioventricular conduction axis through the fibrous insulating plane is the apex of the triangle of Koch (Figure 6.1).[1] The apex is marked by the point at which the tendon of Todaro inserts into the atrioventricular part of the membranous septum, this being the component of the central fibrous body obvious to the surgeon from the right side (Figure 6.2). Just inferior to the apex of this triangle, the components of the atrioventricular node gather themselves together, and enter the insulating tissues of the fibrous body (Figures 6.3, 6.4). Once insulated from the atrial myocardial mass, the conduction axis becomes the penetrating atrioventricular bundle, usually described as the bundle of His. This part of the overall atrioventricular conduction axis is short, but extends leftward as it pierces the fibrous body, having a non-branching component of variable length.[2] As the axis passes through the insulating plane, and divides into its branches, the membranous septum itself is crossed by the septal leaflet of the tricuspid valve, dividing it into atrioventricular and interventricular components. The non-branching component of the conduction axis often occupies

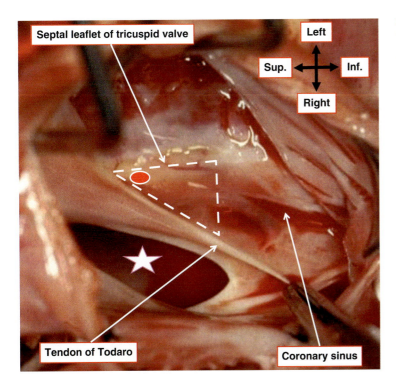

Figure 6.1 The operative photograph shows the surgeon's view through a right atriotomy in a patient with an atrial septal defect in the oval fossa (star). The landmarks defining the triangle of Koch (dashed line) are shown along with the location of the compact atrioventricular node (red oval). Tension has been placed on the Eustachian valve to bring the tendon of Todaro into prominence.

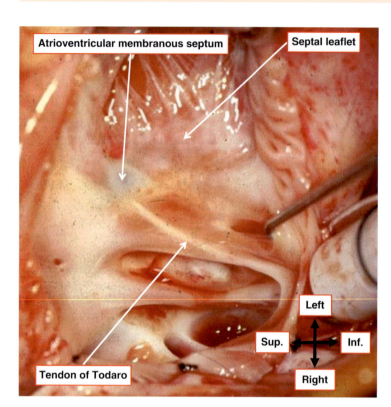

Figure 6.2 Another operative view, in the same orientation as Figure 6.1, shows the tendon of Todaro inserting into the atrioventricular part of the membranous septum.

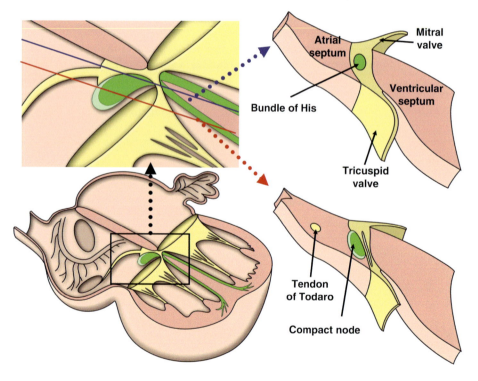

Figure 6.3 The cartoon, drawn in anatomical orientation, shows the location of the conduction tissues within the triangle of Koch, and the mechanism of penetration of the axis of conduction tissue into the central fibrous body to form the bundle of His, the point of penetration serving to delimit the junction of the atrioventricular node with the penetrating bundle. Note the orientation of the bundle branches is purely schematic.

the interventricular component of the septum at its attachment to the crest of the muscular ventricular septum. After extending in non-branching fashion for variable distances, the axis begins to give rise to the fascicles of the left bundle branch, which cascade subendocardially down the left ventricular aspect of the muscular septum (Figure 6.5). When viewed from the left, the axis itself, and the fascicles of the left bundle branch, are intimately related to the subaortic outflow tract, with the inferior and septal fascicles of the trifascicular left bundle taking origin at the base of the fibrous triangle separating the non-coronary and right coronary leaflets of the aortic valve (Figure 6.6). In most instances, the axis is carried on the crest of the muscular septum. It can be found distal to the virtual basal plane of the

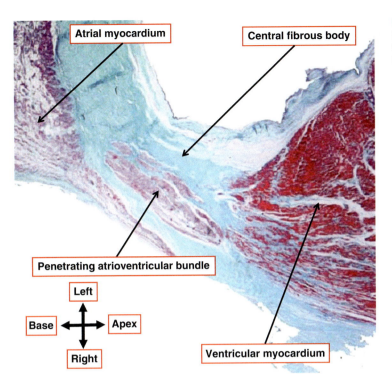

Figure 6.4 The histological section shows the location of the penetrating atrioventricular bundle as an insulated structure within the central fibrous body. The section corresponds to the upper right-hand panel of Figure 6.3.

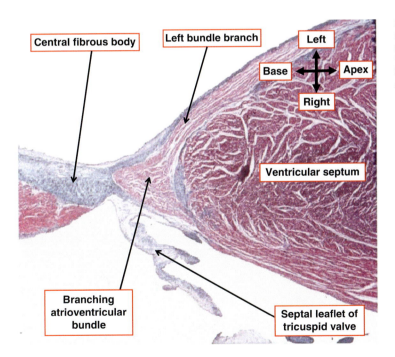

Figure 6.5 The histological section, in the same anatomical orientation as Figure 6.4, shows the branching component of the atrioventricular conduction axis. It lies astride the crest of the muscular ventricular septum, sandwiched between the septum and the central fibrous body. Courtesy of Professor Anton Becker, University of Amsterdam.

aortic root, and hence within the confines of the root (Figure 6.7). In other instances, as it gives rise to the left fascicles, the axis is positioned proximal to the virtual basal ring, and hence more distant from the hinges of the aortic valvar leaflets (Figure 6.8).[3] Irrespective of its adjacency to the aortic root, the conduction axis continues to encircle the subaortic outflow tract as it give rise to the left bundle branches, with the closest relationship to the aortic root being found at the nadir of the right coronary aortic leaflet, as was illustrated by Tawara in his original monograph describing the axis (Figure 6.6). Indeed, on occasion, the superior fascicle of the left bundle can be within one millimetre of the nadir of the leaflet (Figure 6.9A), a finding of obvious significance not only to surgeons, but also to those undertaking transcatheter replacement of the aortic valve. When more distant, the axis can be one centimetre below the virtual basal ring, making it much safer during surgical or interventional procedures (Figure 6.9B). Our recent

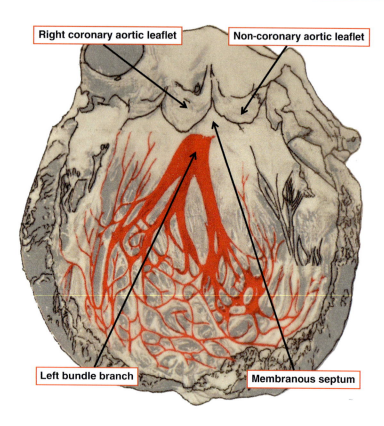

Figure 6.6 The diagram is a reproduction of the original drawing made by Tawara. It shows the location of the left bundle branch (in red) relative to the aortic root. The closest point of the axis is found at the nadir of the right coronary aortic leaflet.

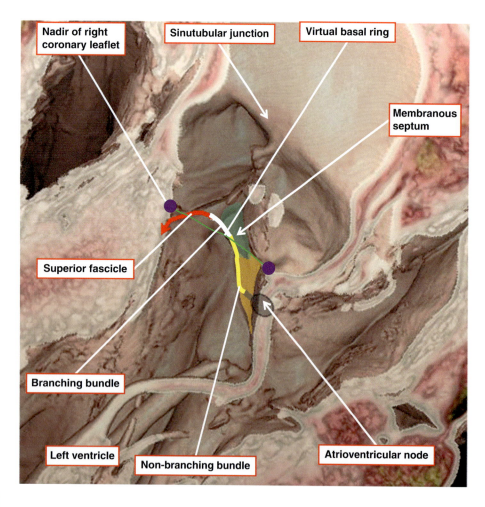

Figure 6.7 The atrioventricular conduction axis has been reconstructed from histological sections and superimposed on the left ventricular aspect of the aortic root. The non-branching bundle is shown in yellow, with the branching part coloured white, and the course of the superior fascicle of the left bundle branch shown in red. The axis is particularly vulnerable in cases such as this, where the proximal margin of the membranous septum is within the aortic root. The virtual basal plane is coloured green, with purple dots showing the nadirs of the hinges of the leaflets of the aortic valve.

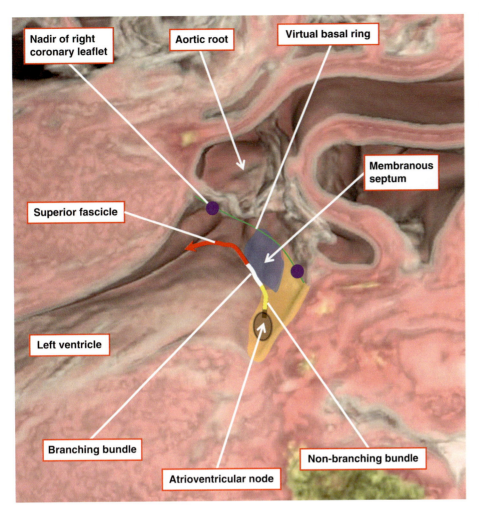

Figure 6.8 In this heart, in which, as for the case shown in Figure 6.7, the conduction axis, coloured as shown in Figure 6.7, was reconstructed from serial histological sections, the arrangement is not as vulnerable, since the axis is proximal to the virtual basal plane, which is coloured green, with the nadirs again shown as purple dots.

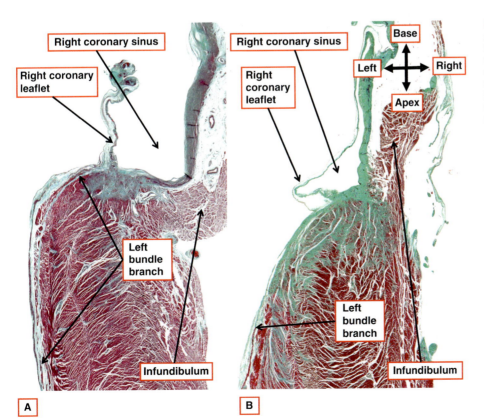

Figure 6.9 The histological sections show, panel A, a heart in which the superior fascicle of the left bundle branch is within 1 millimetre of the nadir of the right coronary aortic leaflet. In contrast, panel B shows an arrangement in which there is a distance of around 1 centimetre between the virtual basal ring and the superior fascicle of the left bundle branch. Courtesy of Professor Damian Sanchez-Quintana.

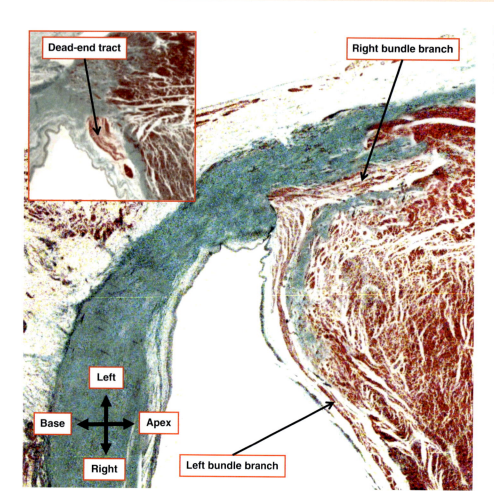

Figure 6.10 The inset shows that, in certain cases, the conduction axis continues beyond the origin of the right bundle branch, which is shown taking origin from the conduction axis in the major part of the figure. Courtesy of Professor Damian Sanchez-Quintana.

investigations suggest that information on the extent of rotation of the aortic root, and the depth and extent of the infero-septal recess, may permit inferences to be made regarding the proximity of the axis to the root.[4]

The right bundle branch takes origin from the axis, burrowing intramyocardially to reach the right side of the septum, and surfacing beneath the medial papillary muscle. The axis itself can continue beyond the origin of the right bundle branch, entering the aortic root as the so-called dead-end tract (Figure 6.10).[5] As viewed from the right side, the site of the conduction axis can be determined by taking a line from the apex of the triangle of Koch to the medial papillary muscle (Figure 6.11). In terms of the atrial components of the axis, the compact atrioventricular node, located within the triangle of Koch, is positioned posterior to the attachment of the septal leaflet of the tricuspid valve and superior to the orifice of the coronary sinus (Figure 6.11).[6]

Ventricular Pre-Excitation

Ventricular pre-excitation is a frequent problem of cardiac rhythm that necessitates knowledge of the pertinent anatomy for its optimal treatment. The arrhythmia occurs when all, or part, of the ventricular myocardium is excited earlier than would be expected had the impulse reached the ventricles by way of the normal atrioventricular conduction system.[7] There are various anatomical pathways, proven and hypothetical, that can produce this phenomenon. Essentially, they are pathways that short-circuit part, or all, of the normal delay induced within the atrioventricular conduction axis. Most of this delay occurs within the atrioventricular node and its zones of transitional cells. Part of the increment of delay reflects the time taken for the impulse to traverse the ventricular bundle branches, since these structures are insulated from the septal myocardium. Accessory pathways can exist between the atrium and the atrioventricular bundle, producing atrio-Hisian tracts, and between the conduction axis and the crest of the ventricular septum, the latter arrangement first being described by Mahaim as paraspecific connections.[8] Mahaim had described his paraspecific pathways, also known as nodoventricular and fasciculoventricular connections, as being ubiquitous. Strong evidence now indicates that he was correct in making these prognostications.[9] An understanding of the extent, location, and dimensions of these pathways will prove crucial to those undertaking specific pacing of the diseased conduction axis.[10] The pathways, however, are not amenable to surgical division. In contrast, the accessory atrioventricular pathways that produce the Wolff–Parkinson–White syndrome, probably the most common form of pre-excitation, are very much amenable to surgical division.[11] Nowadays, nonetheless, if division is

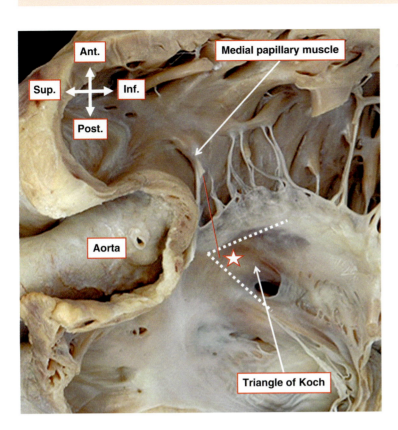

Figure 6.11 The dissection was made by removing the parietal walls of the right atrium and ventricle. It is viewed in surgical orientation, showing the location of the atrioventricular conduction axis (red line). The star shows the position of the atrioventricular node.

necessary, the pathways will almost certainly be ablated in the catheter laboratory. Treatment of this arrhythmia in the operating room remains of significance in that it constituted an important step in the evolution of cardiac surgery. When treatment was first mooted, the bundles were called, inappropriately, bundles of Kent.[11] The atrioventricular muscular strands that are part of the circuit responsible for the abnormal rhythm join together the atrial and ventricular myocardial muscle masses outside the area of the specialized conduction tissues (Figure 6.12). The best initial description of the bundles was given by Ohnell.[12] His illustration (Figure 6.13) shows that the structures, which typically extend through the fat pad on the epicardial aspect of the atrioventricular junctions, bear no resemblance to the node-like remnants described by Kent, and considered inappropriately by him to be part of the normal conduction system (Figure 6.14). The entities that were emphasized by Kent are remnants of the ring of specialized conducting tissue that we have described surrounding the primary interventricular foramen of the developing heart (see Chapter 2). They can be found by careful examination of human hearts.[13] Only in abnormal situations, however, do the node-like remnants give rise to anomalous muscular atrioventricular connections. The abnormal accessory muscular bundles that are much more frequently the substrate for the Wolff–Parkinson–White syndrome (Figure 6.12) can be found anywhere around the atrioventricular junctions. They are best described as being left sided, right sided, and paraseptal. The anatomy of each group shows significant differences.

Left-sided pathways are found at any point around the mural component of the mitral valvar orifice. Pathways can extend through the area of aortic–mitral valvar fibrous continuity, but are exceedingly rare. The pathways almost always cross from the atrial to the ventricular muscle masses outside a well-formed fibrous hinge supporting the mural leaflet of the mitral valve (Figure 6.12). The atrial origins of the connections are very close to the fibrous junction.[14] The bundles themselves usually skirt very close to the fibrous tissue, often branching into several roots, which then insert into the ventricular myocardium. The bundles are rarely thicker than one to two millimetres in diameter. They are made up of ordinary working cardiomyocytes. On occasion, there may be more than one bundle in the same patient.[14] If approached from within the atrium, incisions that divide the atrial myocardium, or ablative lesions placed above the origin of the leaflets of the mitral valve, are unlikely to divide the accessory muscle bundles themselves. In order to ablate surgically the accessory connection, it was usually necessary to dissect within the fat pad on the epicardial aspect of the atrioventricular junction, or to approach the pathway from the epicardium. If approached endocardially, it was necessary to reflect the coronary vessels to expose the accessory muscle bundles. When treated in the catheter laboratory, lesions are usually placed on the ventricular aspect of the hinge point of the mitral valve.

Right-sided accessory pathways may also pass through the fat pad to connect the atrial and ventricular myocardial masses. More frequently, bundles on the right side are found some distance away from the hinges of the leaflets of the tricuspid valve, which are rarely firm and well-formed fibrous structures, as is usually the case on the left side. Right-sided connections can be multiple, and can co-exist with left-sided

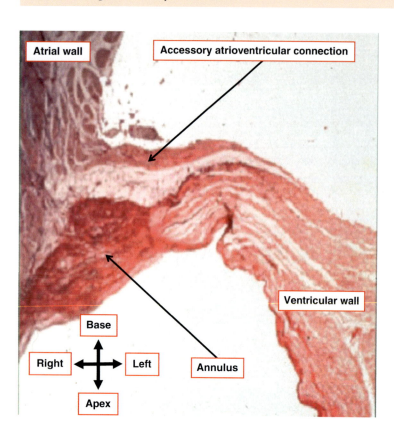

Figure 6.12 The histological section across the atrioventricular junction shows the arrangement of a typical left-sided accessory muscular atrioventricular connection. Courtesy of Professor Anton Becker, University of Amsterdam.

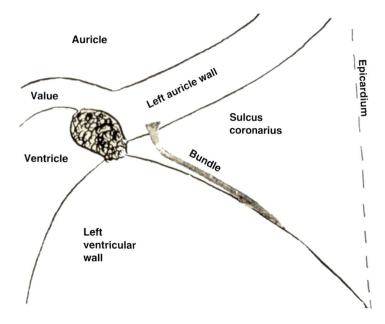

Figure 6.13 The original drawing made by Ohnell shows the arrangement of the typical left-sided accessory muscular atrioventricular connections. Comparison with Figure 6.12 shows the accuracy achieved by Ohnell when making his drawing.

pathways. They are frequently associated with Ebstein's malformation, and may need to be treated concomitantly with repair or replacement of the abnormal tricuspid valve. They can be found at any point within the parietal aspect of the tricuspid orifice, from the site of the membranous septum to the mouth of the coronary sinus (Figure 6.15). The same rules for their ablation apply as discussed for left-sided connections.

It is connections in paraseptal position that constitute the greatest clinical challenge.[15] When viewed from the right atrium, they can cross from the atrial to the ventricular myocardium (Figure 6.16) at any point between the mouth of the coronary sinus and the supraventricular crest. They present problems for ablation, firstly, because they may run deep within the floor of the triangle of Koch as viewed from the right atrium. The second problem is that the atrioventricular node and bundle are also found within this area.[16] The anatomy of the area can be illustrated by dissections that have removed the atrial walls from the base of the ventricular mass

6 Surgical Anatomy of Cardiac Conduction

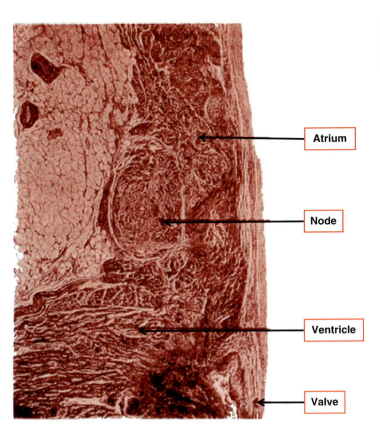

Figure 6.14 The illustration is taken from one of Kent's demonstrations to the Society of Physiology, and re-labelled by us. It shows the structure of remnants of conduction tissue found adjacent to the right atrioventricular junction. The node-like structure bears no resemblance to the accessory connections that produce Wolff–Parkinson–White syndrome (see Figures 6.12 and 6.13), but can rarely give rise to an anomalous connection – see Figure 6.21.

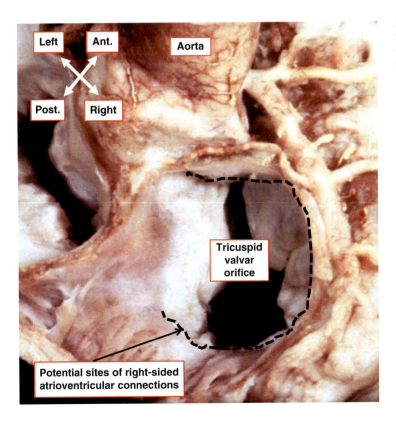

Figure 6.15 The dissection, photographed in anatomical orientation from above and behind, shows the potential sites of atrioventricular connections (dashed line) in the parietal aspect of the right atrioventricular junction.

(Figure 6.17). It is now equally well demonstrated by using virtual dissections of computed tomographic datasets (Figure 6.18). Such dissections, be they virtual or real, reveal the cranial continuation of the inferior atrioventricular groove. The fibro-adipose tissue extends superiorly between the atrial and ventricular muscle masses, reaching the central fibrous

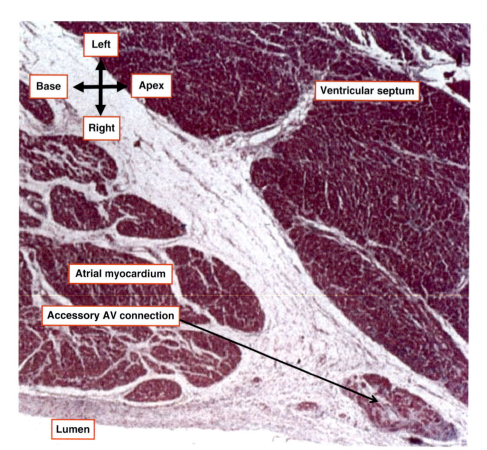

Figure 6.16 The histological section, in anatomical orientation, shows a muscular accessory atrioventricular connection crossing the fibrofatty insulating plane of the right atrioventricular junction. The strand takes its origin from the distal insertion of the atrial myocardium into the area of attachment of the septal leaflet of the tricuspid valve, and crosses the groove to attach to the ventricular myocardium. Courtesy of Professor Anton Becker, University of Amsterdam.

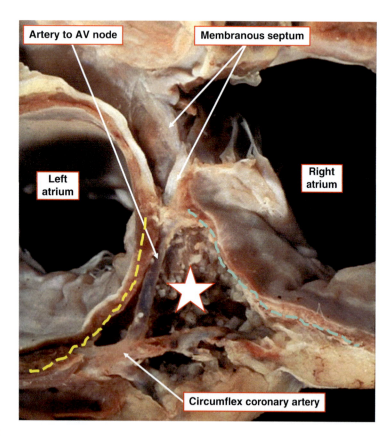

Figure 6.17 The dissection, shown in anatomical orientation, illustrates the plane occupied by adipose tissue that runs superiorly and anteriorly beneath the mouth of the coronary sinus. The right and left atrial walls have been resected (green and yellow dashed lines). The star shows the adipose tissue occupying the inferior atrioventricular groove. The artery to the atrioventricular node runs within the adipose tissue, in this case from a dominant left coronary artery.

6 Surgical Anatomy of Cardiac Conduction

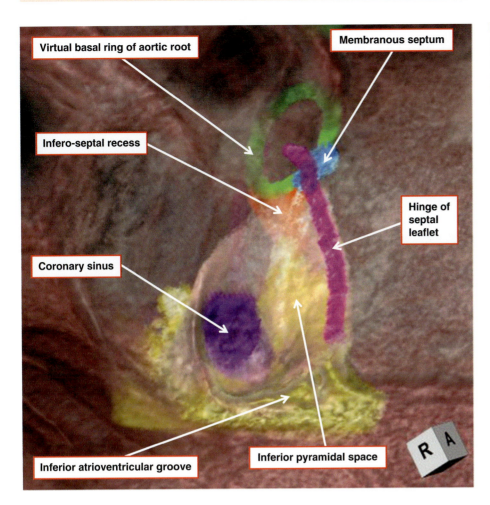

Figure 6.18 The virtual dissection, from a computed tomographic dataset, coloured manually to highlight respective components, shows the extent of the fibro-adipose tissue occupying the inferior pyramidal space, and its relationships to the infero-septal recess. Orientation cube, lower right: R, right, A, anterior.

body when traced cranially. The artery to the atrioventricular node courses forward within this tissue plane (Figure 6.17). The atrioventricular node itself occupies the superior part of the atrial layer of this triangular sandwich, with the fibro-adipose tissue representing the meat between the muscular layers of the sandwich. Accessory muscular connections may cross through this insulating layer at any point from the attachment of the mitral and tricuspid valves at either side of the muscular ventricular septum. Indeed, the only connection of which we are aware that has been identified morphologically within this area was located at the insertion of the tricuspid valve (Figure 6.16).[14] If necessary, the fibro-adipose tissue plane can be entered surgically from the cavity of the right atrium, or can be reached by dissection from the epicardial aspect. Incisions within the atrial component of this atrioventricular sandwich, interrupting the muscular approaches to the atrioventricular node, have also been shown to interrupt reciprocating atrioventricular nodal tachycardias.[11] Treatment of these latter arrhythmias is now also accomplished with efficiency and safety using catheter ablation (Figure 6.19).[17] When treating these arrhythmias, either surgically or by catheter ablation, it should be remembered that the triangle of Koch contains both the atrioventricular node and its nutrient artery. Unless performed with care, there is always the danger that intervention can produce complete atrioventricular dissociation.

Surgeons and catheter ablationists, when attempting to treat arrhythmias, have conventionally referred to the floor of the triangle of Koch as being septal. They also describe an anterior septum in the region cranial to the membranous septum.[18] By this, they mean the area of the right atrioventricular junction that lies adjacent to the supraventricular crest. It is a mistake to describe this part of the right atrioventricular junction as being septal, just as it is incorrect to consider the atrial aspect of the triangle of Koch as representing a septal structure.[19] In reality, the so-called anterior septum is the medial margin of the ventriculo-infundibular fold. If muscular atrioventricular connections exist in this area, they will join the atrial wall to the supraventricular crest of the right ventricle (Figure 6.20).

Experience has shown that muscular connections running to the most lateral margin of the supraventricular crest, at the acute margin of the right ventricle, can produce the electrocardiographic pattern initially attributed to the so-called Mahaim connections.[9] Such connections, when removed surgically from the acute margin, were shown to resemble histologically the tissues of the atrioventricular node.[20] We had previously identified such a pathway running across the right atrioventricular junction (Figure 6.21).[14] The atrial component of these connections is remarkably reminiscent of the illustrations provided by Kent (Figure 6.14). As we have discussed, Kent

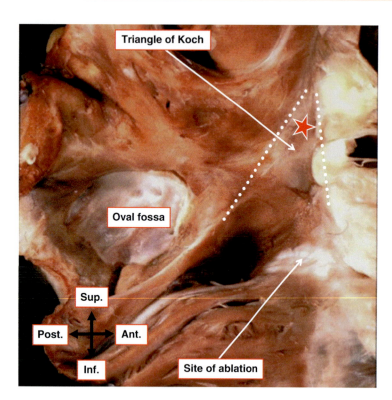

Figure 6.19 The photograph shows the site of ablation at the base of the triangle of Koch, which cured a patient with atrioventricular nodal re-entry tachycardia. It is outside the area occupied by the specialized tissues of the atrioventricular node, shown by the red star with white borders, and its zones of transitional cells. Reproduced by kind permission of Dr Wyn Davies, St Mary's Hospital, London.

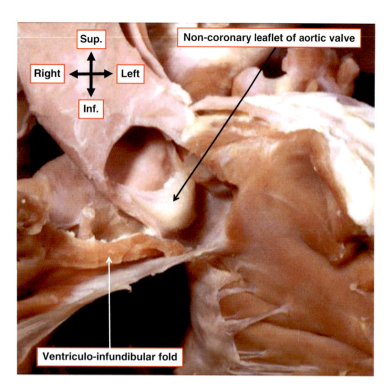

Figure 6.20 The dissection, in anatomical orientation, illustrates how the area anterior to the membranous septum, which was previously considered to represent the anterior septum, is part of the parietal wall of the right atrioventricular junction, specifically the ventriculo-infundibular fold.

himself had argued,[21] incorrectly,[22] that the nodal remnants were pathways for normal atrioventricular conduction. Under abnormal circumstances, nonetheless, these node-like remnants are able to function as the atrial origin of specialized muscular accessory connections. It is these connections that are now known to produce ventricular pre-excitation of the Mahaim type.[9]

Substrates for Other Supraventricular Tachycardias

The attention of both surgeons and interventionists has focused on the substrates of other supraventricular tachycardias, particularly atrial flutter and fibrillation. Atrial flutter of the commonest type has shown itself to be especially amenable

6 Surgical Anatomy of Cardiac Conduction

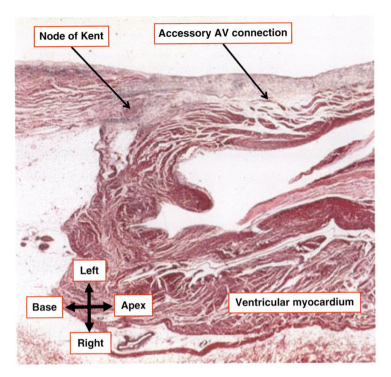

Figure 6.21 The section is taken across the right atrioventricular (AV) junction, and comes from the heart of a patient who had ventricular pre-excitation. The tricuspid valve was deformed by Ebstein's malformation. An accessory muscular connection was identified taking origin from a nodal remnant as identified by Kent, and crossing the insulating plane to run within the muscularized leaflet of the tricuspid valve. Section reproduced by kind permission of Professor Anton Becker, University of Amsterdam.

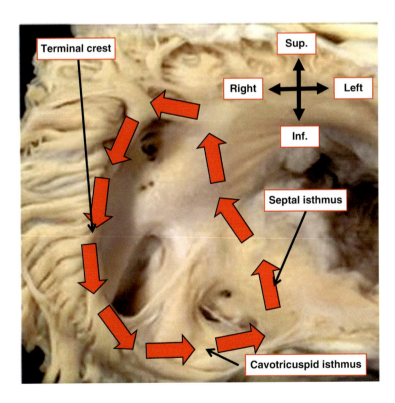

Figure 6.22 The right atrium has been opened and photographed in anatomical orientation to show the circuit (red arrows) known to be responsible for the common variant of atrial flutter. The flutter wave descends the terminal crest, crosses through the inferior cavo-tricuspid isthmus, and then ascends through the septal isthmus to reach the superior aspect of the terminal crest before recommencing the circuit.

to interventional therapy. The usual flutter circuit is known to pass in counterclockwise fashion (Figure 6.22), running down the terminal crest before ascending through the septal isthmus of the tricuspid valvar vestibule.[23] The most inferior part of the circuit passes through another muscular isthmus, this time limited by the orifice of the inferior caval vein and the hinge of the septal leaflet of the tricuspid valve (Figure 6.23). The isthmus has three discrete areas, containing various combinations of fibrous and muscular tissue (Figure 6.24).[24] Interventionists are now able to construct lines of block with great facility so as to divide the circuit. Care should be taken in the vestibular area to avoid damage to the right coronary artery (Figure 6.24). Such lines would obviously be made surgically with equal facility. This is the reasoning behind the surgical

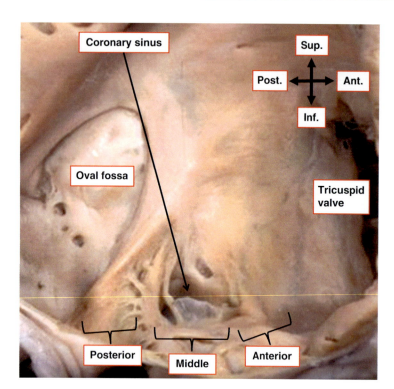

Figure 6.23 The right atrium has been opened through the parietal wall, and photographed in anatomical orientation to show the structure of the inferior cavo-tricuspid isthmus. It has posterior, middle, and anterior components.

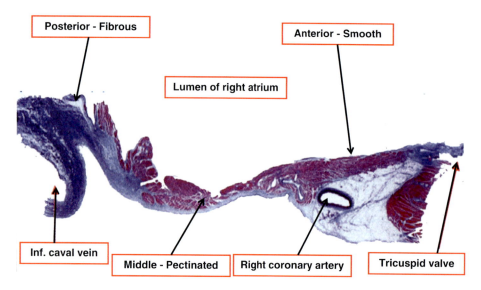

Figure 6.24 This histological section, prepared by Professor Siew Yen Ho, shows the structure of the three components of the inferior cavo-tricuspid isthmus. Note the adjacency of the right coronary artery to the vestibular musculature in the anterior compartment.

manoeuvres performed as part of the treatment of patients with the Fontan circulation, known as the Fontan conversion,[25] to be discussed in greater detail below.

The other arrhythmia now becoming increasingly amenable to interventional therapy is atrial fibrillation. It has long been known that surgical techniques that create mazes[26] or corridors[27] can certainly ameliorate, if not cure, this troublesome entity. The operative procedures are complex and time-consuming. The maze procedure, for example, has undergone many modifications,[28] details of which are beyond the context of our description, although we describe the third iteration designed by Cox when considering treatment of postoperative arrhythmias (see below). More recently, interventionists have shown that it is feasible to construct lines of block within both the left and right atriums, lesions which can provide successful treatment for atrial fibrillation.[29,30] It has now also been shown that a proportion of cases of fibrillation can be cured by making focal lesions in the mouth of the pulmonary veins.[31] This is because the atrial myocardium extends for variable distances along the pulmonary veins from the venoatrial junctions (Figure 6.25). These sleeves of myocardium contain cardiomyocytes aggregated into bundles that run in different directions, along with separating sheaths of fibrous tissue which set the scene for the focal triggering that produces the fibrillation.[32,33] It has been suggested that the cardiomyocytes

6 Surgical Anatomy of Cardiac Conduction

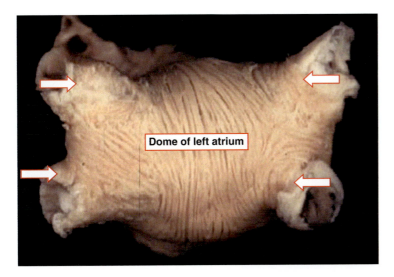

Figure 6.25 The dissection, made by Professor Damian Sanchez-Quintana, shows the dome of the left atrium, having removed the epicardium to illustrate the organization of the aggregated cardiomyocytes. Sleeves of myocardium (arrows) can be seen to extend onto the pulmonary veins for varying distances. These sleeves are now known to be the sources of focal activity in some variants of atrial fibrillation.

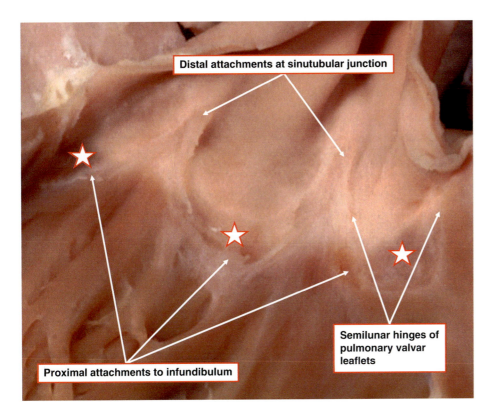

Figure 6.26 The pulmonary root has been opened, and the valvar leaflets removed, to show the muscular crescents (stars) incorporated at the base of the three pulmonary valvar sinuses. These muscular crescents can be the site of substrates for outflow tract tachycardias.

within the sleeves are histologically specialized.[34] This is a spurious claim. The cardiomyocytes are all of working myocardial origin, with the pulmonary venous myocardium never having had the characteristics of conduction tissues.[35]

Substrates for Outflow Tract Tachycardias

Experience shows that some ventricular tachycardias can be cured by placing lesions in the region of the bases of the arterial valvar sinuses.[36,37] Such lesions most frequently are placed in the adjacent sinuses of the aorta and pulmonary trunk. As we have shown in Chapter 3, these sinuses, at their base, contain crescents of ventricular muscle. This is because the semilunar hinges of the valvar leaflets cross the anatomical myocardial–arterial junctions (Figures 6.26, 6.27). It is most likely that the abnormal rhythms producing the outflow tract tachycardias take their origin within these myocardial crescents. It is also known that abnormal rhythms can rarely be cured by ablative lesions placed in the non-adjacent sinus of the aortic root.[38] It is rare to find myocardium within the base of this non-adjacent sinus. Sometimes the aortic valve, like the pulmonary valve, can be supported by a complete muscular infundibulum.[39] If present, such infundibular musculature would then produce a crescent within the non-adjacent sinus. In the absence of such musculature, it must be presumed that the abnormal rhythm has an extraventricular origin. The likely candidate for such a substrate is the retro-aortic node.[38] It is also known that,

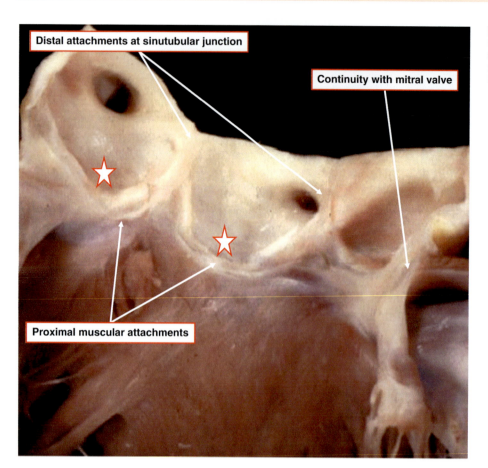

Figure 6.27 The aortic root has been opened, and the valvar leaflets removed. There is muscle at the base of the two aortic valvar sinuses giving rise to the coronary arteries (stars), but not in the non-adjacent sinus.

sometimes, the outflow tract tachycardias are ablated by lesions placed distal to the myocardial–arterial junction.[40] During their development, as we have shown in Chapter 2, the arterial roots are encased within turrets of outflow tract myocardium,[41] which then regress as part of the normal developmental process. Persistence of parts of this sleeve of outflow tract myocardium might provide an explanation should it truly be the case that the arrhythmias are originating distal to the myocardial–arterial junctions found at the bases of the valvar sinuses.

Arrhythmia Surgery in Patients with Congenital Heart Disease

As patients get older subsequent to surgical correction of congenital cardiac lesions, increasing numbers present with arrhythmic problems.[42] The enhanced understanding of the macro-reentrant circuits responsible for the abnormal rhythms has led to modifications of surgical techniques. Advances in the design of pacemakers and implantable cardiac defibrillators have also contributed to improved treatments,[43] but such details are beyond the scope of our current discussion. Knowledge of the anatomical background for the created therapeutic lines of block, nonetheless, now achieves increasing significance. The commonest arrhythmias requiring treatment are macro-reentrant atrial tachycardia, atrial fibrillation, and ventricular tachycardia.

Such problems are themselves encountered most frequently in postoperative patients with functionally univentricular hearts, and those who have undergone surgical treatment of tetralogy of Fallot or transposition. The reasoning behind the therapeutic approach is to transform areas of slow conduction to areas of no conduction.[43] This is achieved by interrupting myocardial corridors or isthmuses between obstacles or scars, while preserving sinus rhythm and normal atrioventricular conduction.

The commonest operations are the right atrial maze, typically performed for those with macro-reentrant tachycardia, and the Cox maze III/IV procedures for patients with atrial fibrillation. The right atrial maze procedure involves the resection of the tip of the right atrial appendage, and part of its anterior surface if the appendage is significantly enlarged, as is often the case in patients with failed Fontan circulations. Lines of block are then created from the edge of the resected appendage to the oval fossa, from the oval fossa across the terminal crest, and then a series of lines to divide the cavotricuspid isthmus (Figure 6.28). The lines dividing the isthmus run from the edge of the oval fossa to the margin of the coronary sinus (Figure 6.29), from the mouth of the coronary sinus to the mouth of the inferior caval vein, and from the inferior caval vein to the hinge of the septal leaflet of the tricuspid valve. The last lesion is obviously not possible in those with tricuspid atresia due to absence of the right atrioventricular

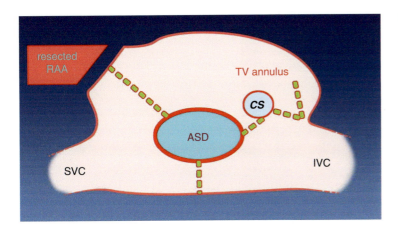

Figure 6.28 The drawing shows the lesions made within the right atrium during the Fontan conversion procedure so as to avoid postoperative problems with rhythm. SVC; IVC: superior and inferior caval veins; ASD: atrial septal defect; TV: tricuspid valve; RAA: right atrial appendage.

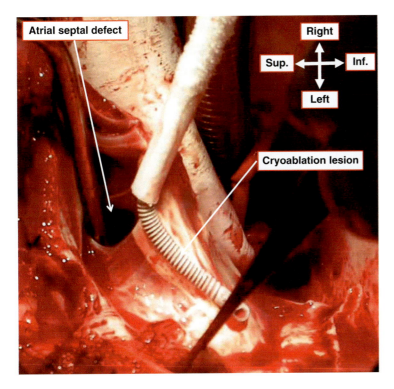

Figure 6.29 The cryoprobe is photographed in position to produce a lesion from the atrial septal defect to the coronary sinus in a patient with tricuspid atresia during a Fontan conversion procedure.

connection, but the other lines can easily be created in this setting (Figure 6.30).

In the third and fourth iterations of the series of procedures designed by Cox for treatment of patients with atrial fibrillation (Figure 6.31),[21] the lines of block can be produced either by surgical incisions or by cryoablation, respectively. An extensive line is created within the roof of the left atrium, encircling the orifices of all pulmonary veins. A line of block is then created to the mouth of the left atrial appendage, which can be excised, or alternatively encircled by another line. A linear lesion is then made from the line encircling the pulmonary veins to the annulus of the mitral valve in the region of the third scallop of the mural leaflet. The final lesion is placed epicardially across the coronary sinus as it runs within the left atrioventricular groove. If using cryoablation, the final lesion is maintained for two minutes, while the other require only one minute of freezing at minus 160 degrees Celsius.

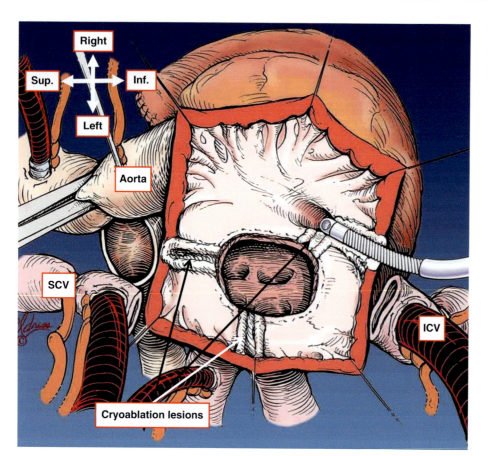

Figure 6.30 The drawing shows the cryoablation lesions producing the right atrial maze procedure as part of the Fontan conversion procedure. SCV, ICV: superior and inferior caval veins.

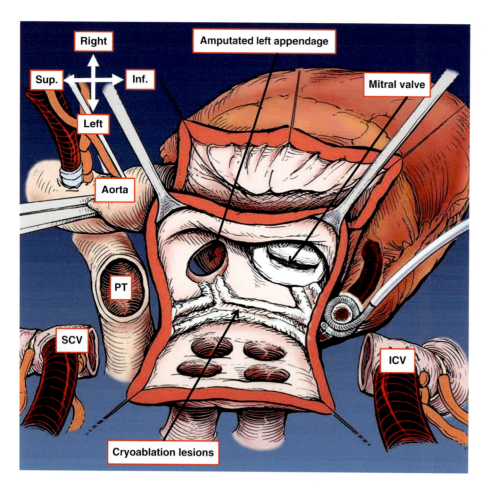

Figure 6.31 The drawing shows the cryoablation lesions produced in the third iteration of the Cox maze procedure for treatment of atrial fibrillation. PT: pulmonary trunk; SCV, ICVs: superior and inferior caval veins.

References Cited

1. Cabrera JÁ, Anderson RH, Macías Y, et al. Variable arrangement of the atrioventricular conduction axis within the triangle of Koch: implications for permanent His bundle pacing. *Clin Electrophysiol* 2020; **6**: 362–377.

2. Macías Y, Tretter JT, Sánchez-Quintana D, et al. The atrioventricular conduction axis and the aortic root – inferences for transcatheter replacement of the aortic valve. *Clinical Anatomy* 2022; **35**: 143–154.

3. Massing GK, James TN. Anatomical configuration of the His bundle and bundle branches in the human heart. *Circulation* 1976; **53**: 609–621.

4. Tretter JT, Spicer DE, Macías Y, et al. Vulnerability of the ventricular conduction axis during transcatheter aortic valvar implantation: a translational pathologic study. *Clin Anat* 2023; **36**: 836–846.

5. Anderson RH, Spicer DE, Mori S. Of tracts, rings, nodes, cusps, sinuses, and arrhythmias – a comment on Szili-Torok et al.'s paper entitled 'The "Dead-End Tract" and Its Role in Arrhythmogenesis'. *J Cardiovasc Dev Dis* 2016; **3**: 11.

6. Anderson RH, Sanchez-Quintana D, Mori S, Cabrera JA, Back Sternick E. Re-evaluation of the structure of the atrioventricular node and its connections with the atrium. *EP Europace* 2020; **22**: 821–830.

7. Durrer D, Schuilenburg RM, Wellens HJJ. Pre-excitation revisited. *Am J Cardiol* 1970; **25**: 690–698.

8. Mahaim I. *Maladies organiques du faisceau de His-Tawara.* Paris: Masson et Cie; 1931.

9. Sternick EB, Sanchez-Quintana D, Wellens HJ, Anderson RH. Mahaim revisited. *Arrhythmia Electrophysiol Rev* 2022; **11**: e14.

10. Cabrera JÁ, Anderson RH, Porta-Sánchez A, et al. The atrioventricular conduction axis and its implications for permanent pacing. *Arrhythmia Electrophysiol Rev* 2021; **10**: 181.

11. Sealy WC, Gallagher JJ, Pritchett ELC. The surgical anatomy of Kent bundles based on electrophysiological mapping and surgical exploration. *J Thorac Cardiovasc Surg* 1978; **76**: 804–815.

12. Ohnell RF. Preexcitation, a cardiac abnormality. Pathophysiological, patho-anatomical and clinical studies of an excitatory spread phenomenon. *Acta Med Scand* 1944; **152** (Suppl.1): 167.

13. Anderson RH, Davies MJ, Becker AE. Atrioventricular ring specialized tissue in the normal heart. *Eur J Cardiol* 1974; **2**: 219–230.

14. Becker AE, Anderson RH, Durrer D, Wellens HJJ. The anatomical substrates of Wolff-Parkinson-White syndrome. A clinicopathologic correlation in seven patients. *Circulation* 1978; **57**: 870–879.

15. Sealy WC, Gallagher JJ. The surgical approach to the septal area of the heart based on experience with 45 patients with Kent bundles. *J Thorac Cardiovasc Surg* 1980; **79**: 542–551.

16. Tretter JT, Spicer DE, Sánchez-Quintana D, et al. Miniseries 1 – part III: 'behind the scenes' in the triangle of Koch. *EP Europace* 2022; **24**: 455–463.

17. Johnson DC, Ross DL, Uther JB. The surgical cure of atrioventricular junctional reentrant tachycardia. In DP Zipes, J Jalife, eds., *Cardiac Electrophysiology from Cell to Bedside.* London: W.B. Saunders; 1990: pp. 921–923.

18. Guiraudon GM, Klein GJ, Sharma AD, et al. Surgical approach to anterior septal accessory pathways in 20 patients with the Wolff-Parkinson-White syndrome. *Eur J Cardio-thorac Surg* 1988; **2**: 201–206.

19. Anderson RH, Sánchez-Quintana D, Mori S, et al. Unusual variants of pre-excitation: from anatomy to ablation: part I – understanding the anatomy of the variants of ventricular pre-excitation. *J Cardiovasc Electrophys* 2019; **30**: 2170–2180.

20. Guiraudon CM, Guiraudon GM, Klein GJ. 'Nodal ventricular' Mahaim pathway: histologic evidence for an accessory atrioventricular pathway with an AV node-like morphology. *Circulation* 1988; **78** (Suppl.2): 1035–1040.

21. Kent AFS. The structure of the cardiac tissues at the auriculo-ventricular junction. *J Physiol* 1913; **47**: 17–18.

22. Anderson RH, Ho SY, Gillette PC, Becker AE. Mahaim, Kent and abnormal atrioventricular conduction. *Cardiovasc Res* 1996; **31**: 480–491.

23. Cosio FG, Lopez-Gil M, Giocolea A, Arribas F, Barroso JL. Radiofrequency ablation of the inferior vena cava-tricuspid valve isthmus in common atrial flutter. *Am J Cardiol* 1993; **71**: 705–709.

24. Cabrera JA, Sanchez-Quintana D, Ho SY, Medina A, Anderson RH. The architecture of the atrial musculature between the orifice of the inferior caval vein and the tricuspid valve: the anatomy of the isthmus. *J Cardiovasc Electrophysiol* 1998; **9**: 1186–1195.

25. Mavroudis C, Backer CL, Deal BJ, Johnsrude C, Strasburger J. Total cavopulmonary conversion and maze procedure for patients with failure of the Fontan operation. *J Thorac Cardiovasc Surg* 2001; **122**: 863–871.

26. Cox JL, Boineau JP, Schuessler RB, Jaquiss RD, Lappas DG. Modification of the maze procedure for atrial flutter and atrial fibrillation. I. Rationale and surgical results. *J Thorac Cardiovasc Surg* 1995; **110**: 473–484.

27. Defauw JJ, Guiraudon GM, van Hemel NM, et al. Surgical therapy of paroxysmal atrial fibrillation with the 'corridor' operation. *Ann Thorac Surg* 1992; **53**: 564–570.

28. Cox JL, Ad N. New surgical and catheter-based modifications of the Maze procedure. *Semin Thorac Cardiovasc Surg* 2000; **12**: 68–73.

29. Goya M, Ouyang F, Ernst S, et al. Electroanatomic mapping and catheter ablation of breakthroughs from the right atrium to the superior vena cava in patients with atrial fibrillation. *Circulation* 2002; **106**: 1317–1320.

30. Pappone C, Oreto G, Rosanio S, et al. Atrial electroanatomic remodelling after circumferential radiofrequency pulmonary vein ablation: efficacy of an anatomic approach in a large cohort of patients with atrial fibrillation. *Circulation* 2001; **104**: 2539–2544.

31. Shah DC, Haissaguerre M, Jais P. Catheter ablation of pulmonary vein foci for atrial fibrillation. PV foci ablation for atrial fibrillation. *Thorac Cardiovasc Surgeon* 1999; **47** (Suppl.3): 352–356.

32. Ho SY, Cabrera JA, Tran VH, et al. Architecture of the pulmonary veins: relevance to radiofrequency ablation. *Heart* 2001; **86**: 265–270.

33. Hocini M, Ho SY, Kawara T, et al. Electrical conduction in canine pulmonary veins. Electrophysiological and anatomical correlation. *Circulation* 2002; **105**: 2442–2448.

34. Perez-Lugones A, McMahan JT, Ratliff NB, et al. Evidence of specialized conduction cells in human pulmonary veins of patients with atrial fibrillation.

J Cardiovasc Electrophysiol 2003; **14**: 803–809.

35. Mommersteeg MT, Christoffels VM, Anderson RH, Moorman AF. Atrial fibrillation: a developmental point of view. *Heart Rhythm* 2009; **6**: 1818–1824.

36. Anderson RH, Mohun TJ, Sánchez-Quintana D, et al. The anatomic substrates for outflow tract arrhythmias. *Heart Rhythm* 2019; **16**: 290–297.

37. Cheung JW, Anderson RH, Markowitz SM, Lerman BB. Catheter ablation of arrhythmias originating from the left ventricular outflow tract. *JACC Clin Electrophysiol* 2019; **5**: 1–2.

38. Bohora S, Lokhandwala Y, Sternick EB, Anderson RH, Wellens HJ. Reappraisal and new observations on atrial tachycardia ablated from the non-coronary aortic sinus of Valsalva. *Europace* 2018; **20**: 124–133.

39. Rosenquist GC, Clark EB, Sweeney LJ, McAllister HA. The normal spectrum of mitral and aortic valve discontinuity. *Circulation* 1976; **54**: 298–301.

40. Timmermans C, Rodriguez LM, Crijns HJ, Moorman AF, Wellens HJ. Idiopathic left bundle-branch block-shaped ventricular tachycardia may originate above the pulmonary valve. *Circulation* 2003; **108**: 1960–1967.

41. Sizarov A, Lamers WH, Mohun TJ, et al. Three-dimensional and molecular analysis of the arterial pole of the developing human heart. *J Anat* 2012; **220**: 336–349.

42. Karamlou T, Silber I, Lao R, et al. Outcomes after late reoperation in patients with repaired tetralogy of Fallot: the impact of arrhythmia and arrhythmia surgery. *Ann Thorac Surg* 2006; **81**: 1786–1793.

43. Mavroudis C, Deal BJ, Backer CL, Tsao S. Arrhythmia surgery in patients with and without congenital heart disease. *Ann Thorac Surg* 2008; **86**: 857–868.

Chapter 7

Analytic Description of Congenitally Malformed Hearts

Systems for describing congenital cardiac malformations have frequently been based on embryological concepts and theories. As useful as these systems have been, they have often had the effect of confusing the clinician, rather than clarifying the basic anatomy of a given lesion. As far as the surgeon is concerned, the essence of a particular malformation lies not in its presumed morphogenesis, but in the underlying anatomy. An effective system for describing this anatomy must be based on the morphology as it is observed. At the same time, it must be capable of accounting for all congenital cardiac conditions, even those that, as yet, might not have been encountered. To be useful clinically, the system must be not only broad and accurate, but also clear and consistent. The terminology used, therefore, should be unambiguous. It should be as simple as possible. The sequential segmental approach provides such a system.[1] This is the more so when the emphasis is placed on its surgical applications.[2] The basis of the system is, in the first instance, to analyse individually the architectural make-up of the so-called cardiac segments. These are the atrial chambers, the ventricular mass, and the arterial segment.[3] Emphasis is then given to the fashion in which the components of the segments are joined or, in some instances, not joined to each other across the atrioventricular and ventriculo-arterial junctions (Figure 7.1). Still further attention is then devoted to the interrelationships of the cardiac structures within each of the individual segments. Such an approach provides the basic framework within which all other associated malformations can then be catalogued.[4]

The Morphological Method

Before getting to grips with the components of the different segments, and going over the features of their connections, or lack of connection, we should discuss our approach to the definition of the entities to be considered. It is no secret that nomenclature remains a contentious issue. Many of the problematic areas relate to the way in which given components are defined. Throughout the evolution of our preferred approach, we have sought to follow the important principle established by Richard Van Praagh fifty years ago.[5] He and his colleagues set out their stall when criticizing one of the early works produced by the European school of morphologists.[6] In that work, we had sought to argue that, when a ventricular chamber lacked its inlet component, it was no longer worthy of ventricular status. Van Praagh and his colleagues[5] pointed to the lack of logic in our approach. They highlighted our mistake in seeking to define one component of the heart on the basis of another component that was itself variable. Instead, the Bostonians

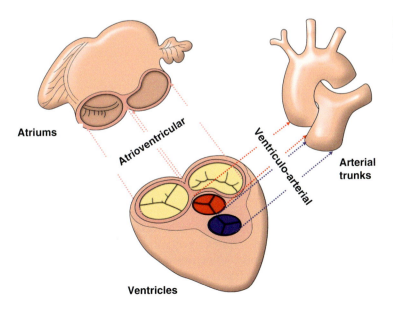

Figure 7.1 The drawing shows the three segments of the heart. These are the atriums, the ventricular mass, and the arterial trunks. The segments are joined together at the atrioventricular and ventriculo-arterial junctions.

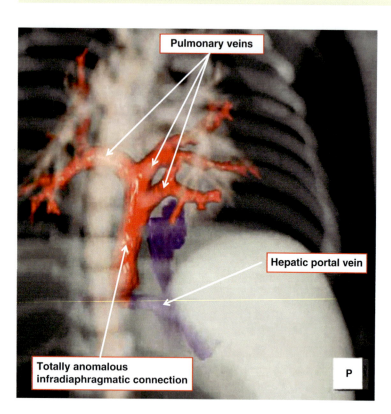

Figure 7.2 The image shows totally anomalous pulmonary venous return to the hepatic portal vein. If the pulmonary veins, in this instance, were being used to define the morphologically right atrium, then the liver perforce would become the right atrium. Orientation cube, lower right: P, posterior.

argued, we should have defined the component on the basis of its own intrinsic anatomy. They dubbed this principle the 'morphological method'.[5] The essence of the approach is exemplified when considering the optimal means of distinguishing between the atrial chambers. The most obvious feature of the atriums is their venous connections. Although most obvious in the normal situation, these features are themselves variable. When most needed, which as we will discuss is in the setting of isomerism, they are themselves usually anomalous. Even when the heart is otherwise normal, the finding of totally anomalous infradiaphragmatic pulmonary venous return (Figure 7.2) points to the inability of using the pulmonary venous connections as a marker for the morphologically right atrium. If the connection of the pulmonary veins was used in the illustrated setting, then the liver would need to be defined as the right atrium. It is for this reason that, following the morphological method, we now define all entities on the basis of their intrinsic morphology. It then transpires that the use of the philosophical concept of the morphological method serves to resolve very many of the ongoing terminological disputes.

Atrial Arrangement

The first step in analysing any malformed heart is to determine the arrangement of the chambers making up the atrial segment. This means that, as our starting point, we must establish how many atrial chambers are present. The literature is replete with descriptions of 'triatrial hearts'. As far as we are aware, all such hearts, in reality, have division of one or other of the morphologically left or the morphologically right atriums.

When the morphological method is used to distinguish between the chambers, as discussed in the previous section, then we can take advantage of the appendage being the most constant atrial component. In our experience, there are only ever two appendages present. On occasion, they can lie alongside one another in the arrangement known as juxtaposition. When juxtaposed, the right appendage itself can be divided. Very rarely, the left appendage can be duplicated. Even in these circumstances, nonetheless, when distinguishing between the appendages on the basis of the extent of the pectinate muscles within them relative to the atrial vestibules,[7] it remains the case that atrial chambers can only be of morphologically right or morphologically left type.

The morphologically right appendage is broad and triangular, whereas the morphologically left appendage is finger-like, and has a much narrower neck (Figure 7.3). In most instances, it is possible to identify the appendages simply on the basis of their shape (Figure 7.4). Only in circumstances of uncertainty will it prove necessary to inspect the extent of the pectinate muscles (Figures 7.5, 7.6), with this feature being readily visible to the surgeon once the atrial chambers have been opened.

When judged on the extent of the pectinate muscles relative to the atrial vestibules, there are only four topological ways in which the appendages can be arranged within the atrial mass (Figure 7.7). Almost always, the atrium possessing the appendage in which the pectinate muscles extend to the crux is right sided, while the one with a smooth infero-posterior vestibule is left sided. This usual arrangement is often called situs solitus. Rarely, the appendages can be disposed in mirror-imaged fashion, so-called situs inversus. More common than the

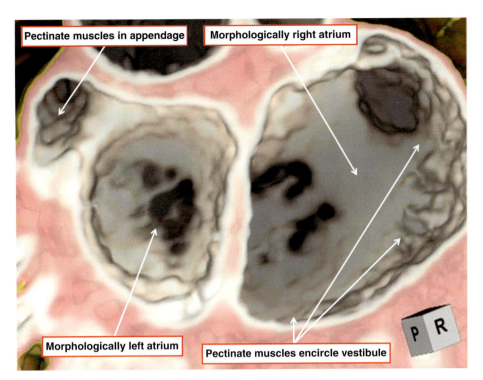

Figure 7.3 The virtual dissection of a computed tomographic dataset shows how, in the usual arrangement, the pectinate muscles of the morphologically right appendage encircle the vestibule of the tricuspid valve, whereas in the morphologically left atrium the pectinate muscles are restricted to the tubular appendage. Orientation cube, lower right: P, posterior, R, right.

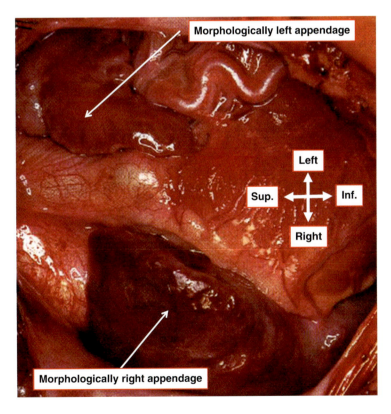

Figure 7.4 This operative view, taken through a median sternotomy, shows the differences between the broad triangular morphologically right atrial appendage, and the narrow finger-like morphologically left atrial appendage.

mirror-imaged topological arrangement, but still relatively rare, is the situation in which the appendages of both atrial chambers have the same morphology. This can occur in two forms, with either bilateral morphologically right (Figure 7.8) or bilateral morphologically left (Figure 7.9) appendages. These bilaterally symmetrical topological patterns, or isomeric arrangements, have traditionally been named according to the arrangement of the abdominal organs, particularly the spleen. This is because they usually exist with jumbled up abdominal arrangement, an arrangement also termed visceral heterotaxy.[8,9] It is far more convenient, as well as more accurate, to designate them in terms of their own intrinsic morphology.[10,11] This is particularly pertinent since the features can readily be determined by the surgeon in the operating room. Isomerism of the right

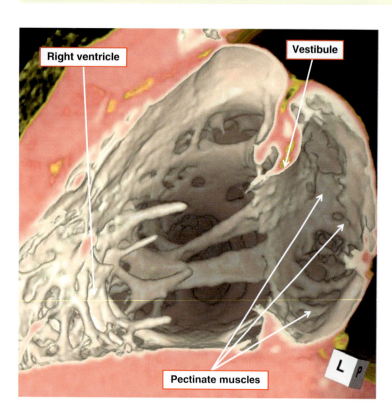

Figure 7.5 The virtual dissection of a computed tomographic dataset shows the pectinate muscles of the morphologically right atrial appendage forming the entirety of the parietal wall of the right atrium, encircling the atrial vestibule. Orientation cube, lower right: L, left.

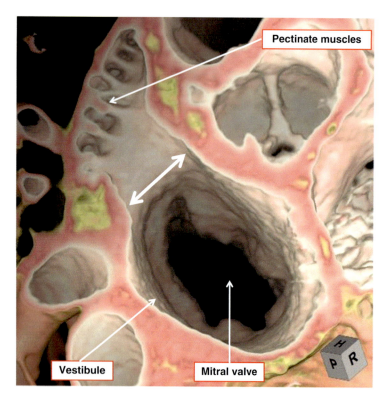

Figure 7.6 As shown in this computed tomogram, the pectinate muscles of the morphologically left appendage are confined within the tubular component, which has a very narrow junction with the body of the atrium (double-headed arrow).

appendages is usually, but not always, found with absence of the spleen. It is almost always associated with right bronchial isomerism. Isomerism of the left appendages is typically found, but again not always, with multiple spleens. The association with left bronchial isomerism is more constant.

The anticipated topological arrangement of the atrial appendages can be predicted preoperatively with a high degree of accuracy by studying the relationships of the abdominal great vessels as determined with cross-sectional ultrasonography.[12] When identified, knowledge of isomerism of the atrial

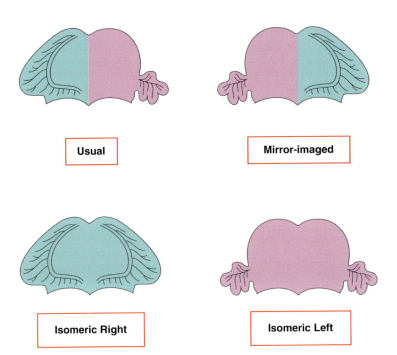

Figure 7.7 The drawing shows the four possible arrangements of the atrial appendages. The appendages cannot always be distinguished on the basis of their shape. The best means of distinguishing between them is to establish the extent of the pectinate muscles. These muscles extend all the way to the crux in the morphologically right atrial appendage, but are confined around the mouth of the appendage in the morphologically left atrial appendage, leaving a smooth posterior vestibule. Using this criterion, all congenitally malformed hearts have appendages fitting within one of the four groups shown in the cartoon.

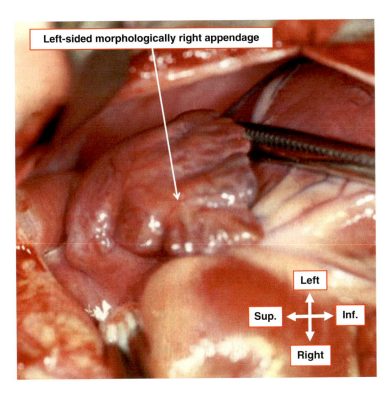

Figure 7.8 This surgical view, through a median sternotomy, shows a left-sided atrial appendage of morphologically right pattern. The right-sided appendage was also of right morphology, so the patient had isomerism of the right atrial appendages. Note the crest of the appendage in relation to the left superior caval vein and the terminal groove. When examined internally, pectinate muscles encircled both atrioventricular junctions.

appendages is of value in two additional ways. First, it alerts the surgeon to unusual dispositions of the sinus node.[13] In right isomerism, the sinus node, being a morphologically right atrial structure, is duplicated. A node is found laterally in each of the terminal grooves.[14] In left isomerism, there are no terminal grooves. In this situation, the sinus node is a poorly formed structure, lacking a constant site. It may even be found in the anterior interatrial groove, close to the atrioventricular junction.[14]

The second advantage of recognizing isomeric appendages is that the arrangements are known to be harbingers of complex intracardiac lesions. Hearts with isomeric appendages of either type tend to have bilateral superior caval veins, an effectively common atrial chamber, albeit with two isomeric

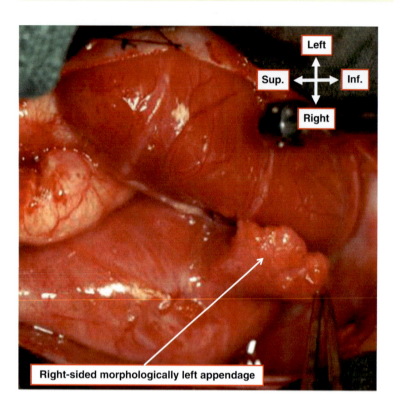

Figure 7.9 This surgical view, through a median sternotomy, shows a right-sided atrial appendage of morphologically left pattern. The left-sided appendage was also of left morphology, so the patient had isomerism of the left atrial appendages. Note the absence of any terminal groove. Internal inspection confirmed the presence of smooth bilateral posterior vestibules.

appendages, and common atrioventricular valves. Right isomerism is always associated with totally anomalous pulmonary venous connection, even if the pulmonary veins are joined to one or other atrium. The coronary sinus is always absent in this variant. It is also seen most frequently with pulmonary valvar stenosis or atresia, and in association with a univentricular atrioventricular connection, typically double inlet ventricle through a common valve. Left isomerism, in the majority of cases, is associated with interruption of the inferior caval vein, with continuation of the venous drainage from the abdomen through the azygos system of veins.

The Atrioventricular Junctions

Having established the arrangement of the atrial appendages, the next step in sequential analysis is to determine the morphology of the atrioventricular junctions. For this, the surgeon needs to know how the atrial chambers are, or are not, connected to the chambers present within the ventricular mass. Almost always, there are two ventricular chambers, which can only be of right or left morphology. The morphological distinction, following again the precepts of the morphological method,[5] is based on the nature of the apical trabeculations. This is because it is the apical components that are most constant. In the morphologically right ventricle, these trabeculations are coarse, in contrast to the fine criss-crossing trabeculations that characterize the morphologically left ventricle (Figure 7.10). The inter-relationships between the two ventricles then permits the description of ventricular topology. This feature is determined according to the way that the palmar surfaces of the hands can be placed on the septal surface of the morphologically right ventricle such that the thumb is within the inlet component, and the fingers in the ventricular outlet. The patterns then reflect the topology of either the right or left hand (Figure 7.11). Once having distinguished between the ventricles, and assessed their topology, it is possible to determine the way in which the atrial chambers are connected, or not connected, to them. In most instances, there are two atrioventricular junctions, although one of the junctions can be absent. Also important is the morphology of the valves that guard the atrioventricular junctions. This is because the paired junctions can be guarded by a common atrioventricular valve. Junctional arrangement and valvar morphology are separate and independent features.

There are five distinct and discrete ways in which the atrial chambers may be connected to the ventricular mass. The fifth variation itself has two subtypes, along with an intriguing further variation. Most often, the cavities of the atrial chambers are connected across the atrioventricular junctions to the cavities of their morphologically appropriate ventricles. This produces concordant atrioventricular connections. When each atrium is connected in this way to its own ventricle, there is rarely any difficulty in distinguishing the morphology of the ventricles, even when the ventricles themselves are unusually related one to the other. In the second pattern, which represents discordant connections, each atrium is connected with a morphologically inappropriate ventricle. In the initial versions of the sequential segmental approach, these connections had been described in terms of 'concordance' and 'discordance'.[1] This was a mistake. When Van Praagh first introduced the concepts of concordance and discordance, he was defining these terms on the basis of segmental harmony or segmental disharmony.[3] Thus, any heart with the segmental combination of {S,D,*}, or {I,L,*} was deemed to represent concordance. This was irrespective of how the cavities of the chambers were joined, or not joined,

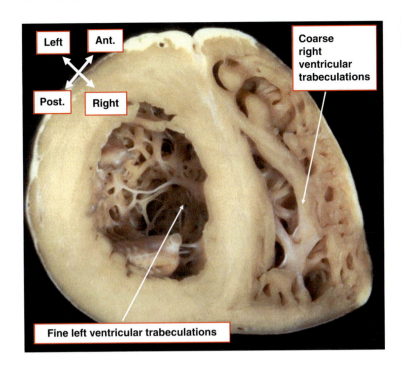

Figure 7.10 The apical part of the normal ventricular mass has been amputated, and is viewed from above. It shows the marked difference between the fine apical trabeculations of the morphologically left ventricle when compared with the coarse right ventricular apical trabeculations.

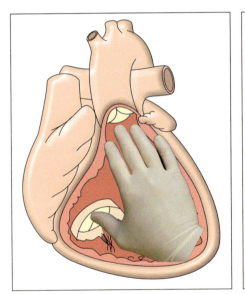

RIGHT HAND TOPOLOGY　　**LEFT HAND TOPOLOGY**

Figure 7.11 The drawing shows how the patterns of ventricular topology can be described, figuratively speaking, in terms of the way that the palmar surface of the hands can be placed on the septal surface of the morphologically right ventricle. The fingers point up the outlet, and the thumb lies in the inlet, giving right-hand and left-hand patterns. In the arrangements shown, the atrioventricular connections are concordant, but the ventriculo-arterial connections can also be discordant, with the aorta arising from the morphologically right ventricle (see Figure 7.29).

across the atrioventricular junctions. In similar fashion, {S,L,*} and {I,D,*} were considered to show atrioventricular discordance. We failed to appreciate, in the early stages of evolving the sequential approach, that Van Praagh was using segmental harmony, rather than the connections between the chambers, as his criterion for distinction of concordance as opposed to discordance.[3] We now do not use 'concordance' or 'discordance'. Instead, we use 'concordant' or 'discordant', in adjectival fashion, so as explicitly to emphasize the fashion of the connections between the components of the cardiac segments.

Concordant and discordant connections can exist with either the usual or mirror-imaged arrangement of the atrial appendages (Figure 7.12). They cannot be found when the atrial appendages are isomeric. When the appendages are isomeric, and each atrium is connected to its own ventricle, then of necessity one junction will be concordantly connected, but the other junction will be discordantly connected (Figure 7.13). This will occur irrespective of the topological pattern of the ventricular mass (see below). The arrangement produces the third discrete pattern, namely biventricular and mixed atrioventricular connections.

In the three connections described thus far, each atrium is connected to its own ventricle. This means that the atrioventricular connections themselves are biventricular. In the remaining two types of atrioventricular connection, the atrial chambers, with one exception, connect to only one ventricle. In the first of these patterns, both atrial chambers connect to the

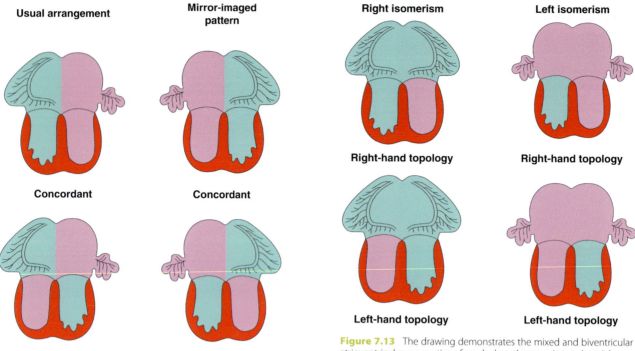

Figure 7.12 The drawing shows how the atrial chambers can be connected to the ventricles in concordant or discordant fashion, with each pattern existing in usual and mirror-imaged variants.

Figure 7.13 The drawing demonstrates the mixed and biventricular atrioventricular connections found when there are isomeric atrial appendages, and each atrium is connected to its own ventricle. In each pattern, half of the heart is concordantly connected, and the other half is discordant. It is essential in these settings, therefore, to describe both the type of isomerism and the specific ventricular topology.

same ventricle. This is double inlet atrioventricular connection (Figure 7.14). In the other variant, one of the atrial chambers is connected to a ventricle, but the other atrium has no connection with the ventricular mass. This latter arrangement can then be divided into two subtypes, depending on whether absence of the connection is right sided (Figure 7.15) or left sided (Figure 7.16). An intriguing variation is then seen when one of the atrioventricular connections is absent. This is when the atrioventricular valve guarding the solitary connection straddles the septum, being attached in both ventricles. This produces a uniatrial, but a biventricular, atrioventricular connection (Figure 7.17). This can be found when the missing connection is either right sided or left sided.[15]

There has been much controversy concerning the description of the hearts in which the atrial chambers connect to only one ventricle. It became conventional to describe them in terms of single ventricle, or common ventricle, or univentricular hearts. It is exceedingly rare, however, to find patients with solitary ventricles. Almost always, in patients described as having univentricular hearts, the ventricular mass contains more than one chamber. By focusing on the fact that the atrioventricular connection is, in reality, joined to only one ventricle, we are able to achieve a satisfactory solution for this dilemma. Thus, the hearts can logically and accurately be described as functionally univentricular. Imbalance between the ventricles in some patients with biventricular atrioventricular connections can produce such a functionally univentricular arrangement, with one ventricle being dominant.[16] In those with univentricular atrioventricular connections, one of the ventricles is dominant because the other ventricle is incomplete, lacking its inlet component. The dominant ventricle, which supports the atrioventricular junction or junctions, can take one of three morphologies: right, left, or indeterminate (Figure 7.18). Most frequently, as judged from the pattern of its apical trabecular component, the dominant ventricle is morphologically left. The complementary ventricle is morphologically right. Such incomplete right ventricles are always found antero-superiorly relative to the dominant left ventricle, irrespective of whether there is double inlet, absent right, or absent left atrioventricular connection. They can be positioned either to the right (Figure 7.19) or to the left (Figure 7.20) relative to the dominant ventricle.

More rarely, the atrial chambers can be connected to a dominant right ventricle. This happens most frequently in the absence of the left atrioventricular connection (Figure 7.21). It can be found with double inlet or, rarely, with absence of the right atrioventricular connection. When only the right ventricle is connected to the atrial chambers, and hence dominant, it is the left ventricle that is incomplete, lacking its atrioventricular connection and its inlet portion. The incomplete left ventricle will always be found in postero-inferior position. Usually it is left sided, although rarely it can be right sided.

In the third morphological configuration found with double inlet or, exceedingly rarely, with absence of either atrioventricular connection, the atrial chambers connect to a solitary ventricle. Such solitary ventricles have particularly coarse and indeterminate apical trabeculations (Figure 7.22). Incomplete second ventricles are never found in this variant of univentricular

7 Analytic Description of Congenitally Malformed Hearts

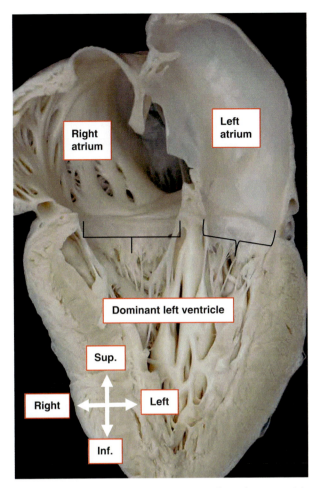

Figure 7.14 When both atriums are connected to only one ventricle, the atrioventricular connection is univentricular. In this heart, showing a four-chamber section in anatomical orientation, there is double inlet to a dominant left ventricle. The brackets show the segments of atrial vestibular myocardium, connected to the dominant left ventricle through separate atrioventricular valves.

atrioventricular connection. The only septal structure in the ventricle is that separating the outflow tracts.

Valvar Morphology

As emphasized, atrioventricular valvar morphology is independent of the way in which the atrial chambers connect with the ventricles. Valvar morphology, therefore, constitutes a separate feature of the atrioventricular junctions. When the connections are concordant, discordant, mixed, or double inlet, then both atrial chambers are connected, actually or potentially, to the ventricular mass. The two atrioventricular junctions can then be guarded by two separate atrioventricular valves (Figure 7.23), or by a common valve (Figure 7.24). When there are two valves, either of them can be imperforate, blocking a potential atrioventricular connection. An imperforate valve, therefore, needs to be distinguished from absence of an atrioventricular connection. Both variations, nonetheless, produce atrioventricular valvar atresia. The essence of the imperforate valve is that the atrioventricular connection has formed, but is blocked by the conjoined valvar leaflets (Figure 7.25). When the connection is absent, the floor of the atrium involved is completely separated from the ventricular mass by the fibro-adipose tissue of the atrioventricular groove (see Figures 7.15 and 7.16).

Either of two valves, or a common valve, can also straddle the ventricular septum. Straddling of the tension apparatus of a valve, when the valvar tension apparatus is attached to both sides of the ventricular septum, should be distinguished from overriding of its supporting atrioventricular junction (Figure 7.26). Overriding is present when the junction is connected to both ventricles. The degree of override, which usually co-exists with straddling, determines the precise atrioventricular connection present. When adjudicating the connection in the presence of overriding, the overriding valve is assigned to the ventricle connected to its greater part (Figure 7.27).

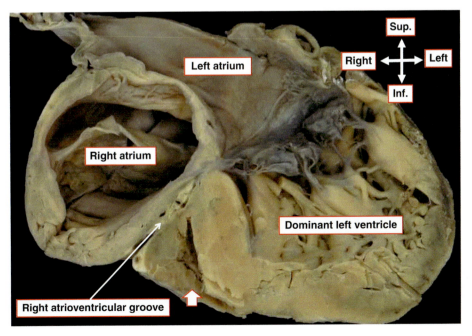

Figure 7.15 This anatomical specimen, seen in four-chamber orientation, shows absence of the right atrioventricular connection, with the fibro-adipose tissue of the right atrioventricular groove interposing between the right atrial floor and the base of the ventricular mass. This arrangement produces another form of univentricular atrioventricular connection. In this case, the morphology is that of classical tricuspid atresia, with the left atrium connected to a dominant left ventricle. Note the presence of the base of the incomplete right ventricle (white arrow with red borders), which has no connection with the atrial chambers.

161

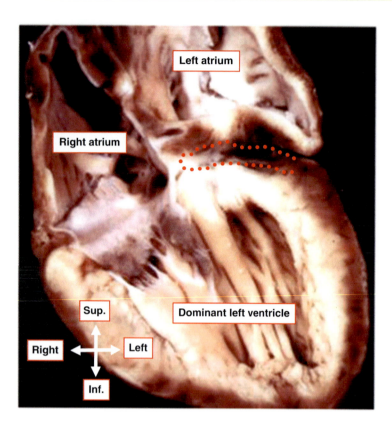

Figure 7.16 This anatomical specimen, again seen in four-chamber orientation (compare with Figures 7.14 and 7.15), shows absence of the left atrioventricular connection (dotted line), giving the third variant of univentricular atrioventricular connection. In this example, the right atrium is connected to a dominant left ventricle through a right-sided atrioventricular valve.

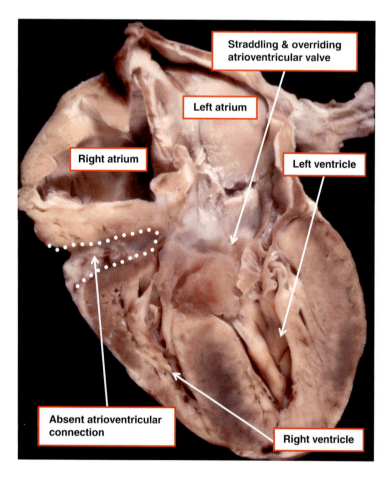

Figure 7.17 This heart shows the arrangement when there is absence of the right atrioventricular connection (dotted line), but with the solitary atrioventricular valve straddling the ventricular septum. This produces a uniatrial but biventricular atrioventricular connection, shown here in the setting of usual atrial arrangement with right hand ventricular topology.

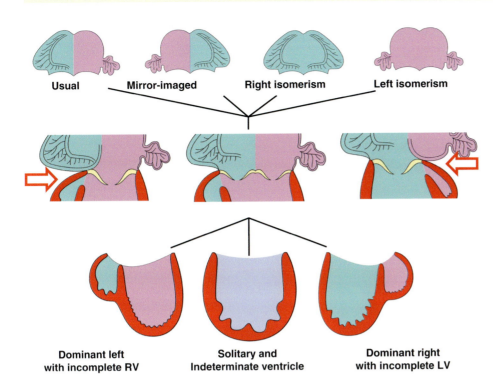

Figure 7.18 This drawing shows the multiple possibilities for univentricular atrioventricular connection that can be produced by combining the variations in atrial morphology, atrioventricular connection, and ventricular morphology. It takes no account of the further variations possible according to ventricular relationships, ventriculo-arterial connections, and so on. The arrows in the middle row emphasize the absence of one of the atrioventricular connections. RV, right ventricle; LV, left ventricle.

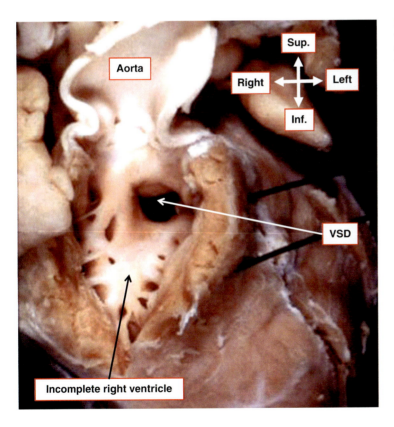

Figure 7.19 In this anatomical specimen with double inlet left ventricle, the incomplete right ventricle is positioned anterosuperiorly and to the right of the dominant left ventricle. VSD, ventricular septal defect.

The possible arrangements are much more limited when one atrioventricular connection is absent. In this situation, the solitary valve can either be committed in its entirety to one ventricle, or else it can straddle and override. When the valve straddles and overrides in this setting, then the atrioventricular connection itself is uniatrial but biventricular (Figure 7.17).

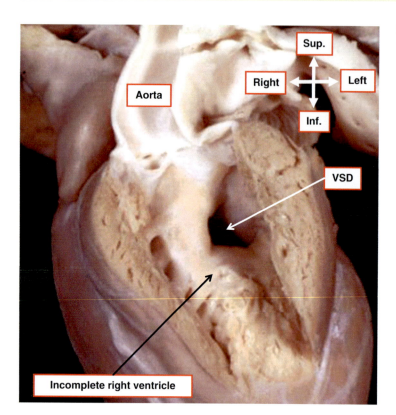

Figure 7.20 This anatomical specimen, again with double inlet left ventricle, has the incomplete right ventricle in anterosuperior and leftward position relative to the dominant left ventricle. VSD, ventricular septal defect.

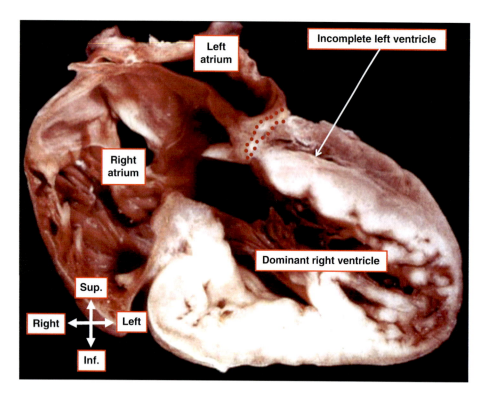

Figure 7.21 This section through a specimen, shown in four-chamber orientation, illustrates absence of the left atrioventricular connection (red dotted line) with the right atrium connected to a dominant right ventricle. This produces one of the variants of the hypoplastic left heart syndrome.

Ventricular Morphology and Topology

The nature of the atrioventricular connections is inextricably linked with the architectural arrangement of the ventricular mass. Biventricular atrioventricular connections, for example, cannot be diagnosed without knowledge of ventricular morphology. Double inlet, and absent connections, in contrast, can all be identified without mention of ventricular morphology. Even in this setting, it is always necessary to give more information concerning the arrangement of the ventricular mass, specifically the morphology and relationships of the dominant and incomplete ventricles. In the case of mixed

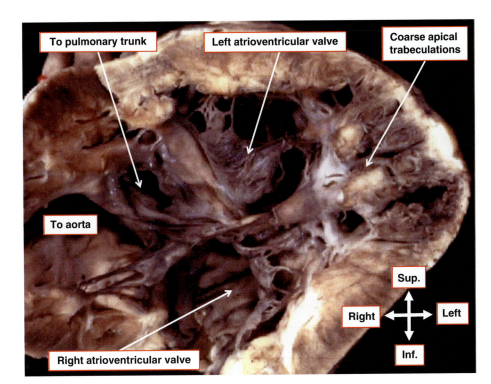

Figure 7.22 This heart, opened in clam-like fashion, has double inlet to, and double outlet from, a solitary and indeterminate ventricle, the ventricle itself having very coarse apical trabeculations.

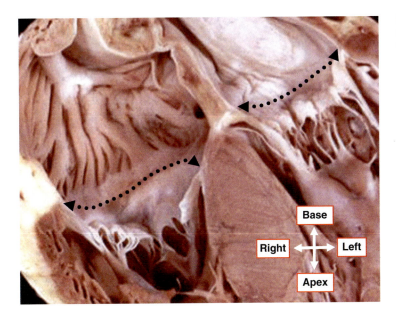

Figure 7.23 This normal heart, sectioned in four-chamber orientation, shows the right and left atrioventricular junctions (dotted lines with double-headed arrows) guarded by separate atrioventricular valves.

and biventricular atrioventricular connections, it is also necessary to describe the pattern in which the morphologically right ventricle is positioned relative to the morphologically left ventricle. This feature can take only one of two topological arrangements. This is because, when their connections are mixed, the right-sided atrium, with either a morphologically right or left appendage, can only be connected to either a morphologically right or a morphologically left ventricle (see Figure 7.13). When there is right isomerism, and the right-sided atrium is connected to a morphologically right ventricle, the ventricular mass is typically as seen in hearts with concordant atrioventricular connections and usual atrial arrangement. In contrast, when there is right isomerism, and the right-sided atrium is connected to a morphologically left ventricle, the ventricular mass is similar to the pattern found with discordant atrioventricular connections and usual atrial arrangement.

As we have already discussed, these two basic patterns of ventricular topology can conveniently be described according to the way in which the hands, figuratively speaking, can be placed palm downward on the septal surface of the morphologically right ventricle. The other hand will then fit in the

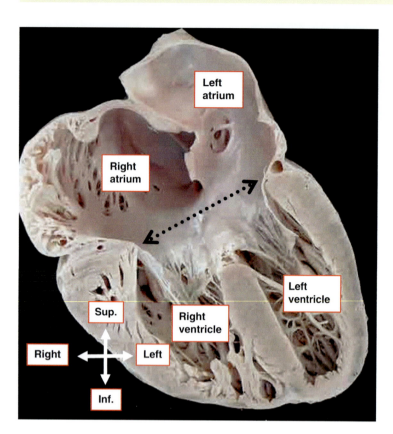

Figure 7.24 This section, again in four-chamber orientation (compare with Figure 7.23), shows that the right and left atrioventricular junctions (dotted line with double-headed arrows) are guarded by a common atrioventricular valve in the setting of an atrioventricular septal defect.

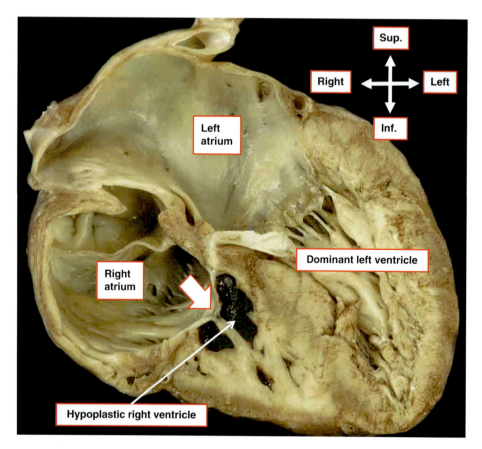

Figure 7.25 This section of a heart, cut in four-chamber orientation, shows an imperforate right atrioventricular valve (white arrow with red borders) connecting to a hypoplastic right ventricle. The atrioventricular connections remain concordant, even though the right valve is imperforate.

7 Analytic Description of Congenitally Malformed Hearts

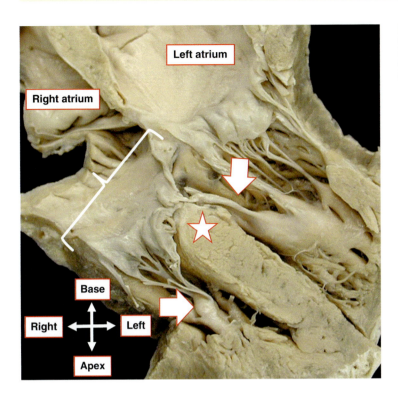

Figure 7.26 This section of a heart, seen in four-chamber orientation, shows how the tension apparatus of the right atrioventricular valve (arrows) is attached to both sides of the ventricular septum (star), while the orifice of the right atrioventricular junction (bracket) is overriding the septal crest (star).

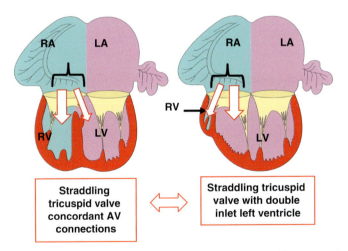

Figure 7.27 In presence of an overriding junction, be it a straddling tricuspid valve, as shown in Figure 7.26, or a ventriculo-arterial valve, the overriding junction (bracket) is assigned to the ventricle supporting its greater part. In the situation illustrated with straddling tricuspid valve, the atrioventricular (AV) connections are then defined accordingly. There is a spectrum between the illustrated extremes (double-headed arrow). The left-hand panel shows the situation with the junction connected primarily to the right ventricle (RV; large arrow), the lesser part joining the left ventricle (LV; small arrow). Hence, the atrioventricular connections are deemed to be concordant. In the right-hand panel, the larger part of the overriding junction is committed to the left ventricle, so that the connection is deemed to be double inlet. This is the essence of the 50% rule. Abbreviations: RA, LA – right and left atriums.

morphologically left ventricle in similar fashion, but it is the arrangement of the morphologically right ventricle that is chosen for the purposes of description (Figure 7.11). In the hearts with biventricular and mixed atrioventricular connections, it is this ventricular topology which determines the disposition of the atrioventricular conduction tissues.[13] When the atrial chambers connect to only one ventricle, the morphology of that ventricle must always be described. This is because the dominant ventricle can be of left ventricular, right ventricular, or solitary and indeterminate pattern. It is also necessary to describe the relationships of the dominant and incomplete ventricles.

Ventricular Relationships

Ventricular relationships, as opposed to ventricular topology, should generally be described as a separate feature of the heart. Where each atrium is connected to its own ventricle, the relationships are almost always in harmony with both the connection and topology present. When the atrial chambers are in their usual position with concordant atrioventricular connections, the relationships described in the setting of the heart within the chest are almost always for the morphologically right ventricle to be right sided, anterior, and superior to the morphologically left ventricle. In mirror-imaged atrial arrangement, with concordant atrioventricular connections, the morphologically right ventricle is almost always left sided and relatively anterior, but frequently more side by side relative to its neighbour.

With the atrial chambers in their usual arrangement, and when the atrioventricular connections are discordant, there is almost always the left-hand pattern of ventricular topology. With this pattern, the morphologically right ventricle is anticipated to be left sided (Figure 7.28). When discordant atrioventricular connections accompany mirror-imaged atrial arrangement, there is usually right-hand topology (Figure 7.29). The ventricular relationships are then similar to

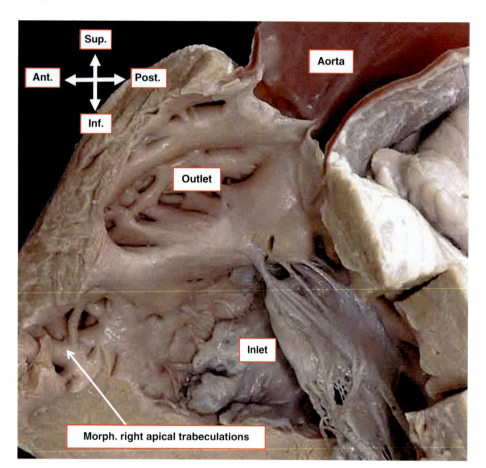

Figure 7.28 The left side of the heart is shown from a patient with discordant atrioventricular and ventriculo-arterial connections, in other words congenitally corrected transposition. It is the palmar surface of only the left hand that can be placed on the septal surface of the morphologically right ventricle so that the fingers occupy the ventricular outlet, and the thumb goes in the tricuspid valve guarding the inlet component.

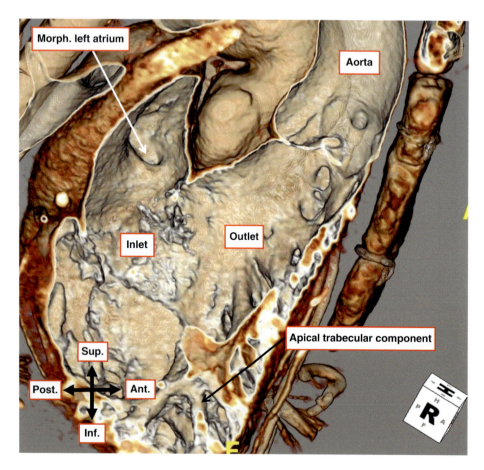

Figure 7.29 The computed tomogram shows the right side of the heart from a patient having congenitally corrected transposition in the setting of mirror-imaged atrial arrangement. The morphologically left atrium is right sided, but connects to a morphologically right ventricle with right-hand topology. It is the palmar surface of the right hand that fits on the septal surface so that the fingers are in the subaortic outlet and the thumb in the inlet component. Orientation cube, right-hand corner: R, right, H, head.

those seen in the normal heart, although the two chambers tend to be more side by side. When the relationships are as anticipated, it is unnecessary to describe them. Very occasionally, the relationships of the ventricles are not as anticipated for the connections present. This disharmony between connections and relationships underscores the anomaly known as the criss-cross heart,[17] better described as twisted atrioventricular connections. In this situation, and also in those with supero-inferior ventricles, connections and relationships must be described separately, using as much detail as is necessary to achieve unambiguous categorization. The essence of the criss-cross heart, and those with supero-inferior ventricles, is that the ventricular relationships are not as expected for the atrioventricular connection present. Even more rarely, the ventricular topology may be disharmonious with the atrioventricular connection.[18] All features must then be described.

In hearts with univentricular atrioventricular connection, it is the relationship of the incomplete ventricle to the dominant ventricle that must be described. When the left ventricle is dominant, the incomplete right ventricle is always antero-superior, but can be right or left sided. The sidedness of the ventricle does not affect the basic disposition of the atrioventricular conduction tissues in these hearts. With dominant right ventricle, the incomplete and rudimentary left ventricle, if present, is always postero-inferior, but again can be right or left sided. In this case, the sidedness of the incomplete ventricle will affect the disposition of the atrioventricular conduction tissue.

When considering the atrioventricular junctions, therefore, there are four different features to take into account. These are, first, the way the atrial myocardium is connected to the ventricular mass, second, the morphology of the atrioventricular valves guarding the junctions, third, the ventricular morphology and topology, and finally the ventricular relationships. All are of importance to the surgeon because they influence the disposition of the atrioventricular conduction axis.

Ventriculo-Arterial Junctions

Analysis of the ventriculo-arterial junctions proceeds as described for the atrioventricular junctions, with the morphology of the connections, the valvar morphology, and the relationships of the arterial trunks all being different facets, and requiring separate description in mutually exclusive terms. It is also necessary to take account of infundibular morphology.

Ventriculo-Arterial Connections

There are four discrete ways in which the arterial trunks can take their origin from the ventricular mass. These are the concordant, discordant, double outlet, and single outlet options. Concordant ventriculo-arterial connections exist when the arterial trunks arise from morphologically appropriate ventricles. Discordant connections account for the trunks being connected with morphologically inappropriate ventricles. Double outlet connections exist when both great arteries take origin from the same ventricle, which may be of right, left, or indeterminate morphology. The single outlet arrangement is seen when only one arterial trunk is connected to the heart. This may be a common trunk, supplying directly the systemic, pulmonary, and coronary arteries, or it may be an aortic or pulmonary trunk when the complementary arterial trunk is atretic, and its connection to a known ventricle cannot be established (Figure 7.30). Rarely, in the absence of intrapericardial pulmonary arteries, it may be more accurate to describe an arterial trunk as solitary rather than common (Figure 7.30).

Arterial Valvar Morphology

The morphological arrangement of the arterial valves is limited because they have no tension apparatus. Furthermore, a common valve can exist only with a common trunk. The different patterns, therefore, involve one or two arterial valves. Usually both valves are perforate, but either or both may override the ventricular septum. When a valvar orifice is overriding, the valve is assigned to the ventricle supporting its greater part, thus avoiding the need for intermediate categories. In the other pattern of valvar morphology, one of the arterial valves is imperforate. As with the atrioventricular junctions, an imperforate arterial valve must be distinguished from absence of one ventriculo-arterial connection, since both produce arterial valvar atresia.

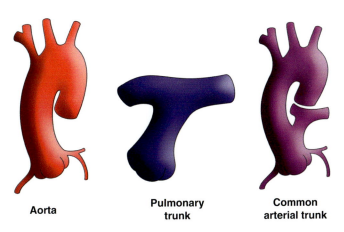
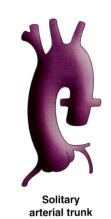

Aorta **Pulmonary trunk** **Common arterial trunk** **Solitary arterial trunk**

Figure 7.30 This drawing shows the patterns that identify the morphology of the arterial trunks. When there is absence of the intrapericardial pulmonary arteries, there is no way of knowing if, had there been an atretic pulmonary trunk, it would have originated from the base of the heart or from the aorta. This pattern, therefore, is best described as a solitary arterial trunk.

Infundibular Morphology

Describing the morphology at the ventriculo-arterial junctions also involves the arrangement of the musculature within the ventricular outflow tracts. This is infundibular morphology. Although the outlet regions are integral parts of the ventricular mass, it is traditional to consider them in concert with the great arteries. The two outflow tracts together make a complete cone of musculature, which has parietal and septal components, along with a component adjacent to the atrioventricular junction (Figure 7.31). The parietal components make up the anterior free wall of the outflow tracts. The septal component is the outlet, or infundibular, septum. This has a body, with septal and parietal insertions, best seen in the setting of tetralogy of Fallot (Figure 7.32). The component adjacent to the atrioventricular junction is the ventriculo-infundibular fold. It separates the leaflets of arterial from atrioventricular valves (Figure 7.33). It is the inner heart curvature.[19] The fold may be attenuated to give arterial–atrioventricular valvar fibrous continuity (Figure 7.34).

The infundibular structures never contain or overlie conduction tissue.[20] They should be distinguished from another structure, namely the septomarginal trabeculation, or septal band. This latter structure is part of the ventricular septum, reinforcing its right ventricular aspect. It has a body that continues apically as the moderator band, and two limbs (Figure 7.35). The antero-cephalad limb, in the normal heart, extends to the pulmonary valve, overlying the medial wall of the infundibulum. The postero-caudal limb runs beneath the interventricular membranous septum. This postero-caudal limb usually overlies the branching part of the atrioventricular bundle, with the right bundle branch passing down to the apex of the right ventricle within the body of the trabeculation.

Although each outflow tract is potentially a complete muscular structure, in most hearts it is only the outflow tract of the right ventricle that is a complete muscular cone. This is because, within the left ventricle, part of the ventriculo-infundibular fold is usually attenuated to permit fibrous continuity between the leaflets of the arterial and atrioventricular valves. In the normal heart, therefore, there is a muscular subpulmonary infundibulum in the right ventricle, and fibrous valvar continuity in the roof of the left ventricle. In congenitally malformed hearts, three other patterns may be found. These are, first, a muscular subaortic infundibulum with pulmonary–atrioventricular continuity, second, a bilaterally muscular infundibulum, which can very rarely be found in the otherwise normal heart, and, third, bilateral deficiency of the infundibulums. In the presence of a common arterial trunk, there may be a complete muscular subtruncal infundibulum, but more often there is truncal-atrioventricular valvar continuity.

Arterial Valvar and Truncal Relationships

The final feature of consideration at the ventriculo-arterial junctions is the relationship of the arterial valves and arterial trunks. Valvar relationships are independent of both ventriculo-arterial connections and infundibular morphology. Of the many methods of description, our preference is to describe the aortic relative to the pulmonary valve in terms of the right–left, antero-posterior and, when necessary, supero-inferior coordinates. This can be done as precisely as required. In our experience, eight coordinates combining lateral and anterior to

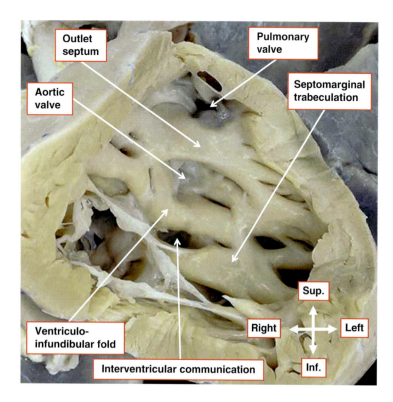

Figure 7.31 This view of a heart with double outlet right ventricle, seen in anatomical orientation, and with a non-committed interventricular communication, shows the muscular components of the ventricular outflow tracts. The hinges of both arterial valves are completed surrounded by outflow musculature.

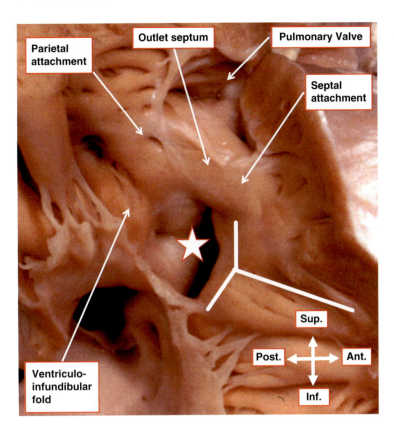

Figure 7.32 The image shows the outflow tracts in a heart with tetralogy of Fallot, viewed from the apex of the right ventricle, with the aortic valve (star) overriding the crest of the muscular ventricular septum, which is reinforced by the septomarginal trabeculation, or septal band (white Y). The septal and parietal attachments of muscular outlet septum are well seen.

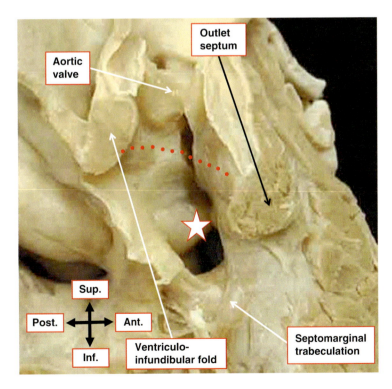

Figure 7.33 In this heart with tetralogy of Fallot, the ventriculo-infundibular fold (red dotted line) interposes between the leaflets of the aortic and mitral valves in the roof of the interventricular communication, producing a completely muscular subaortic infundibulum (white star with red borders).

posterior positions suffice (Figure 7.36). When describing the relationship of the arterial trunks, it is sufficient to account for trunks that spiral around each other as they ascend, and to distinguish them from trunks that ascend in parallel fashion.[21]

Position of the Heart

The system discussed in this chapter establishes the cardiac template. Irrespective of the internal architecture, it is well known that the heart itself can occupy many and varied

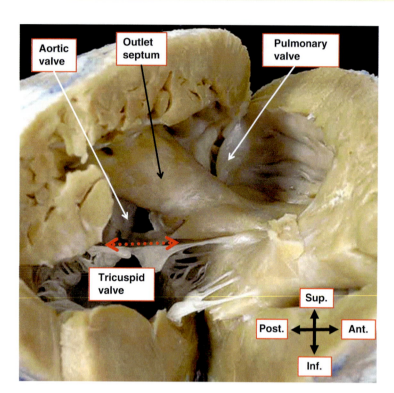

Figure 7.34 This heart has the ventriculo-arterial connection of double outlet right ventricle, but with fibrous continuity between the leaflets of the aortic and tricuspid valves (double-headed red arrow).

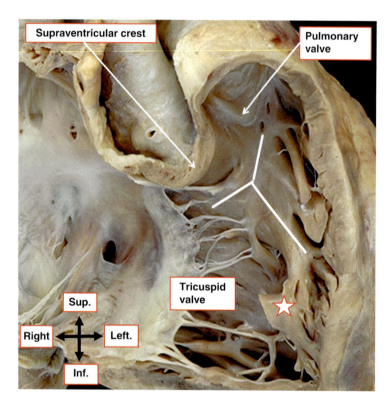

Figure 7.35 The septal surface of the normal right ventricle is photographed to show the extent of the septomarginal trabeculation, or septal band, as shown by the white Y. In the normal heart, the supraventricular crest inserts between the limbs of the trabeculation. The star shows the moderator band, one of the series of septoparietal trabeculations that take origin from the anterior surface of the marginal trabeculation.

positions (see Chapter 11). This is particularly the case when there are complex intracardiac malformations. To describe the position of the heart in unambiguous fashion, account should be taken separately of its site within the thorax, and the orientation of its apex. We describe the heart as being in the left or right side of the chest, or in the midline. Apical orientation is described as being to the left, to the middle, or to the right.

Catalogue of Malformations

Having described the template of the heart, and its position, it is remains to catalogue any septal deficiencies, if

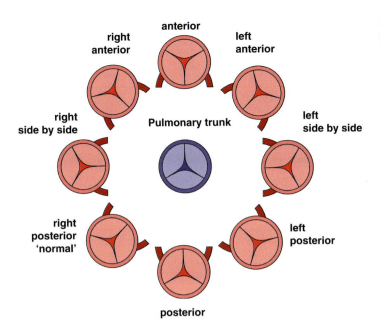

Figure 7.36 The drawing shows the combination of anterior to posterior, and right to left, coordinates that are used to describe the interrelationships of the aortic and pulmonary valves at their origins from the ventricular mass.

present, and to identify all intracardiac malformations. In most cases, it is these features which will require surgical attention. Any lesion, nonetheless, cannot be presumed to be the only lesion present until the rest of the heart has been established as normal. It is these associated lesions which will be emphasized in subsequent chapters, taking particular note, as before, of the features of surgical significance.

References Cited

1. Shinebourne EA, Macartney FJ, Anderson RH. Sequential chamber localization: the logical approach to diagnosis in congenital heart disease. *Br Heart J* 1976; **38**: 327–340.
2. Anderson RH, Wilcox BR. Understanding cardiac anatomy: the prerequisite for optimal cardiac surgery. *Ann Thorac Surg* 1995; **59**: 1366–1375.
3. Van Praagh R. The segmental approach to diagnosis in congenital heart disease. In D Bergsma, ed., *Birth Defects: Original Article Series*, vol. VIII, no. 5. *The Fourth Conference on the Clinical Delineation of Birth Defects. Part XV: The Cardiovascular System*. The National Foundation – March of Dimes. Baltimore: Williams & Wilkins; 1972: pp. 4–23.
4. Anderson RH, Ho SY. Sequential segmental analysis – description and categorization for the millennium. *Cardiol Young* 1997; 7: 98–116.
5. Van Praagh R, David I, Wright GB, Van Praagh S. Large RV plus small LV is not single RV. *Circulation* 1980; **61**: 1057–1059.
6. Keeton BR, Macartney FJ, Hunter S, et al. Univentricular heart of right ventricular type with double or common inlet. *Circulation* 1979; **59**: 403–411.
7. Uemura H, Ho SY, Devine WA, Kilpatrick LL, Anderson RH. Atrial appendages and venoatrial connections in hearts with patients with visceral heterotaxy. *Ann Thorac Surg* 1995; **60**: 561–569.
8. Van Mierop LHS, Gessner IH, Schiebler GL. Asplenia and polysplenia syndromes. In D Bergsma, ed., *Birth Defects: Original Article Series*, vol. VIII, no 5. *The Fourth Conference on the Clinical Delineation of Birth Defects. Part XV: The Cardiovascular System*. The National Foundation March of Dimes. Baltimore: Williams & Wilkins, 1972: pp. 36–44.
9. Ivemark BI. Implications of agenesis of the spleen on the pathogenesis of conotruncus anomalies in childhood. An analysis of the heart; malformations in the splenic agenesis syndrome, with 14 new cases. *Acta Paediatr Scand* 1955; **44** (Suppl.104): 1–110.
10. Loomba RS, Hlavacek AM, Spicer DE, Anderson RH. Isomerism or heterotaxy: which term leads to better understanding? *Cardiol Young* 2015; **25**: 1037–1043.
11. Loomba RS, Ahmed MM, Spicer DE, Backer CL, Anderson RH. Manifestations of bodily isomerism. *Cardiovasc Path* 2016; **25**: 173–180.
12. Huhta JC, Smallhorn JF, Macartney FJ. Two dimensional echocardiographic diagnosis of situs. *Br Heart J* 1982; **48**: 97–108.
13. Smith A, Ho SY, Anderson RH, et al. The diverse cardiac morphology seen in hearts with isomerism of the atrial appendages with reference to the disposition of the specialized conduction system. *Cardiol Young* 2006; **16**: 437–454.
14. Ho SY, Seo J-W, Brown NA, et al. Morphology of the sinus node in human and mouse hearts with isomerism of the atrial appendages. *Br Heart J* 1995; **74**: 437–442.
15. Kiraly L, Hubay M, Cook AC, Ho SY, Anderson RH. Morphologic features of the uniatrial but biventricular atrioventricular connection. *J Thorac Cardiovasc Surg* 2007; **133**: 229–234.

16. Jacobs ML, Anderson RH. Nomenclature of the functionally univentricular heart. *Cardiol Young* 2006; **16** (Suppl.1): 3–8.
17. Anderson RH. Criss-cross hearts revisited. *Pediatr Cardiol* 1982; **3**: 305–313.
18. Anderson RH, Smith A, Wilkinson JL. Disharmony between atrioventricular connections and segmental combinations -unusual variants of 'criss-cross' hearts. *J Am Coll Cardiol* 1987; **10**: 1274–1277.
19. Anderson RH, Becker AE, Van Mierop LHS. What should we call the 'crista'? *Br Heart J* 1977; **39**: 856–859.
20. Hosseinpour A-R, Jones TJ, Barron DJ, Brawn WJ, Anderson RH. An appreciation of the structural variability in the components of the ventricular outlets in congenitally malformed hearts. *Eur J Cardio-thorac Surg* 2007; **31**: 888–893.
21. Cavalle-Garrido T, Bernasconi A, Perrin D, Anderson RH. Hearts with concordant ventriculoarterial connections but parallel arterial trunks. *Heart* 2007; **93**: 100–106.

Chapter 8.1 — Lesions with Normal Segmental Connections

Septal Defects

Understanding the anatomy of septal defects is greatly facilitated if the heart is thought of as having three distinct septal structures: the atrial septum, the atrioventricular septum, and the ventricular septum (Figure 8.1.1). The normal atrial septum is relatively small. It is made up, for the most part, by the floor of the oval fossa. When viewed from the right atrial aspect, the fossa has a floor, surrounded by rims. As we have shown in Chapter 2, the floor is derived from the primary atrial septum, or septum primum. Although often considered to represent a secondary septum, or septum secundum, the larger parts of the rims, specifically the superior, antero-superior, and posterior components, are formed by infoldings of the adjacent right and left atrial walls.[1] Infero-anteriorly, in contrast, the rim of the fossa is a true muscular septum (Figure 8.1.2). This part of the rim, derived by muscularization during development of the mesenchymal cap and the vestibular spine (see Chapter 2), is contiguous with the atrioventricular component of the membranous septum. The buttress is supported by the roof of the infero-septal recess, itself formed by fibrous continuity between the leaflets of the mitral and tricuspid valves. In the normal heart, the atrioventricular component of the fibrous septum is also contiguous with the atrial wall of the triangle of Koch (Figure 8.1.3). In the past, we considered this component of the atrial wall, which overlaps the upper part of the ventricular musculature between the attachments of the leaflets of the tricuspid and mitral valves, as the muscular atrioventricular septum. As we discussed in Chapter 3, we now know that it is better viewed as a sandwich.[2] This is because, throughout the floor of the triangle of Koch, the fibro-adipose tissue of the inferior pyramidal space separates the layers of atrial and ventricular myocardium (Figure 8.1.4).[3] From the stance of understanding septal defects, nonetheless, it is helpful to consider the entire area comprising the fibrous septum and the muscular sandwich as an atrioventricular

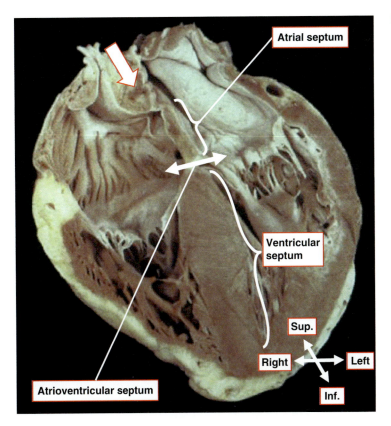

Figure 8.1.1 The four-chamber section through the heart, in anatomical orientation, shows the atrial and ventricular septal components, along with the atrioventricular (AV) component of the membranous septum. These are the three septal structures in the normal heart. There is also an area in which a layer of fibro-adipose tissue interposes between the layers of atrial and ventricular musculature (see Figure 8.1.4). This area, along with the atrioventricular component of the membranous septum, is deficient in the setting of a common atrioventricular junction. Note also that the superior rim of the oval fossa (white arrow with red borders) is an infolding between the right and left atrial walls.

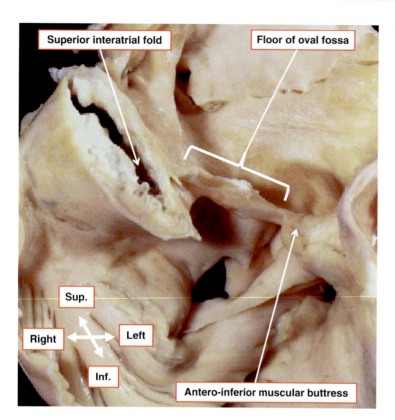

Figure 8.1.2 The heart has been sectioned in a four-chamber plane, showing that the superior rim of the oval fossa is a deep infolding between the origin of the superior caval vein from the right atrium and the entry of the right superior pulmonary vein into the left atrium. It is the floor of the oval fossa, along with the antero-inferior muscular buttress, which are the components of the atrial septum.

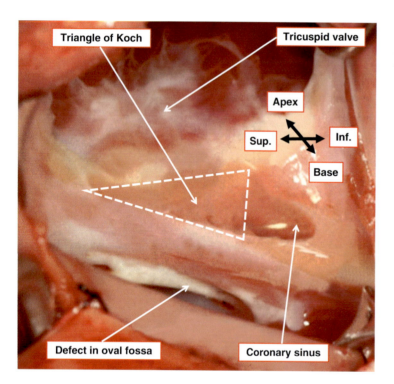

Figure 8.1.3 The surgical view, through a right atriotomy, shows the landmarks of the triangle of Koch (triangle). This area is the atrial aspect of the muscular atrioventricular sandwich. Note that this patient also has a defect within the oval fossa.

separating structure, since the overall area occupied by these components is absent in the hearts we describe as atrioventricular septal defects.

The ventricular septum is usually seen by the surgeon only from its right ventricular aspect. For this reason, and other reasons we will discuss below, holes between the ventricles are best considered in terms of their right ventricular landmarks. Taken overall, the ventricular septum is made up of a small fibrous element, specifically the interventricular part of the membranous septum, and a much larger muscular part. The

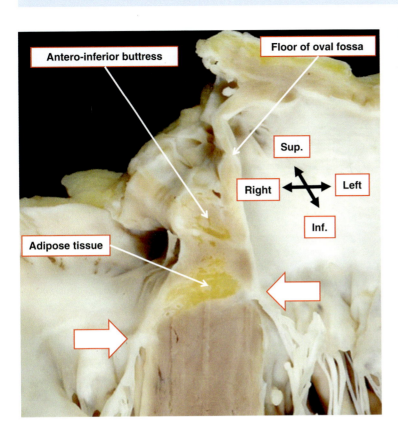

Figure 8.1.4 This four-chamber section of a normal heart, taken across the floor of the triangle of Koch, illustrates the differential attachments of the atrioventricular valves (red-bordered arrows). Note the adipose tissue interposed between the right atrial wall and the crest of the ventricular septum, which forms the 'meat' in the atrioventricular muscular sandwich.

muscular part, which is significantly curved, is more complex geometrically than the other septal structures, which lie almost completely in the coronal plane. In the past, we considered it appropriate to divide the muscular septum into inlet, apical trabecular, and outlet components, each of these parts having reciprocal right and left ventricular surfaces, and abutting centrally on the membranous septum. Closer inspection shows that such analysis is simplistic. We now realize that it is better to describe the septum as seen from its right side and as having inlet, apical trabecular, and outlet components (Figure 8.1.5). This is because, by virtue of the deeply wedged location of the subaortic outflow tract, much of the septum delimited on the right ventricular aspect by the septal leaflet of the tricuspid valve separates the inlet of the right ventricle from the outlet of the left (Figure 8.1.6). And, at first sight, the muscular wall forming the back of the subpulmonary infundibulum seems to be an outlet septum. We now know that none of the free-standing subpulmonary muscular infundibular sleeve interposes between the cavities of the right and left ventricles (Figure 8.1.7). The part we initially considered to represent a 'muscular outlet septum' is no more than the area in which the supraventricular crest inserts between the limbs of the septomarginal trabeculation (Figure 8.1.8). It is the muscular wall separating the apical trabecular components that forms the greater part of the muscular ventricular septum. This part extends to the apex in curvilinear fashion, reflecting the interrelationships of the banana-shaped right ventricle and the conical left ventricle. Reinforcing the right ventricular aspect of this part of the septum is the septomarginal trabeculation, or septal band. This muscular strap has a body and limbs, the latter extending to the base of the heart to clasp the supraventricular crest at the region previously interpreted as a muscular outlet septum. A series of septoparietal trabeculations extend from its antero-cephalad surface and reach the parietal ventricular wall. One of these, the moderator band, is particularly prominent. It crosses from the septomarginal trabeculation to join the anterior papillary muscle (Figure 8.1.9).

Interatrial Communications

There are several lesions which permit interatrial shunting (Figure 8.1.10). Although collectively termed atrial septal defects, not all are within the confines of the normal atrial septum.[1,2] Only the holes within the floor of the oval fossa,[1] and the much rarer vestibular defects found within the muscular antero-inferior buttress,[4] are true deficiencies of the septal components. The ostium primum defect is the consequence of deficient atrioventricular septation. Its cardinal feature is the commonality of the atrioventricular junction.[5] It will be considered in Chapter 8.2. Sinus venosus defects, representing anomalous connection of a pulmonary vein which has retained its left atrial connection,[6] are found at the mouths of the caval veins.[7–9] The rare defect found at the mouth of the coronary sinus is the consequence of the disappearance of the muscular walls that usually separate the component of the coronary sinus running through the left atrioventricular junction from the cavity of the left atrium.[10]

Defects within the oval fossa are often called secundum defects. Since they represent persistence of the secondary atrial foramen, rather than deficiencies of the secondary atrial septum, they should properly be called ostium secundum defects.

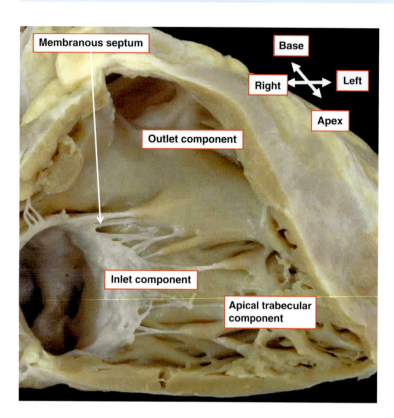

Figure 8.1.5 The right ventricle has been opened to show its septal surface. As we explained in Chapter 3, the cavity has inlet, apical, and outlet components. The surfaces of these components, however, do not match those of the left ventricle. When describing the septum, therefore, it is more accurate to account for its components, noting the location of the membranous septum, rather than suggesting that the muscular septum itself has inlet, apical, and outlet parts.

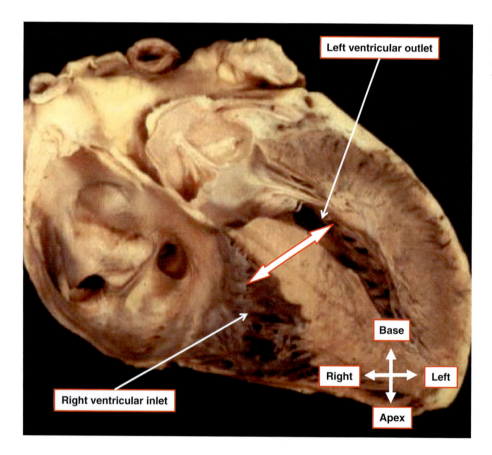

Figure 8.1.6 The section, simulating the oblique subcostal echocardiographic cut, shows how the infero-posterior part of the muscular septum separates the right ventricular inlet from the left ventricular outlet (double-headed arrow).

We prefer to consider them as defects within the oval fossa. They are by far the most common type of interatrial communication. They can be caused by deficiency (Figure 8.1.11), perforation (Figure 8.1.12), or absence (Figure 8.1.13) of the floor of the fossa formed from the primary atrial septum. When the haemodynamics of the shunt across such a defect

8.1 Septal Defects

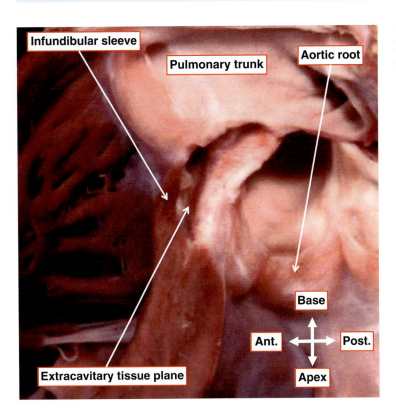

Figure 8.1.7 The dissection of the ventricular outflow tracts, in anatomical orientation, shows the free-standing sleeve of infundibulum that supports the leaflets of the pulmonary valve. The sleeve is not a septal structure. An extensive extracavitary area interposes between the infundibular sleeve and the sinuses of the aortic root.

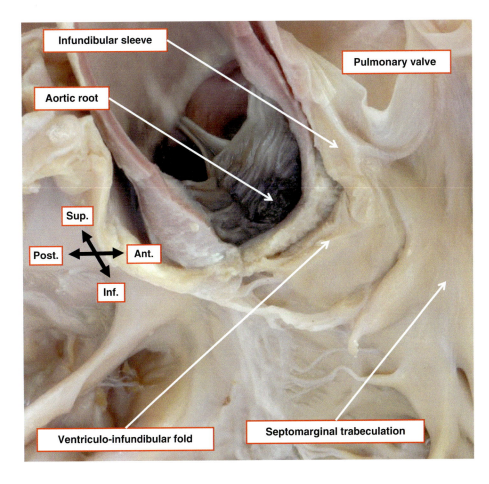

Figure 8.1.8 The dissection, seen in anatomical orientation, shows how the supraventricular crest is formed by the ventriculo-infundibular fold, continuous distally with the subpulmonary infundibular sleeve. There is no obvious part of the area that can uniformly be removed so as to create a track to the left ventricle that might be consistent with the presence of a muscular outlet septum.

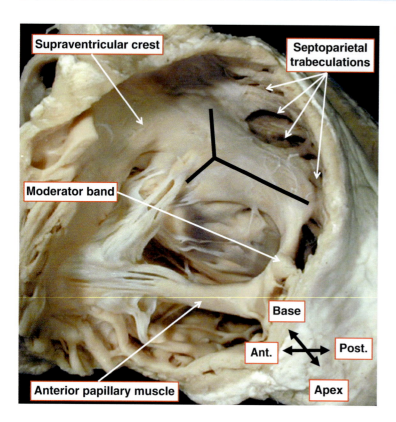

Figure 8.1.9 The septal surface of the right ventricle has been displayed by making a window in the anterior wall to show the septomarginal trabeculation, or septal band (black Y). The supraventricular crest inserts between its basal limbs. The moderator band takes origin from the apical part of its body, crossing the cavity of the ventricle to become continuous with the anterior papillary muscle. The band is but one of a series of septoparietal trabeculations that arise from the anterior margin of the major septomarginal trabeculation.

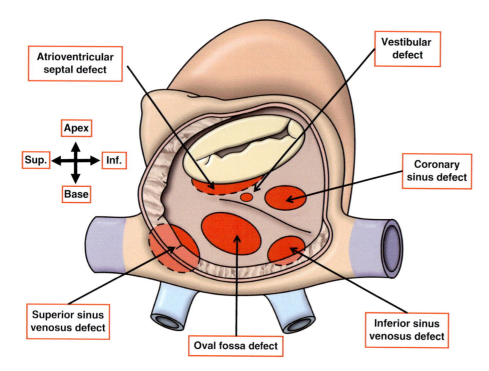

Figure 8.1.10 The cartoon shows the various holes that permit interatrial shunting. Only the holes in the oval fossa, and the rare vestibular defects, are true deficiencies of atrial septal structures.

dictate surgical closure, the hole is rarely likely to be small enough to permit direct suture. Nowadays, all but very large defects within the oval fossa are likely to be closed by the interventional cardiologist. If attempts are made to close directly defects large enough to justify surgical intervention, the results may so distort atrial anatomy as to result in dehiscence. Irrespective of the size of the septal deficiency, it is always possible to secure a patch to the margins of the oval fossa. When placing sutures, the likeliest potential danger relative to the rims is to the artery supplying the sinus node. This artery can either course intramyocardially through the anterior margin of the oval fossa, or lie deep within the

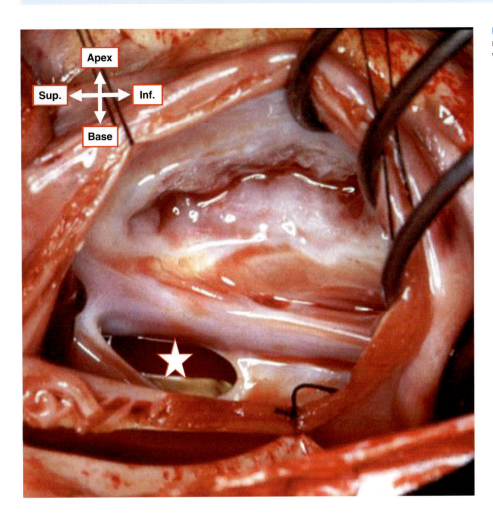

Figure 8.1.11 The surgical view through a right atriotomy shows a deficiency in the flap valve of the oval fossa (star).

superior interatrial fold. There is also a remote chance of damaging the aorta when placing stitches anteriorly, since this part of the rim is related on its epicardial aspect to the aortic root (Figures 8.1.14, 8.1.15). On occasion, deficiency of the postero-inferior rim of the oval fossa permits holes within the fossa to extend into the mouth of the inferior caval vein (Figure 8.1.16). In these circumstances, care must be taken not to mistake a well-formed Eustachian valve for the postero-inferior margin of the defect. A patch attached to the Eustachian valve would connect the inferior caval vein to the left atrium. It is always prudent, therefore, to ensure continuity of the inferior caval vein and right atrium following placement of a patch used to close a deficiency of the floor of the oval fossa.

Sinus venosus defects are rarer than defects within the oval fossa, and present greater problems in repair.[9] The defect adjacent to the inferior caval vein is relatively rare.[6] It opens into the mouth of the inferior caval vein posterior to the confines of the oval fossa (Figures 8.1.17, 8.1.18). Usually, the fossa itself is intact, but it can be deficient or probe patent. The essence of the defect is an anomalous connection of the right inferior pulmonary vein to the inferior caval vein, the pulmonary vein retaining its left atrial connection.[6] It is much more frequent to find sinus venosus defects adjacent to the mouth of the superior caval vein (Figure 8.1.19).[7–9] These defects, again, are due to anomalous connection of one or more of the right pulmonary veins to the superior caval vein, the pulmonary veins retaining their left atrial connection.[9] The defects are outside the confines of the oval fossa, and hence are interatrial communications rather than atrial septal defects (Figure 8.1.10). It follows that, if the inferior sinus venosus defect reflects anomalous connection of the right inferior pulmonary vein, and the superior defect involves the right superior pulmonary vein, then involvement of the right middle pulmonary vein might produce an interatrial communication to the central part of the systemic venous sinus. This proves to be the case, although such intermediate defects (Figure 8.1.20) are the rarest of the sinus venosus variants.

When sinus venosus defects are found in relation to the superior caval vein, the orifice of the vein usually overrides the superior rim of the oval fossa (Figures 8.1.19, 8.1.21). More rarely, such defects can be found when the caval vein is committed exclusively to the right atrium (Figure 8.1.22).[7,9] All the defects are associated with anomalous connection of the right superior pulmonary veins, which drain into the superior caval vein (Figures 8.1.21, 8.1.23, 8.1.24), often through more than one orifice (Figure 8.1.19), but with the crucial feature of retaining their left atrial connection (Figure 8.1.21). The difficulty encountered during surgical repair reflects the need to reconstruct the anatomy so as appropriately to reroute the venous

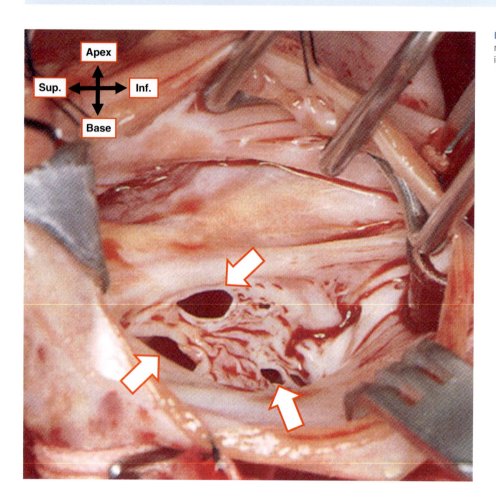

Figure 8.1.12 The surgical view through a right atriotomy shows three perforations (arrows) in the flap valve of the oval fossa.

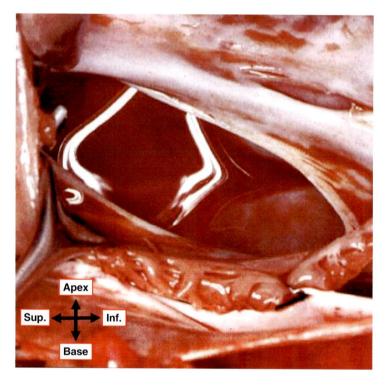

Figure 8.1.13 The surgical view through a right atriotomy shows absence of the entire flap valve of the oval fossa.

return and, at the same time, close the interatrial communication. This must be done without obstructing venous flow or, in the case of a superior defect, damaging the sinus node. The sinus node is related to the antero-lateral quadrant of the cavo-atrial

8.1 Septal Defects

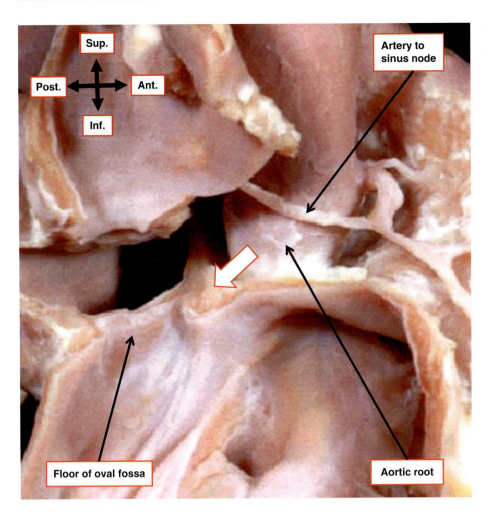

Figure 8.1.14 The dissection, made by transecting the atrial chambers, and illustrated in anatomical orientation, shows the relationship of the artery supplying the sinus node to the antero-superior rim of the oval fossa, which is an infolding of the atrial walls (white arrow with red borders). Note also the proximity of the rim to the aortic root.

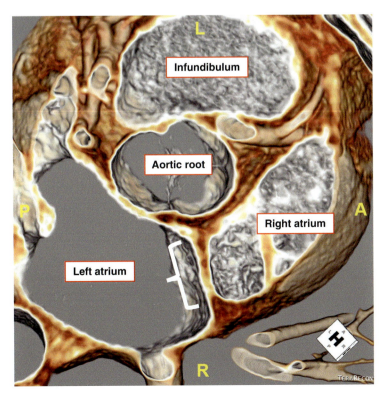

Figure 8.1.15 The computed tomographic angiogram shows the adjacency of the antero-superior margin of the oval fossa (bracket), and the adjacent atrial walls, to the aortic root. Orientation cube, lower right: H, head. L, left; A, anterior; R, right; P, posterior.

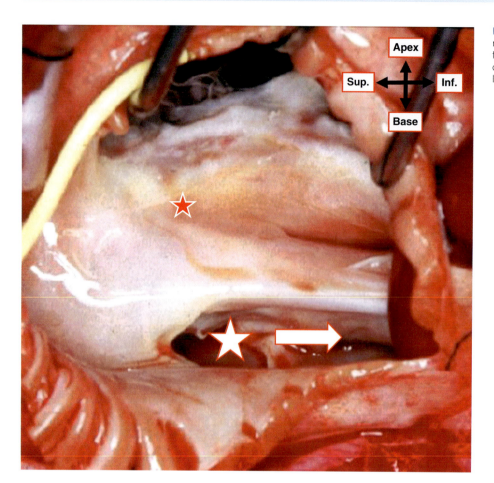

Figure 8.1.16 The surgical view through a right atriotomy shows a defect within the oval fossa (large white star) extending into the mouth of the inferior caval vein (arrow). Note the location of the triangle of Koch (small red star).

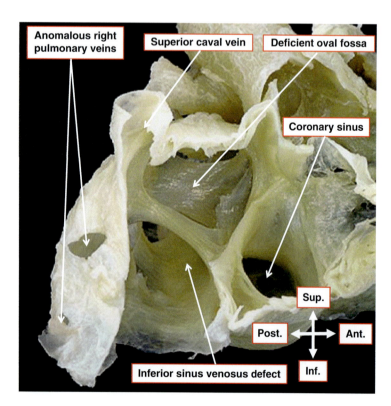

Figure 8.1.17 The specimen, viewed in anatomical orientation, shows the features of an inferior sinus venosus defect. The margins of the oval fossa are intact. The defect is due to anomalous connection of the inferior right pulmonary vein to the inferior caval vein. The anomalously connected veins retain their left atrial connection.

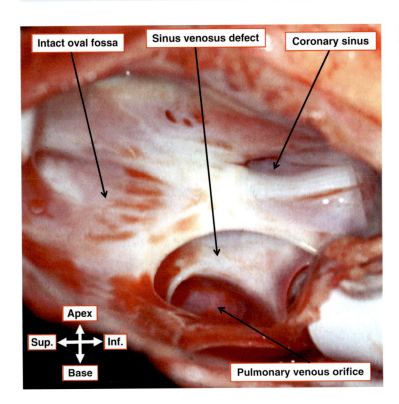

Figure 8.1.18 The surgical view through a right atriotomy shows a defect at the mouth of the inferior caval vein. There is anomalous drainage of the right inferior pulmonary vein, which retains its left atrial connection. The oval fossa is intact. This is a typical example of the inferior sinus venosus defect.

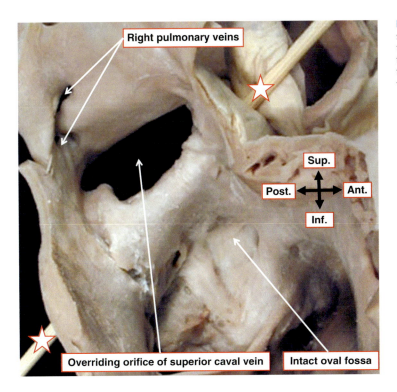

Figure 8.1.19 The specimen, viewed in anatomical orientation, shows a superior sinus venosus defect with overriding of the orifice of the superior caval vein. The probe (stars) has been passed through the fibro-adipose tissue occupying the intact superior margin of the oval fossa. There is anomalous drainage of the two right upper pulmonary veins, which have retained their left atrial connection.

junction. It lies immediately subepicardially within the terminal groove (Figure 8.1.24). Its location should be considered both when making the atriotomy and when placing sutures in the atrial walls. Problems arise should it be necessary either to suture in the area of the node when rerouting the pulmonary venous return, or if there is need to enlarge the orifice of the caval vein.[11] The former risk can be minimized with judicious superficial placement of the sutures. The latter problem is much greater. Because the artery to the sinus node may pass either in front of or behind the caval vein, the entire cavo-atrial junction is a potentially dangerous area. Incisions across the cavo-atrial junction carry a high risk of damaging the artery, or even the

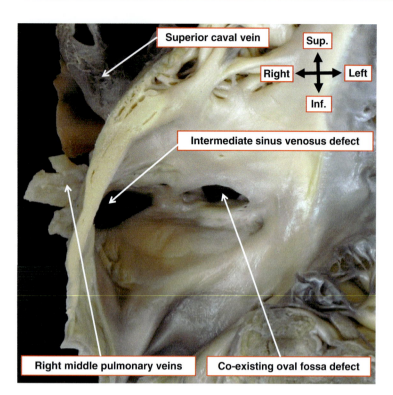

Figure 8.1.20 The specimen, viewed in anatomical orientation, shows the features of an intermediate sinus venosus defect. There is a co-existing defect within the oval fossa. The defect is due to anomalous connection of the right middle pulmonary vein to the systemic venous sinus, with the anomalously connected pulmonary vein again retaining its left atrial connection.

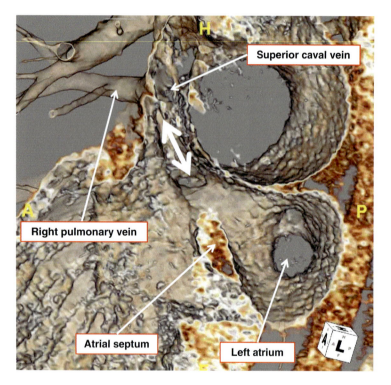

Figure 8.1.21 The computed tomographic angiogram shows how, most frequently, the mouth of the superior caval vein overrides the crest of the atrial septum in the setting of a superior sinus venosus defect. Note that two right pulmonary veins drain anomalously to the superior caval vein while retaining their left atrial connection. Orientation cube, lower right: A, anterior; L, left; H, head.

node itself. Should it be deemed necessary to cut across the junction, a much better option is to perform the Warden operation. This involves detaching the superior caval vein, and re-attaching it to the excised tip of the right atrial appendage.[12]

Another defect which permits interatrial shunting, but which is outside the confines of the true atrial septum, is part of a constellation of lesions termed unroofing of the coronary sinus.[10] In this setting, a persistent left superior caval vein usually drains directly to the left atrial roof (Figure 8.1.25), entering the chamber between the appendage and the left pulmonary veins. Because of the unroofing of the coronary sinus into the cavity of the left atrium (Figure 8.1.26), the mouth of the coronary sinus functions as an interatrial communication (Figure 8.1.27). Evidence is frequently seen of the

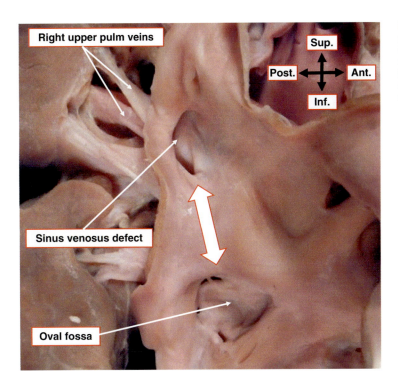

Figure 8.1.22 The specimen, viewed in anatomical orientation, shows a superior sinus venosus defect without overriding of the orifice of the superior caval vein. As in the specimen shown in Figure 8.1.19, there is anomalous drainage of the right upper pulmonary vein, which has retained its left atrial connection. Note the distance between the defect and the oval fossa (double-headed arrow). Note the intact rims of the oval fossa.

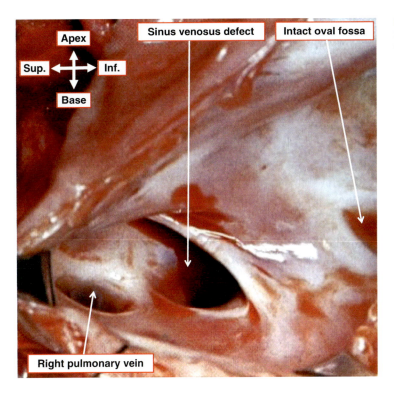

Figure 8.1.23 This surgical view through a right atriotomy shows a superior sinus venosus defect, recognized because it is outside the confines of the intact oval fossa.

walls of the coronary sinus and left atrium along the anticipated course of the left superior caval vein into and through the left atrioventricular groove (Figure 8.1.26). Sometimes the mouth of the coronary sinus can seem to open normally to the right atrium, but in absence of its component usually occupying the left atrioventricular groove, and without persistence of a left superior caval vein draining to the left atrial roof (Figure 8.1.28). In this setting, the left ventricular coronary veins drain directly into the cavity of the left atrium. In these circumstances, the mouth of the coronary sinus again functions as an interatrial communication. The coronary sinus defect is the extreme form of the spectrum of fenestration of the walls of the coronary sinus, providing communications with the cavity of the left atrium (see Chapter 10.1).

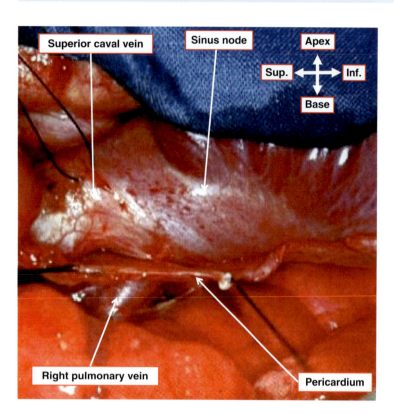

Figure 8.1.24 This surgical view, through a median sternotomy of the heart shown in Figure 8.1.23, illustrates the anomalous connection of the right superior pulmonary vein. Note the site of the sinus node lying in the terminal groove.

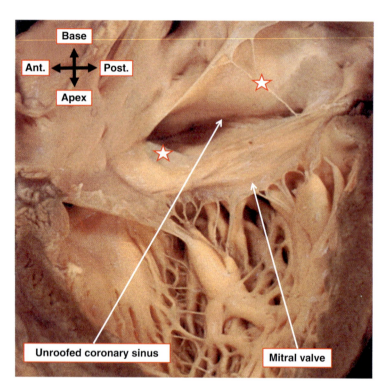

Figure 8.1.25 The heart is shown from the left side in anatomical orientation. There is unroofing of the coronary sinus as it courses through the left atrioventricular groove, draining a persistent left superior caval vein, with filigreed remnants (white stars with red borders) showing the site of the walls that initially separated the vein from the left atrium.

Surgical treatment of interatrial communications through the mouth of the coronary sinus is dictated by the presence, and connections, of the left superior caval vein. If it is present, and in free communication with the right superior caval vein, or if there is no left-sided superior caval vein, the mouth of the coronary sinus can simply be closed. If the right atrial mouth of the sinus is to be closed, decisions must be made concerning the treatment of the left superior caval vein. In the presence of an adequate venous channel communicating with the brachiocephalic vein, the left caval vein can be ligated. If, in contrast, the left-sided channel has no anastomoses with the right side, consideration should be given to construction of a left-sided cavo-pulmonary anastomosis, the Glenn shunt. Alternatively, a channel can be constructed along the postero-inferior wall of the left atrium, connecting the left atrial opening of the left-sided vein with the mouth of the coronary sinus.

8.1 Septal Defects

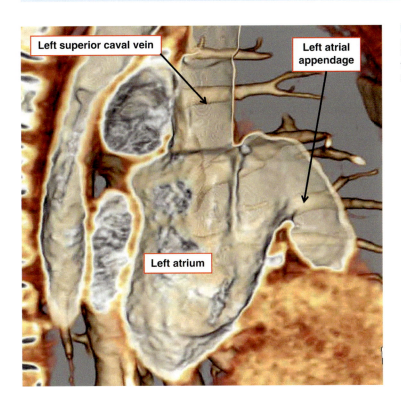

Figure 8.1.26 The computed tomographic angiogram shows a persistent left superior caval vein draining to the roof of the left atrium, in absence of the walls that usually separate the course of the vein through the left atrioventricular groove to the mouth of the coronary sinus.

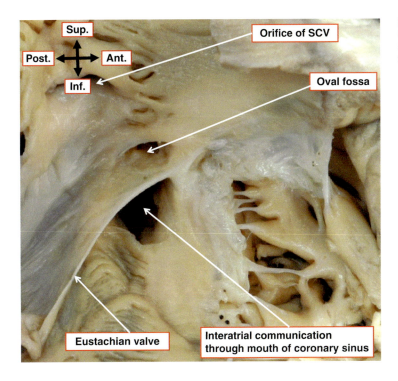

Figure 8.1.27 When the walls separating the coronary sinus from the left atrium are deficient, as in the heart shown in Figure 8.1.25, the orifice of the coronary sinus functions as an interatrial communication. SCV, superior cava vein.

References Cited

1. Jensen B, Spicer DE, Sheppard MN, Anderson RH. Development of the atrial septum in relation to postnatal anatomy and interatrial communications. *Heart* 2017; **103**: 456–462.
2. Anderson RH, Brown NA. The anatomy of the heart revisited. *Anat Rec* 1996; **246**: 1–7.
3. Tretter JT, Spicer DE, Sánchez-Quintana D, et al. Miniseries 1 – part III: 'behind the scenes' in the triangle of Koch. *EP Europace* 2022; **24**: 455–463.
4. Loomba RS, Tretter JT, Mohun TJ, et al. Identification and morphogenesis of vestibular atrial septal defects. *J Cardiovasc Devel Dis* 2020; **7**: 35.
5. Anderson RH, Ho SY, Falcao S, Daliento L, Rigby ML. The diagnostic features of atrioventricular septal

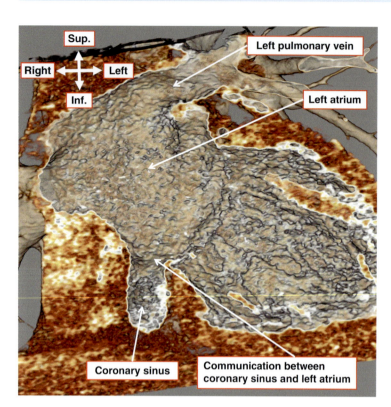

Figure 8.1.28 This computed tomographic angiogram shows a communication between the coronary sinus and left atrium in the absence of a persistent left superior caval vein. The mouth of the coronary sinus again functions as an interatrial communication.

defect with common atrioventricular junction. *Cardiol Young* 1998; **8**: 33–49.

6. Crystal MA, Al Najashi K, Williams WG, Redington AN, Anderson RH. Inferior sinus venosus defect: echocardiographic diagnosis and surgical approach. *J Thorac Cardiovasc Surg* 2009; **137**: 1349–1355.

7. Butts RJ, Crean AM, Hlavacek AM, et al. Veno-venous bridges: the forerunners of the sinus venosus defect. *Cardiol Young* 2011; **21**: 623–630.

8. Ettedgui JA, Siewers RD, Anderson RH, Zuberbuhler JR. Diagnostic echocardiographic features of the sinus venosus defect. *Br Heart J* 1990; **64**: 329–331.

9. Relan J, Gupta SK, Rajagopal R, et al. Clarifying the anatomy of the superior sinus venosus defect. *Heart* 2022; **108**: 689–694.

10. Knauth A, McCarthy KP, Webb S, et al. Interatrial communication through the mouth of the coronary sinus defect. *Cardiol Young* 2002; **12**: 364–372.

11. Stewart RD, Bailliard F, Kelle AM, et al. Evolving surgical strategy for sinus venosus atrial septal defect: effect in sinus node function and late venous obstruction. *Ann Thorac Surg* 2007; **84**: 1651–1658.

12. Warden HE, Gustafson RA, Tarnay TJ, Neal WA. An alternative method for repair of partial anomalous venous connection to the superior vena cava. *Ann Thorac Surg* 1984; **38**: 601–605.

Chapter 8.2 Atrioventricular Septal Defects

It has now become the norm to describe as atrioventricular septal defects anomalies that previously were defined as endocardial cushion defects, atrioventricular canal defects, or persistent atrioventricular canal. This is entirely appropriate since, in anatomical terms, the malformations are due not only to absence of the membranous atrioventricular septum, but also to the overlapping region of atrial and ventricular musculatures which normally forms the floor of the triangle of Koch.[1] The structures are absent because the unifying feature of the group is the commonality of the atrioventricular junction (Figure 8.2.1).[1] The optimal title for the group, therefore, would be atrioventricular septal defect with common atrioventricular junction. This is because, on rare occasions, defects of the membranous atrioventricular septum can be found in the setting of separate right and left atrioventricular junctions. These defects, first described by Gerbode and colleagues,[2] and often called Gerbode defects, can take two forms. The more frequent variant exists when shunting across a ventricular septal defect enters the right atrium through a deficient tricuspid valve (Figure 8.2.2). The rarer variant is a true deficiency of the atrioventricular component of the membranous septum (Figures 8.2.3–8.2.5).[3] The key to differentiating the true defects from those involving passage via a deficient ventricular septum is to demonstrate the competence of the tricuspid valve (Figure 8.2.6).

Although atrioventricular septal defects do exist in the form of the Gerbode defect in the setting of separate right and left atrioventricular junctions, nowadays it is usual to presume the presence of a common atrioventricular junction when considering deficient atrioventricular septation. The presence of the common junction then distorts fundamentally the overall anatomy when compared with the normally separate right and left atrioventricular junctions (compare Figures 8.2.1 and 8.2.7).

Because of the lack of the membranous and muscular atrioventricular structures, there is no septal component separating the atrioventricular junction. Instead, the leading edges of the atrial septum and the ventricular septum,

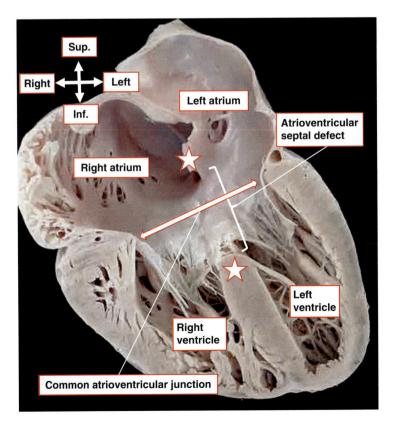

Figure 8.2.1 The section of a specimen, cut in four-chamber orientation, shows a common atrioventricular junction (double-headed arrow) guarded by a common atrioventricular valve in a heart with deficient atrioventricular septation. The bracket shows the atrioventricular septal defect, between the leading edge of the atrial septum and the crest of the muscular ventricular septum (stars).

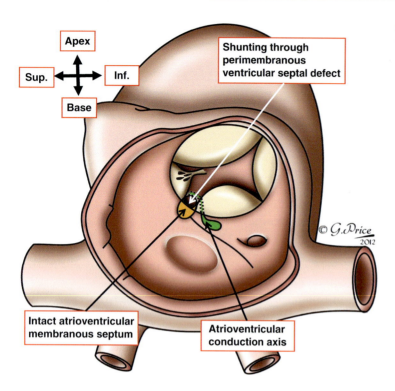

Figure 8.2.2 The drawing shows how, when there is a deficiency of the septal leaflet of the tricuspid valve, shunting across a ventricular septal defect can also produce left ventricular to right atrial shunting. This is the so-called indirect Gerbode defect.

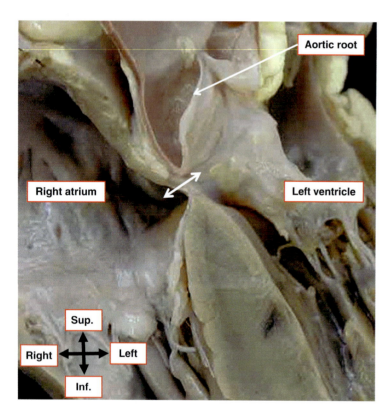

Figure 8.2.3 The section through the heart, replicating the echocardiographic four-chamber cut, shows how the septal leaflet of the tricuspid valve divides the membranous septum into interventricular and atrioventricular components. It is deficiency of the atrioventricular component (double-headed white arrow) that underscores the existence of the direct Gerbode defect.

the latter usually covered by the atrioventricular valvar leaflets, meet at the superior and inferior margins of the common atrioventricular junction (Figure 8.2.8). These meeting points of the septal structures typically divide the common junction into more-or-less equal right and left sides. An eccentric location of the septal structures relative to the junction produces, on the one hand, ventricular imbalance, or if abnormally separating the atriums, the arrangement known as double outlet atrium, on the other hand.

The anatomical arrangement produced by the common atrioventricular junction also distorts the disposition of the

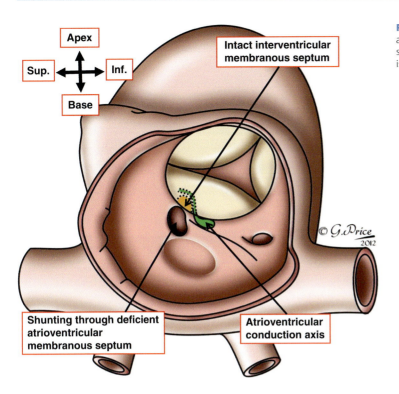

Figure 8.2.4 The cartoon shows how a deficiency of the atrioventricular component of the membranous septum produces the setting for direct shunting from the left ventricle to the right atrium. This is the direct Gerbode defect.

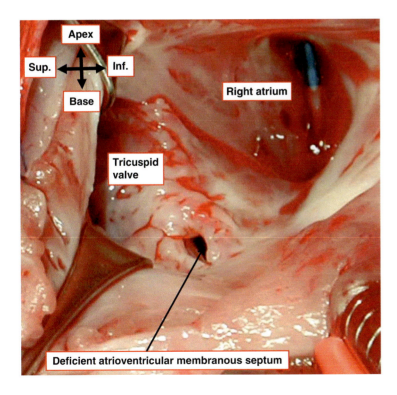

Figure 8.2.5 The image, taken in the operating room, shows a deficiency of the atrioventricular component of the membranous septum.

atrioventricular conduction axis. An analogue of the triangle of Koch can be seen within the leading edge of the atrial septum.[4] Because of the common atrioventricular junction, however, the atrial septal myocardium makes contact with the ventricular myocardium only superiorly and inferiorly (Figure 8.2.8). Usually, the atrioventricular node is displaced inferiorly. It typically lies in a nodal triangle, but not the triangle of Koch. When seen by the surgeon, the nodal triangle has the coronary sinus at its base, with the atrial septum to the left hand, and the attachment of the leaflets of the effectively common atrioventricular valve to the right hand (Figures 8.2.9, 8.2.10). The atrioventricular conduction axis penetrates through the apex of the nodal triangle. It then courses on the crest of the muscular ventricular septum, covered by the inferior bridging leaflet

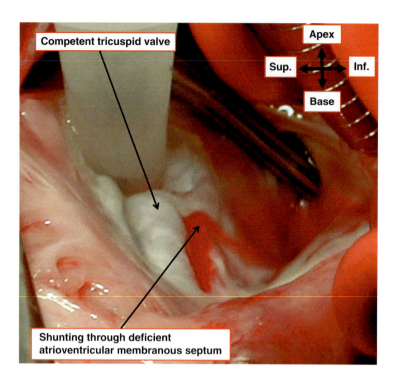

Figure 8.2.6 In the patient illustrated in Figure 8.2.5, insufflations of saline in the right ventricle reveal a competent tricuspid valve, showing that the shunting from left ventricle to right atrium is across a deficiency of the atrioventricular part of the membranous septum, in other words a direct Gerbode defect.

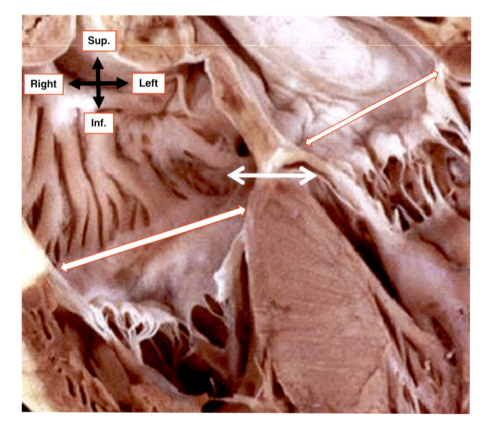

Figure 8.2.7 This normal heart has also been sectioned in four-chamber orientation. It shows the right and left atrioventricular junctions (double-headed arrows with red borders) guarded by separate atrioventricular valves (compare with Figure 8.2.1). The white double-headed arrow shows the separating atrioventricular structures.

of the atrioventricular valve (Figure 8.2.11). The proximity of the coronary sinus to the apex of the nodal triangle is pertinent to surgical closure of the septal defect. Ideally, the surgeon will place a patch so as to leave the coronary sinus draining to the systemic venous atrium. The best option is to deviate the suture line towards the left side of the inferior bridging leaflet at its junction with the atrial septum, using superficial surgical bites (green dashed line in Figure 8.2.9).[4] An alternative is to stay on the right side, but place the suture line within the mouth of the coronary sinus so as to reach the edge of the atrial septum

8.2 Atrioventricular Septal Defects

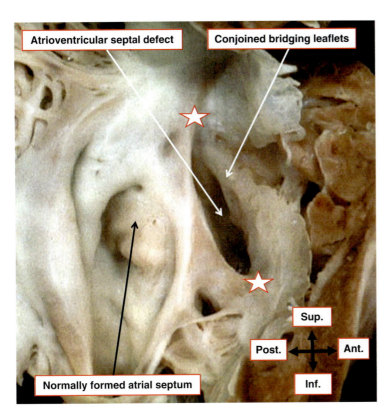

Figure 8.2.8 The specimen, seen in anatomical orientation, has been prepared to show the right side of the heart with deficient atrioventricular septation and separate right and left atrioventricular orifices, the lesion also known as an ostium primum defect. It is the conjoined bridging leaflets that produce the separate valvar orifices. The septal defect occupies the site of the normal atrioventricular separating structures. Note that the atrial septum itself is virtually normal, and the oval fossa is intact, although the leading edge of the septum is bowed from the atrioventricular junction in the margin of the septal defect. The stars show how the meeting points of the septal structures divide the common junction into its right and left sides.

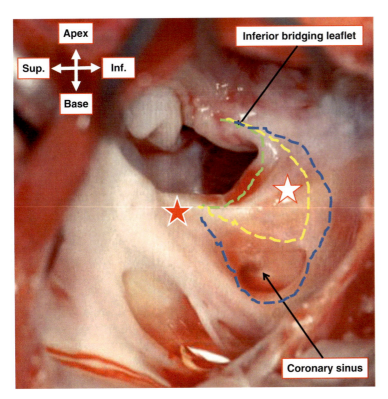

Figure 8.2.9 This view through a right atriotomy shows the surgeon's view of the atrial septal surface in a heart with an atrioventricular septal defect and separate right and left atrioventricular orifices, or the ostium primum defect. Koch's triangle is well formed (red with white border star), but no longer contains the atrioventricular node. The node is displaced postero-inferiorly to the apex of a new nodal triangle (white with red border star). The three dotted lines show the options for placement of sutures so as to avoid traumatizing the atrioventricular conduction axis. The green dashed line runs directly from the inferior bridging leaflet to the inferior margin of the leading edge of the atrial septum. The yellow dashed line courses from the inferior bridging leaflet to the right side of the atrioventricular node and skirts the margins of the coronary sinus, keeping the orifice of the sinus to its right side. The blue dashed line courses to the right side of the atrioventricular node, but is placed so as to leave the coronary sinus draining to the left atrium.

(yellow dashed line in Figure 8.2.9). The safety of this approach depends on the margin between the mouth of the coronary sinus and the apex of the nodal triangle (compare Figures 8.2.9 and 8.2.10). A further alternative is to keep the suture line to the right of the mouth of the coronary sinus, placing the sinus to the left of the atrial patch (blue lines in Figures 8.2.9, 8.2.10). Occasionally, the inferior portion of the atrial septum itself can be deficient. The coronary sinus then opens more posteriorly and medially through the left atrial wall. The conduction axis, however, follows the course of the muscular ventricular

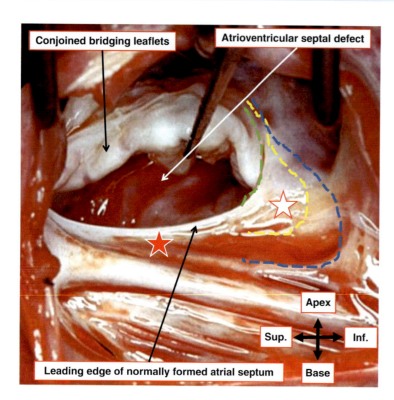

Figure 8.2.10 In this heart, again shown as seen by the surgeon through a right atriotomy, there is less room around the coronary sinus to place a patch so as to leave the sinus draining to the right side (yellow dashed line). The site of the atrioventricular node is again shown by the red-bordered white star (compare with Figure 8.2.9). Note that it is not within the well-formed triangle of Koch (white-bordered red star). The green and blue dashed lines show the alternate options for placement of the suture line, as indicated also in Figure 8.2.9.

septum, with the node formed at the site of its union with the inferior atrioventricular junction (Figure 8.2.10).[5]

The feature that distinguishes between the various forms of atrioventricular septal defects is the morphology of the leaflets of the atrioventricular valve that guards the common atrioventricular junction, together with their relationship to the septal structures bordering the defect.[6] In any heart which lacks the separating atrioventricular structures, the common atrioventricular valve has five leaflets. The arrangement is seen most readily when the valve itself has a common orifice (Figure 8.2.12). Two of the leaflets extend across the ventricular septum, with their tension apparatus attached in both ventricles (Figure 8.2.13). These are the superior and inferior bridging leaflets. Two other leaflets are entirely contained within the right ventricle. They are the antero-superior and inferior mural leaflets. The fifth leaflet is contained exclusively within the left ventricle, and is also a mural leaflet. Although the two leaflets found within the right ventricle are comparable to similar leaflets of the tricuspid valve seen in the normal heart, the left ventricular leaflets of the common atrioventricular valve (Figure 8.2.14) bear no resemblance to a normal mitral valve. In the normal mitral valve, found with separate atrioventricular junctions, the ends of the solitary zone of apposition between the leaflets, and the papillary muscles supporting them, are situated infero-anteriorly and supero-posteriorly within the left ventricle (Figure 8.2.15). With this arrangement, the extensive mural leaflet guards two-thirds of the circumference of the valvar orifice. The left ventricular outflow tract then interposes between the aortic leaflet of the mitral valve and the ventricular septal surface. In atrioventricular septal defects with common atrioventricular junction, in contrast, the left ventricular papillary muscles are deviated laterally, being positioned superiorly and inferiorly.[1,6] Because of this, the mural leaflet is relatively insignificant, and guards much less than one-third of the circumference of the left atrioventricular orifice. The left orifice is, in effect, guarded by a valve possessing three leaflets, these being the small mural leaflet, and the more extensive left ventricular components of the superior and inferior bridging leaflets (Figure 8.2.16).

It had originally been suggested by Rastelli and colleagues[7] that the common valve possessed four rather than five leaflets. They argued that the differing morphology to be found in the setting of a common valvar orifice reflected the morphology of the anterior common leaflet, which is now usually described as the superior bridging leaflet. In the arrangement they described as their Type A, they considered the anterior common leaflet to be divided, with the two components both attached to the ventricular septum. They considered their Type B again to have a divided anterior common leaflet, but with both parts attached to an anomalous papillary muscle in the right ventricle. In their Type C, they interpreted the arrangement in terms of an undivided common anterior leaflet, which was free floating and attached in the right ventricle to an apical papillary muscle. In reality, the purported division of the anterior common leaflet is the site of coaptation between the right ventricular part of the superior bridging leaflet and the antero-superior leaflet of the right ventricle (Figure 8.2.17). In the Rastelli Type A variant, the point of coaptation is supported by the medial papillary muscle of the right ventricle. The variation noted by Rastelli and his colleagues[7] is then readily explained on the basis of increased commitment of the superior bridging leaflet to the right ventricle, with concomitant diminution in size of the antero-superior leaflet of the right ventricle (Figure 8.2.18). As the superior

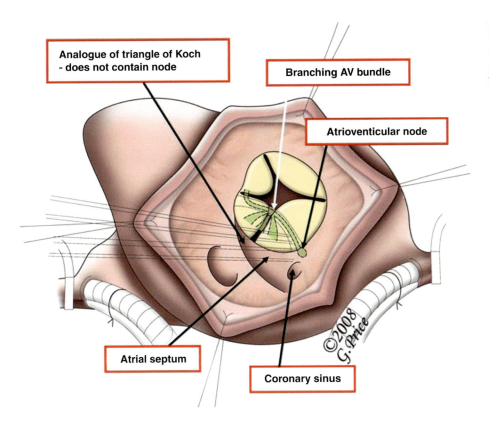

Figure 8.2.11 The drawing shows the usual disposition of the atrioventricular (AV) conduction axis in hearts with atrioventricular septal defect and common atrioventricular junction, here the variant with common valvar orifice.

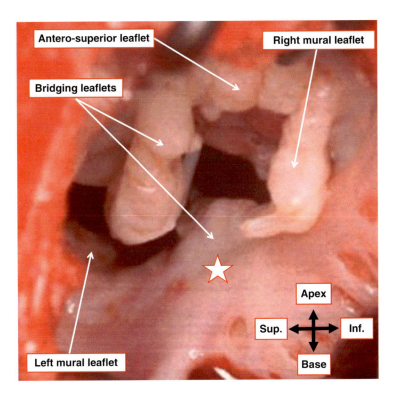

Figure 8.2.12 In this atrioventricular septal defect with separate right and left valvar orifices, the atrial septum is grossly deficient. The atrioventricular node is found at the point where the muscular ventricular septum joins the inferior atrioventricular junction (star).

bridging leaflet becomes increasingly committed to the right ventricle, so its site of coaptation with the antero-superior leaflet moves towards the right ventricular apex (Figures 8.2.19, 8.2.20).[6] A further difference between the hearts at either end of the spectrum identified by Rastelli and colleagues[7] is that, with minimal bridging, the superior bridging leaflet is tethered by cords to the crest of the ventricular septum (Figure 8.2.17). With extreme commitment of the supporting papillary muscle to the right ventricle, in contrast, the superior bridging leaflet is always free floating. The variation noted by Rastelli and colleagues reflected the changing morphology of the superior bridging leaflet. There is also variation in the arrangement of the

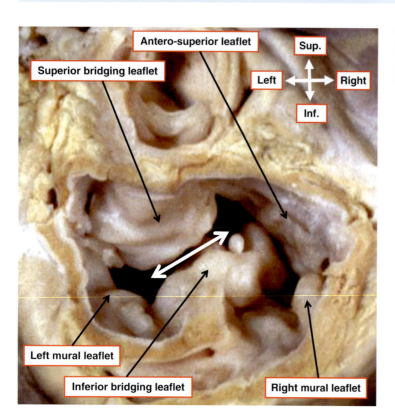

Figure 8.2.13 This atrioventricular septal defect, positioned anatomically and viewed from above, and with a common valvar orifice, has been dissected to show the arrangement of the five leaflets that guard the common atrioventricular junction. The white double-headed arrow shows the zone of apposition between the two bridging leaflets.

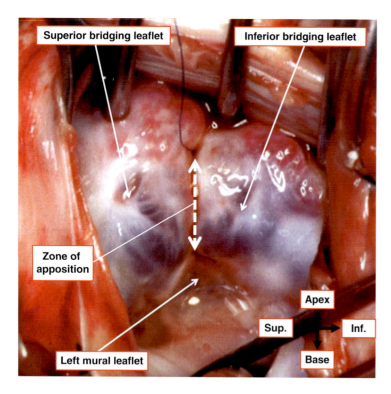

Figure 8.2.14 This operative view through a right atriotomy shows the typical trifoliate formation of the left atrioventricular valve in a heart with deficient atrioventricular septation and common atrioventricular junction. It bears no resemblance to the formation of the leaflets as seen in the normal mitral valve. Note the extensive zone of apposition between the two leaflets that bridge the ventricular septum (white double-headed arrow).

inferior bridging leaflet. This does not, however, reflect its commitment to the two ventricles, which is usually balanced. The leaflet, however, is often divided along the inferior edge of the ventricular septum, with the attachments of the two components providing a relatively clear zone of separation. The edges are most frequently attached to the septal crest, but there can be a ventricular component to the defect through intercordal spaces. Such potential for shunting beneath the inferior bridging leaflet is almost always found when the superior bridging leaflet is free floating.

It is the morphology of the bridging leaflets themselves that accounts for much of the remaining variability in

8.2 Atrioventricular Septal Defects

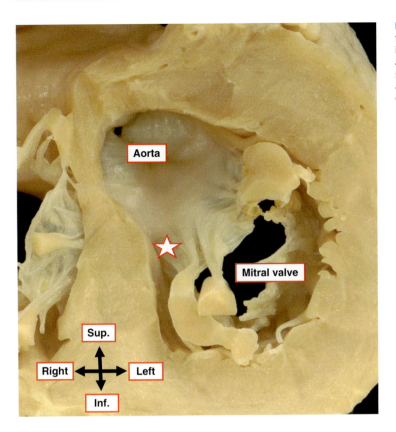

Figure 8.2.15 This view of the left ventricle, taken from the apex with the ventricular mass sectioned in its short axis, shows the interrelationship of the normal mitral valve and the outflow tract to the aorta. Note the oblique position of the papillary muscles supporting the solitary zone of apposition between the leaflets of the mitral valve, along with the extensive infero-septal recess between the aortic leaflet of the mitral valve and the septal surface of the left ventricle (star).

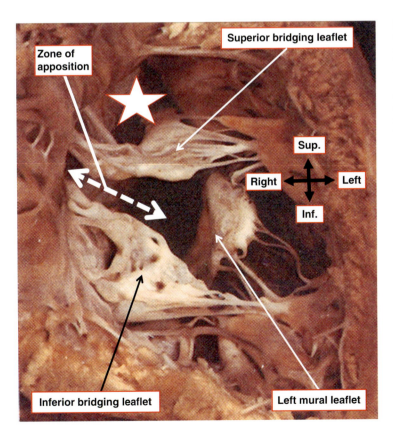

Figure 8.2.16 This view of the left atrioventricular valve and the outflow tract in a heart with atrioventricular septal defect is taken in comparable fashion to the normal heart seen in Figure 8.2.15, showing the short axis of the left ventricle. Note that the left valve in the heart with deficient atrioventricular septation has three leaflets, with papillary muscles positioned directly superiorly and inferiorly, rather than being obliquely positioned as in the normal heart. There is an extensive zone of apposition between the bridging leaflets (white double-headed arrow). Note also the way that the outflow tract is squeezed between the superior bridging leaflet and the superior margin of the left ventricle (star).

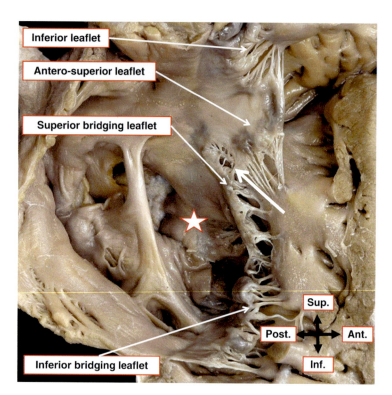

Figure 8.2.17 The image shows the location of the line of coaptation between the superior bridging and antero-superior leaflet of the common atrioventricular valve as seen from the atrial aspect in an atrioventricular septal defect with common valvar orifice (thick white arrow). This arrangement, with minimal bridging of the superior leaflet, produces the so-called Rastelli Type A malformation. The star shows the atrial component of the septal defect. Note that there is the potential for multiple shunts through intercordal spaces to occur at the ventricular level beneath the superior bridging leaflet. Note also that there is an inferior leaflet in the right ventricle. It is a mistake to consider this arrangement to represent a divided common anterior leaflet.

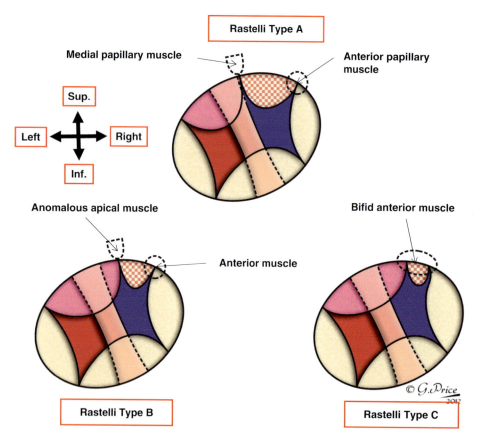

Figure 8.2.18 The drawing is shown as seen in anatomical orientation and viewed from above (compare with Figure 8.2.13). It shows the spectrum of bridging of the superior leaflet in hearts with atrioventricular septal defect and common orifice that underlies the classification introduced by Rastelli and his colleagues.[7] As the superior bridging leaflet (pink) extends further into the right ventricle, so there is concomitant diminution in size of the antero-superior leaflet (pink cross-hatched), and fusion of the anterior and medial papillary muscles of the right ventricle, which are increasingly attached towards the right ventricular apex.

atrioventricular septal defects with common atrioventricular junction. The overall valvar morphology is comparable in all hearts having the phenotypic feature of the common atrioventricular junction. The variability depends on the relationship of the two bridging leaflets to each other, or their relationships, on the one hand, to the lower edge of the atrial septum and, on the other hand, to the crest of the muscular ventricular septum. If these two features are described separately, there is no need

8.2 Atrioventricular Septal Defects

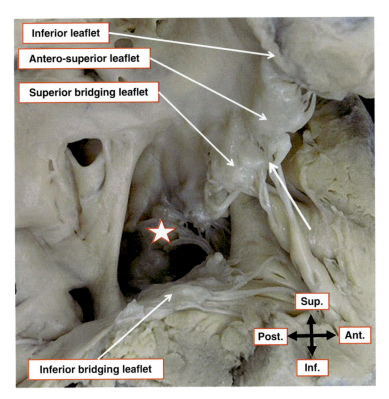

Figure 8.2.19 The image is taken in the same orientation as Figure 8.2.17. It shows how, in the Rastelli Type B variant of common valvar orifice, the line of coaptation between the superior bridging leaflet and the antero-superior leaflet of the right ventricle (thick white arrow) is displaced into the right ventricle. The papillary muscle supporting the zone of coaptation has moved down the ventricular septum towards the apex of the right ventricle. The antero-superior leaflet itself is smaller than in the Rastelli Type A variant, but there is also an inferior leaflet in the right ventricle, displaced upwards because of the opened right atrioventricular junction.

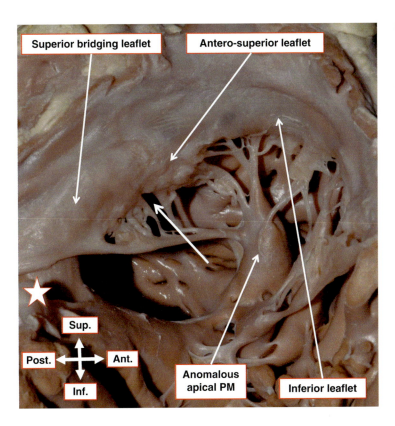

Figure 8.2.20 The image, taken to parallel the views seen in Figures 8.2.17 and 8.2.19, but showing only the right ventricular component of the superior bridging leaflet, illustrates the Rastelli Type C arrangement. Its line of coaptation with the antero-superior leaflet of the right ventricle has moved even further into the right ventricle (thicker white arrow), with concomitant decrease in size of the antero-superior leaflet. The papillary muscle (PM) supporting the line of coaptation is further towards the apex of the right ventricle. The star shows the location of the muscular ventricular septum. The image is reproduced by kind permission of Mr. Bill Devine, Children's Hospital of Pittsburgh.

to use terms such as 'complete', 'partial', and 'intermediate' when seeking to subdivide the group. It is the use of these terms that, in the past, has created most confusion in description. From the surgical stance, if it is possible to visualize a bare area at the mid-portion of the ventricular septal crest, this would constitute a complete lesion. If the crest of the septum is covered by a tongue of tissue that joins together the bridging leaflets, then the lesion is considered either partial or intermediate. The intermediate variant is characterized by the presence of shunting at both atrial and ventricular levels, but with separate valvar orifices within the common atrioventricular junction.

The partial variant, having no potential for ventricular shunting, is well described as the ostium primum variant. The bridging leaflets are joined to each other along the crest of the ventricular septum by a connecting tongue of leaflet tissue (Figure 8.2.21). The essence of the ostium primum defect, therefore, is the presence of separate valvar orifices for the right and left ventricles within the common atrioventricular junction. In essence, it is a double orifice common atrioventricular junction. Because the heart still possesses a common atrioventricular junction, the left valve has three leaflets, with an extensive zone of apposition between the left ventricular components of the superior and inferior bridging leaflets. This area, in the past, was frequently described as a cleft. It has no morphological similarity to the cleft found in the aortic leaflet of the mitral valve in hearts with normal atrioventricular septation and separate right and left atrioventricular junctions.[8] It has been established by surgical experience that it is necessary to close part, or all, of this zone of apposition when repairing ostium primum defects (Figure 8.2.22). The resulting closure, nonetheless, does not recreate a leaflet comparable to the aortic leaflet of the normal mitral valve (Figure 8.2.23).

The options for haemodynamic shunting across the atrioventricular septal defects, which largely colour the clinical features, depend upon the relationship of the bridging leaflets to the septal structures.[1] When there is a common valvar orifice, then it is extremely rare for the leaflets to be attached directly to the crest of the ventricular septum, although the extent of their tethering by tendinous cords can vary markedly. When the bridging leaflets lack direct attachments to the septal structures, the potential exists for shunting at both atrial and ventricular levels, the magnitude of the shunts depending on the prevailing haemodynamic conditions, together with the extent of the tethering. If the leaflets are firmly attached to the ventricular septum, then shunting will be confined at atrial level. This is the arrangement found most frequently in the typical ostium primum defect, with separate right and left valvar orifices within the common junction, but with both bridging leaflets firmly fused to the crest of the ventricular septum (Figure 8.2.24). Much less frequently, the bridging leaflets can be firmly attached to the underside of the atrial septum (Figure 8.2.25). This arrangement will confine the potential for shunting at ventricular level. It produces the true interventricular communication of atrioventricular canal variety, since the valve guarding the common atrioventricular junction will have the characteristics of a common atrioventricular valve, rather than tricuspid and mitral valves (Figures 8.2.25–8.2.29). The potential also exists, nonetheless, for the leaflets to be free floating even in the presence of separate valvar orifices (Figure 8.2.30). Most would consider the lesion shown in Figure 8.2.30 as an intermediate defect. If the variability in terms of attachment of the bridging leaflets is described, along with information concerning the presence of a common valvar orifice or separate right and left orifices, then there is no need to introduce the concept of intermediate or transitional variants. We recognize, nonetheless, the value of

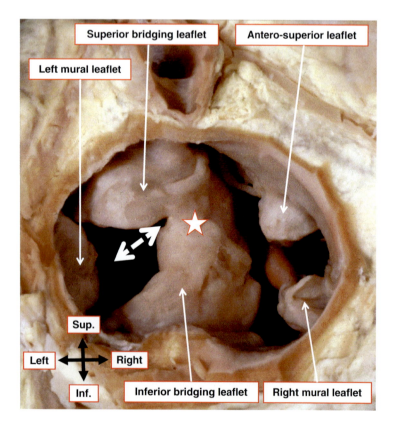

Figure 8.2.21 This heart with atrioventricular septal defect and separate right and left valvar orifices is viewed in anatomical orientation from above, after removal of the atrial chambers and the arterial trunks (compare with Figure 8.2.13). The common atrioventricular junction is now guarded by a valve with separate orifices for the right and left ventricle. This is because a tongue of leaflet tissue (star) joins together the facing surfaces of the bridging leaflets (compare with Figure 8.2.13). The white double-headed arrow shows the zone of apposition between the left ventricular components of the bridging leaflets.

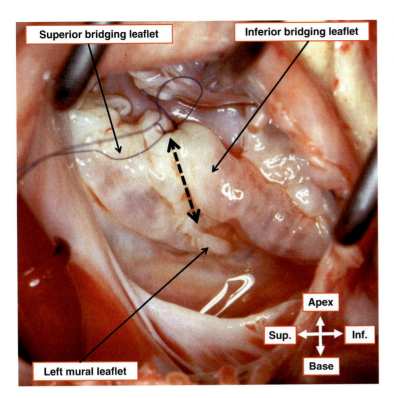

Figure 8.2.22 This view, taken through a right atriotomy, shows the trifoliate configuration of the left atrioventricular valve subsequent to repair of the zone of apposition between the left ventricular components of the bridging leaflets (dashed black arrow). Even after the surgical repair, the valve has no similarity to the normal mitral valve (see Figure 8.2.23).

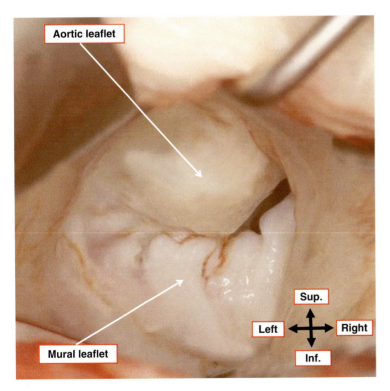

Figure 8.2.23 This view through a right atriotomy shows a normal mitral valve. The structure bears no comparison to the trifoliate valve shown in Figure 8.2.22.

the shorthand terms of partial, intermediate, and complete variants, providing that all working in the same team understand the definitions used for the different types.

Thus, in many patients with so-called partial defects, with separate right and left valvar orifices within the common junction, echo Doppler interrogation reveals the potential for interventricular shunting beneath the tongue that joins together the bridging leaflets, or else through intercordal spaces tethering the bridging leaflets themselves. Such patients are well described as having separate valvar orifices, with predominantly atrial shunting, but with the potential for minimal ventricular shunting (Figures 8.2.31, 8.2.32). The basic morphology of the deficient ventricular septum, therefore, is comparable in all patients having atrioventricular septal

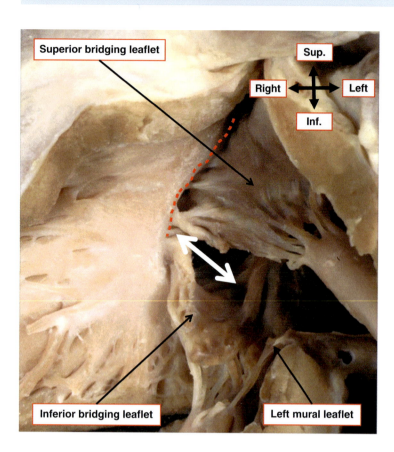

Figure 8.2.24 This heart with common atrioventricular junction and separate right and left valvar orifices is shown from the left side in anatomical orientation. The bridging leaflets are firmly fused to the crest of the ventricular septum (red dashed line), confining shunting through the atrioventricular septal defect at atrial level. This is the essence of the ostium primum defect. The double-headed white arrow shows the zone of apposition between the left ventricular components of the bridging leaflets.

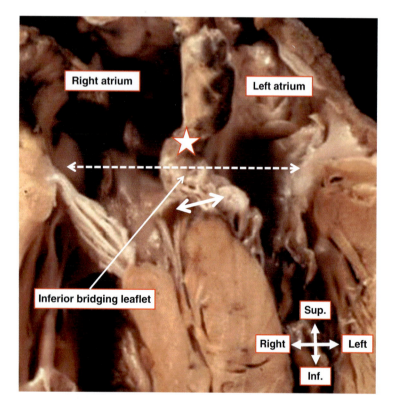

Figure 8.2.25 The four-chamber section is through an anatomical specimen from a patient with deficient atrioventricular septation and common atrioventricular junction (dashed white double-headed arrow). The inferior bridging leaflet is firmly fused to the undersurface of the atrial septum (star), confining shunting through the atrioventricular septal defect at ventricular level (solid white double-headed arrow).

defects with common atrioventricular junction.[1] As already emphasized, it is this disposition which determines the course of the ventricular conduction pathways (Figure 8.2.8).[4,9]

Although the hallmark of the malformation is the common atrioventricular junction, coupled with absence of the atrioventricular membranous septum and the muscular separating

8.2 Atrioventricular Septal Defects

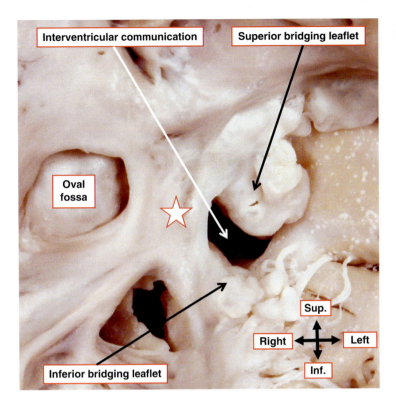

Figure 8.2.26 The specimen is viewed in anatomical orientation from the right side. The defect permits shunting at ventricular level only, since although the leaflets of the atrioventricular valve bridge across the crest of the ventricular septum into the left ventricle, the atrial septum is intact (star).

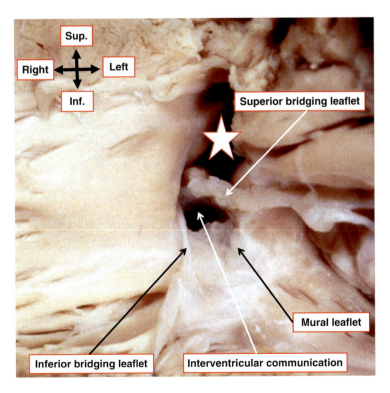

Figure 8.2.27 The image shows the left-sided aspect of another heart with deficient atrioventricular septation and common atrioventricular junction. This picture shows well the attachments of the bridging leaflets to the leading edge of the atrial septum, confining shunting at ventricular level. Note the typical configuration of the left ventricular outflow tract (star).

structures, there is also hypoplasia to a greater or lesser extent of the muscular ventricular septum. This involves disproportion between the inlet and outlet dimensions of the ventricular septum when compared with the normal heart (compare Figures 8.2.33 and 8.2.34). The degree of septal hypoplasia also varies with regard to the extent of scooping of the septum (Figure 8.2.34). The scooping is greater in hearts with common valvar orifice than in those with separate right and left orifices. Although the scooping is greater in hearts with a common valvar orifice, thus increasing the likelihood of there being a ventricular component to the defect, variability is still found among these hearts. When there is minimal scooping, it is possible to close the ventricular component of the septal defect by attaching the bridging leaflets directly to the right

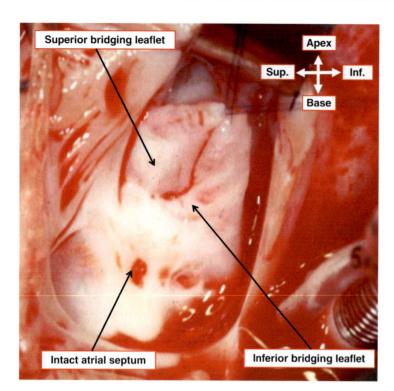

Figure 8.2.28 This picture, taken in the operating room, shows the right atrial aspect of an atrioventricular septal defect with common atrioventricular junction in which shunting is confined at ventricular level because the bridging leaflets are firmly attached to the underside of the atrial septum. In this image, the septal defect itself is not obvious.

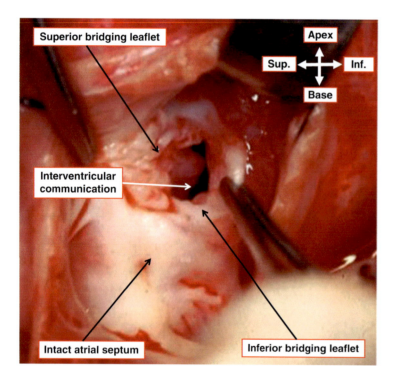

Figure 8.2.29 This image shows how, when the surgeon separated the right ventricular components of the bridging leaflets of the heart shown in Figure 8.2.28, the common atrioventricular junction is seen, with shunting at ventricular level across the atrioventricular septal defect.

ventricular aspect of the ventricular septum.[10] This manoeuvre, in fact, is feasible in all patients with common valvar orifice,[10,11] although not all are convinced of its utility. Thus, the use of the modified single patch approach still remains controversial. Some consider that the technique creates potential narrowing of the left ventricular outflow tract. There may be subtle technical differences that produce the different results.

If the technique is used, care must be taken not to damage the exposed conduction tissues along the septal crest. The non-branching bundle runs down the crest of the scooped-out septum, and is covered by the inferior bridging leaflet.

8.2 Atrioventricular Septal Defects

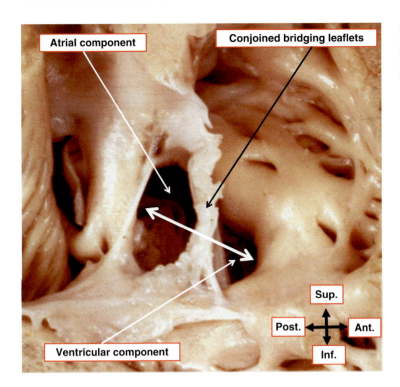

Figure 8.2.30 In this heart from a patient with an atrioventricular septal defect (double-headed arrow), with separate valvar orifices and shown in anatomical orientation, the bridging leaflets and the connecting tongue float free of both atrial and ventricular septal structures so that there are both atrial and ventricular defects.

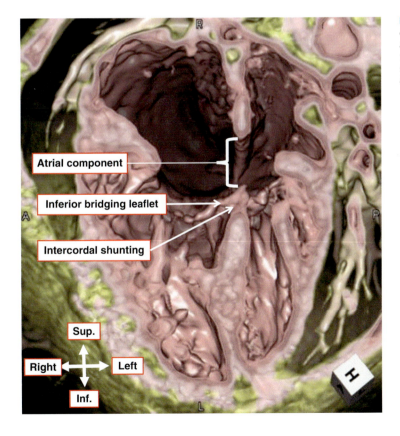

Figure 8.2.31 The virtual dissection shows a four-chamber cut from a computed tomographic dataset prepared from an individual with an atrioventricular septal defect. There are separate valvar orifices, with most of the shunting at atrial level. There is, however, the potential for shunting at ventricular level through intercordal spaces (see Figure 8.2.32). Orientation cube, lower right: H, head.

The inferior leaflet itself is often divided by a midline raphe immediately above the vulnerable non-branching bundle. The branching component of the conduction axis is found astride the midportion of the septal crest. This is usually covered by the connecting tongue and leaflet tissue in hearts with separate right and left valvar orifices. It is exposed in the presence of a common orifice and free-floating leaflets. The right bundle branch then runs towards the medial papillary muscle. Anterior to this point, the septum is devoid of conduction tissue (Figures 8.2.35, 8.2.36).[4,9]

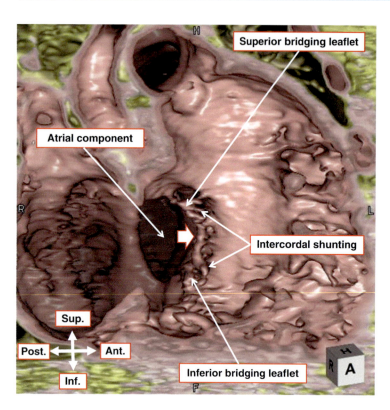

Figure 8.2.32 This virtual dissection, showing the septal aspect of the right-sided chambers, is from the same tomographic dataset as used to prepare Figure 8.2.31. The superior and inferior bridging leaflets are connected together by a tongue of valvar tissue (white arrow with red borders). Although most of the shunting is at atrial level, there is the potential for ventricular shunting through intercordal spaces beneath both bridging leaflets. Orientation cube, lower right: A, anterior; H, head; R, right.

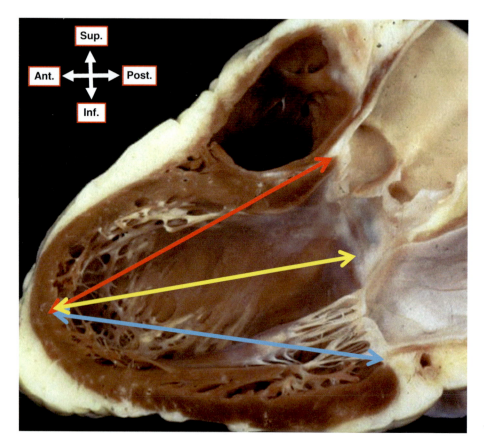

Figure 8.2.33 The normal heart is shown from the left side, the parietal wall of the left ventricle having been removed. There is equality in the inlet (blue arrow) and outlet (red arrow) dimensions of the ventricular septum, along with the midseptal dimension (yellow arrow). Compare with Figure 8.2.34.

8.2 Atrioventricular Septal Defects

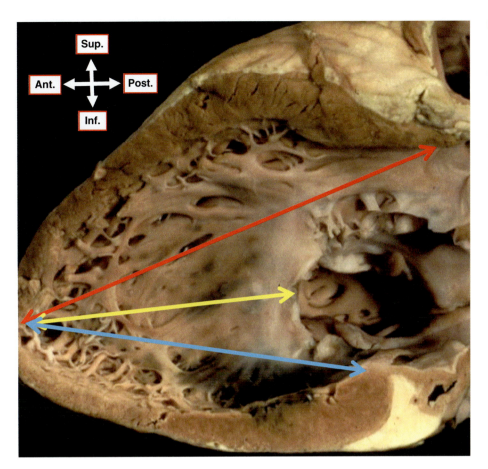

Figure 8.2.34 The valvar leaflets have been removed from the ventricular mass in this heart with deficient atrioventricular septation and common atrioventricular junction. The heart is viewed from the left side and shown in anatomical orientation. Since the leaflets have been removed, there is no way of knowing whether, originally, there was a common atrioventricular orifice, or separate valvar orifices for the right and left ventricles. Note the scooping of the ventricular septum (yellow arrow), and the disproportion between inlet (blue arrow) and outlet (red arrow) dimensions of the ventricular mass.

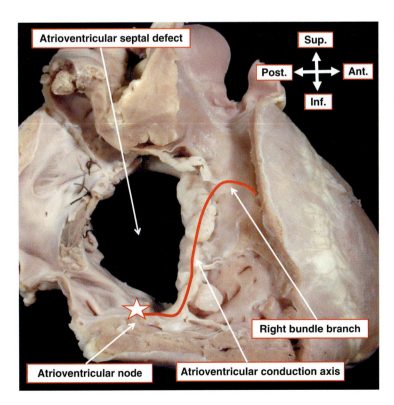

Figure 8.2.35 This heart came from a patient with an atrioventricular septal defect with common atrioventricular junction and shunting confined at atrial level, in other words an ostium primum defect. The disposition of the atrioventricular conduction axis has been superimposed on the picture, as seen from the right side, with the star showing the site of the atrioventricular node, and the red line showing the course of the axis.

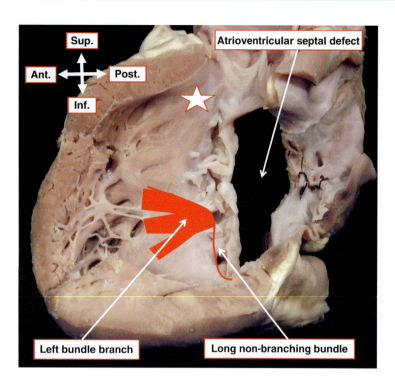

Figure 8.2.36 The photograph shows the left ventricular aspect of the heart illustrated in Figure 8.2.35, again with the location of the atrioventricular conduction axis superimposed on the picture. Note that the left ventricular outflow tract (star) is distant from the conduction tissues.

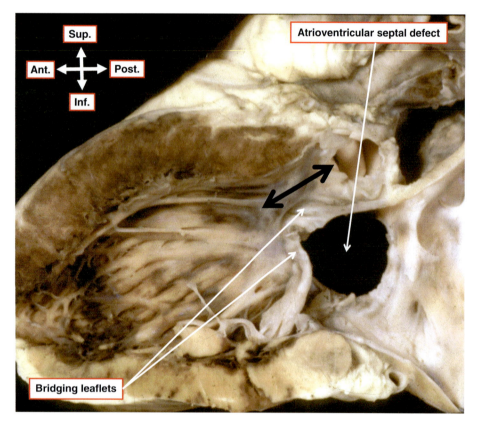

Figure 8.2.37 The heart, shown in anatomical orientation from the left side, has been dissected to show the extent of the narrowed outflow tract in an atrioventricular septal defect with separate right and left atrioventricular valves, and with the potential only for atrial shunting. Because the superior bridging leaflet is firmly attached to the crest of the ventricular septum, the outflow tract has considerable length (double-headed black arrow).

Although not readily evident to the surgeon during operation, the left ventricular outflow tract in atrioventricular septal defects is intrinsically narrow.[12] It is much longer in hearts with separate orifices. This is because of the attachment of the superior bridging leaflet to the ventricular septal crest (compare Figures 8.2.37 and 8.2.38). The area is prone to postoperative obstruction, and surgical enlargement may be necessary. Obstruction may be due to naturally occurring lesions,[13] or to injudicious placement of a prosthesis used to replace the left atrioventricular valve. If a prosthesis must be employed, the anatomy dictates insertion of a model with low profile, or else

8.2 Atrioventricular Septal Defects

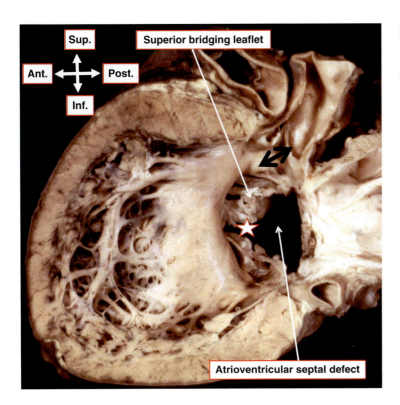

Figure 8.2.38 In this heart, again shown in anatomical orientation from the left side (compare with Figure 8.2.37), the outflow tract (double-headed black arrow in Figure 8.2.37) is much shorter in the presence of a common atrioventricular valvar orifice. The star shows the zone of apposition between the bridging leaflets.

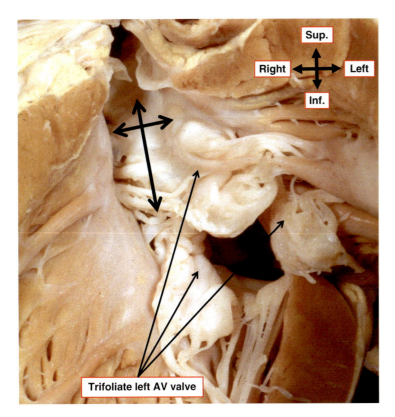

Figure 8.2.39 This heart has an atrioventricular septal defect with common atrioventricular orifice, but with the superior bridging leaflet tethered across the subaortic outflow tract (crossed black arrows). It is photographed in anatomical orientation from the left side.

resection of the shelf that exists between the hinge point of the superior bridging leaflet and the attachment of the aortic valve.[14] The superior bridging leaflet can also be liberated from the septal crest, inserting a gusset to enlarge the outflow tract (Figures 8.2.39, 8.2.40).

Further variability is found in the commitment of the common atrioventricular junction to the ventricular mass. Usually it is shared equally, giving a balanced arrangement (Figure 8.2.1). Should the common junction favour one or other ventricle, producing so-called right or left ventricular

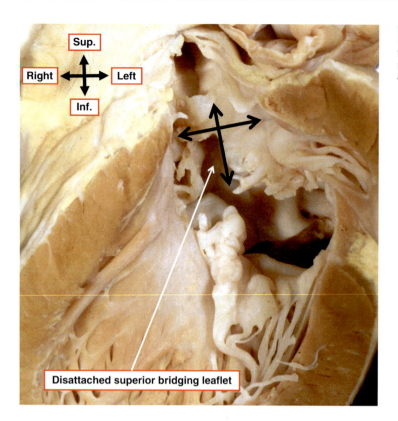

Figure 8.2.40 An incision has been made in the superior bridging leaflet of the heart shown in Figure 8.2.39, at the same time detaching the leaflet from the crest of the ventricular septum. The incision makes it possible to insert a patch so as to widen the outflow tract (crossed black arrows).

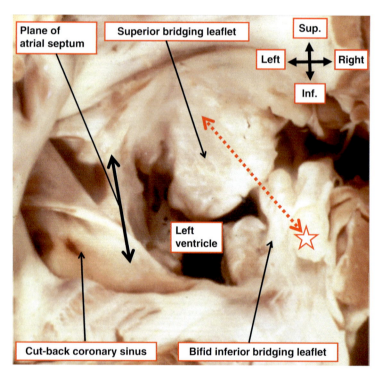

Figure 8.2.41 In this specimen from a patient with atrioventricular septal defect and common atrioventricular junction, shown in anatomical orientation, there is gross malalignment between the muscular ventricular septum (red double-headed arrow) and the atrial septum (black double-headed arrow). As a consequence, the atrioventricular conduction axis originates from an anomalous node (star) in the inferior aspect of the right atrioventricular junction, rather than at the crux of the heart.

dominance, the other ventricle is often severely hypoplastic. This can have a major influence on the outcome of surgery, and should always be assessed preoperatively. In the setting of right ventricular dominance, there is usually alignment between the atrial and ventricular septal structures at the crux. The essence of left ventricular dominance, in contrast, is malalignment between the atrial septum and the muscular ventricular septum (Figure 8.2.41). This produces an arrangement analogous to straddling of the tricuspid valve.[15] As with the straddling tricuspid valve, this has major consequence for the disposition of the atrioventricular conduction axis.[16]

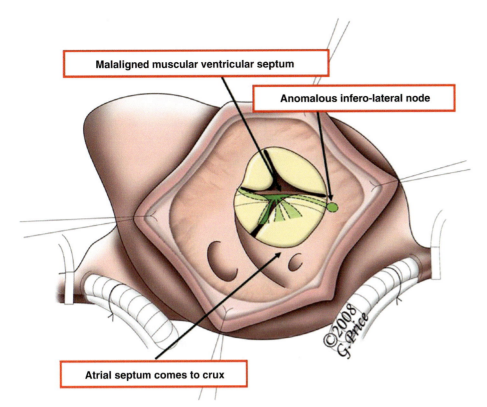

Figure 8.2.42 The drawing shows how, when there is malalignment between the atrial septum and the muscular ventricular septum, with left ventricular dominance, the atrioventricular node is formed at the point where the ventricular septum meets the inferior atrioventricular junction.

Because of the septal malalignment, the connecting atrioventricular node is no longer to be found at the crux. It continues to be formed at the point where the malaligned muscular ventricular septum meets the atrioventricular junction (Figure 8.2.42). This particular arrangement must be identified preoperatively, since it can be exceedingly difficult to recognize during surgery. If unrecognized, it is likely that a standard repair will damage the conduction axis. Septal malalignment, therefore, should be excluded in all cases of atrioventricular septal defect with left ventricular dominance. This arrangement should also be distinguished from those hearts in which the atrial septum is absent, and the coronary sinus terminates in the left atrium.[5]

References Cited

1. Becker AE, Anderson RH. Atrioventricular septal defects. What's in a name? *J Thorac Cardiovasc Surg* 1982; **83**: 461–469.
2. Gerbode F, Hultgren H, Melrose D, Osborn J. Syndrome of left ventricular–right atrial shunt, successful surgical repair of defect in five cases with observation of bradycardia on closure. *Ann Surg* 1958; **148**: 433–446.
3. Kelle AM, Young L, Kaushal S, et al. The Gerbode defect: the significance of a left ventricular to right atrial shunt. *Cardiol Young* 2009; **19** (Suppl.2): 96–99.
4. Lacour-Gayet F, Campbell DN, Mitchell M, Malhotta S, Anderson RH. Surgical repair of atrioventricular septal defect with common atrioventricular junction *Cardiol Young* 2006; **16** (Suppl.3): 52–58.
5. Wilcox BR, Anderson RH, Henry GW, Mattos SS. Unusual opening of coronary sinus in atrioventricular septal defects. *Ann Thorac Surg* 1990; **50**: 767–770.
6. Penkoske PA, Neches WH, Anderson RH, Zuberbuhler JR. Further observations on the morphology of atrioventricular septal defects. *J Thorac Cardiovasc Surg* 1985; **90**: 611–622.
7. Rastelli GC, Kirklin JW, Titus JL. Anatomic observations on complete form of persistent common atrioventricular canal with special reference to atrioventricular valves. *Proc Staff Meet Mayo Clin* 1966; **41**: 296–308.
8. Sigfusson G, Ettedgui JA, Silverman NH, Anderson RH. Is a cleft in the anterior leaflet of an otherwise normal mitral valve an atrioventricular canal malformation? *J Am Coll Cardiol* 1995; **26**: 508–515.
9. Yoshitake S, Kaneko Y, Morita K, et al.; SPring 8 Cardiovascular Structure Analyzing Research Group. Reassessment of the location of the conduction system in atrioventricular septal defect using phase-contrast computed tomography. *Sem Thorac Cardiovasc Surg* 2020; **32**: 960–968.
10. Wilcox BR, Jones DR, Frantz EG, et al. An anatomically sound, simplified approach to repair of 'complete' atrioventricular septal defect. *Ann Thorac Surg* 1997; **64**: 487–494.
11. Nicholson IA, Nunn GR, Sholler GF, et al. Simplified single patch technique for the repair of atrioventricular septal defect. *J Thorac Cardiovasc Surg* 1999; **118**: 642–646.
12. Karl TR, Provenzano SC, Nunn GR, Anderson RH. The current surgical perspective to repair of atrioventricular septal defect with common atrioventricular junction.

13. Ebels T, Ho SY, Anderson RH, Meijboom EJ, Eigelaar A. The surgical anatomy of the left ventricular outflow tract in atrioventricular septal defect. *Ann Thorac Surg* 1986; **41**: 483–488.

    Cardiol Young 2010; **20** (Suppl.3): 120–127.

14. Piccoli GP, Ho SY, Wilkinson JL, et al. Left sided obstructive lesions in atrioventricular septal defects. *J Thorac Cardiovasc Surg* 1982; **83**: 453–460.

15. Pillai R, Ho SY, Anderson RH, Shinebourne EA, Lincoln C. Malalignment of the interventricular septum with atrioventricular septal defect: its implications concerning conduction tissue disposition. *Thorac Cardiovasc Surgeon* 1984; **32**: 1–3.

16. Milo S, Ho SY, Macartney FJ, et al. Straddling and overriding atrioventricular valves morphology and classification. *Am J Cardiol* 1979; **44**: 1122–1134.

Chapter 8.3: Ventricular Septal Defects

When asked to close a clinically significant hole between the ventricles, the primary concern of the surgeon is to ensure that the task can be achieved in safe and secure fashion. The important anatomical features to be considered reflect the location of the defect relative to the landmarks of the right ventricle. These features, when assessed relative to the leaflets of the atrioventricular and arterial valves, determine the proximity of the defect to the atrioventricular conduction axis. One categorization of the defects[1] was designed specifically to focus the attention of the surgeon on these pertinent features. The essence of the system was that, according to the anatomical features of the margins of the defects as seen from the morphologically right ventricle, all the holes fitted into one of three groups.

The first group included all those holes that, when viewed from the right ventricle, had exclusively muscular borders (Figure 8.3.1). The phenotypic feature of the second group was that part of the border of the defect, as viewed from the morphologically right ventricle, was composed of fibrous continuity between the leaflets of the atrioventricular valves (Figure 8.3.2). The initial chosen criterion was continuity between the leaflets of an atrioventricular and an arterial valve.[1] We have now become aware that defects within this category can be found with atrioventricular-arterial valvar discontinuity. All defects falling within the group, however, do have fibrous continuity between the leaflets of the mitral and tricuspid valves.[2] The patients falling in the third group were unified because part of their borders, as viewed from the morphologically right ventricle, was made up of fibrous continuity between the leaflets of the aortic and pulmonary valves (Figure 8.3.3). Defects of this third type were found to show additional variability depending on whether the fibrous continuity extended to include continuity between the leaflets of the atrioventricular valves. The defects in the patients making up the third group, of necessity, open between the outflow tracts of the ventricles. Defects within the other groups, however, need further description depending on whether they open primarily to the inlet, to the apical, or to the outlet components

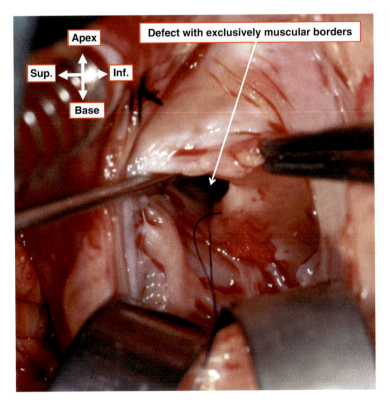

Figure 8.3.1 This view through a right atriotomy, and across the orifice of the tricuspid valve, shows a hole between the ventricles that is enclosed by the walls of the muscular ventricular septum.

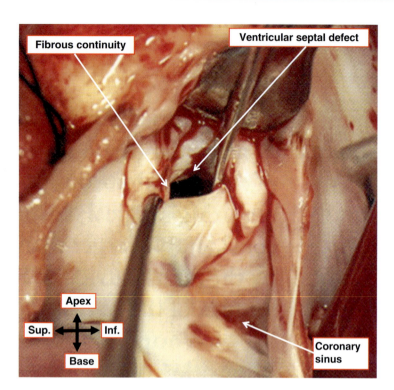

Figure 8.3.2 This view, again through a right atriotomy with retraction of the leaflets of the tricuspid valve, shows the fibrous tissue of the atrioventricular septum forming part of the right ventricular border as viewed by the surgeon. This is the criterion that permits the defect to be categorized as being perimembranous.

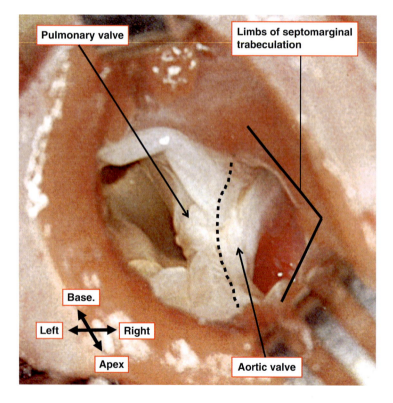

Figure 8.3.3 This surgical view shows a hole between the ventricles that, at its cranial border, has fibrous continuity between the leaflets of the aortic and pulmonary valves (black dotted line). The defect, opening to the ventricular outlets between the limbs of the septomarginal trabeculation directly juxta-arterial, and also doubly committed.

of the right ventricle. There is then an additional feature which always requires description, if present, namely malalignment between the septal components.[3]

Other categorizations have been used for distinguishing between the types of holes shown above. One time-honoured system identified four variants, and grouped them in numeric fashion.[4] Another popular system used developmental considerations so as to distinguish between the different holes.[5] The problem with the system allegedly based on embryology is that the concepts used to explain septal development are unequivocally wrong. Our recommended system, which was initially designed specifically to emphasize the surgical considerations (Figure 8.3.4), as we will show, has now proved also to be entirely compatible with the account of cardiac

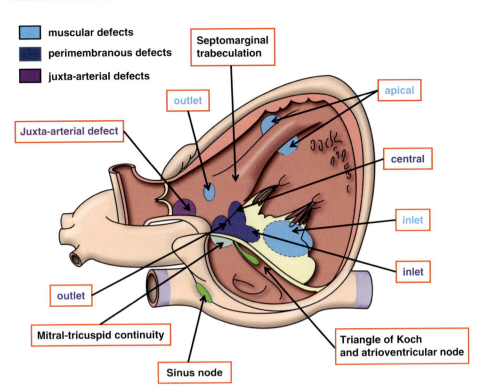

Figure 8.3.4 The drawing, shown in surgical orientation, illustrates the categorization used for differentiating the phenotypic variations for holes between the ventricles. It combines the phenotypic features shown in the previous three figures with the location of the hole relative to the components of the right ventricle.

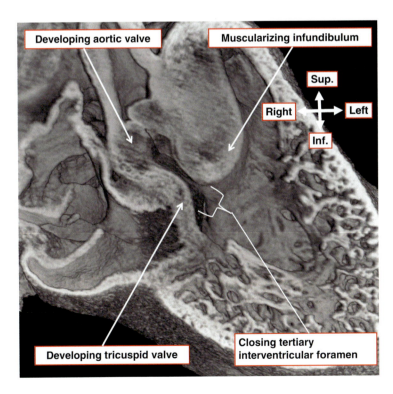

Figure 8.3.5 The image is a section taken from a dataset prepared from a mouse embryo at embryonic day 13.5. It shows the margins of the closing tertiary interventricular foramen, formed dorsally by continuity between the cushions forming the leaflets of the mitral and tricuspid valves. Perimembranous defects reflect failure to close this embryonic interventricular communication.

development provided in Chapter 2. The system, nonetheless, depends on descriptions of the borders of the holes between the ventricles as seen by the surgeon working through the morphologically right ventricle (Figures 8.3.1–8.3.3).

The essence of the largest group of defects requiring surgical closure is that an area of fibrous continuity between the leaflets of the mitral and tricuspid valves forms a direct part of the rim of the defect as seen from the right ventricle (Figure 8.3.2). This is because the holes in question represent the final area of the septum to be closed during development. This is the so-called tertiary interventricular communication (Figure 8.3.5), which is closed by the tubercles of the superior and inferior atrioventricular cushions. These cushions, of course, become the membranous septum. The holes exist simply because these cushions are

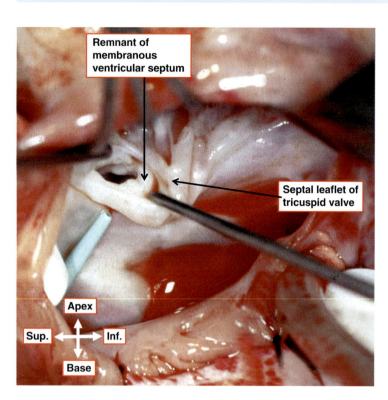

Figure 8.3.6 In this heart, viewed through a right atriotomy and through the orifice of the tricuspid valve, a remnant of the interventricular membranous septum is present in the postero-inferior margin of the perimembranous defect.

unable to achieve closure. This explains why the fibrous area incorporates the atrioventricular component of the membranous septum. The defects, therefore, surround the membranous part of the septum, and are justifiably described as being perimembranous. In many instances, furthermore, the interventricular component of the membranous septum is found as a fold of fibrous tissue in the postero-inferior margin of the defect (Figure 8.3.6). We presume that the foramen persists as a communication between the aortic root and the right ventricle because of deficiency of the muscular ventricular septum, which forms the apical and cranial rims of the persisting hole. Defects requiring surgical closure will always be considerably larger than the area occupied by the interventricular membranous septum of the normal heart.

The extent of the deficiency of the muscular rims has important consequences for the disposition of the axis of atrioventricular conduction tissue.[6] When development proceeds normally, the conduction axis penetrates through the junction between the roof of the infero-septal recess and atrioventricular membranous septum to reach the crest of the muscular septum. Having penetrated, it is sandwiched between the crest of the muscular septum and the interventricular component of the membranous septum (Figure 8.3.7). In perimembranous defects, when the atrioventricular connections are concordant, so as to reach the crest of the muscular ventricular septum, the axis penetrates through the area of continuity between the leaflets of the tricuspid and mitral valves (Figure 8.3.8). When a remnant of the interventricular membranous septum is present, it lies immediately on top of the atrioventricular bundle (Figure 8.3.8). If such a remnant is seen at operation (Figure 8.3.6), and is substantial, it may safely be used for anchorage of sutures placed superficially to anchor a surgical patch.

The location of the medial papillary muscle, together with the apex of the triangle of Koch, provides the guide for predicting the location of the conduction axis in almost all holes that are perimembranous, in other words the holes bordered postero-inferiorly by fibrous continuity between the leaflets of the tricuspid and mitral valves (Figure 8.3.9). The only exceptions to this rule are the defects associated with straddling and overriding of the tricuspid valve.[7] The proximity of the conduction tissues to the leaflets of the aortic and atrioventricular valves, however, varies depending upon the precise area of deficiency of the muscular septum. It is likely that all parts are deficient to a certain extent. It can usually be determined, nonetheless, which part is most affected. When a perimembranous defect extends to open mostly into the inlet of the right ventricle, its atrial margin, as viewed through the tricuspid valve, is the area of fibrous continuity between the leaflets of the mitral and tricuspid valves that supports the base of the atrial septum, and forms the roof of the infero-septal recess (Figure 8.3.10). In this setting, the apex of the triangle of Koch is usually deviated inferiorly towards the coronary sinus. It is then to the right hand of the surgeon working through the atrium. The axis of atrioventricular conduction tissue penetrates through this corner of the defect. The non-branching and branching components of the conduction axis are then carried on the left ventricular aspect of the muscular septum as they descend the right-hand margin of the defect. The right bundle branch courses intramyocardially, surfacing beneath the medial papillary muscle, which is usually at the left-hand margin of the defect. The non-coronary leaflet of the aortic valve is more to the left, and usually distant from the rim of the defect, although it often maintains fibrous continuity with the septal leaflet of the tricuspid valve (Figure 8.3.10).

8.3 Ventricular Septal Defects

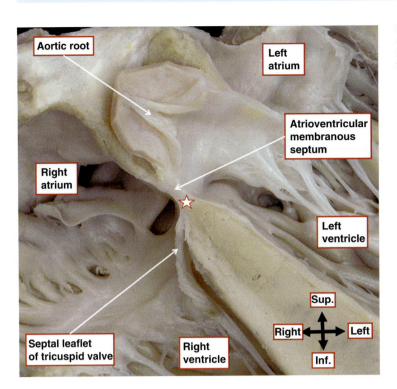

Figure 8.3.7 This four-chamber section, shown in anatomical orientation, reveals the position of the penetrating atrioventricular bundle (star) in the normal heart. It is sandwiched between the central fibrous body and the crest of the muscular ventricular septum.

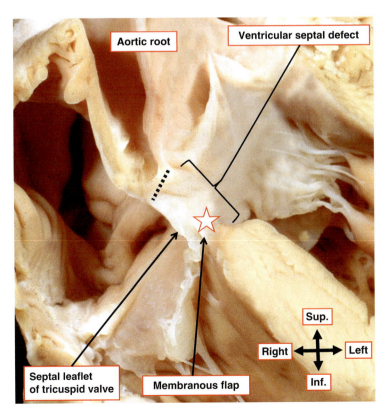

Figure 8.3.8 This 'four-chamber' section, again seen in anatomical orientation, shows the position of the penetrating atrioventricular bundle (star) in a heart with a perimembranous ventricular septal defect.

When perimembranous defects requiring surgical closure are located so as to open mostly towards the ventricular apex, they are large. They typically open additionally towards the inlet and outlet components, and hence are well described as being confluent. The triangle of Koch is not deviated as far towards the coronary sinus in such defects as when they open primarily to the right ventricular inlet, but the right-hand rim is still the major area at risk. The medial papillary muscle tends to be at the apex of such defects. The non-coronary leaflet of the aortic valve is more closely related to the atrial margin. The septal leaflet of the tricuspid valve is often cleft or deficient, an

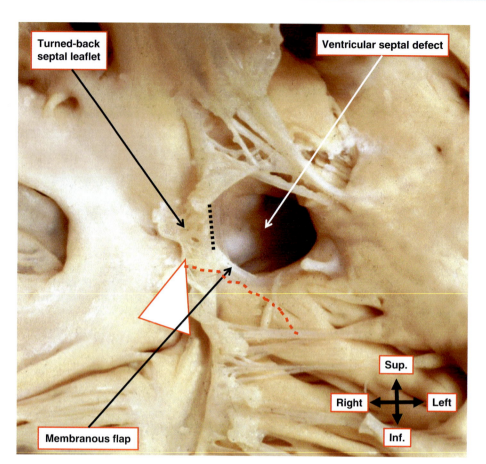

Figure 8.3.9 This hole between the ventricles, shown in anatomical orientation, is viewed from its right ventricular aspect. The postero-inferior margin of the defect is made up of fibrous continuity between the leaflets of the mitral and tricuspid valves (black dotted line). In this setting, which makes the defect perimembranous, the course of the conduction axis, shown by the red dotted line originating from the triangle of Koch, is always positioned postero-inferiorly. Note that the axis lies directly beneath a membranous flap. The septal leaflet of the tricuspid valve has been retracted.

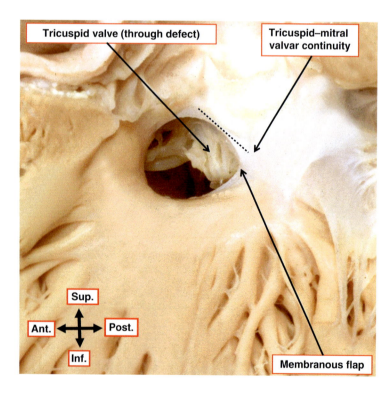

Figure 8.3.10 This illustration, seen in anatomical orientation, shows the left ventricular aspect of the perimembranous defect that opened primarily to the inlet of the right ventricle shown in Figure 8.3.9. The black dotted line shows the fibrous continuity between the leaflets of the tricuspid and mitral valves, via the membranous flap.

arrangement which may permit shunting from left ventricle to right atrium, and hence producing an indirect Gerbode defect (see Figure 8.2.2). If the cleft in the septal leaflet of the tricuspid valve requires surgical closure, it should be remembered that the penetrating atrioventricular bundle is located at its apex.

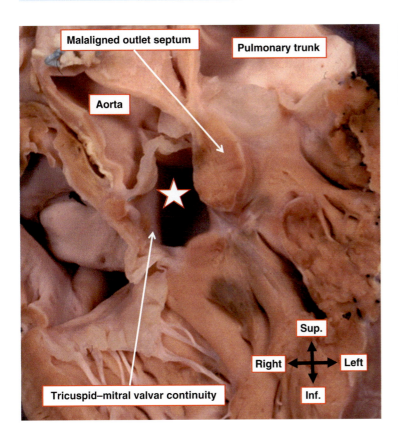

Figure 8.3.11 This heart, shown in anatomical orientation, has been sectioned to replicate the subcostal oblique long-axis echocardiographic projection. The perimembranous defect (star) opens towards the outlet of the right ventricle. The muscular outlet septum is now recognized in its own right. It is malaligned relative to the muscular ventricular septum, and attached antero-cephalad relative to the septomarginal trabeculation.

The third type of perimembranous defect extends mostly so as to open into the outlet of the right ventricle. The outlet septum, along with the free-standing subpulmonary infundibulum, can then be recognized separating the leaflets of the aortic and pulmonary valves, being malaligned relative to the rest of the septum (Figure 8.3.11). It is this type of defect that others describe as being conoventricular.[5] In the presence of antero-cephalad malalignment of the muscular outlet septum, the aortic root overrides the crest of the muscular ventricular septum (Figures 8.3.12, 8.3.13). The medial papillary muscle is on the right-hand margin of the defect, and the axis of atrioventricular conduction tissue is more distant from the edge, being carried well down on the left surface of the ventricular septum. The non-coronary and right coronary leaflets of the aortic valve are much more closely related to the left-hand margin (Figure 8.3.13), and may prolapse towards the right ventricle.[8,9]

The essential feature of muscular defects is that, when viewed from the right ventricle, they have exclusively muscular borders (Figure 8.3.1). They can open to the inlet, apical, or outlet parts of the right ventricle.[1] Of necessity, nonetheless, ventricular musculature must interpose between the edges of the defect and the attachments of the leaflets of the valves. When a muscular defect opens to the inlet of the right ventricle (Figure 8.3.14), it is inferior to the atrioventricular axis of conduction tissue. When viewed by the surgeon through the tricuspid valve (Figures 8.3.15, 8.3.16), the conduction axis is located on the left-hand margin of the defect. The proximity of the axis to the edge depends on the adjacency of the defect to the intact membranous septum. The basal margin of the muscular septum, interposing between the edge of the defect and the atrial septum, separates the septal leaflet of the tricuspid valve from the mitral valve, preserving the off-setting of the valvar hinges. Its size will determine whether it is suitable to be an anchorage for sutures.

Defects opening through the apical part of the septum can be single (Figure 8.3.17) or double, or seem to be multiple (Figure 8.3.18).[10] They are unrelated to the proximal parts of the conduction tissue axis, but may be related to ramifications of the distal bundle branches. It can be difficult to recognize the right ventricular openings of apical muscular defects because of the normal coarse apical trabeculations of the right ventricle. This is particularly the case when there is a so-called swiss-cheese septum (Figure 8.3.19). The multiple perforations in the setting of the swiss-cheese lesion reflect the fact that, during development, the muscular septum is formed by coalescence of the initial trabecular layers of the ventricular walls. If multiple and small, it may not be possible to identify all the defects through a right ventriculotomy. The septal deficiencies are much more readily identified from the left ventricular aspect. Inspection from the left side will often demonstrate that the seemingly multiple defects (Figure 8.3.18) reflect the presence of a solitary hole (Figure 8.3.20). The swiss-cheese variant will more readily be identified from the left ventricular aspect, with the features demonstrating why the arrangement that can be notoriously difficult to close surgically (Figure 8.3.21).[11]

Muscular defects opening to the outlet of the right ventricle are relatively rare in patients with concordant atrioventricular and ventriculo-arterial connections. If small, the endocardium may appear to be heaped up at the edges to produce a fibrous rim (Figure 8.3.22). Larger defects opening

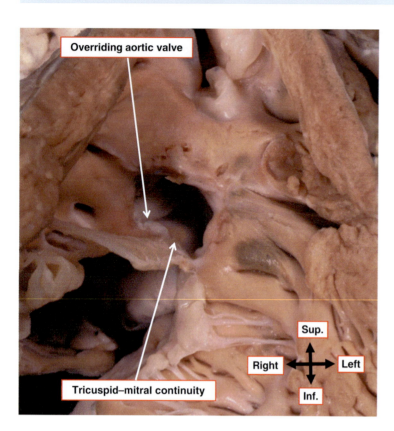

Figure 8.3.12 This is the heart shown in Figure 8.3.11 prior to making the section to correlate with the echocardiographic plane. The ventricular septal defect opens to the outlet of the right ventricle, with the aortic valve overriding the crest of the ventricular septum.

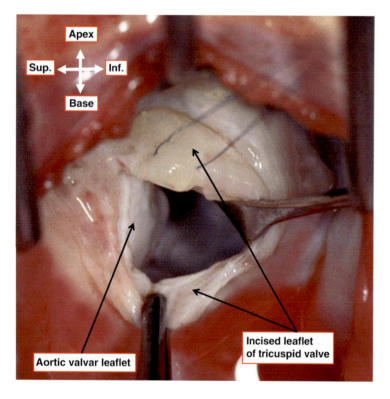

Figure 8.3.13 This view is through a right atriotomy, subsequent to making an incision at the junction of the septal and antero-superior leaflets of the tricuspid valve. It shows a perimembranous defect opening to the outlet of the right ventricle. The leaflets of the aortic valve are overriding the ventricular septal crest to the left-hand margin of the defect.

to the right ventricular outlet typically show malalignment of the muscular outlet septum (Figure 8.3.23). Close inspection will show whether the postero-caudal limb of the septomarginal trabeculation is fused with the ventriculo-infundibular fold to form a muscular postero-inferior rim to the defect, thus distinguishing the hole from a perimembranous defect with outlet extension. When present, the fusion of these muscle bars separates the edge of the defect from the axis of atrioventricular conduction tissue. The superior rim is the muscular outlet septum, combined with the free-standing

8.3 Ventricular Septal Defects

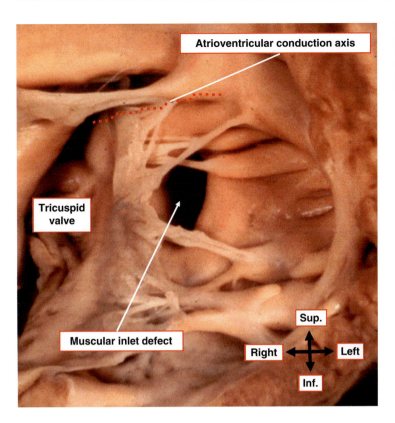

Figure 8.3.14 This heart, photographed from the right side in anatomical orientation, has a muscular ventricular septal defect opening to the inlet of the right ventricle. The atrioventricular conduction axis (red dotted line) runs antero-cephalad relative to the defect. In this instance, it is well removed from the superior margin of the hole.

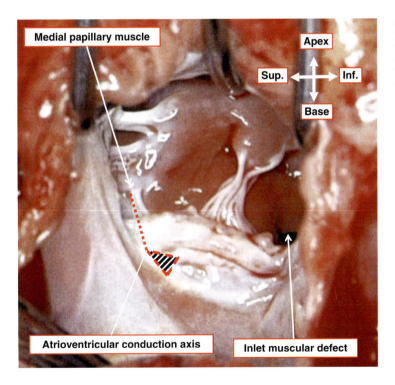

Figure 8.3.15 This surgical view shows a muscular defect opening to the inlet of the right ventricle, viewed through the orifice of the tricuspid valve. The conduction axis (red dotted area, with the black cross-hatched area showing the site of the atrioventricular node), arising from the apex of the triangle of Koch, is seen to the left hand of the surgeon working through the tricuspid valve.

subpulmonary infundibulum. These myocardial tissues separate the leaflets of the pulmonary valve from the right coronary leaflet of the aortic valve, the latter attached to its left ventricular surface. If this superior muscular rim is attenuated, then the leaflet of the aortic valve may again prolapse through the defect (Figure 8.3.23).

The third type of ventricular septal defect is the one which is juxta-arterial. In the past these have also been called doubly committed, but keeping to the borders approach, juxta-arterial describes these defects most accurately. Commitment of a defect to an arterial trunk or to both arterial trunks (doubly committed) is then a subsequent level of categorization. The phenotypic

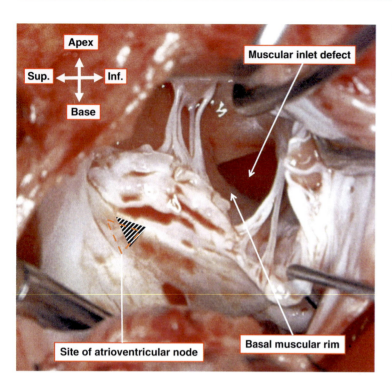

Figure 8.3.16 This view of the heart shown in Figure 8.3.15, again seen through a right atriotomy and the orifice of the tricuspid valve, shows the musculature of the ventricular septum interposing between the basal margin of the defect and the hinge of the septal leaflet of the tricuspid valve. The triangle of Koch is to the left hand of the surgeon relative to the defect.

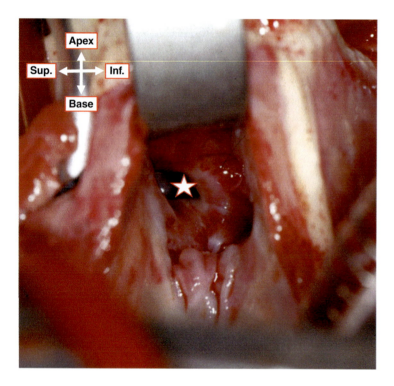

Figure 8.3.17 This defect is seen through a right atriotomy with the tricuspid valve retracted. It shows a muscular defect (star) opening into the outlet of the right ventricle.

feature of this defect is absence of both the muscular outlet septum, and the posterior aspect of the free-standing subpulmonary infundibulum. It reflects the failure of muscularization, during development, of the proximal outflow cushions (see Chapter 2). Because of the absence of the muscularized cushions, the adjacent leaflets of the aortic and pulmonary valves are in fibrous continuity, producing a fibrous raphe which forms the superior rim of the defect (Figure 8.3.24). The leaflets are attached at the same level, albeit that in some hearts part of the aortic sinus may interpose between them, producing a degree of valvar off-setting. In either event, sutures can be secured in the region of fibrous continuity.[12] The juxta-arterial defect can also be found with overriding of the orifice of the aortic valve (Figure 8.3.25). In most instances, the inferior rim of the defect is similar to that found in the muscular defect which opens to the outlet part of the right ventricle, the postero-caudal limb of the septo-marginal trabeculation fusing with the ventriculo-infundibular fold (Figure 8.3.24). When present, this muscular rim separates

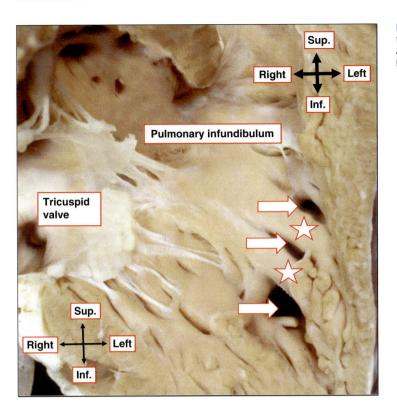

Figure 8.3.18 In this heart, viewed in anatomical orientation, it seems that there are three muscular defects (red-bordered arrows) opening anteriorly into the apical trabecular component of the right ventricle. Note, however, the presence of the septoparietal trabeculations (stars).

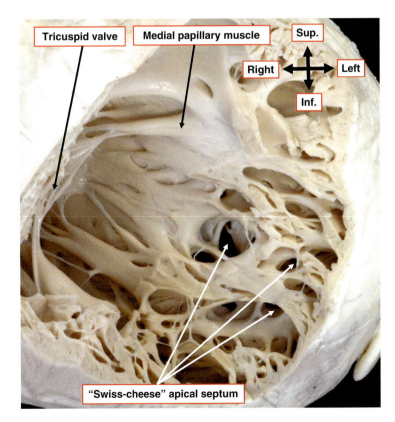

Figure 8.3.19 In this heart, the muscular septum failed completely to coalesce during development, leaving the so-called swiss-cheese septum.

the axis of atrioventricular conduction tissue from the edge of the defect. Occasionally, the muscular bundles do not fuse. The defect then extends to be bordered by fibrous continuity between the leaflets of the mitral and tricuspid valves, making it perimembranous as well as juxta-arterial (Figure 8.3.26). The conduction axis is then much closer to its inferior corner. It is the juxta-arterial variant that is particularly prone to set the scene for prolapse of the leaflets of the aortic valve.[8,9] Such

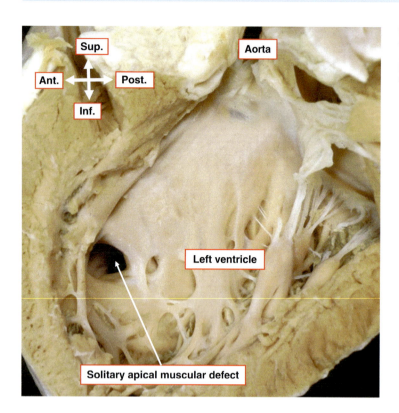

Figure 8.3.20 The left ventricular view, seen in anatomical orientation, shows the left ventricular aspect of the heart illustrated in Figure 8.3.18. In reality, there is a solitary defect in the muscular septum but it is crossed by on the right side by the septoparietal trabeculations, giving the spurious impression of multiple defects.

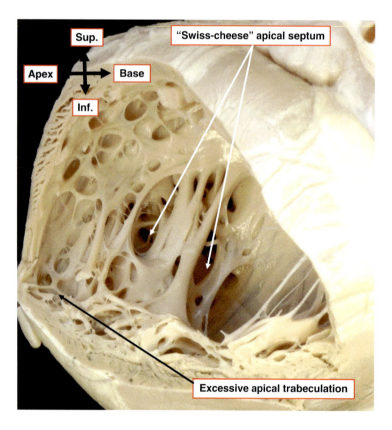

Figure 8.3.21 This shows the left ventricular aspect of the heart with the swiss-cheese septum (Figure 8.3.19). It is obvious, when viewed from the left side, that the septum has failed to coalesce. Note also the excessive apical trabeculations, often incorrectly diagnosed as 'non-compaction'.

defects are also much more frequent in Asian as opposed to European populations.

Although the descriptions thus far have related to ventricular septal defects in patients having concordant atrioventricular and ventriculo-arterial connections, this topology, and the guidance it gives to the site of the conduction axis, is equally valid for patients with concordant atrioventricular connections, but abnormal

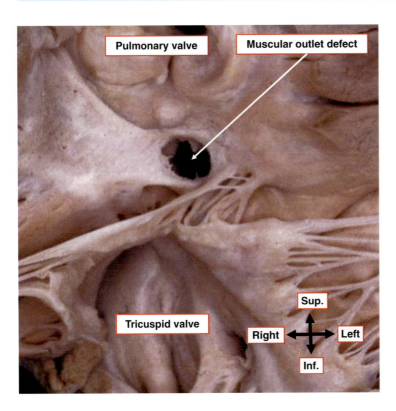

Figure 8.3.22 The heart is photographed in anatomical orientation, showing a muscular defect opening to the outlet of the right ventricle. Note the accretion of fibrous tissue at the edges of the defect, reducing its size.

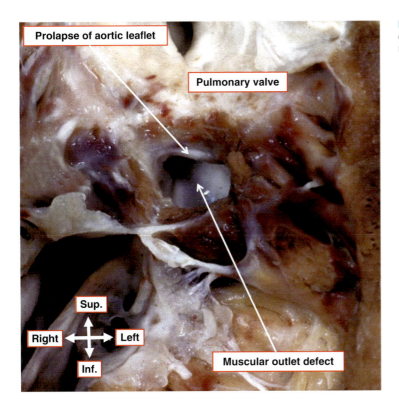

Figure 8.3.23 In this heart, viewed in anatomical orientation, the right coronary leaflet of the aortic valve prolapses minimally through a muscular defect that opens to the outlet of the right ventricle.

ventriculo-arterial connections (see Chapter 9.5). The only exception to the rules we have described for recognition of the location of the atrioventricular conduction axis is produced by overriding and straddling of the tricuspid valve (see below). This arrangement results in a particular type of defect that opens to the inlet of the right ventricle. As we have described, defects with markedly different phenotypic features, and with markedly different dispositions of the atrioventricular conduction axis, can open towards the inlet of the morphologically right ventricle. This is why it is insufficient simply to describe them as inlet defects.[7] The commonest defects opening to the right ventricular inlet

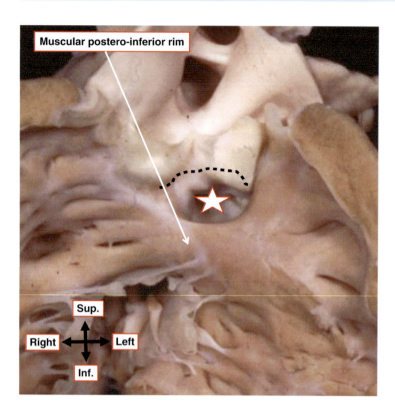

Figure 8.3.24 In this heart, the defect opening to the outlet of the right ventricle (star) is juxta-arterial and also doubly committed, due to failure of muscularization of the subpulmonary infundibulum. The roof of the defect is made up of fibrous continuity between the leaflets of the aortic and pulmonary valves (black dotted line). Note the extensive muscular postero-inferior rim to the defect that protects the atrioventricular conduction axis.

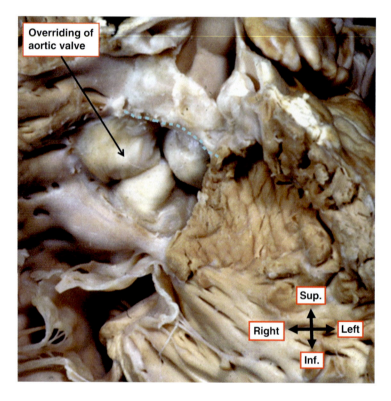

Figure 8.3.25 This heart, photographed in anatomical orientation, also has a juxta-arterial ventricular septal defect opening to the outlet of the right ventricle in absence of muscularization of the muscular subpulmonary infundibulum. There is fibrous continuity between the leaflets of the arterial valves (blue dotted line). Note the extensive overriding of the orifice of the aortic valve which makes the defect more subaortic than doubly committed in this instance.

are probably the ones that are perimembranous (Figure 8.3.6). These, and the ones associated with straddling and overriding of the tricuspid valve, have been described as being of atrioventricular canal type. It is certainly the case that hearts with a common atrioventricular junction can exist with shunting exclusively at the ventricular level (Figure 8.2.26). Patients with this morphology, however, must be distinguished from those with either perimembranous defects opening to the right ventricular inlet, or those associated with straddling and overriding of the tricuspid valve. This is because both of the latter variants are found in the setting of separate atrioventricular junctions. As

8.3 Ventricular Septal Defects

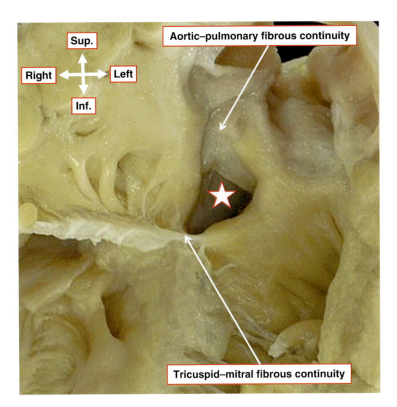

Figure 8.3.26 This juxta-arterial ventricular septal defect (star), shown in anatomical orientation, extends so that its postero-inferior margin in formed by fibrous continuity between the leaflets of the tricuspid and mitral valves, making it additionally perimembranous. The pathognomonic feature is the fibrous continuity between the leaflets of the aortic and pulmonary valves.

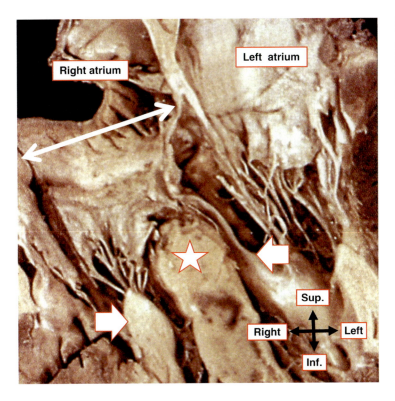

Figure 8.3.27 This heart has been sectioned to replicate the 'four-chamber' echocardiographic view, and is shown in anatomical orientation. There is overriding of the orifice of the tricuspid valve (double-headed arrow), and straddling of its tension apparatus (red-bordered arrows). Note the gross malalignment between the atrial and ventricular septal structures, the star marking the crest of the muscular ventricular septum.

such, therefore, they will have a bifoliate left atrioventricular valve, as opposed to the trifoliate variant found in the setting of a common atrioventricular junction. All of these variants, furthermore, must then be distinguished from muscular defects opening to the inlet of the right ventricle (Figure 8.3.14). This is because the location of the atrioventricular conduction axis is markedly different in these four lesions, all of which appropriately can be described as inlet defects. That is why we recommend using borders, rather than geography, as the starting point for differentiation of the multiple types of ventricular septal defect.[13]

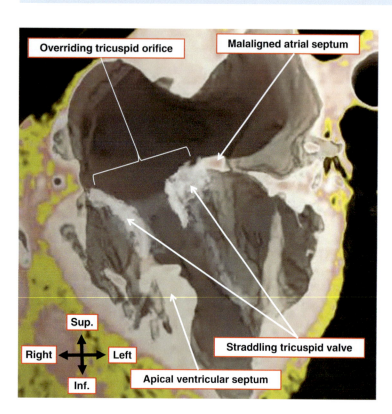

Figure 8.3.28 The image is taken from a computed tomographic dataset prepared from an individual with a perimembranous inlet defect associated with straddling and overriding of the tricuspid valve. It shows well the atrioventricular septal malalignment.

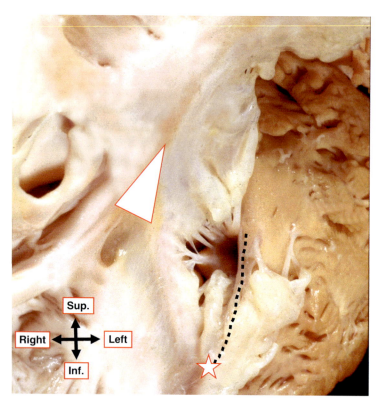

Figure 8.3.29 The heart is photographed in anatomical orientation. It shows the right atrial aspect of a straddling and overriding tricuspid valve in the setting of concordant atrioventricular connections. There is gross malalignment between the muscular ventricular septum, which carries the atrioventricular conduction axis (black dotted line), and the atrial septum. Because of this, the connecting atrioventricular node is formed inferiorly in the atrioventricular junction (star), and is not in the regular triangle of Koch (outlined in red).

The essence of the defect with a straddling tricuspid valve is the malalignment between the atrial septum and the apical ventricular septum (Figures 8.3.27, 8.3.28). In consequence, the inferior component of the muscular ventricular septum joins the right atrioventricular junction along its diaphragmatic aspect (Figures 8.3.29, 8.3.30). Almost always, such overriding of the orifice of the tricuspid valve is accompanied by straddling of its tension apparatus (Figure 8.3.27). It is the abnormal inferior insertion of the muscular ventricular septum to the atrioventricular

8.3 Ventricular Septal Defects

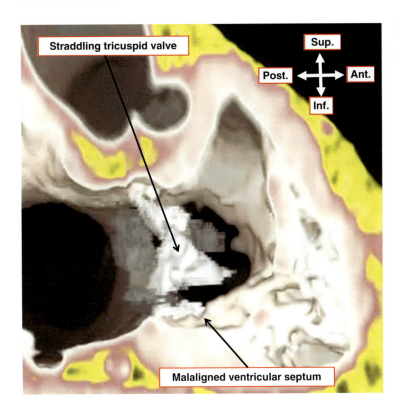

Figure 8.3.30 The image comes from the same computed tomographic dataset as used to prepare Figure 8.3.28. It shows the defect from the right side, illustrating how the malaligned muscular ventricular septum inserts inferiorly to the atrioventricular junction, underscoring the abnormal location of the atrioventricular node (see Figures 8.3.31 and 8.3.32).

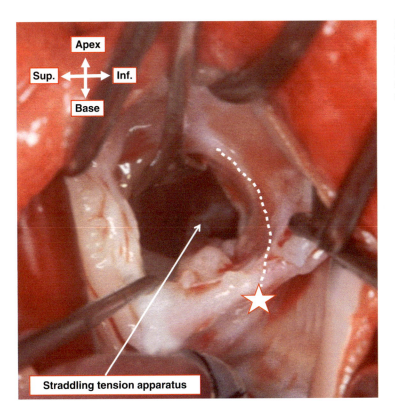

Figure 8.3.31 The image shows an operative picture through a right atriotomy in a patient with concordant atrioventricular connections complicated by straddling and overriding of the tricuspid valve with basically concordant atrioventricular connections. Note the malalignment of the muscular ventricular septum, which carries the atrioventricular conduction axis (white dotted line). The axis arises from an anomalous postero-inferior atrioventricular node (star).

junction, rather than the atrial septum, however, that underscores the abnormal location of the atrioventricular conduction axis. The conduction axis is carried on the crest of the muscular ventricular septum (Figure 8.3.31), and when deviated inferiorly in consequence of the overriding, can no longer make contact with the regular atrioventricular node in the triangle of Koch (Figure 8.3.32). It was likely the failure to recognize this abnormal disposition of the atrioventricular conduction axis that contributed to the frequent occurrence of iatrogenic heart

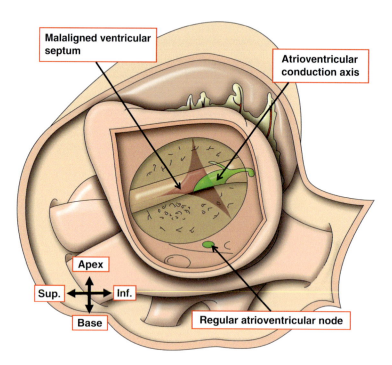

Figure 8.3.32 The drawing shows the anomalous location of the atrioventricular conduction axis as seen by the surgeon operating through a right atriotomy in the setting of straddling and overriding of the tricuspid valve. The rudimentary node (green oval) found at the apex of the regular triangle of Koch does not make contact with the ventricular musculature.

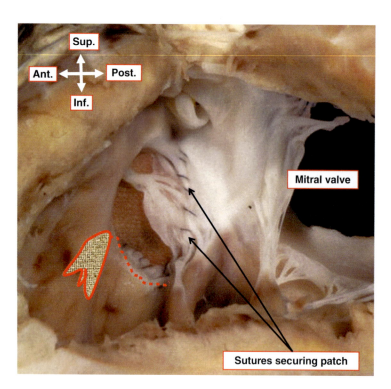

Figure 8.3.33 This picture, taken in anatomical orientation, shows the left ventricular aspect of the heart with straddling and overriding of the tricuspid valve. It shows how the atrioventricular conduction axis (shown in red, with the left bundle shown in brown hatching) is carried on the malaligned muscular ventricular septum.

block after attempts surgically to correct straddling and overriding of the tricuspid valve.[14] When the surgeon is armed with appropriate knowledge of the arrangement of the conduction axis, nonetheless, it is possible to place a patch so as to restore the tricuspid valve to the right ventricle, and at the same time avoid the atrioventricular conduction axis (Figures 8.3.31, 8.3.33). Similar phenotypic variability as seen for inlet defects can also be found amongst defects opening to the right ventricular outlet. The major feature of surgical significance in this latter setting is to determine whether or not a muscular bar interposes between the caudal rim of the defect and the atrioventricular conduction axis (compare Figures 8.3.24 and 8.3.26).

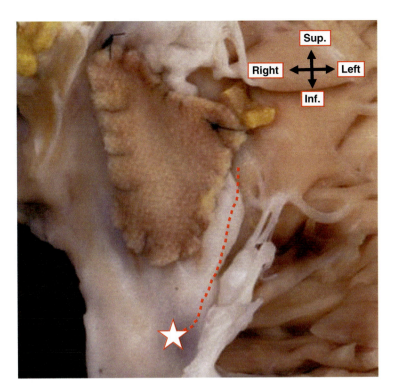

Figure 8.3.34 The image shows the right atrial aspect of the heart seen also in Figure 8.3.33. It is photographed in anatomical orientation, demonstrating how the surgeon was able successfully to close the ventricular septal defect, at the same time avoiding the atrioventricular conduction axis (red dotted line). The site of the abnormal atrioventricular node is shown by the star.

References Cited

1. Soto B, Becker AE, Moulaert AJ, Lie JT, Anderson RH. Classification of ventricular septal defects. *Br Heart J* 1980; **43**: 332–343.
2. Tretter JT, Tran VH, Gray S, et al. Assessing the criteria for definition of perimembranous ventricular septal defects in light of the search for consensus. *Orphanet J* 2019; **14**: 1.
3. Lopez L, Houyel L, Colan SD, et al. Classification of ventricular septal defects for the eleventh iteration of the International Classification of Diseases – striving for consensus: a report from the International Society for Nomenclature of Paediatric and Congenital Heart Disease. *Ann Thor Surg* 2018; **106**: 1578–1589.
4. Wells WJ, Lindesmith GG. Ventricular septal defect. In E Arciniegas, ed., *Pediatric Cardiac Surgery*. Chicago: Year Book Medical Publishers; 1985: pp. 133–139.
5. Van Praagh R, Geva T, Kreutzer J. Ventricular septal defects: how shall we describe, name and classify them? *J Am Coll Cardiol* 1989; **14**: 1298–1299.
6. Milo S, Ho SY, Wilkinson JL, Anderson RH. The surgical anatomy and atrioventricular conduction tissues of hearts with isolated ventricular septal defects. *J Thorac Cardiovasc Surg* 1980; **79**: 244–255.
7. Spicer DE, Anderson RH, Backer CL. Clarifying the surgical morphology of inlet ventricular septal defects. *Ann Thor Surg* 2013 **95**: 236–241.
8. Van Praagh R, McNamara JJ. Anatomic types of ventricular septal defect with aortic insufficiency. Diagnostic and surgical considerations. *Am Heart J* 1968; **75**: 604–619.
9. Kawashima Y, Danno M, Shimizu Y, Matsuda H, Miyamoto T. Ventricular septal defect associated with aortic insufficiency: anatomic classification and method of operation. *Circulation* 1973; **47**: 1057–1064.
10. Spicer DE, Anderson RH, Chowdhury UK, et al. A reassessment of the anatomical features of multiple ventricular septal defects. *J Card Surg* 2022; **37**: 1353–1360.
11. Chowdhury UK, Anderson RH, Spicer DE, et al. A review of the therapeutic management of multiple ventricular septal defects. *J Card Surg* 2022; **37**: 1361–1376.
12. Devlin PJ, Russell HM, Mongé MC, et al. Doubly committed and juxtaarterial ventricular septal defect: outcomes of the aortic and pulmonary valves. *Ann Thor Surg* 2014; **97**: 2134–2141.
13. Edgar LJ, Anderson RH, Stickley J, Crucean A. Borders as opposed to so-called geography: which should be used to classify isolated ventricular septal defects? *Eur J Cardio-Thorac Surg* 2020; **58**: 801–808.
14. Pacifico AD, Soto B, Bargeron LMJ. Surgical treatment of straddling tricuspid valves. *Circulation* 1979; **60**: 655–664.

Chapter 8.4: Malformations of the Valves of the Heart

The pathological lesions which affect the atrioventricular valves, be they acquired or congenital, are legion. Not all are amenable to surgical repair. We will concentrate on features of immediate surgical relevance.

The anatomy of atrioventricular valves themselves indicates that problems may be encountered at the atrioventricular junction, where the leaflets are hinged at the so-called annulus, within the leaflets themselves, or in the tension apparatus. Sometimes all the components of the valve, along with the entire atrioventricular connection, are totally absent. This produces the commonest variant of atrioventricular valvar atresia, which we will discuss as a separate entity, since no longer can the heart be considered normally connected in this setting. The lesions to be considered in this section can involve either the morphologically tricuspid or mitral valves. Because the tricuspid valve usually functions in an environment of low pressure, the lesions are more frequently manifest when affecting the mitral valve. We will deal with the respective lesions in turn, indicating their proclivity towards one or the other valve.

Of considerable surgical significance is overriding of the atrioventricular junction.[1] This means that the valvar orifice is looking into both ventricles, positioned astride a septal defect (Figure 8.4.1). Almost always, such overriding of the junction is associated with straddling of the valvar tension apparatus, with the tendinous cords attached to both sides of the muscular ventricular septum (Figure 8.4.1).[1] Although it is the mode of insertion of the tension apparatus across the septum that determines the surgical options, the degree of override is also important. Overriding of the tricuspid valve, as shown in Figure 8.4.1, is typically associated with malalignment between the atrial and ventricular septums. This is also associated with a particular type of perimembranous inlet ventricular septal defect, as we discussed in the previous chapter. And, as we emphasized, this has major consequences in terms of arrangement of the conduction tissues (Figure 8.4.2). Straddling and overriding, nonetheless, can also affect the morphologically mitral valve.[1] Irrespective of the valve involved, the spectrum in terms of override can occur in various segmental

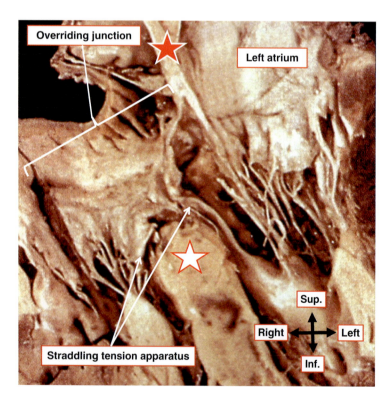

Figure 8.4.1 The image shows a four-chamber section through a straddling and overriding tricuspid valve. The phenotypic feature of the lesion is the malalignment between the atrial and ventricular septums (white star with red borders and red star with white borders). This particular example was from a patient with tetralogy of Fallot.

8.4 Malformations of the Valves of the Heart

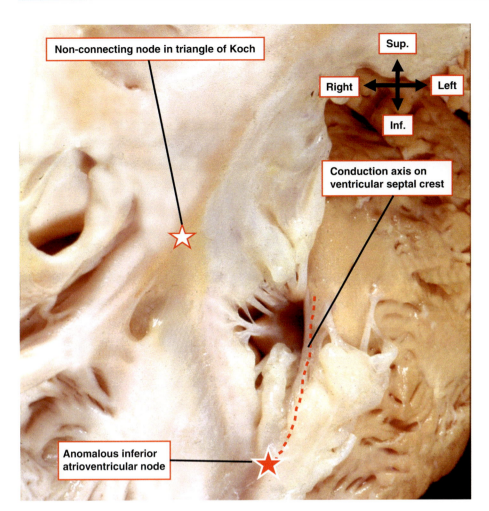

Figure 8.4.2 The image shows the right ventricular aspect of an isolated example of straddling an overriding of the tricuspid valve. It illustrates the abnormal location of the atrioventricular node in consequence of the atrioventricular septal malalignment. There is a hypoplastic node found at the apex of the triangle of Koch, but it is unable to make contact with the atrioventricular conduction axis.

combinations. Straddling in the setting of the double inlet ventricle, and with discordant atrioventricular connections, is considered in subsequent chapters. Here, our concern is with straddling and overriding valves co-existing with concordant atrioventricular connections.

As shown in our previous chapter, straddling of the tricuspid valve is one of the features of the perimembranous inlet ventricular septal defect found with atrioventricular septal malalignment. Although found as an isolated lesion (Figure 8.4.2), it can complicate tetralogy of Fallot (Figure 8.4.1), or be found in association with other abnormal ventriculo-arterial connections such as transposition. Because of the atrioventricular septal malalignment, the conduction axis, carried on the crest of the muscular ventricular septum, originates from an anomalous node formed at the site of union between the malaligned septum and the inferior margin of the right atrioventricular junction (Figure 8.4.2). A mini-septation procedure is often necessary for complete ventricular repair, and can carry a high risk of producing heart block if the surgeon is unaware of the abnormal arrangement of the conduction axis.[2] As we showed in Chapter 8.3, nonetheless, a patch can be secured by sewing the stitches exclusively in the straddling leaflet of the tricuspid valve (Figures 8.3.33, 8.3.34), thus ensuring avoidance of the conduction tissues. An alternative option is always to convert the patient to the Fontan circulation.

Straddling of the tricuspid valve is associated with an inlet ventricular septal defect. When the mitral valve straddles, it does so through a ventricular septal defect, or interventricular communication, which opens to the outlet of the right ventricle (Figure 8.4.3).[1] This arrangement does not produce atrioventricular septal malalignment, so that the muscular ventricular septum is normally related to the atrial septum at the crux, and the atrioventricular conduction axis is normally disposed. It is the superior papillary muscle of the mitral valve that is abnormally attached within the right ventricle. It is typically tethered to the limbs of the septomarginal trabeculation alongside, but separate from, the tension apparatus of the tricuspid valve. The arrangement is rare in hearts with concordant ventriculo-arterial connections (Figure 8.4.3), but is seen more frequently with either discordant ventriculo-arterial connections, or double outlet right ventricle with subpulmonary defect, being a frequent association of the Taussig–Bing malformation. When present, it can seriously compromise surgical repair. We discuss the problems in greater detail in our subsequent sections devoted to hearts with abnormal segmental combinations.

Dilation of the atrioventricular junction occurs almost exclusively as an acquired lesion. A dilated mitral valvar orifice is most

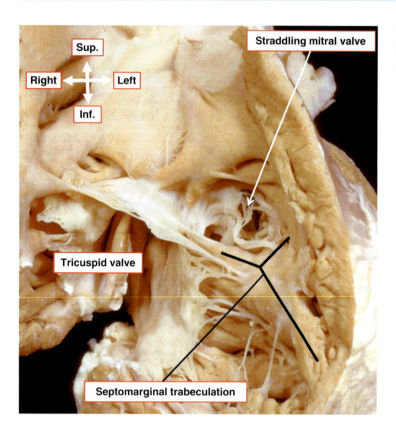

Figure 8.4.3 The image shows the right ventricular aspect of a heart with concordant atrioventricular and ventriculo-arterial connections, but with straddling and overriding of the mitral valve. The valve straddles through a perimembranous outlet ventricular septal defect, with the straddling tension apparatus attached to the limbs of the septomarginal trabeculation.

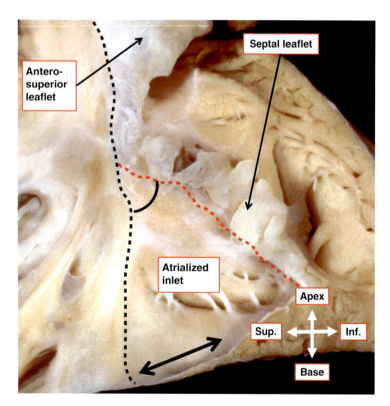

Figure 8.4.4 The heart is photographed from the right side in anatomical orientation. The hinge line of the septal leaflet of the tricuspid valve has been displaced rotationally (red dotted line) away from the atrioventricular junction, shown by the black dotted line. This feature, incorrectly described as 'downwards displacement', is the hallmark of Ebstein's malformation. It is better considered as rotational displacement (curved line). The double-headed arrow shows the so-called atrialization of the inlet of the right ventricle. Note also the marked dysplasia of the septal leaflet.

frequently secondary to myocarditis. When surgical narrowing of the orifice is indicated, it can be accomplished using various annuloplasty techniques, without resorting to replacement of the valve. Dilation of the tricuspid valvar orifice is seen most frequently as a result of right heart failure.

More of a challenge surgically is the dilation that accompanies Ebstein's malformation.[3] The crucial feature of this anomaly is the attachment of the hinge point of the septal and mural leaflets of the tricuspid valve towards the junction of the inlet and apical trabecular components of the right ventricle, rather than at the atrioventricular junction (Figure 8.4.4).[4] The displacement is usually described as being downwards. In reality, there is rotational displacement of the valvar orifice around the area of the membranous septum.[4] The antero-superior leaflet is less affected in terms of its junctional attachment, but shows important variations in its distal attachments.[5] These can be focal (Figure 8.4.5). In more severe cases, the leading edge of the leaflet is attached in linear fashion, severely restricting antegrade flow into the pulmonary trunk (Figure 8.4.6). In essence, the tricuspid valve then closes in bifoliate rather than trifoliate fashion. In the most severe form, the keyhole orifice looking into the infundibulum can

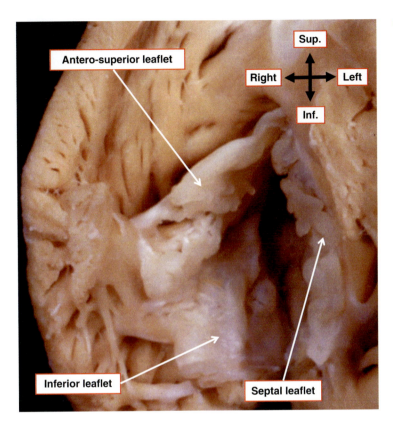

Figure 8.4.5 This picture, photographed in anatomical orientation from the right ventricle, shows the ventricular aspect of the heart shown in Figure 8.4.4. The antero-superior leaflet of the abnormal tricuspid valve is tethered in focal fashion, with normal attachments to the medial and anterior papillary muscles. The rotational displacement has produced a bifoliate valve hinged at the junction of the inlet and apical trabecular components of the right ventricle.

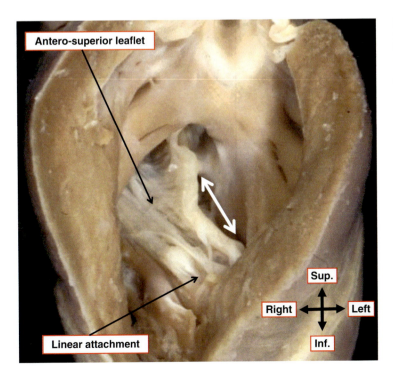

Figure 8.4.6 This heart also has Ebstein's malformation, and is again photographed in anatomical orientation to show the ventricular aspect of the abnormal tricuspid valve. In this example, the antero-superior leaflet has grossly abnormal linear attachments towards the apex of the right ventricle. The valvar orifice is now a mere keyhole (double-headed white arrow), opening directly to the subpulmonary infundibulum.

become imperforate, producing tricuspid atresia in the setting of Ebstein's malformation (see also Chapter 9.1).

Ebstein's malformation requires surgical treatment when there is significant dilation of the true atrioventricular junction, and when the wall of the inlet component of the right ventricle is both dilated and thinned. Surgical repair has now been revolutionized by the description of the cone operation.[6] This involves detaching the leaflets of the valve in cone-like fashion, and re-attaching them at the level of the atrioventricular junction. This will require placement of sutures in the area of thinning of walls of the inlet component of the right ventricle (Figure 8.4.4). Particular care should be taken to avoid the right coronary artery and its branches. In the septal area, the triangle of Koch remains the guide to the atrioventricular conduction axis (Figure 8.4.7). Ebstein's malformation involving the left-sided morphologically tricuspid valve when the atrioventricular connections are discordant is discussed in the section devoted to congenitally corrected transposition. Rarely, the normally located morphologically mitral valve can show Ebstein's malformation. It is then the hinge of the mural leaflet that is displaced away from the atrioventricular junction.[7,8]

Malformations of the leaflets can be summarized in terms of dysplasia, prolapse, and cleftings. Dysplastic valves show thickening and heaping up of the substance of the leaflets, usually with either shortened cords or obliteration of the intercordal spaces. A dysplastic valve may pose a significant surgical problem. It is frequently seen with atresia of the outflow tract, and is an integral part of Ebstein's malformation.[9] Isolated dysplasia (Figure 8.4.8) is exceedingly rare except in neonatal life,[10] when it is often a fatal lesion.

Prolapse occurs more frequently, and usually involves the mitral valve (Figure 8.4.9). It is usually associated with deficiency of the tension apparatus,[11] particularly elongation of the tendinous cords (Figure 8.4.10). It may be sufficiently severe to warrant valvar replacement, but the prolapsing leaflets can be repaired by various techniques, including cordal shortening (Figure 8.4.11), and insertion of annular rings (Figure 8.4.12).

The true cleft of the aortic leaflet of the mitral valve can be repaired simply by reconstituting its edges. Such an isolated cleft of the aortic leaflet (Figure 8.4.13) has to be distinguished from the lesion often described as a cleft in the setting of atrioventricular septal defects. When found with a common atrioventricular junction (Figure 8.4.14), the space is the zone of apposition between the left ventricular components of the bridging leaflets of the common atrioventricular valve. Along with the short mural leaflet, the bridging leaflets guard the left side of the common atrioventricular junction in trifoliate fashion.

We have already discussed some of the abnormalities of the tension apparatus that accompany malformations of the atrioventricular junction or the leaflets, such as straddling of the tension apparatus. Of those which remain, the so-called parachute deformity is probably the most worrisome lesion, apart from rare anomalies such as arcade lesions.[12] Some confusion exists about the definition of a parachute valve. It is logically considered to represent fusion of the papillary muscle groups (Figure 8.4.15), so that all the cords insert into a common muscle mass.[13] In the original description,[14] in contrast, the parachute lesion was defined on the basis of gross hypoplasia of one end of the zone of apposition between the leaflets, together with absence of its supporting papillary muscle. Irrespective of how the lesion is defined, surgical

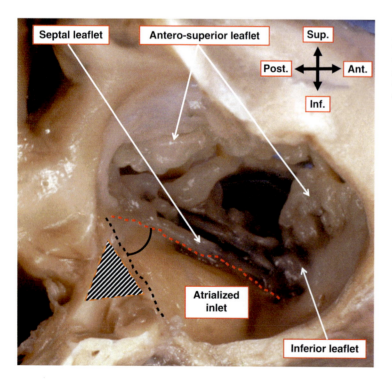

Figure 8.4.7 This heart with Ebstein's malformation, viewed in anatomical orientation as seen from the right atrium, shows how the triangle of Koch (cross-hatched triangle) remains the guide to the atrial components of the atrioventricular conduction tissue axis, despite the abnormal attachments of the septal leaflet. Note again the rotational displacement (curved black line) of the hinge of the septal leaflet (red dotted line) relative to the atrioventricular junction (black dotted line).

8.4 Malformations of the Valves of the Heart

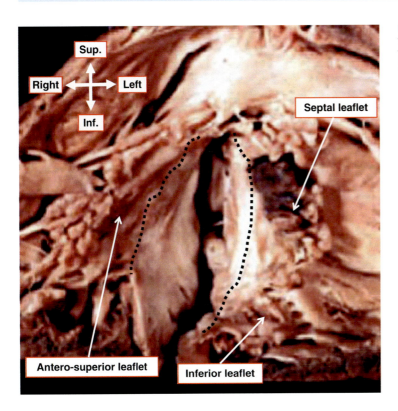

Figure 8.4.8 The right ventricle in this heart is opened in clam-like fashion and photographed from the ventricular apex. The tricuspid valve, although grossly dysplastic, has normal junctional attachments (black dotted lines). This is not Ebstein's malformation.

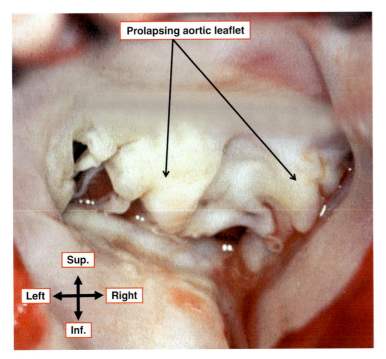

Figure 8.4.9 This surgical view of the mitral valve, taken through the dome of the left atrium, shows prolapse of its aortic leaflet.

reconstruction is difficult, and valvar replacement is likely to be necessary. Parachute deformity of the mitral valve may be further complicated by other lesions, such as the supravalvar left atrial stenosing ring, and coarctation of the aorta. The combinations are known as Shone's syndrome.[14] Parachute malformation of the tricuspid valve can occur, but is rarely of clinical significance.[15]

Abnormalities of the arterial valves are usually considered along with the associated aspects of subvalvar and supravalvar obstruction. In the normally connected heart, obstruction in the outflow tract of the left ventricle produces problems in the systemic circulation. It must then be remembered that the same anatomical lesions will produce subpulmonary obstruction should the ventriculo-arterial

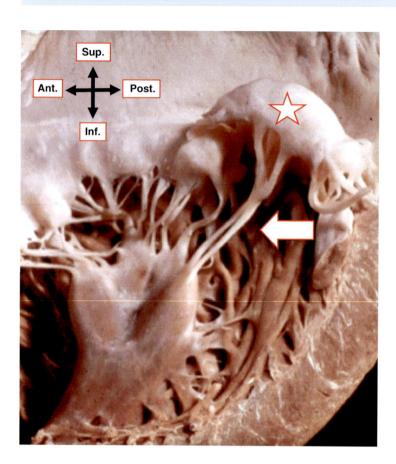

Figure 8.4.10 In this specimen, photographed in anatomical orientation, there is gross elongation of the cords supporting the middle scallop of the mural leaflet of the mitral valve (arrow), which is prolapsed (star).

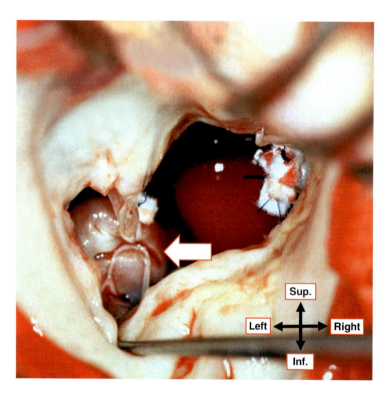

Figure 8.4.11 As shown in Figure 8.4.10, when the leaflets of the mitral valve are prolapsed, then the cords supporting them are usually elongated. This view shows how the surgeon has shortened the elongated cords by incising the papillary muscle and suturing the cords within the muscle (arrow).

connections be discordant. Similarly, obstruction within the right ventricular outflow tract produces pulmonary problems in the heart with normal segmental connections, but systemic problems when the ventriculo-arterial connections are discordant. When both outflow tracts are connected to the same ventricle, the anatomical problems are more discrete. These are considered separately in our sections dealing with double outlet ventricles.

8.4 Malformations of the Valves of the Heart

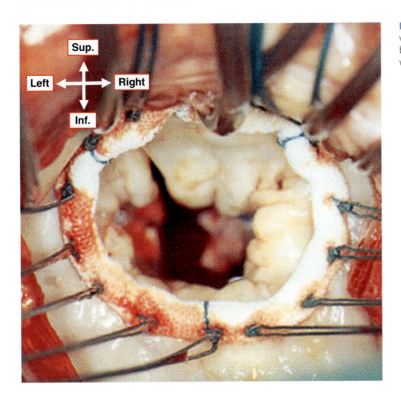

Figure 8.4.12 Having shortened the cords of the prolapsed mitral valve, as shown in Figure 8.4.11, the surgeon has completed the repair by inserting an annular ring to support the atrioventricular junction, which has been reduced by annuloplasty.

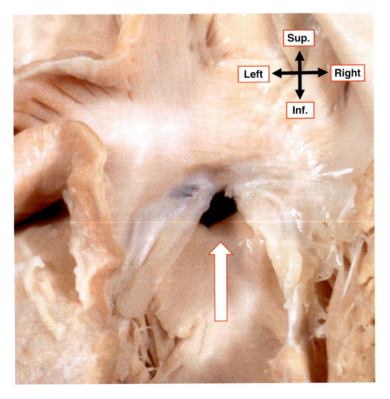

Figure 8.4.13 This specimen, seen from the inlet aspect of the left ventricle in anatomical orientation, has a cleft (white arrow with red borders) in the aortic leaflet of an otherwise normally structured mitral valve. This lesion should be distinguished from the space between the left ventricular bridging leaflets, or the so-called cleft, found in the left atrioventricular valve of hearts with deficient atrioventricular septation and common atrioventricular junction (see Figure 8.4.14).

Narrowing of the outflow tract of the left ventricle, therefore, can occur at valvar, subvalvar, and supravalvar levels. Aortic regurgitation is ultimately a valvar problem, and the perivalvar anatomy is often of great importance. To understand fully the substrates for stenosis and regurgitation across the arterial valves, it is essential to have a firm grasp of the arrangement of the valvar leaflets at the ventriculo-arterial junction. As described in Chapters 3 and 4, the arterial valves do not possess an 'annulus' in the sense of a circular ring of collagen that supports the leaflets in the fashion of a circle. The obvious anatomical ring within the valvar complex is the sinutubular junction. The other circular area over which

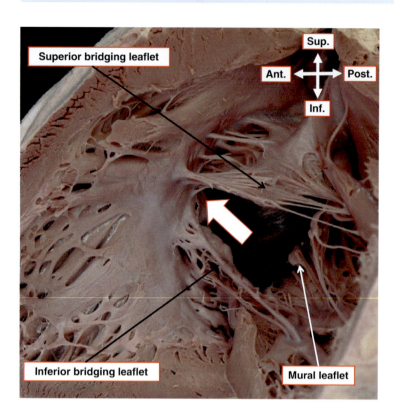

Figure 8.4.14 This heart with deficient atrioventricular septation, common atrioventricular junction, and shunting exclusively at ventricular level, the so-called ostium primum defect, is photographed from the left side in anatomical orientation. Note the difference between the zone of apposition between the left ventricular components of the bridging leaflets, the so-called cleft (white arrow with red borders), and the true cleft of the aortic leaflet of an otherwise normal mitral valve shown in Figure 8.4.13.

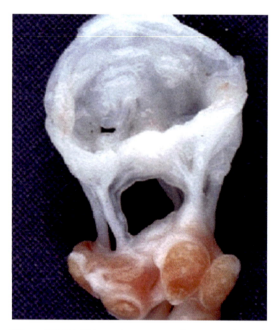

Figure 8.4.15 This specimen, removed at surgery, shows the so-called parachute arrangement of the mitral valve. There is fusion of the papillary muscles, along with thickening and fusion of the tendinous cords.

the fibrous wall of the great arterial trunk is supported by the underlying ventricular structures is found only in the pulmonary root (Figure 8.4.16).[16] Surgeons, however, do not define this myocardial–arterial junction as the annulus.[17] As we demonstrated in Chapter 4, the myocardial–arterial junctions in the aortic root are found only in the valvar sinuses that give rise to the coronary arteries (Figure 8.4.17).[18] The attachments of the leaflets are semilunar, with their nadirs attached at the level of the virtual basal ring, and their zeniths attached to the fibrous wall of the arterial trunk at the sinutubular junction. When seen in closed position, the three leaflets then coapt snugly along their zones of apposition, which extend from the circumferential margins of the arterial wall to the centre of the valve (Figure 8.4.18). It is on the basis of perturbation of this coaptation of the leaflets under pressure of the diastolic column of blood that stenosis or regurgitation occurs within the valvar complex.

Analysis of valvar aortic stenosis is greatly simplified by taking note separately of the number of sinuses as opposed to functional leaflets found within the malformed root.[19,20] Most usually, the root retains its trisinuate scaffold, but depending on the fusion of the leaflets supported within the scaffold, the valve itself can be functionally trifoliate, bifoliate, or unifoliate. More rarely, the bifoliate, or bicuspid, variant can be found with only two sinuses.[21] Very rarely, the overall root may be quadrisinuate and quadricuspid.[22] Dysplastic lesions are also seen in the aortic valve, but only rarely can surgery provide the answer to this problem. The so-called unicuspid and unicommissural valve has a trisinuate scaffold, with two raphes at the ends of abortive zones of apposition (Figures 8.4.19–8.4.21). The leaflets are also abnormally attached in linear rather than semilunar fashion (Figure 8.4.22). Surgical opening of the raphes in the conjoined leaflets typically results in valvar incompetence. The creation of new interleaflet triangles, supplementing the leaflet tissue so as to create new semilunar hinges, is likely to produce greater clinical success.

A trisinuate root with a functionally bileaflet valve is most frequently seen in the adult patient. Perhaps this is because such a valve, usually described as being bicuspid, is not usually in itself intrinsically stenotic. It is only with the effects of time and

8.4 Malformations of the Valves of the Heart

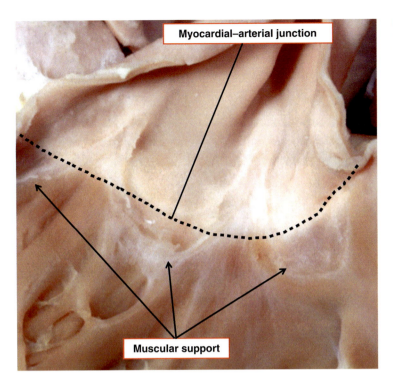

Figure 8.4.16 In this anatomical specimen, the subpulmonary infundibulum has been opened and photographed in anatomical orientation having removed the leaflets of the pulmonary valve. Note that the semilunar attachments of the leaflets cross the circular myocardial–arterial junction (dashed black line). This is more obvious than in the subaortic outflow tract (see Figure 8.4.17), but the basic arrangement is comparable.

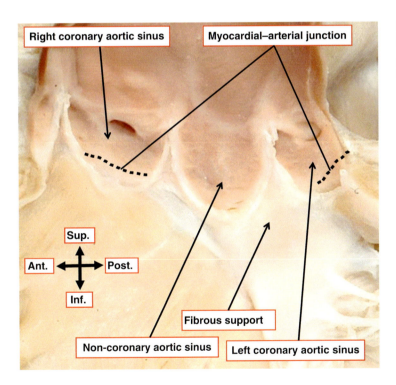

Figure 8.4.17 The aortic outflow tract has been spread open and is photographed from the ventricular aspect in anatomical orientation. The arterial valvar leaflets are attached in semilunar fashion, taking their origin in part from fibrous tissue, and in part from the muscular ventricular septum.

turbulence that the bicuspid valves become manifestly obstructive. If the valvar morphology has not been totally obscured by calcific deposits, a functionally bifoliate valve seen at operation will usually take one of two forms. The leaflets are unequal, with the large, or conjoined, leaflet usually exhibiting a raphe, which can be eccentrically placed (Figure 8.4.23) or centrally positioned (Figures 8.4.24, 8.4.25) within the conjoined leaflet. If the conjoined leaflet is produced by fusion of the leaflets guarding the aortic sinuses giving rise to the coronary arteries (Figure 8.4.24), then both arteries will arise from the conjoined sinus. Alternatively, when the conjoined sinus is formed from the right coronary and non-coronary aortic sinuses, the coronary arteries will be positioned so that one coronary artery arises from the conjoined sinuses, and the other from the third sinus. It is increasingly becoming recognized that the two phenotypes carry significant differences with regard to anticipated problems during follow-up. When the conjoined leaflet is made up of the right and non-coronary aortic leaflets, it is frequent to find

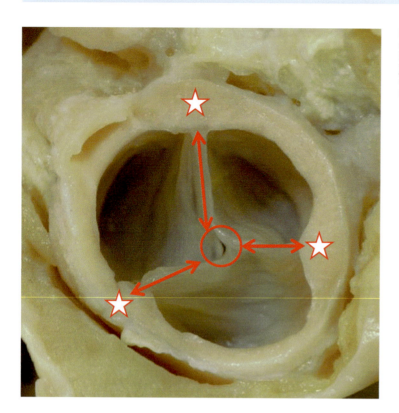

Figure 8.4.18 In this specimen, the aortic valve is photographed from above in its closed position. The three zones of apposition between the leaflets (double-headed red arrows) extend from the sinutubular junction at the periphery (stars) to the centre of the valvar orifice (red circle). The leaflets are closed by the hydrostatic pressure of the column of blood they support.

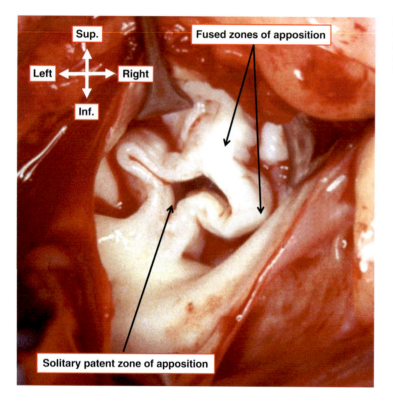

Figure 8.4.19 This view of an abnormal aortic valve seen through an aortotomy shows the so-called unicuspid and unicommissural arrangement. Fusion of two of the putative zones of apposition during development leaves the persisting zone of apposition as the eccentric valvar orifice.

degenerative disease of the aortic walls. If valves with two effective leaflets are seen before they become rigid and distorted by calcification, some relief from the stenosis can be obtained by careful enlargement of the ends of the solitary zone of apposition. Careful follow-up is essential, especially when the phenotype points towards degenerative disease. It is possible to find the functionally bileaflet valve formed with fusion between the left coronary and the non-coronary leaflets, but this is the least common of the phenotypic variants. It is also possible, however, to find aortic roots with the two leaflets of equal size, the solitary zone of apposition between them then bisecting the aortic root (Figure 8.4.26). This type of valve is frequently found in patients

8.4 Malformations of the Valves of the Heart

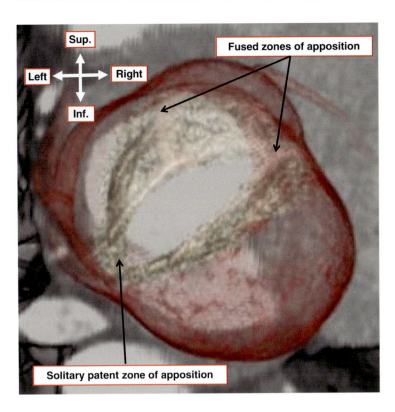

Figure 8.4.20 The image is a virtual dissection, viewed from above, of a computed tomographic dataset prepared from an individual with a unicuspid and unicommissural aortic valve, with the valve seen during ventricular systole. There is a solitary zone of apposition opening to the sinutubular junction.

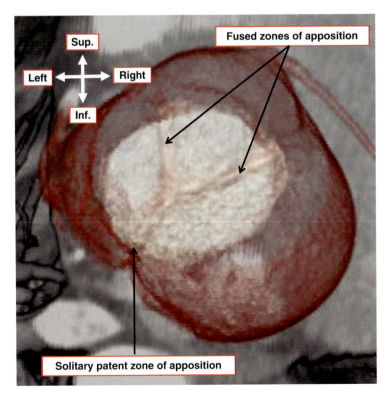

Figure 8.4.21 The same valve as seen in Figure 8.4.20 is shown during ventricular diastole. It can now be seen that the unicuspid valve is formed within a trisinuate root.

with coarctation of the aorta, or those with Turner syndrome. When examined carefully, such valves can be found within a bisinuate root, with no raphes, and absence of a hypoplastic interleaflet triangle. The prognostic significance of this phenotype has yet to be established. The aortic root with four sinuses can be found with varying arrangement of the origins of the coronary arteries and of the leaflets. These lesions are sufficiently rare that a descriptive approach provides a better understanding, rather than seeking to compress the variants into a procrustean classification.[22]

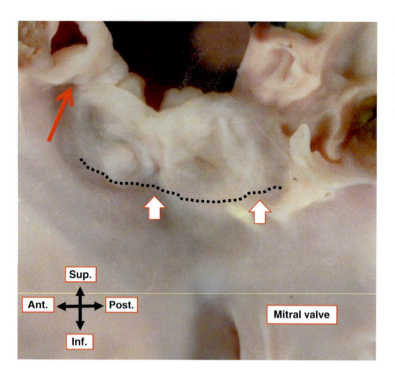

Figure 8.4.22 This picture of the aortic valve, taken in a specimen having opened the left ventricular outflow tract, shows the unicuspid and unicommissural arrangement as shown in Figure 8.4.19. There is loss of the semilunar suspension of the leaflets, so that paradoxically they are attached in true annular fashion (black dotted line), with reduction in size of the interleaflet triangles (white arrows). The solitary zone of apposition points backwards towards the mitral valve, and is associated with a better formed interleaflet triangle (red arrow).

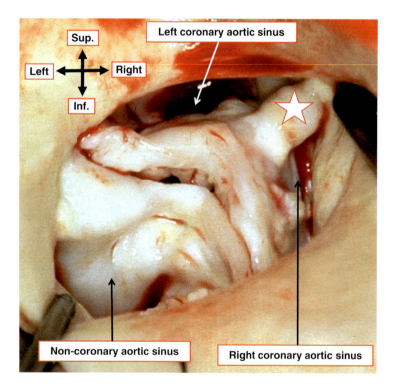

Figure 8.4.23 This picture, taken in the operating room through an aortotomy, show a bicuspid aortic valve with an eccentric raphe in one of the leaflets.

Aortic stenosis also occurs in patients with valves having a trisinuate root with three discrete leaflets, but is not usually-seen until later in life. A possible cause of such stenosis is the unequal size of the leaflets in the otherwise normal aortic valve. This, coupled with the high pressure in the aortic root, may lead to the development of calcification and stenosis in the elderly (Figure 8.4.27).[23]

Subvalvar stenosis may be fibrous, fibromuscular, or muscular, reflecting the fact that the left ventricular outflow tract is partly muscular and partly fibrous. The muscular portion comprises the ventriculo-infundibular fold antero-laterally, the small outlet component of the muscular septum anteriorly, and the upper edge of the apical part of the muscular septum posteriorly. The fibrous part comprises the membranous septum, the roof of the infero-septal recess, the right fibrous trigone, the area of continuity between the leaflets of the aortic and mitral valves, and the left fibrous trigone. Subvalvar stenoses may also be either fixed or dynamic in nature.

8.4 Malformations of the Valves of the Heart

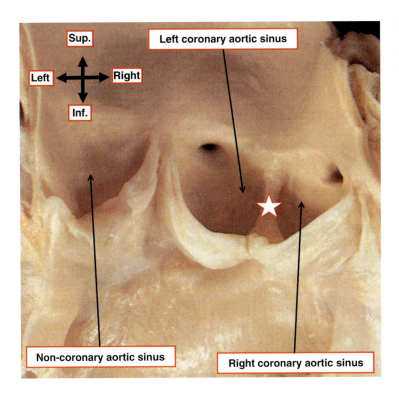

Figure 8.4.24 In this specimen, the aortic valve is photographed from behind in anatomical orientation having opened the left ventricular outflow tract through the mitral valve. The two leaflets arising from the sinuses giving rise to the coronary arteries have fused, with the line of fusion represented by the raphe (star).

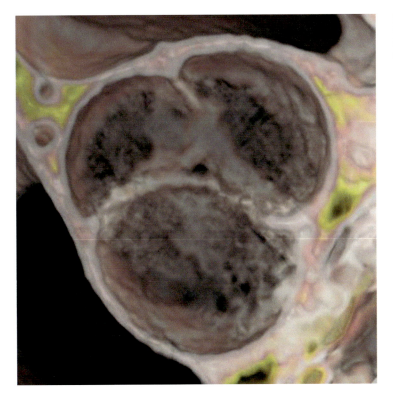

Figure 8.4.25 The virtual dissection of a computed tomographic dataset shows a functionally bileaflet aortic valve in a trisinuate root. The raphe is equally positioned within the conjoined right and left coronary aortic leaflets.

Of the variants producing fixed stenosis, a subvalvar fibrous shelf is perhaps most easily approached surgically. It appears circular when viewed through the usually normal aortic valve (Figure 8.4.28). Indeed, it can be circular. This is not always the case. A relatively thin shelf of tissue sometimes runs from beneath the non-coronary leaflet of the aortic valve, originating over the site of the penetrating bundle, then extending to the septal musculature, eventually coursing over the ventriculo-infundibular fold. The shelf can also extend laterally to involve the aortic leaflet of the mitral valve (Figure 8.4.29). If dissection is performed carefully,[24] a circumferential lesion can be completely removed (Figure 8.4.30). Particular care is required where the shelf intimately overlies the conduction tissues. Too vigorous an attack on the side of

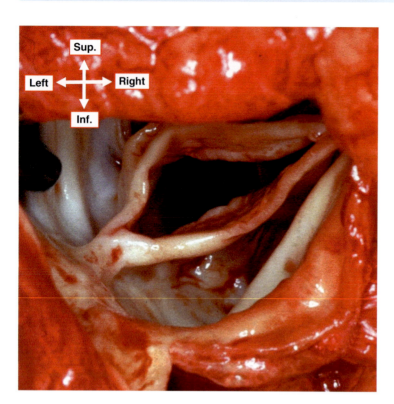

Figure 8.4.26 This picture, taken in the operating room through an aortotomy, shows an aortic valve with two leaflets of comparable size.

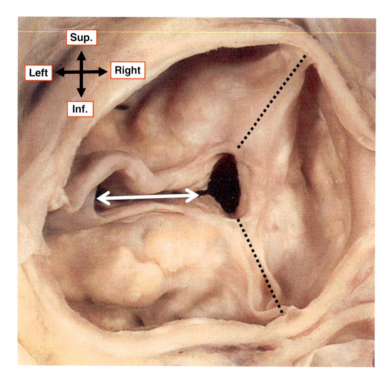

Figure 8.4.27 This abnormal aortic valve, photographed from the aortic aspect, has fusion of two of the zones of apposition (black dotted lines) between the leaflets, with only one remaining open (white double-headed arrow). Leaflet calcification is also present. This is the typical substrate of aortic stenosis as seen in the elderly.

the mitral valve may lead to detachment of that structure. In cases where the ventricular septum appears to be playing a part in causing the stenosis, it may be prudent to remove a segment of muscle (Figure 8.4.31).

In cases where complete removal proves difficult, interruption of the fibrous shelf in the safe area over the ventriculo-infundibular fold will result in a safe and satisfactory relief of the stenosis. The same rules apply when resecting the variant of aortic stenosis producing a fibromuscular tunnel. Surgical correction, however, may be less successful than with a simple shelf, since the tunnel extends farther into the left ventricle, making the obstruction it produces more difficult to relieve.

A much rarer form of fixed subaortic obstruction is produced by hypertrophy of the usually inconspicuous

8.4 Malformations of the Valves of the Heart

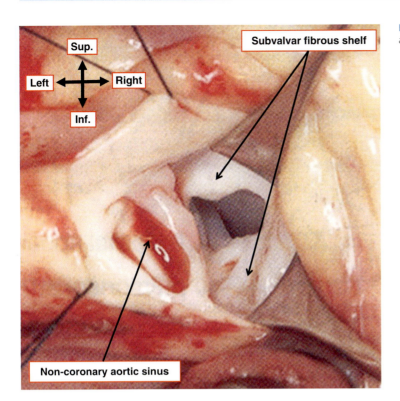

Figure 8.4.28 This view, taken in the operating room through the aortic valve, shows a circular fibrous shelf producing subaortic stenosis.

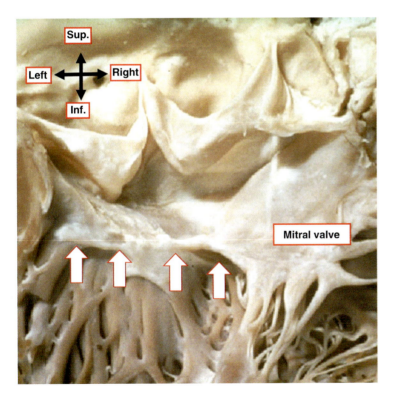

Figure 8.4.29 This specimen is opened anteriorly through the subaortic outflow tract, and is photographed in anatomical orientation. Note the extensive shelf-like lesion producing subvalvar stenosis and extending onto the aortic leaflet of the mitral valve (arrows).

antero-lateral muscle bundle.[25] This muscle runs down the outflow tract from the ventriculo-infundibular fold to the ventricular septum. In its course over the parietal wall, it would not be expected to involve the conduction tissues.

Anomalous attachment of the left atrioventricular valve can also cause fixed obstruction, as can a deviated muscular outlet septum. The former is usually seen with atrioventricular septal defect. The latter occurs only in the presence of a ventricular septal defect (Figure 8.4.32).

The fixed type of subaortic obstruction is also produced by so-called tissue tags. These can herniate from any

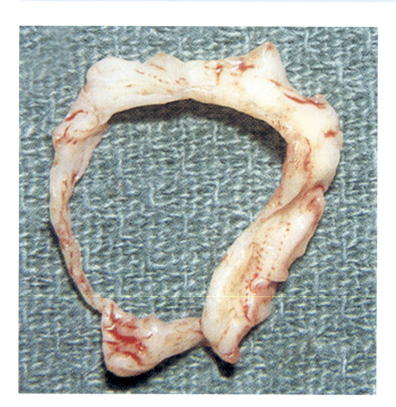

Figure 8.4.30 This specimen is the subaortic shelf shown in Figure 8.4.28 subsequent to its surgical removal. Note the horseshoe configuration.

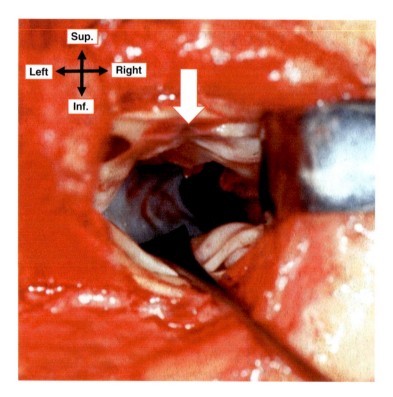

Figure 8.4.31 This view, taken in the operating room through the aorta, shows how a segment of ventricular muscle (white arrow with red borders) can safely be removed to relieve the shelf-like fibrous obstruction of the left ventricular outflow tract.

adjacent fibrous tissue structure, but are exceedingly rare as an isolated lesion in the normally connected heart.[26] They can produce significant obstruction of the left ventricular outflow tract in hearts with an atrioventricular septal defect (Figure 8.4.33), or with discordant ventriculo-arterial connections (see subsequent sections).

Dynamic subvalvar obstruction is a result of thickening of the septal musculature abutting the aortic leaflet of the mitral valve during ventricular systole. This usually creates a ridge of thickened endocardium easily seen through the aortic valve. If an operation becomes necessary, the hypertrophied muscle bundle can be resected, offering satisfactory relief of the

8.4 Malformations of the Valves of the Heart

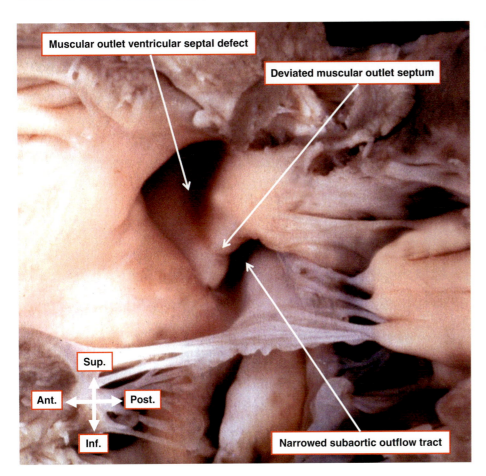

Figure 8.4.32 This anatomical specimen shows the left ventricle opened in clam-like fashion, and viewed from the apex of the left ventricle. There is fixed subaortic obstruction produced by posterior deviation of the muscular outlet septum through a ventricular septal defect.

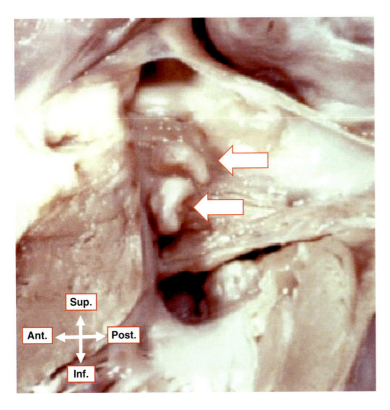

Figure 8.4.33 This heart is opened through the subaortic outflow tract, and photographed in anatomical orientation. There is an atrioventricular septal defect with common atrioventricular junction, with subaortic obstruction due to tissue tags (arrows).

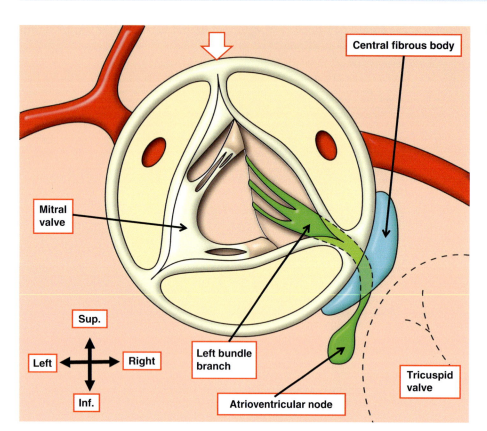

Figure 8.4.34 The drawing shows the location of the atrioventricular conduction axis as it would be visualized by the surgeon working through the aortic valve. The axis is located rightward from the interleaflet triangle between the two coronary aortic valvar sinuses (white arrow with red borders), but may be within a millimetre of the nadir of the right coronary leaflet.

obstruction.[27] Again, the surgeon must scrupulously avoid the conduction tissue as it emerges beneath the zone of apposition between the right and non-coronary leaflets and descends on the muscular ventricular septum (Figure 8.4.34). Interventionists are now able to offer alternative therapy by injecting alcohol into the first septal perforating artery.

Supravalvar aortic stenosis occurs in hourglass, membranous, and more diffuse tubular variants. All forms are rare. Fortunately, the severe tubular type is extremely unusual. Two problems are shared by all three varieties because of narrowing of the aorta at the junction of the sinuses with the ascending tubular aorta.[28] First, the aortic sinuses, which usually contain the coronary arteries, may be converted into high-pressure zones, in which the arteries provide the only run-off other than through the distal stenosis. This can produce marked dilation of both the sinuses and the coronary arteries. Second, the circumferential narrowing at the sinutubular junction (Figure 8.4.35) tends to tether the three aortic leaflets at the ends of their zones of apposition in such a way that it is rarely enough to perform a simple aortoplasty.[29] If possible, all three sinuses should be opened to release the tethering of the leaflets. This can be accomplished by resecting the thickened sinutubular junction, and inserting pericardial patches in each sinus (Figures 8.4.36–8.4.40).

Aortic valvar insufficiency may be due to congenital malformation of the valve (Figure 8.4.41), its supporting structures, or both. It may also be secondary to an infectious process in the aortic root (Figure 8.4.42), or to degenerative disease of the aortic walls. Occasionally, aortic insufficiency may be due to trauma. Its frequent association with the doubly committed and juxta-arterial ventricular septal defect suggests that deficiency in the structures supporting the leaflets plays some role in these problems. Prolapse of the leaflets, and insufficiency, may occur with other types of ventricular septal defect (Figure 8.4.43). Prolapse can be found even when the ventricular septum is intact, the latter situation usually being associated with a bicuspid aortic valve.

The critical importance of the anatomy of this region is perhaps best demonstrated by the problems exhibited by patients with endocarditis of the aortic valve.[30] Because the valve is the keystone to all the other valves and chambers of the heart (Figure 8.4.44), an eroding abscess in the aortic root may lead to formation of a fistula involving any of these adjacent structures. The patient may present with findings of left heart failure, left-to-right shunting, complete heart block, or any combination of these, in addition to the usual signs of sepsis. Surgical management requires a detailed knowledge of this area, since the surgeon may be faced with virtual disruption of the ventriculo-arterial connection.[30] A similar problem can occur when the aortic root, or the fibrous coronet, is severely damaged by dissection or marked degeneration of its fibrous structure.

As with aortic stenosis, stenosis of the right ventricular outflow can occur at the valvar, supravalvar or subvalvar levels. The latter is discussed in association with tetralogy of Fallot (Chapter 8.5). Dysplasia of the valvar leaflets is most often seen as marked distortion and thickening, although three discrete leaflets can sometimes be recognized (Figure 8.4.45). It can be associated with insufficiency as well as stenosis.

8.4 Malformations of the Valves of the Heart

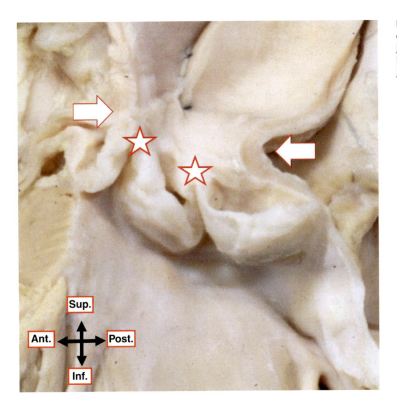

Figure 8.4.35 In this specimen, photographed in anatomical orientation, there is severe narrowing at the level of the sinutubular junction (arrows). Although usually termed 'supravalvar', the obstruction involves the attachment of the valvar leaflets (stars) at the sinutubular junction.

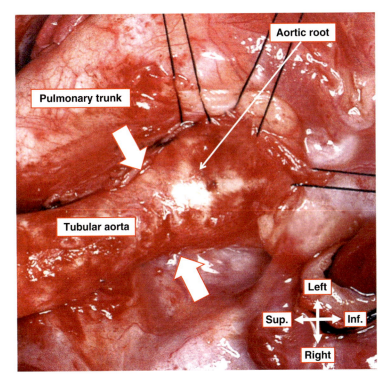

Figure 8.4.36 This picture, taken in the operating room through a median sternotomy, shows narrowing (arrows) of the aorta at the level of the sinutubular junction.

Isolated pulmonary stenosis is typically found in the form of a dome-shaped valve with three well-developed but fused commissures (Figure 8.4.46). The leaflets are typically attached to the wall of the pulmonary trunk along the peripheral ends of the zones of apposition between them, leaving only a restricted central opening (Figure 8.4.47). The arterial root is then narrowed at the sinutubular junction. This is an integral part of the valvar mechanism, although such narrowing is often described as being supravalvar. These areas of tethering can be dissected from the arterial wall and incised, providing a particularly satisfactory relief of the obstruction. The effectiveness of surgery is best measured six to nine months after operation,

253

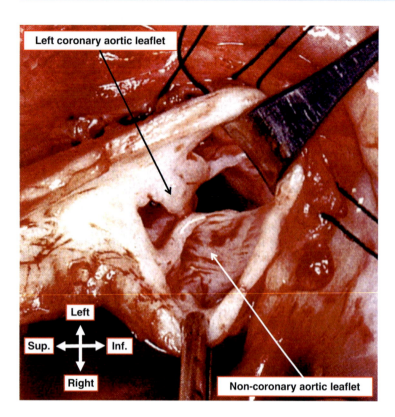

Figure 8.4.37 In the patient shown in Figure 8.4.36, the surgeon has made an extensive vertical excision into the non-coronary sinus or the aortic root, revealing the marked constriction at the sinutubular junction, with a particularly narrow entry to the left coronary aortic sinus, which is guarded by the edge of the valvar leaflet.

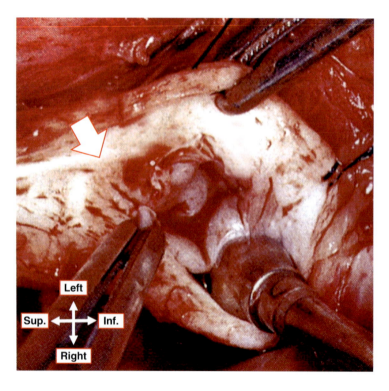

Figure 8.4.38 The attachments of the left and non-coronary leaflets at the thickened sinutubular junction, as shown in Figure 8.4.37, have been liberated (arrow), thus releasing the left coronary leaflet so as to allow its full excursion.

since significant secondary muscular obstruction at the subvalvar level may maintain a pressure gradient across the outflow tract. This muscular hypertrophy will almost always regress with time.[31] Despite the excellent results of surgery, treatment of congenital pulmonary valvar stenosis has largely become the province of the interventional cardiologist. It is doubtful, however, whether inflation of a balloon will ever rival the anatomical precision achieved by the competent surgeon.

True supravalvar stenosis usually takes the form of a waist-like narrowing of the pulmonary trunk distal to the sinutubular junction (Figure 8.4.48), though it may occur at the sinutubular junction, or anywhere at one or more

8.4 Malformations of the Valves of the Heart

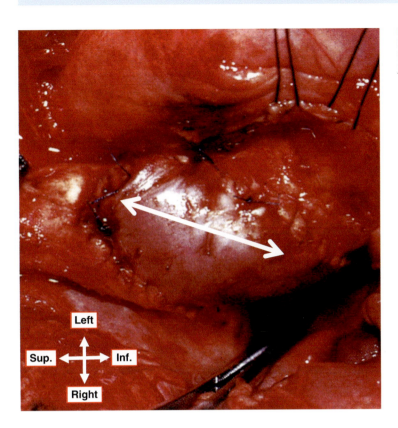

Figure 8.4.39 In the patient shown in Figures 8.4.36 and 8.4.37, a helical pericardial patch (double-headed arrow) has been inserted in the incision to the non-coronary sinus, thus enlarging the sinutubular junction and the ascending aorta.

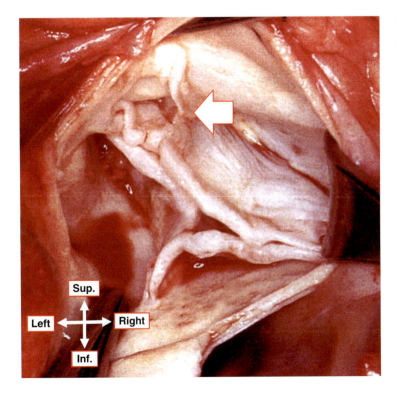

Figure 8.4.40 This view, taken in the operating room through an aortotomy, shows a regurgitant aortic valve as the consequence of tethering of one of its leaflets (arrow).

locations within the pulmonary arterial tree. Narrowing has also been reported within collateral arteries supplying the lung directly from the aorta in cases of tetralogy of Fallot with pulmonary atresia.[32] Very rarely, the obstructions may be membrane-like, but the usual lesion is more akin to a segment of tubular hypoplasia. These lesions, if anatomically accessible, are amenable to enlargement using a simple patch.

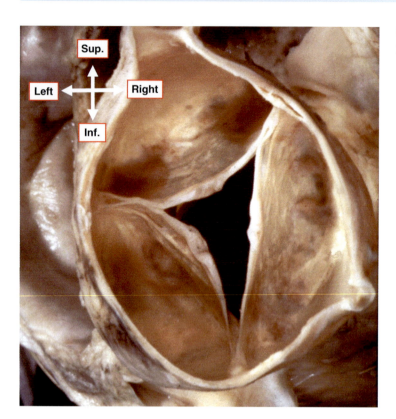

Figure 8.4.41 This anatomical specimen is photographed from above, showing failure of central coaptation of the leaflets of the aortic valve because of dilation at the sinutubular junction.

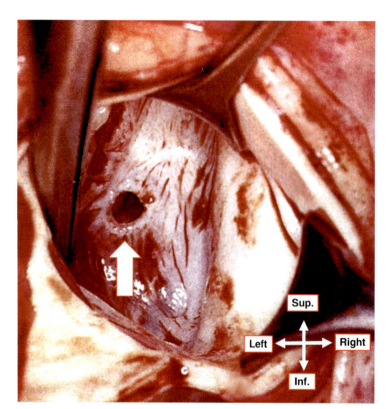

Figure 8.4.42 This operative view, taken through an aortotomy, shows a perforation (arrow) in one leaflet of a bicuspid aortic valve due to infective endocarditis.

8.4 Malformations of the Valves of the Heart

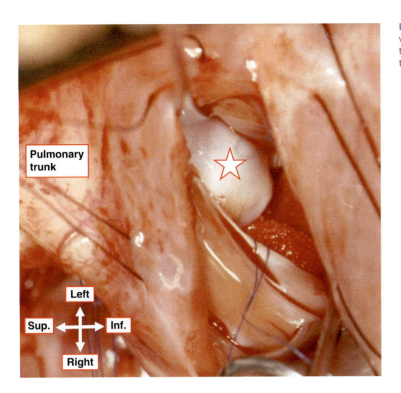

Figure 8.4.43 This operative view, seen through a right ventriculotomy, shows prolapse of the leaflets of the aortic valve (star) in the setting of a perimembranous ventricular septal defect opening to the outlet of the right ventricle.

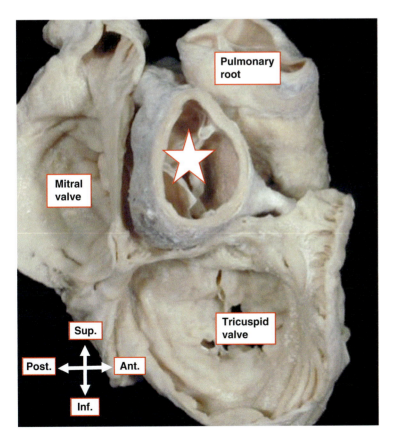

Figure 8.4.44 The short axis of the ventricular mass has been displayed by removing the atrial musculature and the arterial trunks, showing the 'keystone' location of the centrally positioned aortic valve (star).

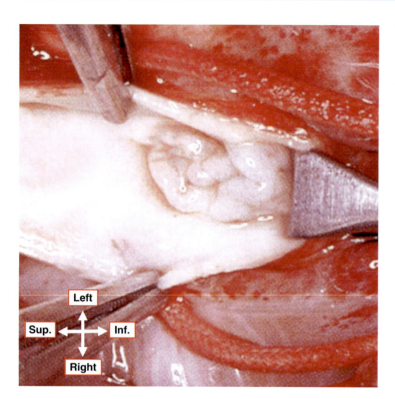

Figure 8.4.45 This operative view, taken through an incision in the pulmonary trunk, shows gross dysplasia of the leaflets of the pulmonary valve.

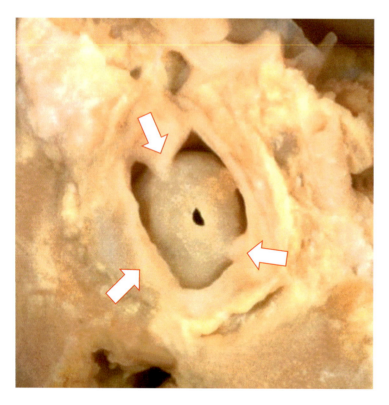

Figure 8.4.46 This pulmonary valve is viewed from above in anatomical orientation. There is extensive fusion of the zones of apposition between the leaflets, leaving a domed membrane with a central orifice the size of a pinhole. Note the tethering of the domed valvar tissue to the walls of the pulmonary trunk at the sites of fusion of the leaflets (arrows).

References Cited

1. Milo S, Ho SY, Macartney FJ, et al. Straddling and overriding atrioventricular valves morphology and classification. *Am J Cardiol* 1979; **44**: 1122–1134.
2. Pacifico AD, Soto B, Bargeron LMJ. Surgical treatment of straddling tricuspid valves. *Circulation* 1979; **60**: 655–664.
3. Chauvaud SM, Mihaileanu SA, Gaer JAR, Carpentier AC. Surgical treatment of Ebstein's malformation – the 'Hôpital Broussas' experience. *Cardiol Young* 1996; **6**: 4–11.
4. Schreiber C, Cook A, Ho SY, Augustin N, Anderson RH. Morphologic spectrum of Ebstein's malformation: revisitation

8.4 Malformations of the Valves of the Heart

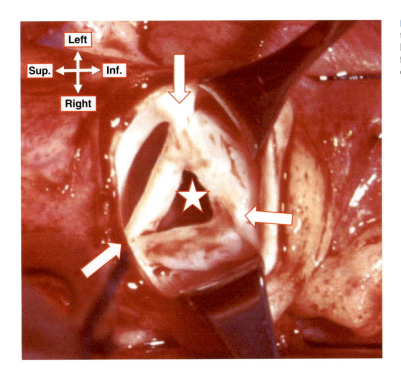

Figure 8.4.47 This operative view, taken through an incision in the pulmonary trunk, shows fusion of the zones of apposition between the leaflets of the pulmonary valve, with tethering of the fused leaflets to the wall of the pulmonary trunk (arrows), leaving a constricted central opening (star).

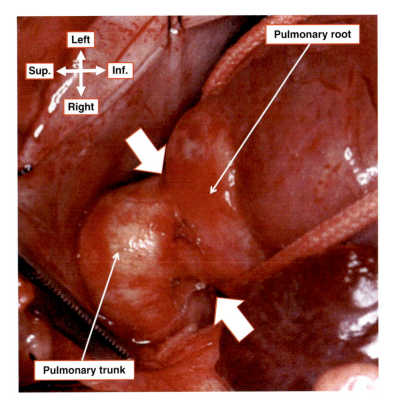

Figure 8.4.48 The view, taken in the operating room, shows the external narrowing (large arrows) at the sinutubular junction of the pulmonary valve shown in Figure 8.4.47.

relative to surgical repair. *J Thorac Cardiovasc Surg* 1999: **117**: 148–155.

5. Leung MP, Baker EJ, Anderson RH, Zuberbuhler JR. Cineangiographic spectrum of Ebstein's malformation: its relevance to clinical presentation and outcome. *J Am Coll Cardiol* 1988; **11**: 154–161.

6. da Silva JP, da Silva LD. Ebstein's anomaly of the tricuspid valve: the cone repair. *Sem Thorac Cardiovasc Surg* 2012; **15**: 38–45.

7. Ruschhaupt DG, Bharati S, Lev M. Mitral valve malformation of Ebstein type in absence of corrected transposition. *Am J Cardiol* 1976; **38**: 109–112.

8. Leung M, Rigby ML, Anderson RH, Wyse RKH, Macartney FJ. Reversed off-setting of the septal attachments of the atrioventricular valves and Ebstein's malformation of the morphologically mitral valve. *Br Heart J* 1987; **57**: 184–187.

9. Becker AE, Becker MJ, Edwards JE. Pathologic spectrum of dysplasia of the tricuspid valve, features in common with Ebstein's malformation. *Arch Pathol* 1971; **91**: 167–178.

10. Oberhoffer R, Cook AC, Lang D, et al. Correlation between echocardiographic and morphological investigations of lesions of the tricuspid valve diagnosed during fetal life. *Br Heart J* 1992; **68**: 580–585.

11. Van der Bel-Kahn J, Duren DR, Becker AE. Isolated mitral valve prolapse: chordal architecture as an anatomic basis in older patients. *J Am Coll Cardiol* 1985; **5**: 1335–1340.

12. Layman TE, Edwards JE. Anomalous mitral arcade: a type of congenital mitral insufficiency. *Circulation* 1967; **35**: 389–395.

13. Rosenquist GC : Congenital mitral valve disease associated with coarctation of the aorta. A spectrum that includes parachute deformity of the mitral valve. *Circulation* 1974; **49**: 985–993.

14. Shone JD, Sellers RD, Anderson RC, et al. The developmental complex of 'parachute mitral valve', supravalvular ring of left atrium, subaortic stenosis, and coarctation of the aorta. *Am J Cardiol* 1963; **11**: 714–725.

15. Milo S, Stark J, Macartney FJ, Anderson RH. Parachute deformity of the tricuspid valve (case report). *Thorax* 1979; **34**: 543–546.

16. Stamm C, Anderson RH, Ho SY. Clinical anatomy of the normal pulmonary root compared with that in isolated pulmonary valvular stenosis. *J Am Coll Cardiol* 1998; **31**: 1420–1425.

17. Sievers HH, Hemmer G, Beyersdorf F, et al. The everyday used nomenclature of the aortic root components: the Tower of Babel? *Eur J Cardiothoracic Surg* 2012; **41**: 478–482.

18. Anderson RH. Clinical anatomy of the aortic root. *Heart* 2000; **84**: 670–673.

19. Tretter JT, Spicer DE, Mori S, et al. The significance of the interleaflet triangles in determining the morphology of congenitally abnormal aortic valves: implications for noninvasive imaging and surgical management. *JASE* 2016; **29**: 1131–1143.

20. Tretter JT, Spicer DE, Franklin RCG, et al. Describing the normal and congenitally malformed aortic root – the view from specialists in Congenital Cardiac Disease. *Ann Thor Surg* 2023; **116**: 6–16.

21. Angelini A, Ho SY, Anderson RH, et al. The morphology of the normal aortic valve as compared with the aortic valve having two leaflets. *J Thorac Cardiovasc Surg* 1989; **98**: 362–367.

22. Tretter JT, Mori S, Spicer DE, Anderson RH. The aortic valve with four leaflets: how should we best describe this blue moon? *Eur Heart J-Cardiovasc Imag* 2021; **22**: 777–780.

23. Vollebergh FEMG, Becker AE. Minor congenital variations in cusp size in tricuspid aortic valves. Possible link with isolated aortic stenosis. *Br Heart J* 1977; **39**: 1006–1011.

24. McKay R, Ross DN. Technique for the relief of discrete subaortic stenosis. *J Thorac Cardiovasc Surg* 1982; **84**: 917–920.

25. Moulaert AJ, Oppenheimer-Dekker A. Anterolateral muscle bundle of the left ventricle, bulboventricular flange and subaortic stenosis. *Am J Cardiol* 1976; **37**: 78–81.

26. Anderson RH, Lenox CC, Zuberbuhler JR. Morphology of ventricular septal defect associated with coarctation of the aorta. *Br Heart J* 1983; **50**: 176–181.

27. Morrow AG. Hypertrophic subaortic stenosis: operative methods utilised to relieve left ventricular outflow obstruction. *J Thorac Cardiovasc Surg* 1978; **76**: 423–430.

28. Stamm C, Li J, Ho SY, Redington AN, Anderson RH. The aortic root in supravalvar aortic stenosis: the potential surgical relevance of morphologic findings. *J Thorac Cardiovasc Surg* 1997; **114**: 16–24.

29. Doty DB, Polansky DB, Jenson CB. Supravalvular aortic stenosis. Repair by extended aortoplasty. *J Thorac Cardiovasc Surg* 1977; **74**: 362–371.

30. Frantz PJ, Murray GF, Wilcox BR. Surgical management of left ventricular–aortic discontinuity complicating bacterial endocarditis. *Ann Thorac Surg* 1980; **29**: 1–7.

31. Gilbert JW, Morrow AG, Talbert JW. The surgical significance of hypertrophic infundibular obstruction accompanying valvar pulmonary stenosis. *J Thorac Cardiovasc Surg* 1963; **46**: 457–467.

32. Haworth SG, Macartney FJ. Growth and development of pulmonary circulation in pulmonary atresia with ventricular septal defect and major aortopulmonary collateral arteries. *Br Heart J* 1980; **44**: 14–24.

Chapter 8.5
Tetralogy of Fallot and Pulmonary Atresia with an Intact Ventricular Septum

One form of obstruction of the right ventricular outflow tract is so clearly demarcated that it constitutes an entity in its own right, namely tetralogy of Fallot. When there is extreme overriding of the aortic valvar orifice, it can also show the abnormal ventriculo-arterial connection of double outlet right ventricle, but it is convenient to discuss tetralogy at this point in our narrative. Its anatomical hallmark is antero-cephalad deviation of the insertion of the muscular or fibrous outlet septum, combined with subpulmonary obstruction due to a squeeze between the deviated outlet septum and the septoparietal trabeculations (Figure 8.5.1).[1] In the normal heart, it is not possible to recognize the muscular outlet septum as a discrete entity. Instead, the myocardium created by muscularization of the proximal outflow cushions (see Chapter 2) has been remodelled to form the free-standing subpulmonary infundibular sleeve. This tissue fuses with the much more extensive ventriculo-infundibular fold to form the supraventricular crest (Figure 8.5.2).

In tetralogy of Fallot, as in double outlet right ventricle, the building blocks of the normal outflow tract are divorced one from the other.[2] Each is then recognizable in its own right (Figure 8.5.3). The septomarginal trabeculation, formed by coalescence of the initial right ventricular trabeculations, reinforces the septal surface of the muscular ventricular septum. The tissues derived from the proximal cushions, be they myocardial or fibrous, can be seen to be malaligned antero-cephalad to the cranial limb of the septomarginal trabeculation. The inner heart curvature, or ventriculo-infundibular fold, now supports the leaflets of the aortic valve that have retained their origin from the right ventricle. The deviated position of

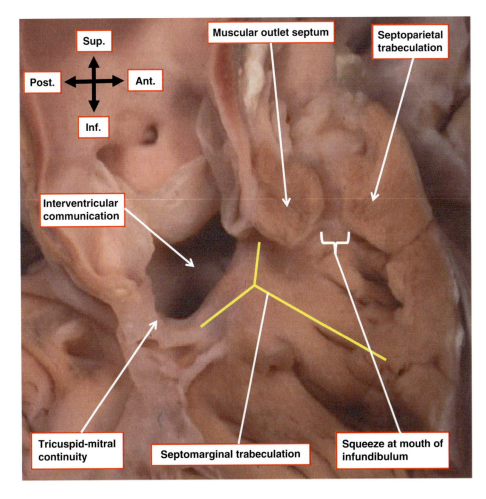

Figure 8.5.1 The image shows the right ventricular septal aspect of a typical example of tetralogy of Fallot, having bisected the aortic root. The phenotypic feature is the squeeze provided between the muscular outlet septum and the septoparietal trabeculations (yellow lines).

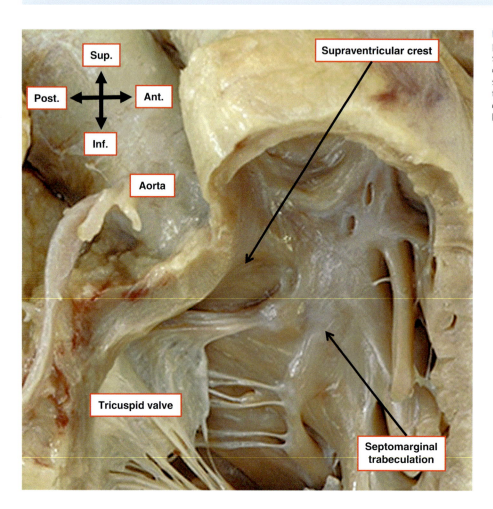

Figure 8.5.2 The normal right ventricle is photographed in anatomical orientation, showing the septal aspect. The supraventricular crest inserts between the limbs of the septomarginal trabeculation. It is not possible, in the normal heart, to distinguish where the septal component finishes, and where the musculature becomes that of the parietal ventricular wall.

the outlet septum, combined with the septoparietal trabeculations, then serves to narrow the subpulmonary outflow tract (Figure 8.5.1). By virtue of the separation of these various components, there is, perforce, an interventricular communication, which is overridden by the leaflets of the aortic valve (Figure 8.5.3).

The interventricular communication, therefore, is positioned beneath the aortic root. It is then the rightward margin of the cone of space subtended by the overriding valvar leaflets that should be defined as the ventricular septal defect (Figure 8.5.4).[1] As with regular ventricular septal defects, this area represents the tertiary embryonic interventricular communication, in other words the aorto-right ventricular communication (see Chapter 2). In the majority of cases, there is fibrous continuity between the leaflets of the tricuspid and mitral valves in the inferior-caudal quadrant of the defect, thus making it perimembranous (Figure 8.5.4). In a minority of cases, around one-fifth in Caucasian populations, the infero-caudal rim can be muscular when the ventriculo-infundibular fold fuses with the caudal limb of the septomarginal trabeculation (Figure 8.5.6).[3] These features have the same implications for protection of the axis of atrioventricular conduction tissue as they do in isolated ventricular septal defects (Chapter 8.3). When the infero-caudal margin is fibrous, the atrioventricular conduction axis penetrates beneath the atrioventricular membranous component of this area (Figure 8.5.7). Often, this is overlain by the membranous flap, or pseudo-flaps derived from the tricuspid valve.[4] In tetralogy, the non-branching and the branching components of the atrioventricular bundle are usually carried down the left ventricular side of the septum, being positioned some distance from the septal crest. In a minority of cases, the bundle can branch directly astride the septum.[5,6] It can then be traumatized (Figure 8.5.8) by sutures placed directly through the septal crest (Figure 8.5.9). In the cases in which the caudal limb of the septomarginal trabeculation has fused with the ventriculo-infundibular fold, the interventricular membranous septum is intact, with the postero-inferior myocardial tissues (Figure 8.5.6) protecting the atrioventricular conduction tissues. This variant is found in about one-fifth of Caucasian populations with tetralogy. It follows that, in this setting, superficial sutures can be placed along the entire muscular margin of the right ventricular aspect of these defects without fear of traumatizing the conduction axis.

In a very small minority of cases found in the Caucasian population, but more frequently encountered in Asia or South America,[7] the outlet septum is fibrous rather than muscular, with failure of formation of the posterior aspect of the freestanding subpulmonary infundibular sleeve. The defect is then juxta-arterial (Figure 8.5.10).[8] These defects can exist with or without mitral-to-tricuspid valvar continuity in the inferoposterior margin of the defect, with the same implications as discussed above regarding the relationship of the conduction axis.

While it is clearly important to close securely the ventricular septal defect in patients with tetralogy, thus committing the

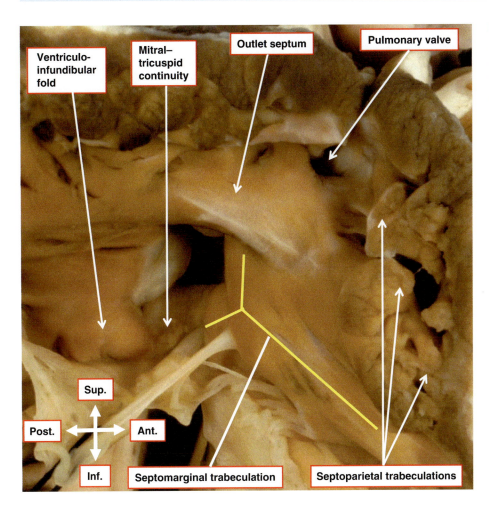

Figure 8.5.3 This view of the outlet of the right ventricle of the heart from a patient with tetralogy of Fallot, taken in anatomical orientation, shows the divorce of the muscular structures that combine to form the normal subpulmonary outflow tract. The yellow 'Y' shows the septomarginal trabeculation.

aorta to the left ventricle, probably the most important feature for a successful surgical outcome is relief of the subpulmonary obstruction. One of the major determinants of this success is the size of the pulmonary trunk. Tables are available for preoperative evaluation to select those patients who can successfully be corrected without incising across the ventriculo-arterial junction.[9,10] Such incisions are usually described as being transannular. An understanding of the precise anatomy of the subpulmonary outflow tract is also vital if the surgeon is to plan accurately a reproducible operation for successful relief of the muscular obstruction. This is the consequence of the formation of a constrictive muscular ring at the mouth of the subpulmonary infundibulum, with its parietal segment produced by hypertrophy of free-standing septoparietal trabeculations (Figure 8.5.11). Knowledge of this feature is important to the surgeon when deciding which muscle to resect so as to widen the narrowed outflow tract. The major limiting structure is always the hypertrophied septal insertion of the outlet septum, which can be incised without fear of damaging vital structures. At the same time, any free-standing septoparietal trabeculations should be identified and removed (Figures 8.5.12, 8.5.13). They, too, never contain vital structures. The body of the outlet septum usually contributes to obstruction, and it is tempting also to resect this structure. Excessive resection, however, may lead to damage to the leaflets of the aortic valve arising from its left ventricular aspect (Figure 8.5.5). It is also usual to resect the parietal insertion of the outlet septum. This fuses with the ventriculo-infundibular fold, which is the inner curvature of the heart. Care must be taken not to perforate through to the right-sided atrioventricular groove in this region. Dissection, or injudicious placement of sutures, can damage the right coronary artery.[11] It is very unusual for the septomarginal trabeculation itself to contribute to the subpulmonary obstruction. Thus, it is usually unnecessary to resect its limbs. Its body, and the moderator band, nonetheless, may be hypertrophied, particularly when the latter structure has a high take-off. Severe hypertrophy produces a two-chambered right ventricle (Figure 8.5.14).[12] The intervening muscle band may then require resection. The anterior papillary muscle of the tricuspid valve often arises from the inlet aspect of the obstructing shelf. Care must be taken, therefore, not to damage this muscle should resection be deemed necessary. When planning surgical relief of subpulmonary obstruction, one must also heed the presence of an anomalous origin of the anterior interventricular coronary artery from the right coronary artery, which is more common in patients with tetralogy of Fallot and often courses anterior to the right ventricular outflow tract (Figures 8.5.15, 8.5.16).[13]

The final variable in tetralogy of Fallot is the connection of the leaflets of the overriding aortic valve. Depending on this feature, the aorta can be connected mostly to the left ventricle, making the ventriculo-arterial connection concordant, or connected mostly to the right ventricle, and hence producing a

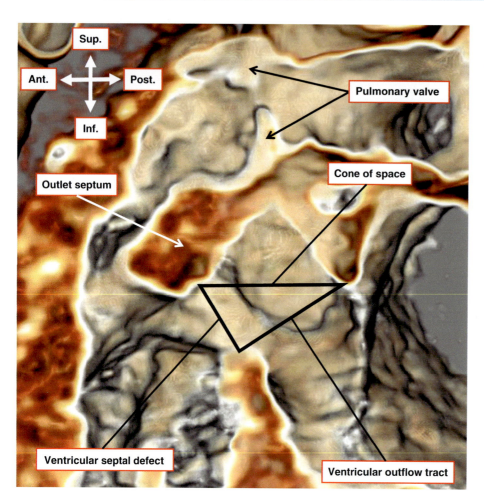

Figure 8.5.4 This virtual dissection of a computed tomographic angiogram from a patient with tetralogy of the Fallot shows the cone of space subtended beneath the leaflets of the overriding aortic valve. It is the right ventricular margin of the cone that represents the ventricular septal defect. The left ventricular margin is the outflow tract for the left ventricle.

double outlet connection. The degree of override should not markedly affect the surgical procedure. With greater commitment of the aorta to the right ventricle, nonetheless, the placement of the patch tunnelling the aorta to the left ventricle, and thus closing the ventricular septal defect, becomes more important. The internal conduit constructed from the left ventricle to the aorta may further complicate relief of the obstruction to the right ventricular outflow tract, since it is always necessary to ensure an adequate outlet from the left ventricle, this being provided by the left ventricular border of the cone of space subtended beneath the overriding aortic valve (Figure 8.5.4). Although the primary obstruction in tetralogy is at the infundibular level, the pulmonary valve is frequently stenotic, being bifoliate in the majority of patients. Any stenosis must be relieved during operative repair. The sequels of postoperative pulmonary regurgitation are only now becoming evident. It could be that, in the long term, they will be just as troublesome as residual pulmonary stenosis, and less easy to relieve.

Patients with tetralogy of Fallot can have multiple associated lesions, such as straddling and overriding of the tricuspid valve, or deficient atrioventricular septation (Figure 8.5.17). The end point is then a combination of the anatomical lesions already discussed. One of the most important associated lesions is the presence of pulmonary atresia rather than pulmonary stenosis. This combination is often described as pulmonary atresia with ventricular septal defect, which is not an incorrect designation. The variant found with the intracardiac anatomy of tetralogy, however, is so distinctive that it should be described as tetralogy of Fallot with valvar or infundibular pulmonary atresia.[14] The intracardiac anatomy includes deviation of the muscular outlet septum sufficient to block completely the subpulmonary infundibulum (Figure 8.5.18). The anatomy of the ventricular septal defect can vary as in tetralogy, with the same surgical connotations. The feature that dominates the surgical options is the morphology of the pulmonary arteries. Exceedingly rarely, the pulmonary arteries may be supplied through an aortopulmonary window, or coronary arterial fistulas.[15,16] In about half of cases, nonetheless, the lungs are supplied through a persistently patent arterial duct (Figures 8.5.19, 8.5.20), which itself may take an unexpected origin from the aortic arch. In the past, such unusual origins were frequently interpreted as representing a persistent artery of the fifth pharyngeal arch. Since we now know that there is never a fifth pharyngeal arch (see Chapter 2), this cannot be a rational explanation. Remodelling of the distal insertion of the artery of the pulmonary arch provides a better explanation of such findings. When the arterial supply is through the arterial duct, then almost always the confluent pulmonary arteries supply all the pulmonary parenchyma (Figure 8.5.21).

In the remainder of the cases, the pulmonary arterial supply is provided by major systemic-to-pulmonary collateral

8.5 Tetralogy of Fallot and Pulmonary Atresia with an Intact Ventricular Septum

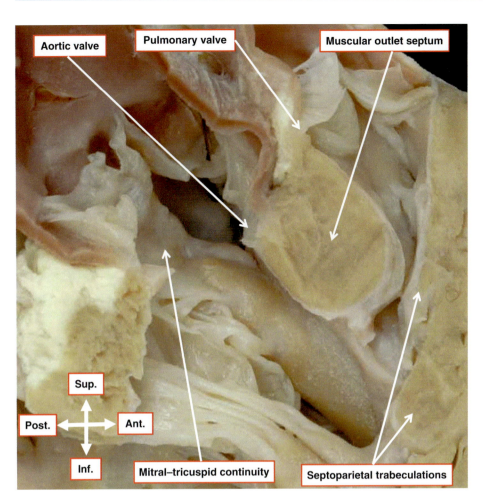

Figure 8.5.5 This view of an anatomical specimen, photographed in anatomical orientation, shows the usual variant of ventricular septal defect in tetralogy of Fallot, in which the postero-inferior border is formed by fibrous continuity between the leaflets of the mitral and tricuspid valves, thus making it perimembranous. The deviated muscular outlet septum supports a sleeve of free-standing subpulmonary infundibular musculature. Note the off-set of the valvar leaflets on either side of the muscular outlet septum and the infundibulum. Note also the tight fibrous ring formed at the mouth of the infundibulum.

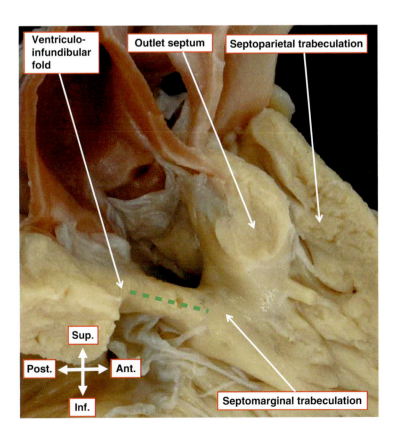

Figure 8.5.6 In this specimen with tetralogy of Fallot, photographed in anatomical orientation, the defect, as seen from the right ventricle, has exclusively muscular borders because of fusion postero-inferiorly between the caudal limb of the septomarginal trabeculation and the ventriculo-infundibular fold (green dashed line).

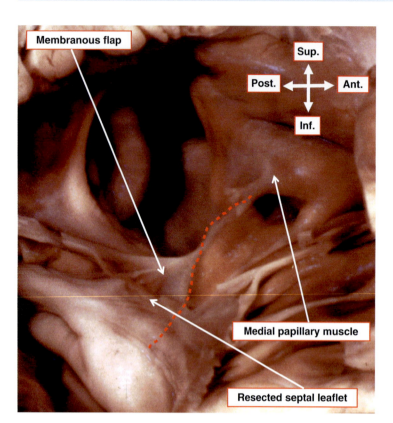

Figure 8.5.7 This anatomical specimen with tetralogy of Fallot, photographed in anatomical orientation, has been prepared by removal of the septal leaflet of the tricuspid valve. It shows the site of the remnant of the interventricular membranous septum, known as the membranous flap, and illustrates the relationships of the atrioventricular conduction axis (red dotted line) when the ventricular septal defect is perimembranous.

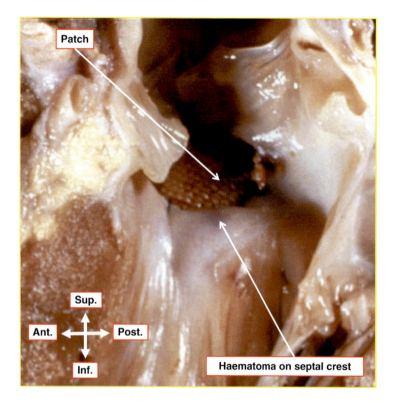

Figure 8.5.8 In this heart, viewed in anatomical orientation from the left ventricle, the defect in a patient with tetralogy of Fallot was repaired by placing sutures directly through the crest of the muscular ventricular septum. Note the haemorrhage produced at the septal crest.

arteries.[17] It is rare to find such collateral arteries supplying the pulmonary circulation except when the intracardiac anatomy is that of tetralogy. And only very rarely will a duct and collateral arteries supply the same lung, although these two sources of flow can supply separate lungs (Figure 8.5.22). As emphasized, when a duct is present, and the pulmonary arteries are confluent, the arteries supply the entirety of the lung parenchyma (Figure 8.5.21), although they may be variably developed. The degree of hypoplasia determines whether total correction is feasible.

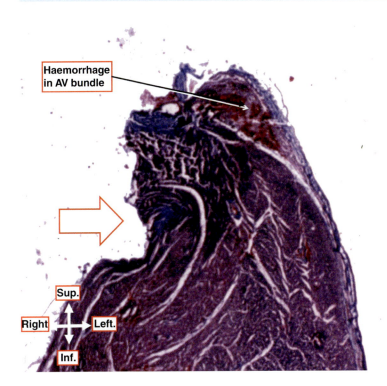

Figure 8.5.9 The histological section is taken across the ventricular septum in the heart shown in Figure 8.5.4. The atrioventricular conduction tissue axis in this heart branched directly astride the septum. The atrioventricular (AV) bundle was traumatized by a suture securing the patch, producing atrioventricular block. The white arrow with red borders shows the site of the suture.

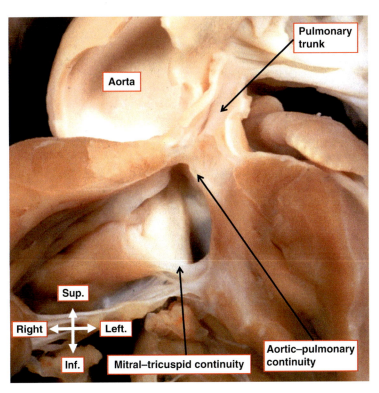

Figure 8.5.10 This specimen, viewed in anatomical orientation from the apex of the right ventricle, shows tetralogy of Fallot with a juxta-arterial defect, due to failure of formation of the muscular subpulmonary infundibulum. Note the fibrous continuity between the leaflets of the mitral and tricuspid valves, showing that the defect is also perimembranous.

When the right and left pulmonary arteries are not confluent, or when major systemic-to-pulmonary collateral arteries are present, the situation is more complex. Non-confluent pulmonary arteries can be supplied independently by bilateral ducts, or one lung can be supplied by a duct and the other through collateral arteries (Figure 8.5.22). It is more usual for the collateral arteries to supply both lungs, with no duct being present. Even when there are collateral arteries, nonetheless, well-developed confluent pulmonary arteries usually co-exist within the pericardial sac (Figure 8.5.23). It is important to establish how much of the pulmonary parenchyma is connected to the intrapericardial pulmonary arteries, and how much is supplied directly by collateral arteries. The collateral arteries can anastomose with the pulmonary arteries at the hilum (Figure 8.5.24), or extend into the parenchyma to supply lobar or segmental arteries directly. Intersegmental anastomoses also occur. The object of preoperative evaluation, therefore, should be to establish precisely

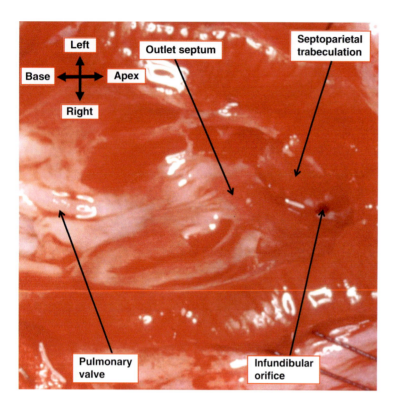

Figure 8.5.11 This view, taken in the operating room through a right infundibulotomy, shows the stenotic orifice of the subpulmonary infundibulum in a patient with tetralogy of Fallot. The stenosis is formed in part by the hypertrophied outlet septum, and also by septoparietal trabeculations.

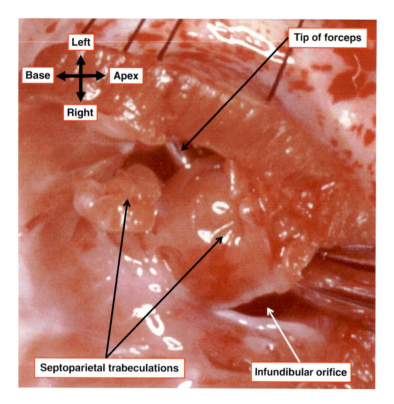

Figure 8.5.12 In the patient shown in Figure 8.5.11, the surgeon was able to liberate the septoparietal trabeculations. They could then be excised.

how much of each lung is supplied by the intrapericardial pulmonary arteries, since this feature is the ultimate determinant of the success of any attempted total correction. Cases can be found with supply exclusively from collateral arteries (Figure 8.5.25). In this setting, the arterial trunk arising from the heart is best described as a solitary structure, although it still functions as an aorta.

In contrast to tetralogy with pulmonary atresia, where initial survival is good, and the results of surgery are continually improving, attempted surgical correction of patients with pulmonary atresia and an intact ventricular septum continues to be disappointing. The anatomy of the lesion itself accounts for the dismal outcome.[18-20] The atresia can be due either to an imperforate pulmonary valvar membrane

8.5 Tetralogy of Fallot and Pulmonary Atresia with an Intact Ventricular Septum

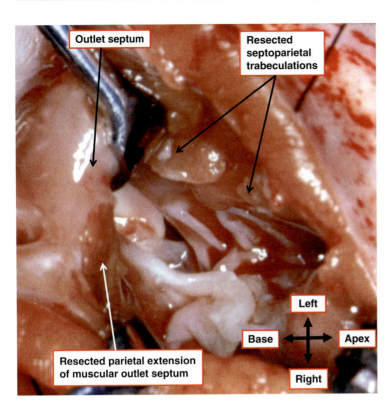

Figure 8.5.13 In the patients shown in Figures 8.5.11 and 8.5.12, the obstruction at the mouth of the infundibulum was completely relieved by resecting the parietal extension of the outlet septum.

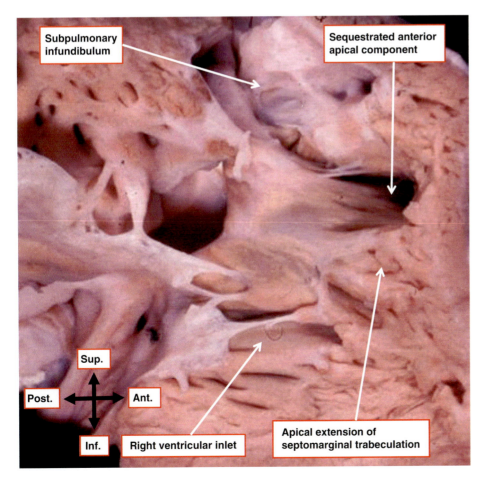

Figure 8.5.14 In this heart from a patient with tetralogy of Fallot, shown in anatomical orientation, there is hypertrophy of the body of the septomarginal trabeculation, separating the apical trabecular component into two parts. This is the so-called two-chambered right ventricle.

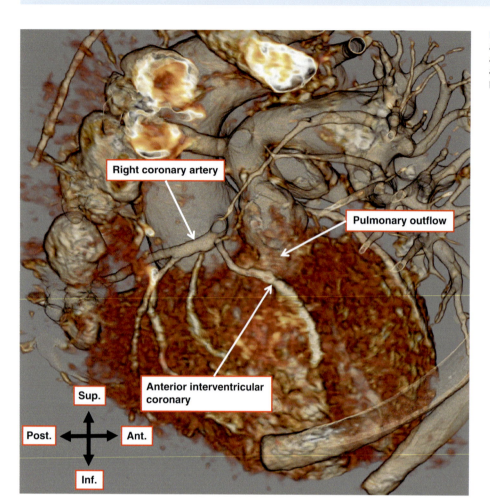

Figure 8.5.15 This computed tomographic angiogram shows anomalous origin of the anterior interventricular coronary artery travelling anterior to the right ventricular outflow tract in a patient with tetralogy of Fallot.

(Figure 8.5.26), or to muscular infundibular atresia. In the latter situation, the pulmonary trunk is blind-ending, with no vestiges of leaflets of the pulmonary valve (Figure 8.5.27). In the setting of the blind-ending trunk, it is usually the case that the cavities of the outlet and apical components of the right ventricle are more-or-less completely obliterated by gross hypertrophy of the ventricular wall. In consequence, the cavity is effectively represented only by the hypoplastic inlet portion (Figure 8.5.28). This cavity is unlikely ever to perform a useful function, particularly when fistulous communications extend to the coronary arteries. The right ventricle should probably be disregarded when deciding surgical treatment. When there is a pulmonary valve present, but its leaflets are imperforate, a spectrum is seen in terms of the size of the right ventricular cavity.[21] In some hearts, the hypertrophy of the walls of the right ventricle can obliterate only the apical trabecular part of the cavity (Figure 8.5.29). It is questionable whether these ventricles will ever grow and become useful, although attempts have been made to resect apical trabeculations and rehabilitate the ventricle.[22] In the most favourable situation, the cavity is less hypoplastic, and has well-developed inlet, apical, and outlet components (Figure 8.5.30). These cases are those that are most amenable to total operative correction, although increasingly they are treated by the interventional cardiologist, who will perforate the valvar membrane before dilating it with balloons. Whatever the intracardiac anatomy, it is rare that one finds the thread-like pulmonary arteries seen so frequently with tetralogy and pulmonary atresia. Furthermore, the flow of pulmonary blood is almost always duct-dependent. With prostaglandins now available to improve ductal flow, the pulmonary arteries are almost always of sufficient size to permit construction of a systemic-pulmonary shunt. Other options, such as the need for pulmonary valvotomy, should be decided after assessment of the precise anatomy of the individual case.

Pulmonary valvar insufficiency may be congenital or acquired, the latter usually secondary to surgical intervention or pulmonary hypertension. Congenital pulmonary valvar insufficiency may be associated with marked deformity of the valvar tissue, as in valvar dysplasia, or with purported absence of the valvar tissue altogether. In reality, rudimentary leaflets are almost always present in the so-called absent pulmonary valve syndrome. This can rarely be seen with an intact ventricular septum,[23,24] but more usually in combination with a ventricular septal defect (Figure 8.5.31). It is another of the associated lesions found in combination with tetralogy of Fallot. While gross pulmonary valvar insufficiency may be relatively well-tolerated by the right heart, it can result in marked enlargement of the pulmonary trunk and arteries, and is usually associated with absence of the arterial duct.[24]

8.5 Tetralogy of Fallot and Pulmonary Atresia with an Intact Ventricular Septum

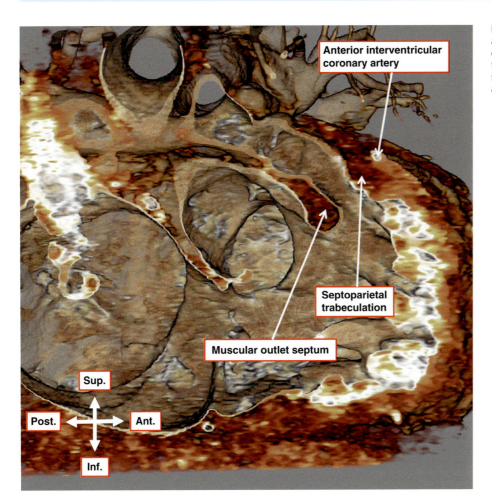

Figure 8.5.16 The computed tomographic angiogram shown in Figure 8.5.15 has been cropped to show the right ventricular outflow tract. Note the relationship between the subpulmonary obstruction and the anomalous anterior interventricular coronary artery.

Compromise of the tracheobronchial tree by these grossly enlarged vessels (Figures 8.5.32–8.5.36) results in most patients presenting with symptoms of respiratory distress. Because only a limited number of cases have come to surgical correction, the efficacy of replacement of the valve with or without arterial plication has not been proved. Perhaps fortunately, so-called absence of the pulmonary valvar leaflets is a rare condition.

References Cited

1. Anderson RH, Tynan M. Tetralogy of Fallot – a centennial review. *Int J Cardiol* 1988; **21**: 219–232.
2. Aiello VD, Spicer DE, Anderson RH, Brown NA, Mohun TJ. The independence of the infundibular building blocks in the setting of double-outlet right ventricle. *Cardiol Young* 2017; **27**: 825–836.
3. Anderson RH, Allwork SP, Ho SY, Lenox CC, Zuberbuhler JR. Surgical anatomy of tetralogy of Fallot. *J Thorac Cardiovasc Surg* 1981; **81**: 887–896.
4. Suzuki A, Ho S Y, Anderson RH, Deanfield JE. Further morphologic studies on tetralogy of Fallot, with particular emphasis on the prevalence and structure of the membranous flap. *J Thorac Cardiovasc Surg* 1990; **99**: 528–535.
5. Titus JL, Daugherty GW, Edwards JE. Anatomy of the atrioventricular conduction system in ventricular septal defect. *Circulation* 1963; **28**: 72–81.
6. Anderson RH, Monro JL, Ho SY, Smith A, Deverall PB. Les voies de conduction auriculo–ventriculaires dans le tetralogie de Fallot. *Coeur* 1977; **8**: 793–807.
7. Neirotti R, Galindez E, Kreutzer G, et al. Tetralogy of Fallot with sub-pulmonary ventricular septal defect. *Ann Thorac Surg* 1978; **25**: 51–56.
8. Griffin ML, Sullivan ID, Anderson RH, Macartney FJ. Doubly committed subarterial ventricular septal defect: new morphological criteria with echocardiographic and angiocardiographic correlation. *Br Heart J* 1988; **59**: 474–479.
9. Blackstone EH, Kirklin JW, Bertranou EG, et al. Preoperative prediction from cineangiograms of post–repair right ventricular pressure in tetralogy of Fallot. *J Thorac Cardiovasc Surg* 1979; **78**: 542–552.
10. Kirklin JW, Blackstone EH, Pacifico AD, Brown RN, Bargeron LM Jr. Routine primary repair versus two-stage repair of tetralogy of Fallot. *Circulation* 1979; **60**: 373–385.
11. McFadden PM, Culpepper WS, Ochsner J. Iatrogenic right ventricular failure in tetralogy of Fallot repairs: reappraisal of a distressing problem. *Ann Thorac Surg* 1982; **33**: 400–402.
12. Alva C, Ho SY, Lincoln CR, et al. The nature of the obstructive muscular bundles in double–chambered right ventricle. *J Thorac Cardiovasc Surg* 1999; **117**: 1180–1189.

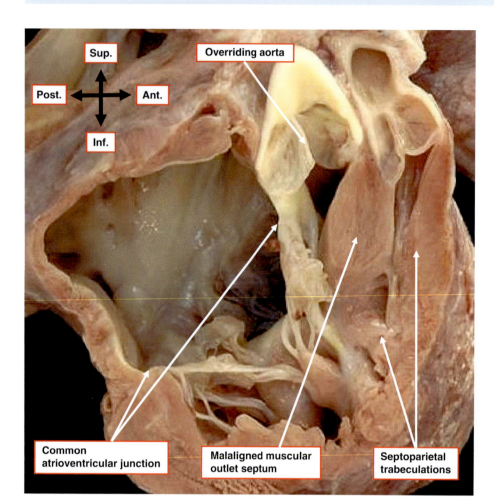

Figure 8.5.17 The image shows the combination of tetralogy of Fallot and an atrioventricular septal defect.

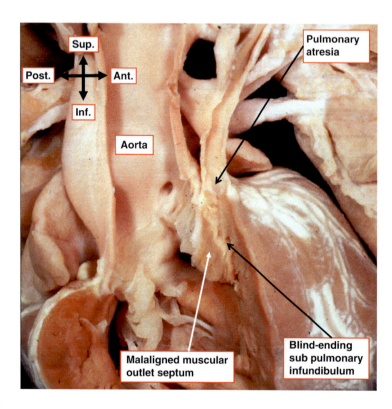

Figure 8.5.18 In this heart from a patient with tetralogy of Fallot with pulmonary atresia, viewed in anatomical orientation, there are confluent pulmonary arteries supplied by an arterial duct. Note the extreme antero-cephalad deviation of the muscular outlet septum, with muscular atresia at the ventriculo-arterial junction.

8.5 Tetralogy of Fallot and Pulmonary Atresia with an Intact Ventricular Septum

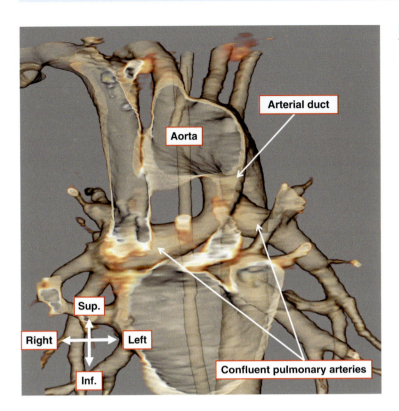

Figure 8.5.19 The computed tomographic angiogram from a patient with tetralogy of Fallot and pulmonary atresia shows confluent pulmonary arteries fed through a persistently patent arterial duct.

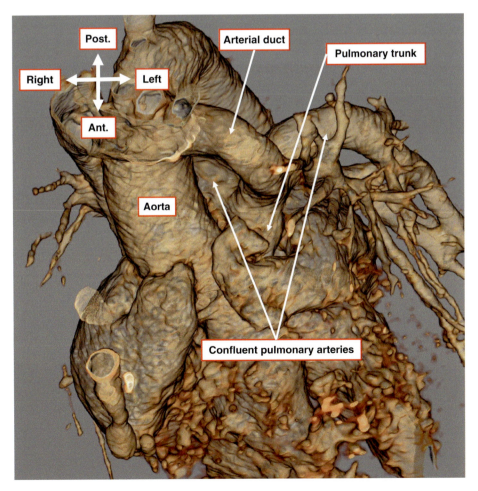

Figure 8.5.20 This computed tomographic angiogram from a patient with tetralogy of Fallot and pulmonary atresia shows confluent pulmonary arteries fed through a patent arterial duct. Unlike Figure 8.5.19, there is a small, atretic pulmonary trunk present.

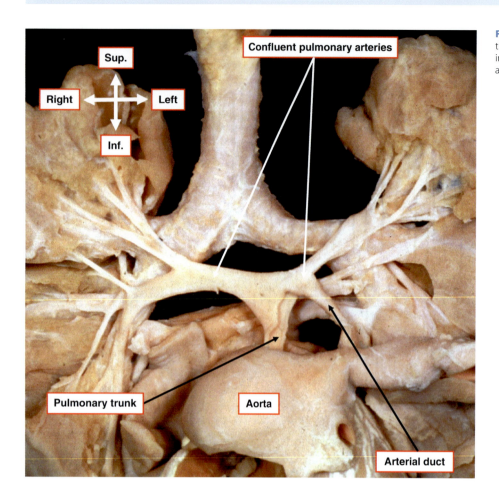

Figure 8.5.21 The dissection shows how, in the setting of a patent arterial duct, the intrapericardial pulmonary arteries usually supply all the pulmonary broncho-pulmonary segments.

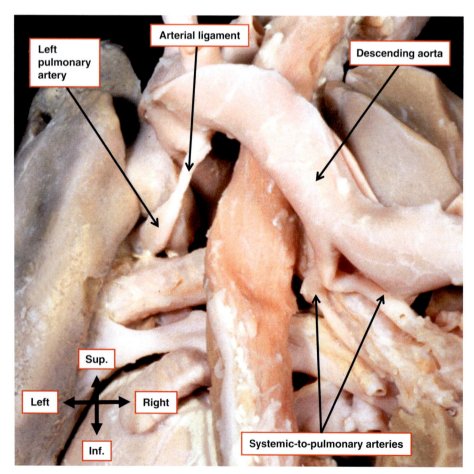

Figure 8.5.22 In this specimen of tetralogy of Fallot with pulmonary atresia, viewed from behind, the pulmonary arteries are discontinuous. The left pulmonary artery was initially supplied by an arterial duct, which has become ligamentous. The right lung is supplied through systemic-to-pulmonary collateral arteries.

8.5 Tetralogy of Fallot and Pulmonary Atresia with an Intact Ventricular Septum

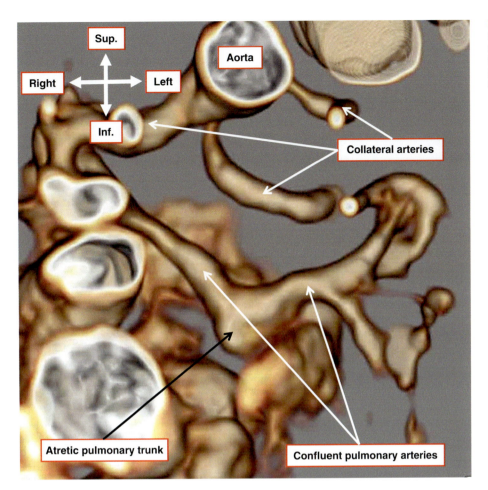

Figure 8.5.23 The computed tomographic angiogram from a patient with tetralogy of Fallot and pulmonary atresia shows presence within the pericardial cavity of both systemic-to-pulmonary collateral arteries and pulmonary arteries.

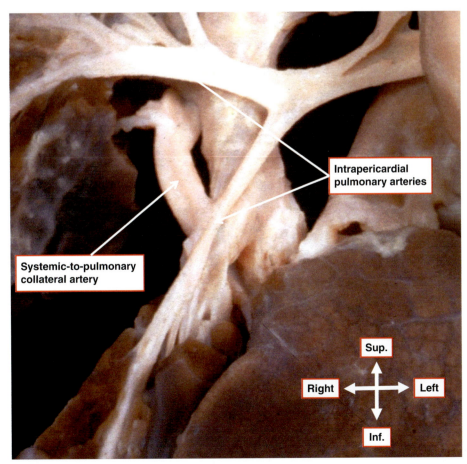

Figure 8.5.24 In this heart from a patient with tetralogy of Fallot and pulmonary atresia, shown in anatomical orientation, the intrapericardial pulmonary arteries in the right lung are supplied through a hilar anastomosis by a large systemic-to-pulmonary collateral artery.

275

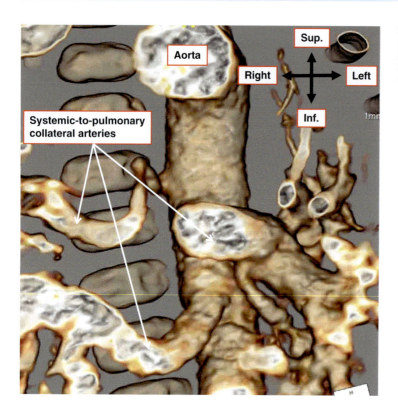

Figure 8.5.25 The computed tomographic angiogram from a patient with tetralogy of Fallot and pulmonary atresia shows the systemic-to-pulmonary collateral arteries arising from the descending aorta that supply the entirety of the pulmonary parenchyma. In this patient, there was absence of the intrapericardial pulmonary arteries.

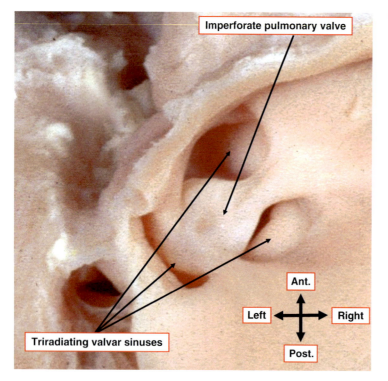

Figure 8.5.26 In this heart from a patient with pulmonary atresia and an intact ventricular septum, viewed from above, dissection of the ventriculo-pulmonary junction shows an imperforate pulmonary valvar membrane.

13. Pandey NN, Bhambri K, Verma M, et al. Anomalies of coronary arteries in tetralogy of Fallot: evaluation on multidetector CT angiography using dual-source scanner. *J Card Surg* 2021; **36**: 2373–2380.

14. Alfieri OA, Blackstone EH, Kirklin JW, et al. Surgical treatment of tetralogy of Fallot with pulmonary atresia. *J Thorac Cardiovasc Surg* 1978; **76**: 321–335.

15. Macartney FJ, Scott O, Deverall PB. Haemodynamic and anatomical characteristics of pulmonary blood supply in pulmonary atresia with ventricular septal defect–including a case of persistent fifth aortic arch. *Br Heart J* 1974; **36**: 1049–1060.

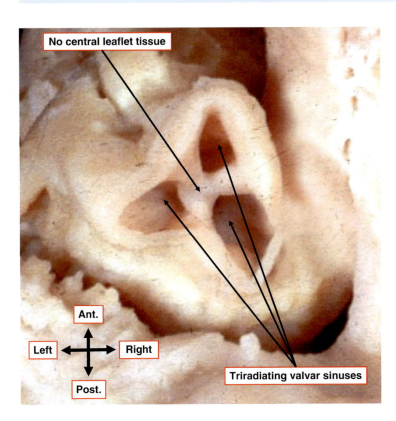

Figure 8.5.27 In this heart from a patient with pulmonary atresia and an intact ventricular septum, there is no evidence of valvar tissue in the blind-ending pulmonary root (compare with Figure 8.5.26).

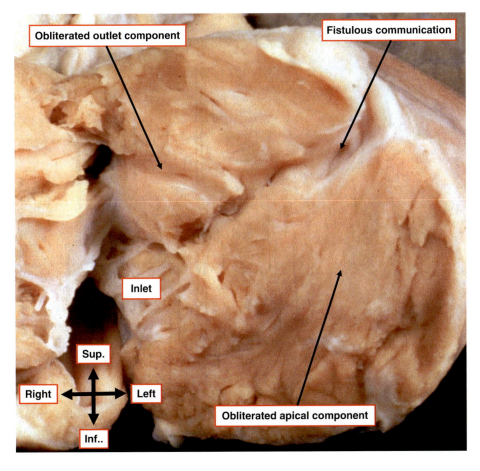

Figure 8.5.28 In this heart from a patient with pulmonary atresia and an intact ventricular septum, viewed anatomically, the cavity of the right ventricle is effectively represented by the inlet component alone, due to gross hypertrophy of the walls of the apical trabecular and outlet components. Note the fistulous communication extending through the wall to the anterior interventricular coronary artery.

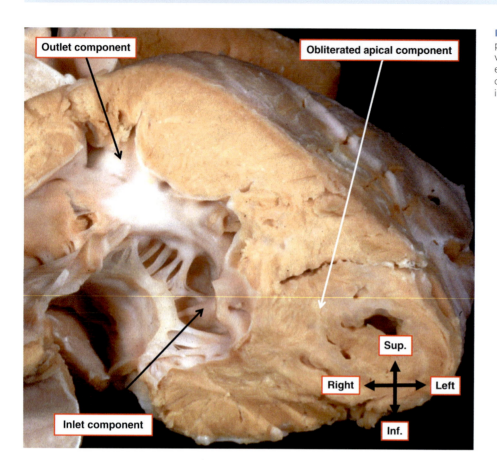

Figure 8.5.29 In this heart, again from a patient with pulmonary atresia and an intact ventricular septum, mural hypertrophy has effectively obliterated the apical trabecular component of the cavity, while leaving narrowed inlet and outlet components.

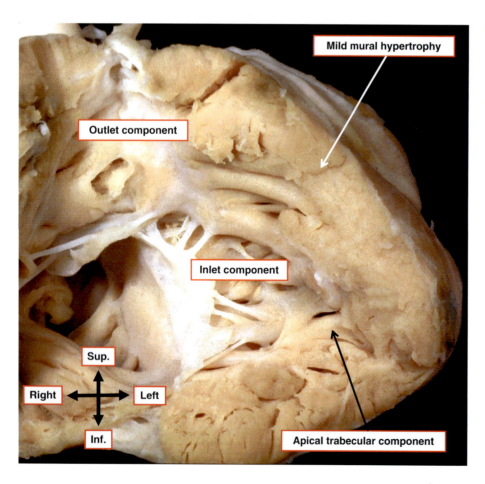

Figure 8.5.30 This heart is once more from a patient having pulmonary atresia with an intact ventricular septum. It shows the most favourable variant, in which the pulmonary valve is imperforate, but the mural hypertrophy has barely obliterated any of the right ventricular cavity.

8.5 Tetralogy of Fallot and Pulmonary Atresia with an Intact Ventricular Septum

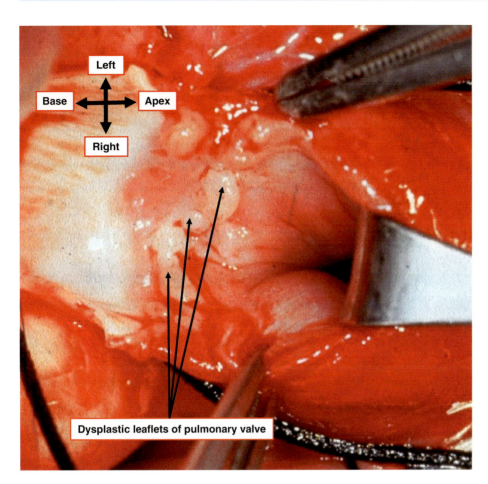

Figure 8.5.31 This operative view shows the right ventriculo-pulmonary arterial junction in a patient with tetralogy of Fallot and so-called absence of the leaflets of the pulmonary valve. In fact, there are grossly abnormal and dysplastic leaflets formed in annular fashion at the ventriculo-arterial junction.

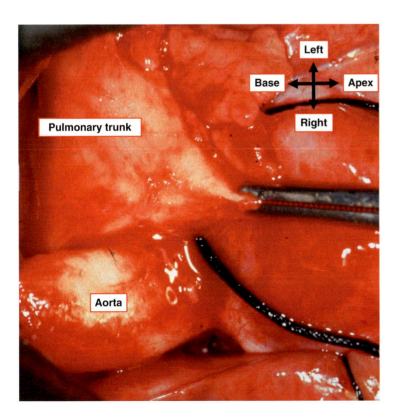

Figure 8.5.32 In the patient shown in Figure 8.5.31, there was gross dilation of the pulmonary trunk and the pulmonary arteries.

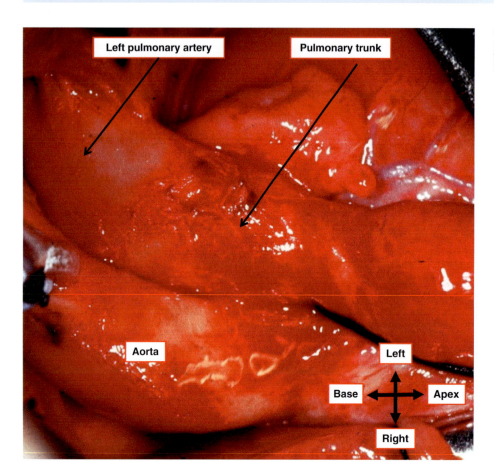

Figure 8.5.33 This operative view of the patient shown in Figures 8.5.31 and 8.5.32 shows the grossly enlarged left pulmonary artery, which is as large as the aorta.

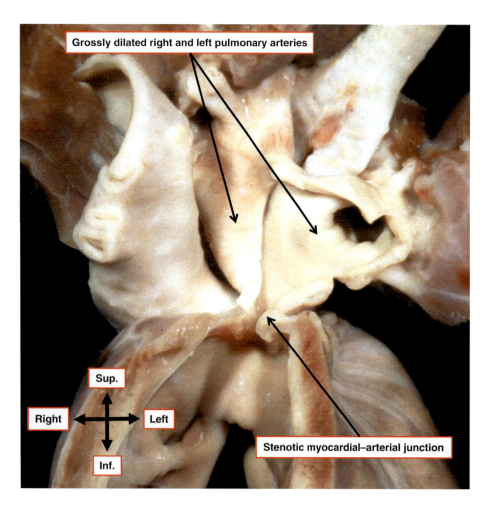

Figure 8.5.34 The image shows a specimen with so-called absent pulmonary valve syndrome in the setting of tetralogy of Fallot. There is gross stenosis at the level of the myocardial–arterial junction of the right ventricle, with gross dilation of the pulmonary trunk and the right and left pulmonary arteries.

8.5 Tetralogy of Fallot and Pulmonary Atresia with an Intact Ventricular Septum

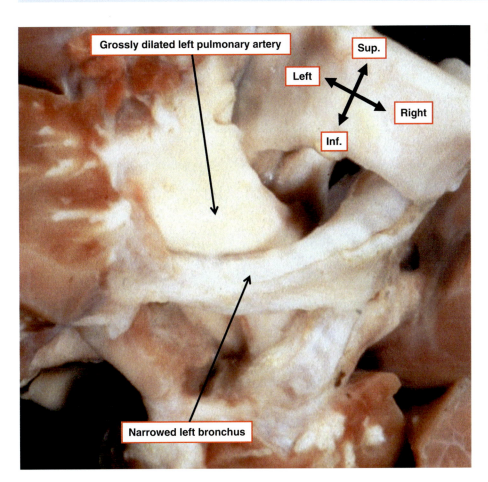

Figure 8.5.35 This posterior view of the hilum of the left lung of the heart from the patient seen in Figure 8.5.34 shows the obstruction produced by the gross dilation of the left pulmonary artery as it crosses the narrowed bronchus.

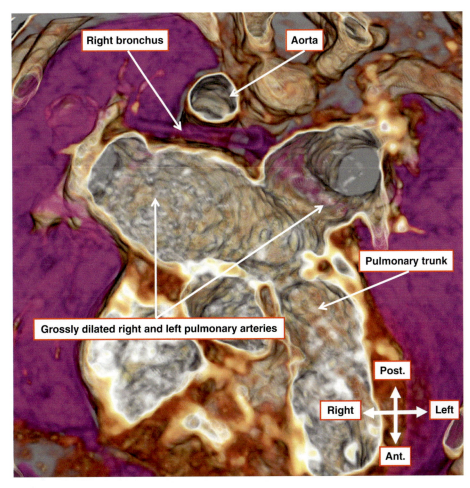

Figure 8.5.36 This computed tomographic angiogram from a patient with tetralogy of Fallot and 'absent pulmonary valve' shows gross dilation of the right and left pulmonary arteries. Note the compression of the right bronchus between the right pulmonary artery and the descending aorta.

16. Pahl E, Fong L, Anderson RH, Park SC, Zuberbuhler JR. Fistulous communications between a solitary coronary artery and the pulmonary arteries as the primary source of pulmonary blood supply in tetralogy of Fallot with pulmonary valve atresia. *Am J Cardiol* 1989; **63**: 140–143.

17. Rossi RN, Hislop A, Anderson RH, Maymone Martins F, Cook AC. Systemic-to-pulmonary blood supply in tetralogy of Fallot with pulmonary atresia. *Cardiol Young* 2002; **12**: 373–388.

18. Freedom RM, Dische MR, Rowe RD. The tricuspid valve in pulmonary atresia with intact ventricular septum. A morphological study of 60 cases. *Arch Pathol Lab Med* 1978; **102**: 28–31.

19. Zuberbuhler JR, Anderson RH. Morphological variations in pulmonary atresia with intact ventricular septum. *Br Heart J* 1979; **41**: 281–288.

20. Anderson RH, Anderson C, Zuberbuhler JR. Further morphologic studies on hearts with pulmonary atresia and intact ventricular septum. *Cardiol Young* 1991; **1**: 105–114.

21. Bull C, de Leval MR, Mercanti C, Macartney FJ, Anderson RH. Pulmonary atresia with intact ventricular septum: a revised classification. *Circulation* 1982; **66**: 266–271.

22. Pawade A, Capuani A, Penny DJ, Karl TR, Mee RB. Pulmonary atresia with intact ventricular septum: surgical management based on right ventricular infundibulum. *J Card Surg* 1993; **8**: 371–383.

23. Macartney FJ, Miller GAH. Congenital absence of the pulmonary valve. *Br Heart J* 1970; **32**: 483–490.

24. Emmanouilides GC, Thanopoulos B, Siassi B, Fishbein M. Agenesis of ductus arteriosus associated with the syndrome of tetralogy of Fallot and absent pulmonary valve. *Am J Cardiol* 1976; **37**: 403–409.

Chapter 8.6

Hypoplastic Left Heart Syndrome

In the chapters relating to the congenital malformations we have discussed thus far, we have described hearts in which the associated cardiac malformation was found in the setting of the usual atrial arrangement and concordant connections between the cardiac segments. All those associated lesions can also be found in hearts with abnormal segmental connections. It is these abnormal connections that will be our focus in the series of chapters to follow. In those chapters, we will emphasize the associated anomalies that are particularly frequent with any given abnormal segmental arrangement. There is, however, a group of lesions that, when put together, constitute another specific phenotype. The hearts provide a transition from the hearts having normal as opposed to those having abnormal segmental connections. They are the lesions well described as making up the hypoplastic left heart syndrome.[1] The term was introduced by Noonan and Nadas. When used by these authors, it accounted for those patients presenting with a similar clinical profile, which reflected the influence of severe hypoplasia of the morphologically left ventricle. The hearts had previously been described by Lev in terms of hypoplasia of the aortic outflow tract.[2] In his initial analysis, Lev had included examples with deficient ventricular septation,[2] as had Noonan and Nadas when describing their syndrome.[1] In a subsequent account, however, Lev suggested that the definition would be strengthened by including only those hearts with an intact ventricular septum, and with potentially concordant atrioventricular and ventriculo-arterial connections.[3] It is the latter definition offered by Lev that we believe best encapsulates the phenotypic features of the syndrome. When analysed in this fashion, the findings permit the inference to be made that the lesions exhibit the features of an acquired disease of fetal life.[4,5] The morphologically left ventricle, of course, can be grossly hypoplastic in the setting of a deficient ventricular septum, or when there is an atrioventricular septal defect. The left ventricle can similarly be incomplete and grossly hypoplastic when there is mitral atresia and a patent aortic root, but again when there is an interventricular communication.[6] In all these settings with deficient ventricular septation, the hypoplastic left ventricle of necessity is markedly different in its morphology when compared with the arrangement found in the hearts making up the hypoplastic left heart syndrome as defined by Lev in his second account.[3,7] As we will show, the left ventricle can still exhibit significant differences within the hearts appropriately defined as belonging to the syndrome. These differences are well explained on the basis of the time, during gestation, that the left ventricle stopped its normal growth. Since the embryonic interventricular communication is normally closed during the seventh or eighth week of gestation, it follows that the stimulus for normal left ventricular growth must have occurred after this point in time.

The morphological features of the hearts making up the syndrome are of importance to the cardiac surgeon, since it is now well recognized that it is patients with these lesions that make up the majority of those coming forward for conversion to the Fontan circulation.[8] From the anatomical stance, despite the fact that it is always possible to recognize all four cardiac chambers in the hearts, the arrangement is almost always functionally univentricular.[9] Hardly ever is the hypoplastic left ventricle capable of supporting the systemic circulation. In a small minority of hearts justifiably included as belonging to the syndrome, nonetheless, it may be possible to achieve biventricular surgical repair. These are the hearts identified as representing the hypoplastic left heart complex.[10] The morphology found in these patients suggests that the factors involved in cessation of normal left ventricular growth occurred relatively late. It is the morphology of the left ventricle, therefore, that best provides the inferences as to when, during gestation, the chamber ceased its normal growth.

At the most severe end of the spectrum are the hearts with combined aortic and mitral atresia. The mitral atresia in this setting can either be due to absence of the left atrioventricular connection (Figure 8.6.1) or to presence of an imperforate left atrioventricular valve (Figure 8.6.2). The presence of rudimentary tension apparatus in the tiny left ventricle, along with the presence of a hypoplastic but imperforate vestibule in the floor of the left atrium (Figure 8.6.3), indicates that the left atrioventricular connection must have been initially been present. Indeed, on the basis of our knowledge of normal cardiac development, it is difficult to believe that the connection was not initially present (see Chapter 2). The presence of a dimple in the floor of the left atrium, and the findings histologically of a fibrous connection between the left atrium and the hypoplastic left ventricle, supports this interpretation.[11] The inference can be made, therefore, that in cases with mitral atresia the left ventricle stopped its normal growth soon after the closure of the embryonic interventricular communication, with subsequent growth of the heart then obliterating the left atrioventricular connection. This inference is supported still further by the finding that the left ventricle has a marginally larger cavity when the mitral valve is imperforate. The left ventricle in the setting of all examples of mitral atresia is slit-like, and found on the diaphragmatic surface of the ventricular mass. It can be

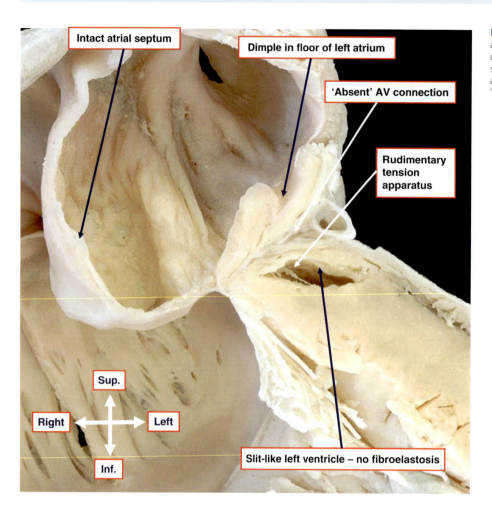

Figure 8.6.1 The close-up image of the left atrioventricular junction from a heart fulfilling the criteria for inclusion as hypoplastic left heart syndrome shows effective absence of the left atrioventricular connection. Note the rightward 'ballooning' of the intact atrial septum.

found in the autopsy room by dissecting between the branches of the so-called delimiting coronary arteries (Figure 8.6.4). Because of the presence of mitral atresia, no blood will have entered the left ventricle for the larger part of fetal life. Although the left ventricle is slit-like and hypoplastic, its walls are smooth, lacking the fibroelastotic changes that are the features of the majority of hearts making up the syndrome. The aortic outflow tract is always atretic in this setting, with the ascending aorta usually being thread-like (Figure 8.6.5). The blood enters the ascending aorta in retrograde fashion, having passed through the arterial duct and entered the isthmus of the transverse arch in retrograde fashion (Figure 8.6.6). In the combination of aortic and mitral atresia, the ascending aorta is essentially a conduit feeding the coronary arteries, often from a bulb that is larger than the ascending aorta itself (Figures 8.6.7, 8.6.8). One of the major 'howlers' of diagnosis is the description of the arrangement in combined aortic and mitral atresia of the anomalous origin the coronary arteries from the brachiocephalic artery, with the pulmonary trunk then incorrectly identified as a common arterial trunk.[12]

The second phenotypic variant to be found making up the syndrome is the combination of aortic atresia with mitral stenosis, rather than atresia. The feature of this subset is that the left ventricle is globular and thick walled, and with a dense layer of endocardial fibroelastosis (Figure 8.6.9). The inference can be made that normal growth of the ventricle occurred later in gestation, so that the mitral valve did not become atretic. It is the flow of blood into the left ventricle, but with no exit because of the aortic atresia (Figure 8.6.10), that provides the stimulus for the development of thickening of the ventricular walls and gross fibroelastosis. Since the left ventricle grew for a longer period, the ascending aorta is typically larger in this setting, albeit still feeding the coronary arteries in retrograde fashion. Continuing towards the milder end of the spectrum of ventricular size, the next variant is the combination of mitral and aortic stenosis (Figure 8.6.11). In this subset, the ascending aorta tends to be still larger (Figure 8.6.12). The aortic valve, although patent, is typically unicuspid and unicommissural. It is built on a trisinuate scaffold, but with only the commissure between the left coronary and non-coronary leaflets extending to the sinutubular junction. The zones of apposition between the left and right coronary leaflets, and between the right coronary leaflet and the non-coronary leaflet, are represented by raphes, with hypoplastic interleaflet triangles on their ventricular aspect (Figure 8.6.13). The left ventricle is often larger, but is unable to function so as to support the systemic circulation because of the gross fibroelastosis. Another of the potentially deleterious features found in the setting of mitral stenosis, with either aortic atresia or aortic stenosis, is the presence of fistulous communications between the cavity of

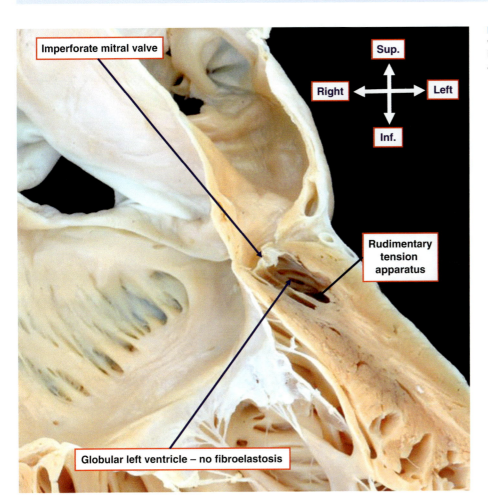

Figure 8.6.2 In this heart, again from a patient with hypoplastic left heart syndrome, there is an imperforate mitral valve blocking the left atrioventricular junction to produce mitral atresia.

the left ventricle and the coronary arteries. When searched for in autopsy specimens using histological sections, such communications are frequent, but usually are very small, and blocked at their left ventricular end by the layer of endocardial fibroelastosis.[13] It is the rare large communications (Figure 8.6.14) that will create problems, since then the coronary arteries themselves become ectatic (Figure 8.6.15), compromising the flow to the entirety of the ventricular cone.

In a small minority of hearts diagnosed at autopsy as belonging within the syndrome, the left ventricle can extend almost to the apex of the ventricular cone, with the size of the aortic and mitral valves, both patent, being commensurate with the size of the left ventricle.[4,7] The aortic arch in these cases often shows significant tubular hypoplasia along with coarctation. Significantly, in hearts of this type, the left ventricle also lacks a fibroelastotic lining, or else any fibroelastosis present is limited (Figure 8.6.16). These are the hearts that are potentially suitable for biventricular repair, and are described as representing the hypoplastic left heart complex.[10]

Although it is the morphology of the left ventricle that provided the pathognomonic features of the hearts to be included within the syndrome, and also permits sub-categorization, it is the features of the remainder of the heart that are of greater significance to the cardiac surgeon. The right ventricle inevitably is the dominant ventricle, and is called upon to drive both circulations subsequent to conversion to the Fontan circulation as the ultimate operation in the Norwood sequence of procedures.[14] It is frequent to find variations in the structure of the ventricle, such as a free-standing septomarginal trabeculation (Figure 8.6.17).[15] This can produce problems during diagnosis, since the free-standing myocardial strap can be misdiagnosed as the muscular ventricular septum. Of more functional significance is the finding of lesions such as dysplastic valvar leaflets, since the tricuspid valve is called upon to withstand the full force of the systemic circulation subsequent to the creation of the Norwood sequence.[16]

Also of significance is the arrangement of the atrial septum. The function of the oval foramen is to permit the passage of blood from right-to-left during fetal lie. In the setting of mitral atresia, or severe mitral stenosis, a functioning oval foramen is deleterious, since it is harder for pulmonary venous blood to reach the right side of the heart. A patent oval foramen is found in the majority of cases of hypoplastic left heart syndrome, although often with deviation leftward of the flap valve, derived from the primary atrial septum.[17] Of far greater concern is finding an intact atrial septum (Figure 8.6.18).[18] This is now well-recognized as a poor prognostic feature for those diagnosed with the syndrome. It has bad consequences, including 'arterialization' and thickening of the pulmonary veins (Figure 8.6.19), with

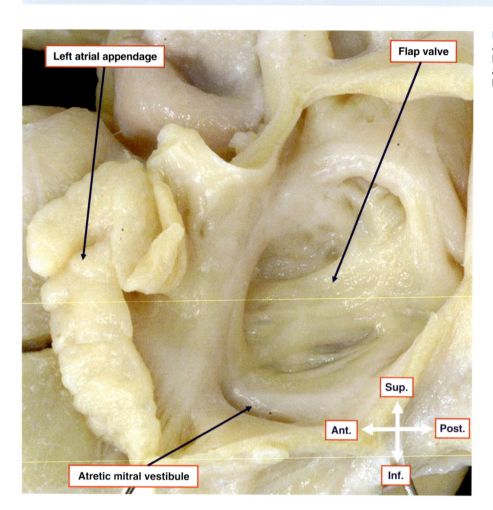

Figure 8.6.3 Examination of the floor of the left atrium in hearts from patients with hypoplastic left heart syndrome characterized by combined aortic and mitral atresia shows the presence of a hypoplastic vestibule.

'cobble-stoning' of the surfaces of the lungs in consequence of gross lymphangiectasia (Figure 8.5.20). On occasion, nonetheless, the consequences of atrial septal integrity can be ameliorated by still further lesions that unload the left atrium, such as fenestrations of the walls between the atrium and the coronary sinus (Figures 8.6.21, 8.6.22), or presence of a so-called levoatrial cardinal vein.

Also of concern is the presence of aortic coarctation. It is now well established that the coarctation lesion is itself the consequence of encirclement of the aortic isthmus or transverse arch by ductal tissue.[19] The presence and severity of such lesions (Figure 8.6.23) also relates to the morphology of the left ventricle, and thereby the timing of aortic atresia or stenosis with subsequent reversal of flow in the aortic arch via the arterial duct. Coarctation shelves were found in half of one series of autopsied examples of the syndrome, usually in preductal position (Figure 8.6.24).[20]

References Cited

1. Noonan JA, Nadas AS. The hypoplastic left heart syndrome: an analysis of 101 cases. *Ped Clin North Am* 1958; **5**: 1029–1056.
2. Lev M. Pathologic anatomy and interrelationship of the hypoplasia of the aortic tract complex. *Lab Invest* 1952; **1**: 61–70.
3. Lev ML. Some newer concepts of the pathology of congenital heart disease. *Med Clin North Am* 1966; **50**: 3–14.
4. Stephens EH, Gupta D, Bleiweis M, et al. Pathologic characteristics of 119 archived specimens showing the phenotypic features of hypoplastic left heart syndrome. *Semin Thorac Cardiovasc Surg* 2020; **32**: 895–903.
5. Anderson RH, Spicer DE, Crucean A. Clarification of the definition of hypoplastic left heart syndrome. *Nature Reviews Cardiol* 2021; **18**: 147–148.
6. Mickell JJ, Mathews RA, Anderson RH, et al. The anatomical heterogeneity of hearts lacking a patent communication between the left atrium and the ventricular mass ('mitral atresia') in presence of a patent aortic valve. *Eur Heart J* 1983; **4**: 477–486.
7. Crucean A, Alqahtani A, Barron DJ, et al. Re-evaluation of hypoplastic left heart syndrome from a developmental and morphological perspective. *Orphanet J* 2017; **12**: 1.
8. Fontan F, Baudet E. Surgical repair of tricuspid atresia. *Thorax* 1971; **26**: 240–248.
9. Jacobs ML, Anderson RH. Nomenclature of the functionally univentricular heart. *Cardiol Young* 2006; **16** (Suppl.1): 3–8.

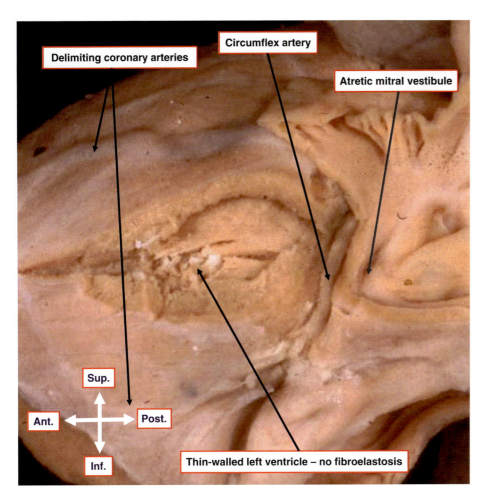

Figure 8.6.4 The slit-like left ventricle found in the variant of hypoplastic left heart syndrome with combined aortic and mitral atresia is found on the diaphragmatic surface of the ventricular mass, and is revealed by dissecting between the delimiting coronary arteries.

10. Tchervenkov CI, Tahta SA, Jutras LC, Béland MJ. Biventricular repair in neonates with hypoplastic left heart complex. *Ann Thor Surg* 1998; **66**: 1350–1356.

11. Gittenberger-de Groot AC. Wenink A. Mitral atresia. Morphological details. *Br Heart J* 1984; **51**: 252–258.

12. Li W, Li J, Chen X. A rare case of congenital heart disease: anomalous origin of coronary artery from innominate artery with coronary fistula and truncus arteriosus. *Cardiol Young* 2021; **31**; 1345–1347.

13. O'Connor WN, Cash JB, Cottrill CM, Johnson GL, Noonan JA. Ventriculocoronary connections in hypoplastic left hearts: an autopsy microscopic study. *Circulation* 1982; **66**: 1078–1086.

14. Norwood WI, Lang P, Hansen DD. Physiologic repair of aortic atresia-hypoplastic left heart syndrome. *NEJM* 1983; **308**: 23–26.

15. Stamm C, Anderson RH, Ho SY. The morphologically tricuspid valve in hypoplastic left heart syndrome. *Eur J Cardio-thorac Surg* 1997; **12**: 587–592.

16. Barber G, Helton JG, Aglira BA, et al. The significance of tricuspid regurgitation in hypoplastic left-heart syndrome. *Am Heart J* 1988; **116**: 1563–1567.

17. Weinberg PM, Chin AJ, Murphy JD, Pigott JD, Norwood WI. Postmortem echocardiography and tomographic anatomy of hypoplastic left heart syndrome after palliative surgery. *Am J Cardiol* 1986; **58**: 1228–1232.

18. Rychik J, Rome JJ, Collins MH, DeCampli WM, Spray TL. The hypoplastic left heart syndrome with intact atrial septum: atrial morphology, pulmonary vascular histopathology and outcome. *J Am Coll Cardiol* 1999; **34**: 554–560.

19. Ho SY, Anderson RH. Coarctation, tubular hypoplasia, and the ductus arteriosus. Histological study of 35 specimens. *Br Heart J* 1979; **41**: 268–274.

20. Aiello VD, Ho SY, Anderson RH, Thiene G. Morphologic features of the hypoplastic left heart syndrome – a reappraisal. *Ped Pathol* 1990; **10**: 931–943.

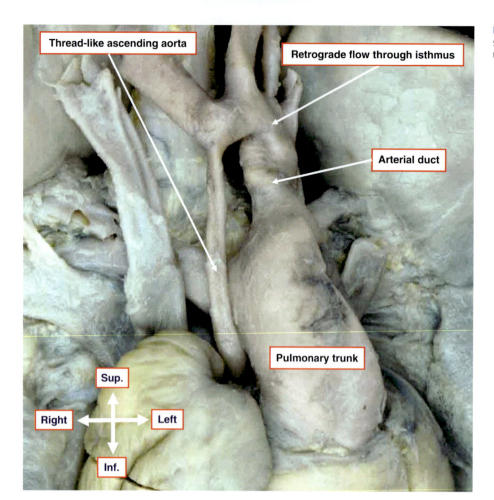

Figure 8.6.5 The ascending aorta, as in this specimen from a heart with combined aortic and mitral atresia, is typically thread-like.

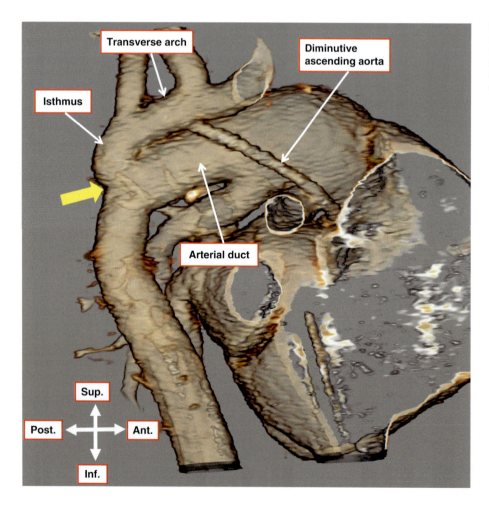

Figure 8.6.6 As shown in this computed tomographic angiogram viewed from the right, the thread-like ascending aorta is fed in retrograde fashion through the arterial duct and the isthmus. Note the coarctation at the junction of the isthmus with the duct (yellow arrow).

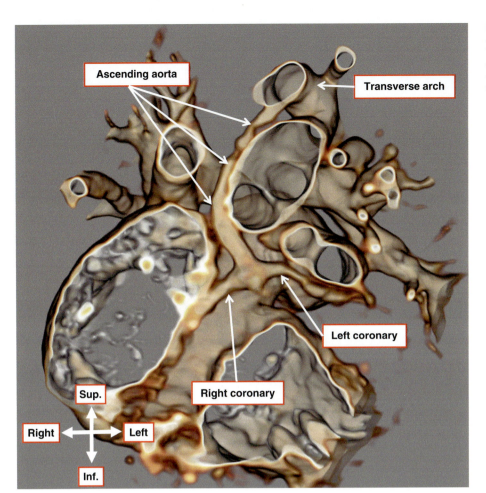

Figure 8.6.7 This computed tomographic angiogram, viewed from the front, reveals the thread-like ascending aorta in a heart with mitral and aortic atresia. Note that portions of the ascending aorta are smaller than the proximal coronary arteries.

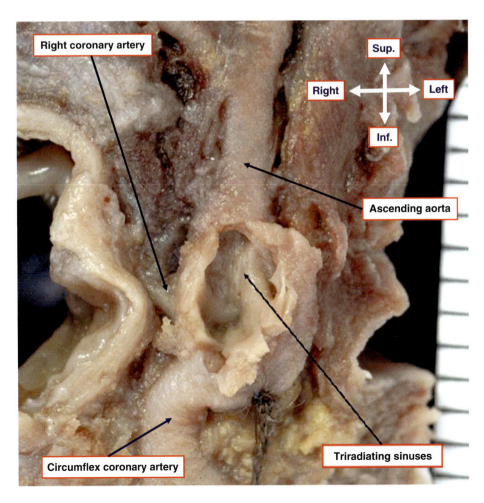

Figure 8.6.8 In the setting of hypoplastic left heart syndrome with aortic atresia, the ascending aorta feeds the coronary arteries in retrograde fashion.

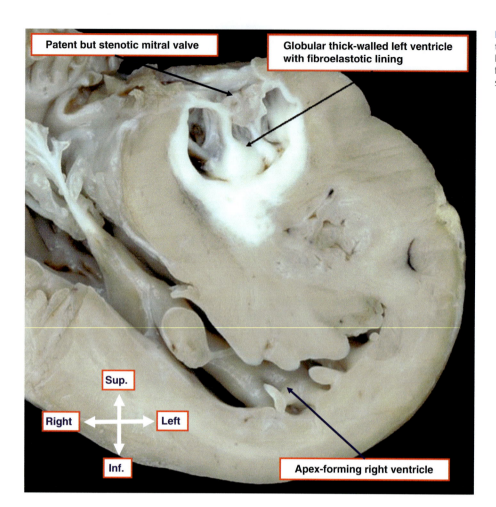

Figure 8.6.9 The four-chamber section through an explanted heart from a patient with hypoplastic left heart syndrome shows the features of combined aortic atresia with mitral stenosis.

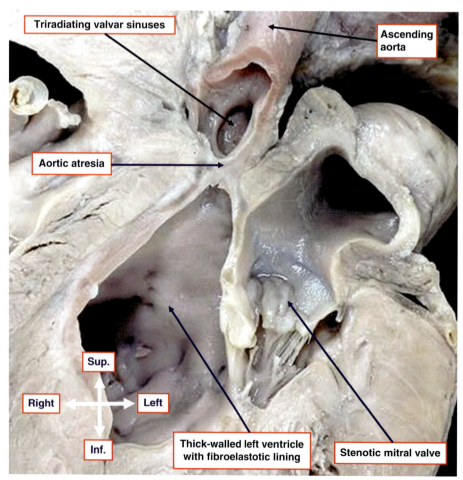

Figure 8.6.10 When aortic atresia co-exists with mitral stenosis in the setting of hypoplastic left heart syndrome, the left ventricle is lined by a dense layer of endocardial fibroelastosis.

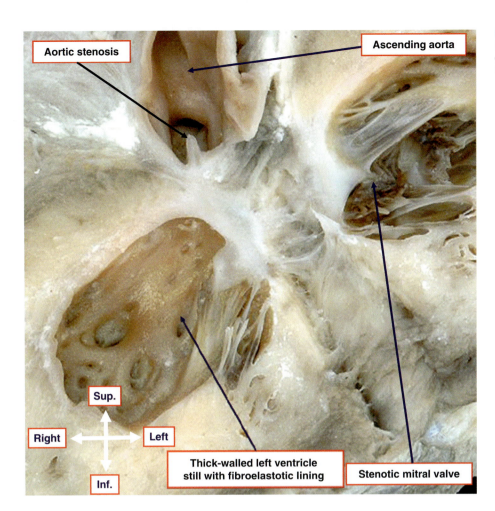

Figure 8.6.11 The third subset of hypoplastic left heart syndrome, as seen in this heart, is characterized by the combination of aortic and mitral stenosis.

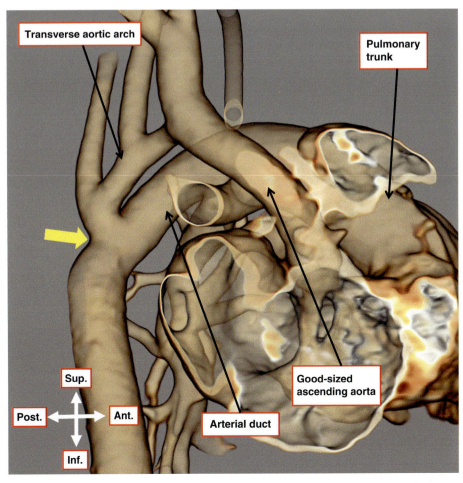

Figure 8.6.12 As shown by the computed tomographic angiogram viewed from the right, the ascending aorta is larger when there is a combination of mitral and aortic stenosis in the setting of hypoplastic left heart syndrome. Note the hypoplastic transverse arch and coarctation at the junction of the isthmus with the duct (yellow arrow).

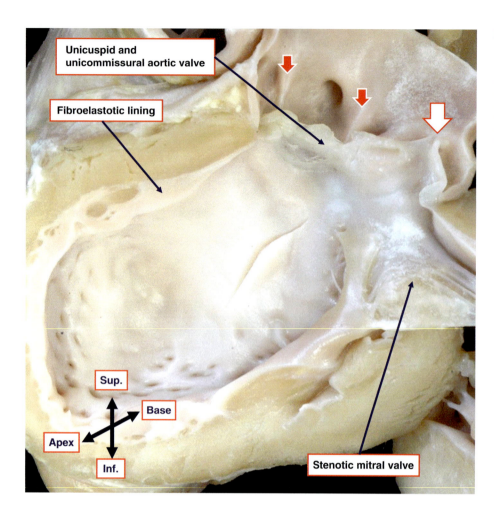

Figure 8.6.13 The stenotic aortic valve in the setting of hypoplastic left heart syndrome is usually a functionally unileaflet entity, but built on a trisinuate aortic root. The left ventricle is of good size, but still lined by a dense layer of endocardial fibroelastosis. The white arrow with red borders shows the solitary commissure extending to the sinutubular junction, while the red arrows with white borders show the raphes representing the putative zones of apposition.

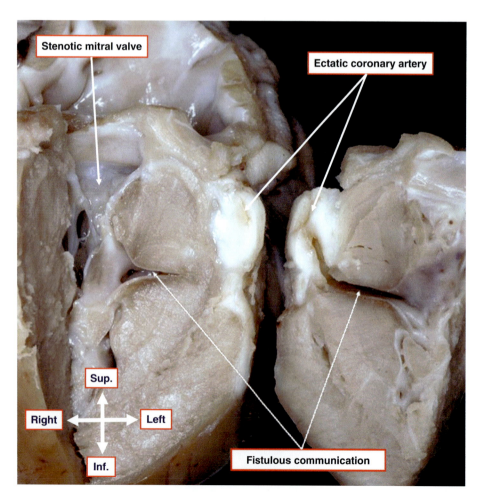

Figure 8.6.14 The explanted heart has been sectioned to show a large fistulous communication extending from the left ventricle into an ectatic coronary artery. In this case, the extent of endocardial fibroelastosis is not severe and the communication is still patent.

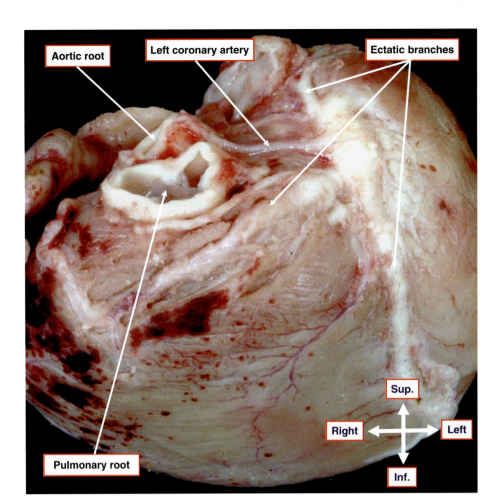

Figure 8.6.15 The image shows the epicardial surface of the explanted heart shown in sectioned form in Figure 8.6.14. Note the extent of the ectatic coronary arteries.

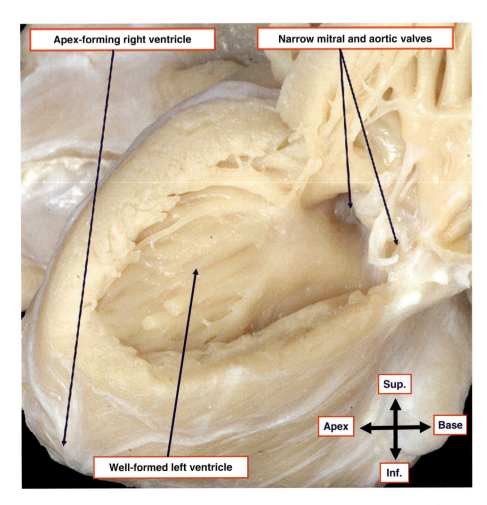

Figure 8.6.16 This heart was diagnosed by the pathologist as exhibiting hypoplastic left heart syndrome. The aortic and mitral valves are both patent, but narrow and smaller than normal. There is no fibroelastosis in the left ventricle. This is an example of the so-called hypoplastic left heart complex.

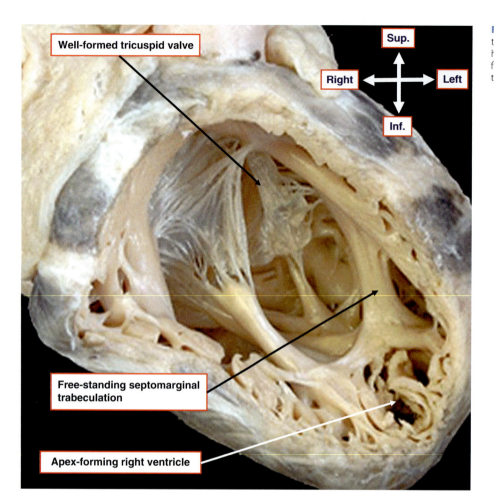

Figure 8.6.17 The image shows an example of the right ventricle from the heart of a patient with hypoplastic left heart syndrome. There is a free-standing septomarginal trabeculation, but the tricuspid valve itself is well-formed.

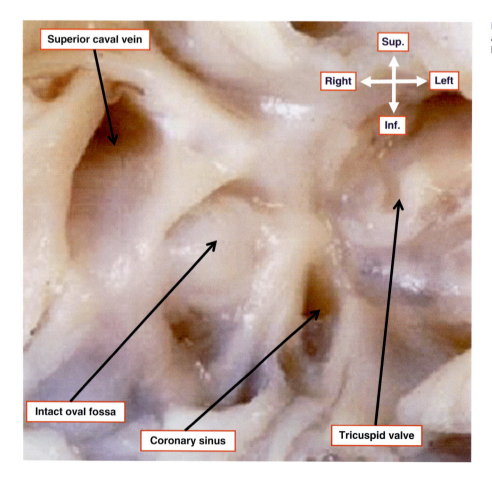

Figure 8.6.18 The right atrium in a heart from a patient with hypoplastic left heart syndrome has been opened to show an intact atrial septum.

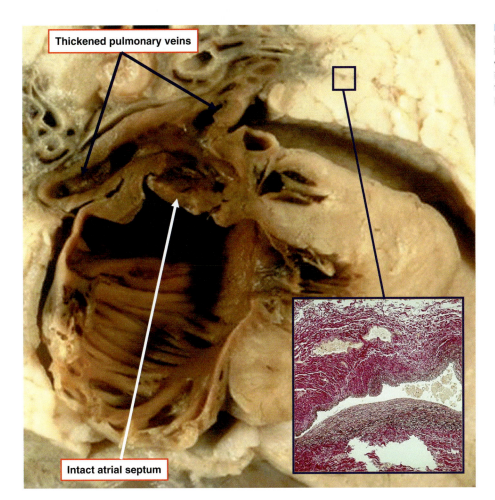

Figure 8.6.19 This heart is from a patient with hypoplastic left heart syndrome, but with an intact atrial septum. There is thickening of the walls of the left atrium with overgrowth of an imperforate mitral valve. The inset shows how this spreads to 'arterialize' the walls of the pulmonary veins.

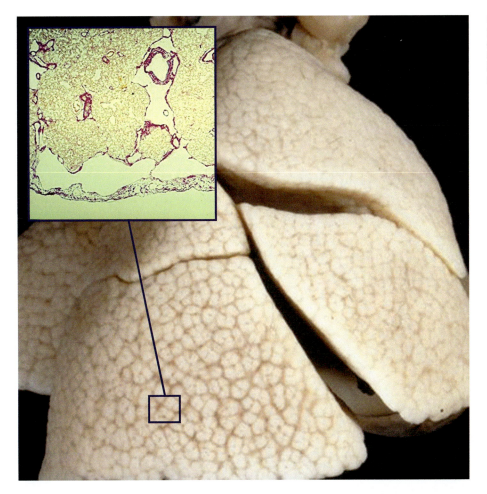

Figure 8.6.20 The right lung is shown from the patient with hypoplastic left heart and intact atrial septum seen in Figure 8.6.19. The surfaces of the lung show the 'cobble-stone' appearance, in consequence of gross lymphangiectasia, as shown in the histological section (inset).

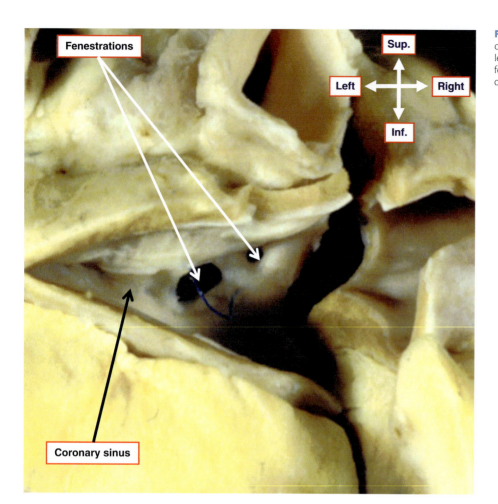

Figure 8.6.21 The coronary sinus has been opened in the heart of a patient with hypoplastic left heart syndrome and intact atrial septum. The fenestrations provide an overflow for the obstructed left atrium.

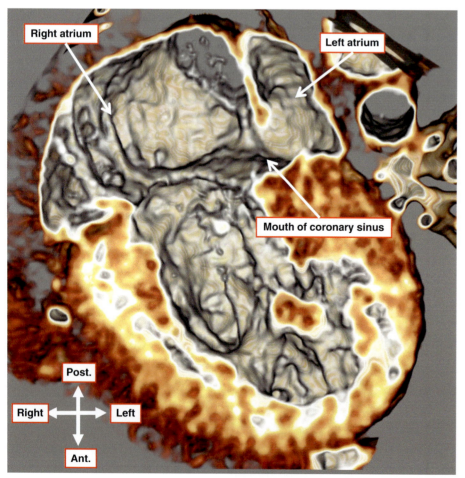

Figure 8.6.22 In this computed tomogram performed on a patient with hypoplastic left heart syndrome and intact atrial septum, the wall separating the coronary sinus and left atrium is absent. The mouth of the coronary sinus functions as the only interatrial communication.

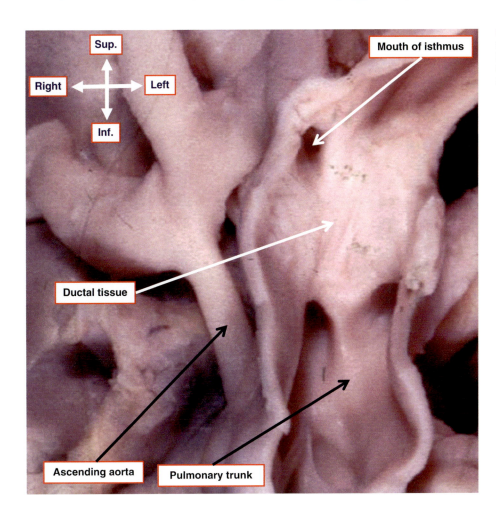

Figure 8.6.23 The pulmonary trunk has been opened in the heart from a patient with hypoplastic left heart syndrome. The walls of the arterial duct extend into the descending aorta, surrounding the mouth of the aortic isthmus.

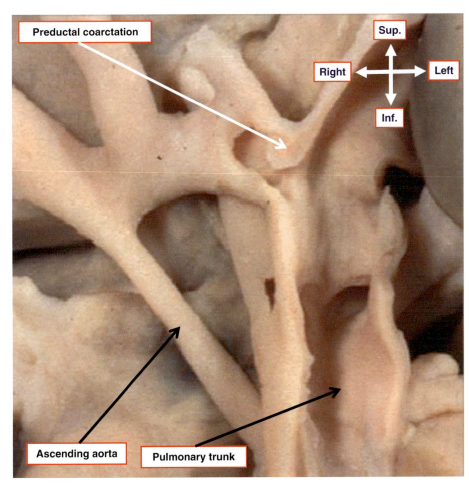

Figure 8.6.24 The junction between the aortic isthmus, the arterial duct, and the descending aorta has been sectioned in the heart from a patient with hypoplastic left heart syndrome, showing how the ductal tissue as shown in Figure 8.6.23 produces preductal coarctation.

Chapter 9
Lesions in Hearts with Abnormal Segmental Connections

9.1 Functionally Univentricular Heart

Over the years, so-called univentricular hearts represented one of the greatest challenges for surgical correction. All this changed with the advent of the Fontan procedure,[1] along with the realization that it could become the final stage of the sequence of procedures used to correct lesions such as those included in the hypoplastic left heart syndrome,[2] which previously had been beyond surgical repair. The overall group of lesions also posed significant problems in adequate description and categorization. Even these days, many continue to describe patients with a double inlet left ventricle as having a single ventricle, despite the fact that, with the availability of clinical diagnostic techniques producing three-dimensional datasets, patients with this lesion can be seen to have two chambers within their ventricular mass, one being large and the other small (Figure 9.1.1). The semantic problems with description can now be resolved by the simple expedient of describing the patients as having functionally univentricular hearts.[3] This approach also accounts for other lesions dominated by ventricular imbalance, many of these having biventricular atrioventricular connections, such as those making up the hypoplastic left heart syndrome (see Chapter 8.6). In this chapter, we concentrate on the relevant anatomical characteristics of the hearts unified by the presence of a univentricular atrioventricular connection.[4,5] Almost all of these hearts also have one big and one small ventricle. The hearts are unified because their atrial chambers are connected to only one of the ventricles, meaning that a second ventricle, if present is incomplete.

Previous problems with description had centred on whether the small chamber in hearts with ventricular imbalance should be described as a ventricle.[6] As we indicated in Chapter 7, we describe all chambers possessing characteristic apical components as ventricles. We then recognize them as

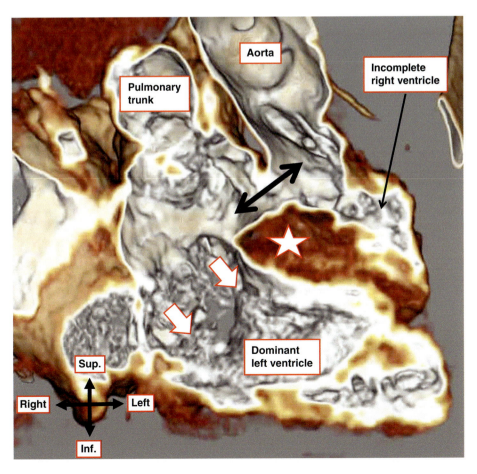

Figure 9.1.1 The reconstructed computed tomographic angiogram shows in exemplary fashion the essential anatomy of the heart that, in the past, was considered to represent a 'single ventricle'. Both atrioventricular junctions open to the dominant left ventricle (white arrows with red borders), which gives rise to the pulmonary trunk. The aorta arises from the incomplete right ventricle, which is separated from the dominant ventricle by the apical ventricular septum. The hole between the ventricles is a ventricular septal defect (double-headed black arrow). The star indicates the apical muscular ventricular septum.

being complete or incomplete, depending on their component make-up. This form of analysis greatly simplifies the description of the communications between the dominant and incomplete ventricles, which are no more and no less than ventricular septal defects (Figure 9.1.1). The lesions to be discussed in this chapter are those with double inlet ventricle, and those with absence of either the right-sided or left-sided atrioventricular connection. We also mention briefly the anatomy of other variants of atrioventricular valvar atresia.

Hearts exhibit double inlet atrioventricular connection whenever the greater parts of both atrioventricular junctions, which belong to the right-sided and left-sided atrial chambers, are connected to the same ventricle. This definition holds good irrespective of whether the connections are guarded by two separate atrioventricular valves, as is usually the case (Figure 9.1.2), or by a common valve (Figure 9.1.3). The double inlet connection can also be found in the presence of overriding and straddling atrioventricular valves, but only when the degree of overriding is such as to leave the greater part of both junctions connected to the same ventricle, again either through two valves (Figure 9.1.4) or a common valve. When there is a straddling common valve, it becomes moot as to whether the hearts should also be considered as possessing atrioventricular septal defects with gross ventricular imbalance (see Chapter 8.3). In all these instances, it is the precise atrioventricular connections that determine the surgical approach.

Whenever patients are found with double inlet connection as here defined, their hearts inevitably will be functionally univentricular. The chosen surgical therapeutic option will almost certainly be to create the Fontan circulation, although rarely it can be possible to septate the dominant ventricle.[7] It will be exceedingly rare for patients to be encountered with a truly solitary ventricle (Figure 9.1.5). Most usually, there will be two ventricles in the setting of double inlet, one being dominant and the other incomplete, the smaller ventricle lacking at least the greater part of its inlet component (Figure 9.1.6). Although the surgical options are the same for all patients with a double inlet atrioventricular connection,[7] the hearts themselves can show marked anatomical variation. They can exist with any arrangement of the atrial chambers, with one of three ventricular morphologies, with the variations in valvar morphology discussed above, with any ventriculo-arterial connection, and with varied associated malformations. From the anatomical stance, and probably from the stance of long-term follow-up, the most important differentiating feature is the morphology of the dominant ventricle. There are three possibilities. The first, and most common, is the arrangement in which the atrial chambers are connected to a dominant left ventricle in the presence of an incomplete right ventricle (Figures 9.1.1, 9.1.2). The second group comprises those with

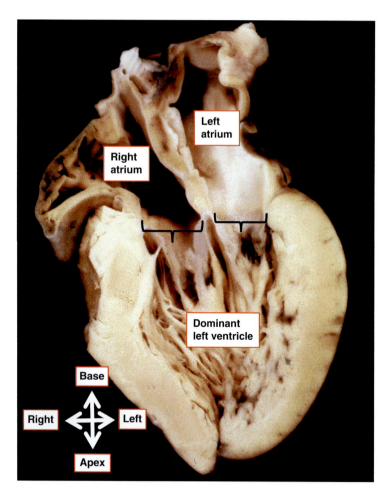

Figure 9.1.2 This specimen, prepared by slicing the heart in 'four-chamber' projection, shows the essence of the double inlet atrioventricular connection. Note that the cavity of only one ventricle is visible. It possesses fine criss-crossing apical trabeculations, identifying it as a dominant left ventricle. Both atrioventricular junctions (brackets) are connected to the dominant ventricle through separate atrioventricular valves.

9.1 Functionally Univentricular Heart

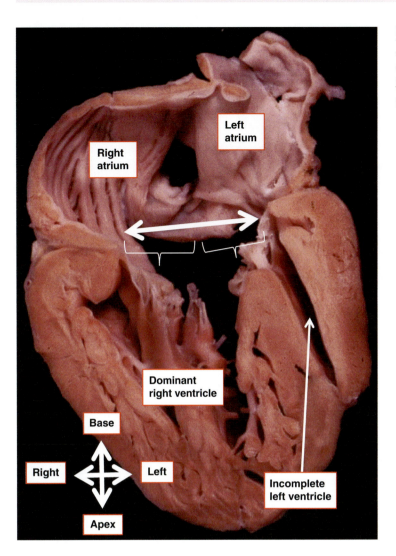

Figure 9.1.3 This specimen is also prepared by making a section in 'four-chamber' plane. It shows double inlet to a dominant right ventricle, since both atrioventricular junctions (brackets) drain to the dominant ventricular chamber. In this heart, however, the junctions are guarded by a common atrioventricular valve (double-headed arrow). The section also demonstrates the incomplete left ventricle, which lacks its inlet component.

a dominant right and an incomplete left ventricle (Figures 9.1.3, 9.1.6). The final small set is made up of those patients having a solitary ventricle of indeterminate morphology (Figure 9.1.5). These three variants must then be distinguished from other hearts that, in essence, represent huge ventricular septal defects (Figure 9.1.7).

A potential means of correcting surgically these hearts with double inlet is to septate the dominant or solitary ventricle.[7] The overall morphological arrangement, however, usually conspires to defeat this option. The most frequent surgical tactic, therefore, is to produce the Fontan circulation. We will concentrate, therefore, on those anatomical features influencing the Fontan procedure, and its several variations, although we will discuss the morphologies that lend themselves to, or compromise, septation. In most examples of double inlet ventricle, both atrioventricular junctions are connected to a dominant left ventricle, in the presence of an incomplete morphologically right ventricle (Figure 9.1.1).[8] The small ventricle lacks its inlet component, either completely when the atrial chambers are exclusively connected to the dominant left ventricle (Figures 9.1.8, 9.1.9), or for the greater part when there is overriding of one (Figure 9.1.4), or rarely both atrioventricular

junctions. The incomplete ventricle can be positioned to the right (Figure 9.1.8) or the left (Figure 9.1.9) or, rarely, directly in front of the dominant ventricle. The small ventricle is always located antero-superiorly, close to the arterial segment, with the atrioventricular connections opening posteriorly relative to the septum (Figures 9.1.1, 9.1.10). This makes sense in terms of cardiac development, as we know that the morphologically right ventricle is added to the arterial end of the left ventricle from the secondary heart field. In most instances, the small incomplete ventricle gives rise to the aorta. It then has a very short infundibular component. The morphology is markedly different when the ventriculo-arterial connections are concordant, and it supports the pulmonary trunk (Figures 9.1.4, 9.1.11). In all instances, nonetheless, the incomplete chambers possess an apical component of morphologically right ventricular pattern. They are separated from the dominant ventricle by the apical muscular ventricular septum (Figure 9.1.10), which carries the atrioventricular conduction axis, and which is nourished by septal perforating arteries.[9]

The crucial feature in terms of surgical corrections is the dimensions of the ventricular septal defect, since this must be of adequate size to support the systemic circulation irrespective of

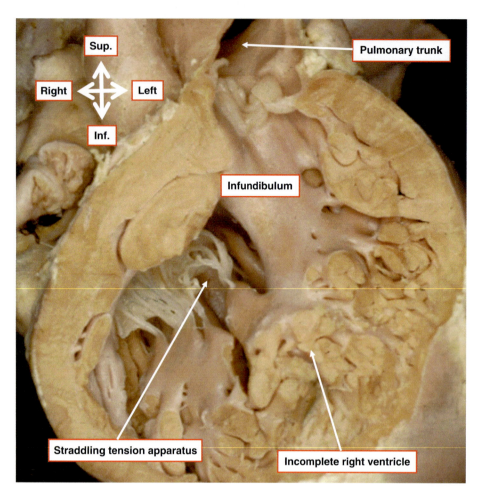

Figure 9.1.4 In this specimen with double inlet left ventricle, the incomplete right ventricle is photographed from the front with the heart positioned anatomically. The ventriculo-arterial connections are concordant, with the pulmonary trunk seen supported by an infundibulum and arising from the incomplete right ventricle. The right atrioventricular valve straddles and overrides, but its greater part remains connected within the dominant left ventricle, so the connection remains one of double inlet.

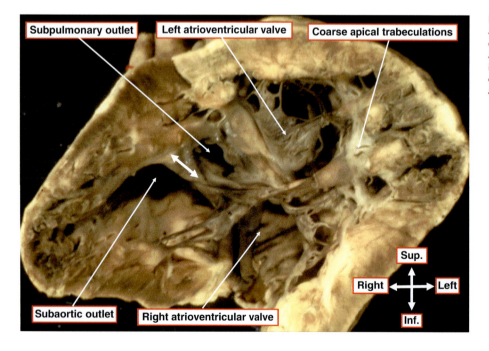

Figure 9.1.5 This specimen, seen in anatomical orientation, with the ventricle opened in clam-like fashion, has double inlet to and double outlet from a solitary ventricle of indeterminate morphology, which has very coarse apical trabeculations. This is the true anatomically univentricular heart.

the precise surgical tactics to be adopted. If it is restrictive (Figure 9.1.12), then it may need to be surgically enlarged, although more frequently the option is to bypass the restrictive area by opting for the Norwood approach, or performing a Damus–Kaye–Stansel procedure. Should the surgeon opt to enlarge the ventricular septal defect, the major anatomical feature of concern is the course of the axis of atrioventricular conduction tissue.[10] The axis always originates from an

9.1 Functionally Univentricular Heart

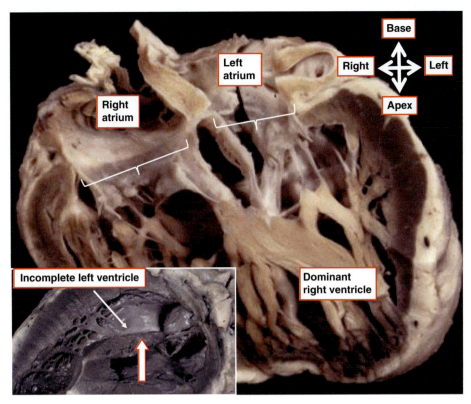

Figure 9.1.6 This specimen, windowed and viewed in anatomical orientation, also has double inlet to a dominant right ventricle, but through two separate atrioventricular valves. The inset, photographed from behind, shows that one papillary muscle of the left atrioventricular valve (arrowed) retains its position within the incomplete left ventricle.

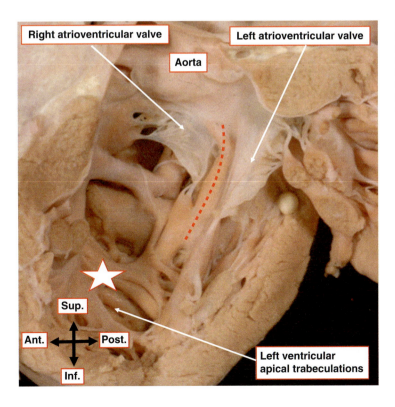

Figure 9.1.7 This view, in anatomical orientation, shows the left ventricle in a heart with concordant atrioventricular connections and a huge ventricular septal defect. The site of the axis of atrioventricular conduction tissue has been marked in red dots on the left ventricular aspect of the hypoplastic ventricular septum, which runs to the apex (star), where it separates the apical ventricular components. The right atrioventricular valve is connected within the right ventricle, hence the concordant nature of the atrioventricular connections.

anomalously located atrioventricular node, as described in more detail below. Irrespective of the relationship of the small ventricle to the dominant left ventricle, the axis always extends postero-inferior to the defect when viewed from the incomplete right ventricle, being carried on the left ventricular aspect of the septal crest (Figure 9.1.13). When the ventriculo-arterial

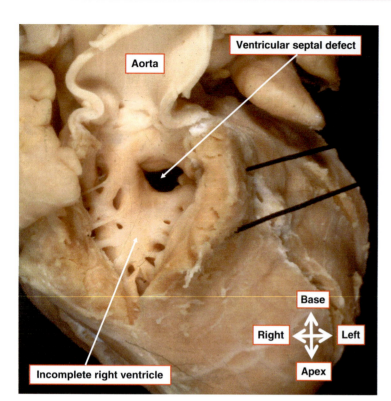

Figure 9.1.8 In this specimen with double inlet left ventricle and discordant ventriculo-arterial connections, viewed anatomically, the incomplete right ventricle, supporting the aorta, is right sided.

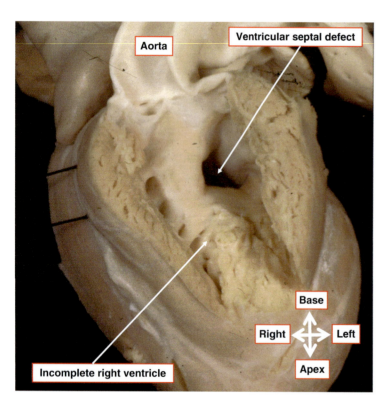

Figure 9.1.9 In this specimen, again with double inlet left ventricle and discordant ventriculo-arterial connections, and viewed anatomically, the incomplete rudimentary right ventricle, supporting the aorta, is left sided.

connections are discordant, the incomplete right ventricle usually has a very short outlet portion (Figures 9.1.8, 9.1.9), making it difficult to remove any tissue cephalad to the defect. The safest way surgically to enlarge the defect, therefore, is to remove a wedge of the muscular ventricular septum closest to the obtuse margin of the heart (Figure 9.1.12).[10]

In a small proportion of patients with double inlet left ventricle, the ventriculo-arterial connections may be concordant (Figure 9.1.11), or there can be double outlet from the dominant left or incomplete right ventricle. The variant with concordant ventriculo-arterial connections is of significant anatomical interest. The lesion is described eponymously as

9.1 Functionally Univentricular Heart

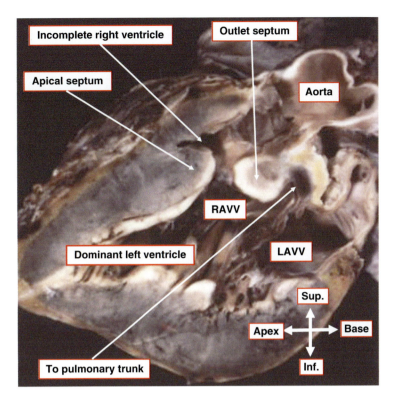

Figure 9.1.10 This specimen with double inlet left ventricle and discordant ventriculo-arterial connections has been sectioned to replicate the parasternal long-axis view, and is photographed in anatomical orientation. The apical ventricular septum separates the apical components of the dominant left and incomplete right ventricles. It carries the conduction axis, and is nourished by the septal perforating arteries. LAVV, left atrioventricular valve; RAVV, right atrioventricular valve.

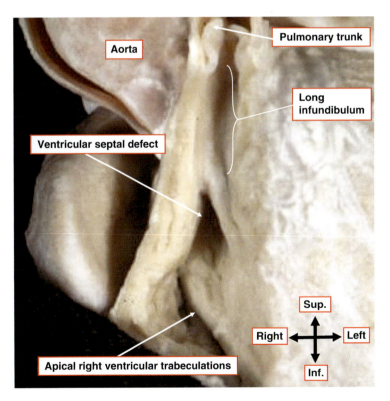

Figure 9.1.11 In this specimen, again with double inlet left ventricle, but now with concordant ventriculo-arterial connections, as with the heart shown in Figure 9.1.4, the right-sided incomplete right ventricle supports the pulmonary trunk, with the aorta arising from the dominant left ventricle. This is the so-called Holmes heart. Note the length of the infundibulum of the incomplete ventricle when it supports the pulmonary trunk, compared with those supporting the aorta (Figures 9.1.8, 9.1.9).

the Holmes heart.[11] In this setting, the incomplete right ventricle, when seen in isolation, can be virtually indistinguishable from the incomplete right ventricle seen in hearts with tricuspid atresia (compare Figures 9.1.11 and 9.1.14). The ventricular septal defect is often restrictive in this form of double inlet left ventricle (Figure 9.1.11). The same rules pertain should it require surgical enlargement. This is unlikely to be performed, however, unless a septation is also attempted. The more likely approach will be to perform a Fontan procedure. The incomplete right ventricle will then be excluded from the circulation.

Taken overall, the Fontan procedure, or one of its modifications, will be the likely operation of choice for most patients with double inlet left ventricle. It can successfully be used for all the various anatomical variants, providing that the

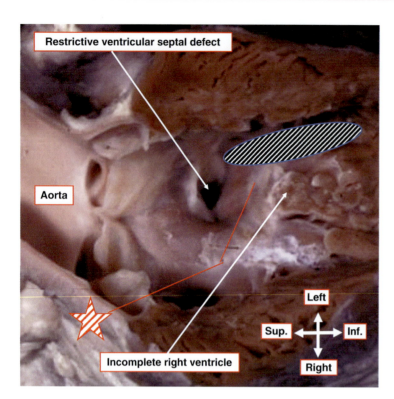

Figure 9.1.12 This specimen, photographed in surgical orientation, shows the relationship of the axis of atrioventricular conduction tissue to the ventricular septal defect in the double inlet left ventricle with discordant ventriculo-arterial connections when viewed from the incomplete right ventricle. The ventricular septal defect is restrictive. The course of the conduction axis is superimposed in red, with the site of the anomalous atrioventricular node shown by the star, with the cross-hatched oval showing the area that can be removed without inflicting trauma to the conduction tissues.

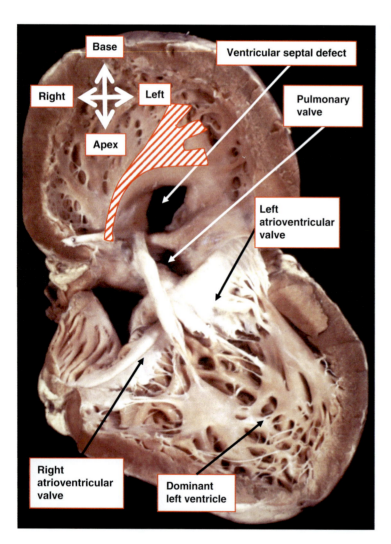

Figure 9.1.13 This heart is an example of the commonest form of double inlet left ventricle. The dominant left ventricle has been opened in clam-like fashion, and the specimen is shown in anatomical orientation. The abnormal course of the conduction axis, which is carried on the left ventricular aspect of the septum, has been superimposed on the picture as the red cross-hatched area.

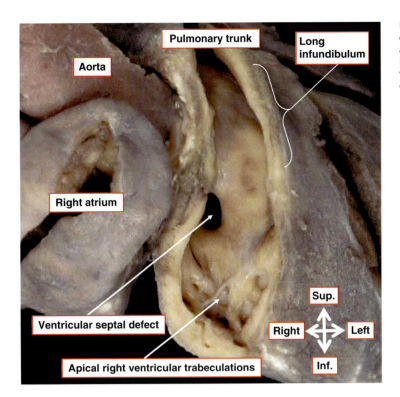

Figure 9.1.14 This specimen has classical tricuspid atresia with concordant ventriculo-arterial connections, and is photographed in anatomical orientation. Note the similarity in the morphology of the incomplete right ventricle in this setting, with its long infundibulum, with that seen in double inlet left ventricle when the ventriculo-arterial connections are concordant.

haemodynamic criteria are satisfactory.[12] Almost always, the procedure includes connecting the systemic venous returns, in one way or another, to the pulmonary arteries. This is now usually achieved either by creating a conduit within the right atrium to produce a so-called total cavo-pulmonary connection,[13] or else inserting an extracardiac conduit that connects the inferior caval vein to the pulmonary arteries, combining this with a Glenn procedure.[14] In the past, the roof of the right atrium at its junction with the appendage was often connected directly to the pulmonary trunk. Such an atriopulmonary connection still remains a surgical option. When there is juxtaposition of the atrial appendages, a not infrequent associated malformation with double inlet left ventricle, this anastomosis becomes even simpler. If the atrium is to be connected to the pulmonary arteries, either directly or by construction of an internal conduit, it is crucial for the surgeon to avoid the sinus node and its arterial supply. In this respect, the key area is the superior interatrial groove, through which courses the artery to the sinus node irrespective of its arterial origin (Figure 9.1.15). Use of an internal or external conduit obviously obviates the need to isolate surgically the systemic venous return from the right atrioventricular valve, an added manoeuvre that is essential if attempting an atriopulmonary connection. If this has to be done, there are at least two options open to the surgeon. It can be done by securing a patch across the vestibule of the valve. It can also be achieved by deviating the atrial septum to the parietal border of the right atrium, thus leaving both valves draining to the dominant ventricle. With both of these options, it is important to avoid the atrioventricular node, which in double inlet left ventricle is no longer located at the apex of the triangle of Koch.[15] This is because the muscular ventricular septum, carrying the ventricular conduction tissues, does not reach to the crux of the heart, rising instead to the acute margin of the ventricular mass (Figure 9.1.13). The atrioventricular node, therefore, is located within the quadrant of the junction related to the mouth of the right atrial appendage (Figure 9.1.16). This area is the major site of danger. Irrespective of its precise location, nonetheless, the node can be avoided by securing the patch above the vestibule of the right atrioventricular valve.

The features discussed above, however, are less pertinent to the modern-day surgeon, since it is now the rule to insert an extracardiac conduit so as to direct the inferior caval venous blood to the lungs or to the superior caval vein. Like an internal baffle, this procedure produces the total cavo-pulmonary connection,[13] with the extracardiac conduit also having advantages in terms of the pattern of flow into the pulmonary arteries. Should it be decided to construct an internal baffle, the major areas to be avoided are again the sinus node and its arterial supply. Such problems are avoided when inserting an extracardiac conduit.

Relatively few surgeons nowadays choose septation for patients with double inlet left ventricle, even though it is, perhaps, the most logical surgical option.[7] Relatively few patients, however, have anatomy suitable for successful septation. Both atrioventricular valves must be competent structures, and the relationships of dominant and incomplete ventricles must permit the construction of a patch to channel flow from the left atrioventricular valve to the ventricular septal defect. This means that the incomplete right ventricle should be left sided (Figure 9.1.9) or, at worst, directly anterior. The dominant ventricle also needs to be of good size, which means that septation is unlikely to be attempted in infancy. If the pulmonary circulation is not protected by naturally occurring stenosis, this must be achieved

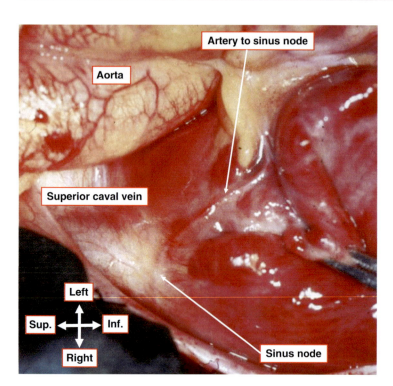

Figure 9.1.15 In this heart, photographed in the operating room, the artery to the sinus node, arising from the right coronary artery, is seen coursing through the interatrial groove to cross the cavo-atrial junction at the crest of the right atrial appendage. The sinus node is visible as a pale area within the terminal groove.

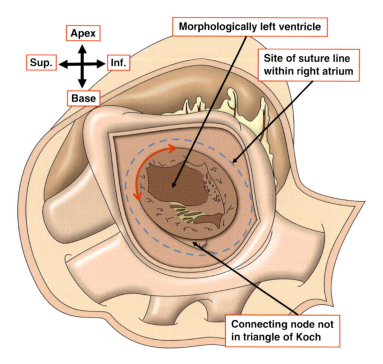

Figure 9.1.16 This drawing, shown in surgical orientation, indicates the danger area of the right atrioventricular orifice (red double-headed arrow) in hearts with double inlet left ventricle relative to the location of the anomalous anterior atrioventricular node, and the way the conduction tissue can be avoided by suturing above the level of the atrioventricular junction (blue dotted line).

immediately after birth by banding the pulmonary trunk. Banding itself tends to promote additional hypertrophy of the ventricular myocardium, and narrowing of the ventricular septal defect. It may also be necessary, therefore, to combine enlargement of the defect (Figure 9.1.12) with septation. The presence of naturally occurring subpulmonary stenosis may dictate the insertion of a conduit from the dominant ventricle to the pulmonary arteries. Remarkably few patients will match all these criteria, and become suitable candidates for septation. In those that are, the major consideration during surgery will be to avoid the axis of atrioventricular conduction tissue, thus avoiding iatrogenic heart block. It is also necessary, of course, to preserve the sinus node and its arterial supply (Figure 9.1.15).

The atrioventricular conduction axis in hearts with double inlet left ventricle takes its origin from an anomalous node located antero-cephalad within the right atrioventricular junction, beneath the mouth of the appendage

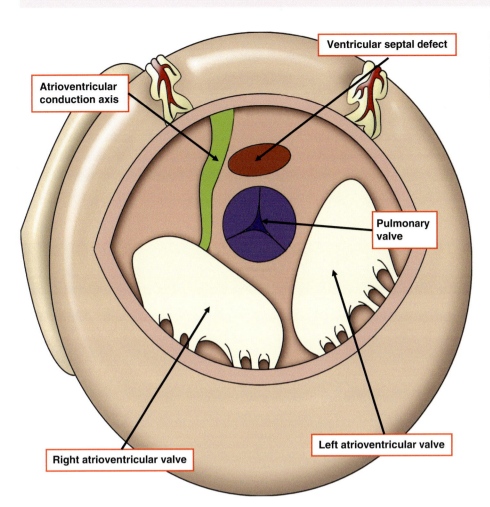

Figure 9.1.17 This drawing shows the path of the atrioventricular conduction axis, in green, relative to the right atrioventricular valve, the pulmonary valve and the ventricular septal defect, as seen through a fishmouth incision in the apex of the left ventricle.

(Figure 9.1.16). From this anterior node, the atrioventricular bundle penetrates through the lateral end of the area of fibrous continuity between the leaflets of the pulmonary and the right atrioventricular valves. When the incomplete right ventricle is left sided, as it will be in most cases suitable for septation, the non-branching atrioventricular bundle then encircles the anterior quadrants of the pulmonary orifice to reach the rightward margin of the muscular ventricular septum (Figures 9.1.13, 9.1.17, 9.1.18). The left bundle branch then cascades down the left ventricular aspect of the septum, the axis of conduction tissue itself being located antero-cephalad to the ventricular septal defect when viewed either through a fish-mouth incision in the dominant left ventricle (Figure 9.1.17), or through the right atrioventricular valve (Figure 9.1.18). Unless a conduit is also placed from the dominant left ventricle to the pulmonary arteries, the line of sutures used to septate the dominant ventricle must cross this course of the axis of conduction tissues. The axis itself is relatively narrow as it emerges from the area of fibrous continuity between the pulmonary and right atrioventricular valves. If this site is known with precision, the sutures can be placed so as to avoid the axis. All of these considerations, taken together, indicate that septation is a formidable surgical procedure if the pathways through the dominant ventricle are to be separated without insertion of a conduit, or involuntary induction of atrioventricular dissociation. Septation can be a potentially feasible option for patients with double inlet left ventricle and concordant ventriculo-arterial connections. If attempted, the same rules hold good for the disposition of the axis of conduction tissue, but a potential caveat is that the ventricular septal defect is most frequently restrictive or obstructed.

The other variants of double inlet ventricle are much rarer, and hardly ever are suitable for septation. Double inlet right ventricle is seen most frequently along with double outlet from the dominant right ventricle (Figure 9.1.19), often with straddling and overriding of the left atrioventricular valve (Figure 9.1.6).[16] The incomplete left ventricle, usually found in left-sided position, although sometimes found to the right, is then nothing more than a pouch with left ventricular apical trabeculations (Figure 9.1.20). It is always found postero-inferiorly relative to the atrioventricular valves, occupying the diaphragmatic surface of the ventricular mass. The Fontan procedure is the most likely therapeutic surgical option, in which case the landmarks within the atrial chambers, together with the surgical caveats, are as discussed for double inlet left ventricle. Sometimes, double inlet right ventricle can be found with concordant ventriculo-arterial connections (Figure 9.1.21), usually with a common valve guarding the atrioventricular junctions (Figure 9.1.22). The axis of atrioventricular conduction in this setting descends from a node located within its usual position in the triangle of Koch. The exception is when the incomplete left ventricle is right sided, the conduction axis then

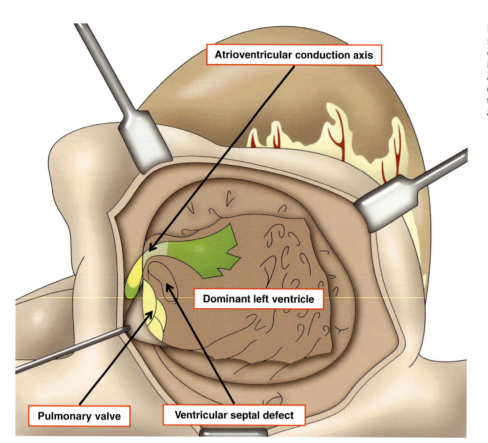

Figure 9.1.18 This drawing, again drawn in surgical orientation, shows the view of the dominant left ventricle in the setting of double inlet left ventricle with discordant ventriculo-arterial connections, and the course of the conduction axis, in green, as it would be seen by the surgeon working through the right atrioventricular valve.

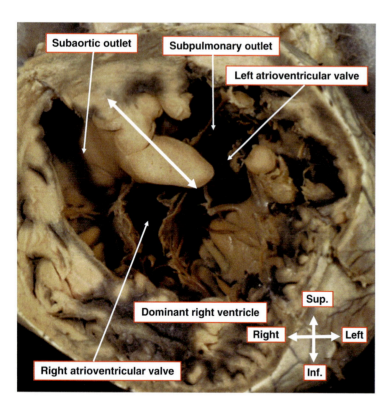

Figure 9.1.19 This specimen with double inlet and double outlet right ventricle is photographed in anatomical orientation. Both atrioventricular valves connect exclusively to the dominant right ventricle, while the extensive outlet septum (white double-headed arrow) separates the origins of the two arterial trunks.

arising from an anomalous node,[17] as in congenitally corrected transposition (see Chapter 9.2).

Those rare hearts with double inlet to a solitary and indeterminate ventricle usually co-exist with isomerism of the atrial appendages, when the multiple associated malformations, particularly the anomalous venoatrial connections, dominate the picture. Rare examples can be found with usual arrangement of the atrial appendages (Figure 9.1.5). In this setting, the crossing

9.1 Functionally Univentricular Heart

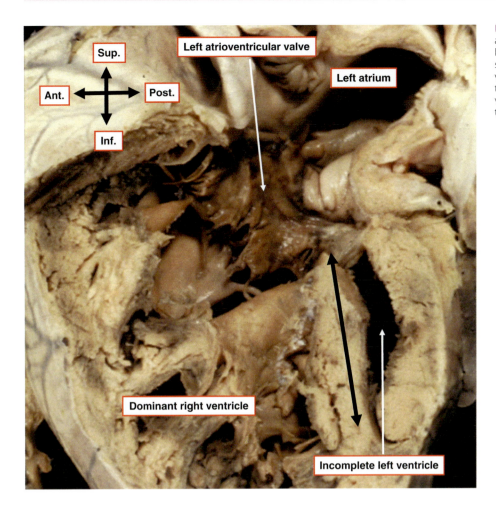

Figure 9.1.20 This picture, again viewed in anatomical orientation, shows the location of the left-sided incomplete left ventricle in the heart shown in Figure 9.1.19 with double inlet right ventricle. The incomplete ventricle is no more than an outpouching from the dominant ventricle. The black double-headed arrow shows the hypoplastic apical ventricular septum.

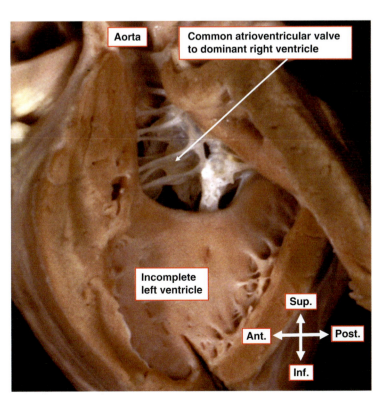

Figure 9.1.21 In this picture, again in anatomical orientation, an example is seen of double inlet right ventricle in which the incomplete left ventricle gives rise to the aorta. There is a common atrioventricular valve joining both atriums to the dominant right ventricle, shown in cross-section in Figure 9.1.3.

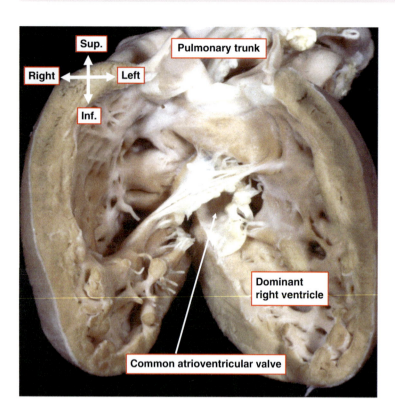

Figure 9.1.22 This picture shows the dominant right ventricle in the heart illustrated in Figure 9.1.21. Both atriums drain to the dominant ventricle through the common atrioventricular valve. The ventriculo-arterial connections are concordant, with the pulmonary trunk arising from the dominant ventricle.

of tension apparatus from the atrioventricular valves, along with the particularly coarse indeterminate apical trabeculations, tend to conspire against septation. Patients with solitary ventricles, therefore, are also most likely to undergo repair by means of the Fontan option, and the same rules apply as discussed above.

Hearts with huge ventricular septal defects can sometimes be confused with double inlet to a solitary and indeterminate ventricle. Even in those with huge septal defects, septation remains a formidable undertaking. In these rare patients, it is the persisting rim of muscular septum separating the apical trabecular components, together with the inlet septum rising to the crux, which provide the anatomical landmarks. The axis of conduction tissue descends from the regular atrioventricular node when the atrioventricular connections are concordant in this setting (Figure 9.1.7).

The other hearts making up the group with univentricular atrioventricular connection have absence of either the right-sided or the left-sided atrioventricular connection. It is absence of the right-sided atrioventricular connection, in the setting of usual atrial arrangement, that is the substrate for the lesion most usually described as tricuspid atresia (Figure 9.1.23). The lesion exists because of failure of expansion of the atrioventricular canal during embryonic life (see Chapter 2). Some of the hearts with mitral atresia also exist because of seeming absence of the left atrioventricular connection. These are the worst end of the spectrum of hypoplastic left heart syndrome, but a connection had been formed initially in these hearts (see Chapter 8.6). Morphologically, nonetheless, the appearance remains that of an absent connection (Figure 9.1.24). Because of the absence of one of the atrioventricular connections, it follows that, in most instances, only one of the atrioventricular junctions is able to make contact with the ventricular mass. The ventricular morphology, in terms of dominant and incomplete ventricles, is then comparable to that seen with double inlet. On rare occasions, nonetheless, when there is absence of one of the atrioventricular connections, the solitary atrioventricular valve can straddle and override. This produces a uniatrial, but biventricular, atrioventricular connection.[18] Both of the ventricles are then incomplete to greater or lesser degree, but one can still usually be recognized as being dominant (Figure 9.1.25).

Although the variations in terms of ventricular morphology are the same as for double inlet ventricle when one atrioventricular connection is absent, most examples fall into what can be considered to represent classical types of atrioventricular valvar atresia. We will concentrate our attention, therefore, on these anticipated variants, while drawing attention to the less familiar formats. In tricuspid atresia, it is the morphologically right atrium which is blind-ending, usually with no vestige of the tricuspid valve in its floor (Figure 9.1.26). Because of the absent connection, the right ventricle is incomplete, lacking its inlet component.[19] The apical part of the incomplete ventricle, as with double inlet left ventricle, is separated from the dominant ventricle by the apical muscular ventricular septum (Figure 9.1.27). As in double inlet left ventricle, the apical ventricular septum does not extend to the crux, but rather extends to the acute margin of the ventricular mass (Figure 9.1.28). Surgical palliation involves the Fontan operation, or one of its modifications. In hearts with concordant ventriculo-arterial connections, attempts were often made during the early

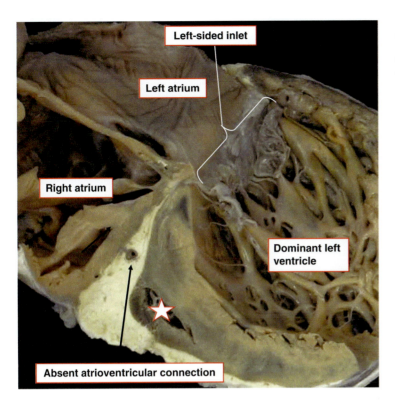

Figure 9.1.23 The heart has been sectioned to replicate the four-chamber echocardiographic view. It shows complete absence of the right atrioventricular connection, the atrioventricular groove being filled with adipose tissue, and containing the right coronary artery. This is the essence of the usual variant of tricuspid atresia. The section passes mostly through the dominant left ventricle, but the posterior part of the incomplete right ventricle is just visible (star).

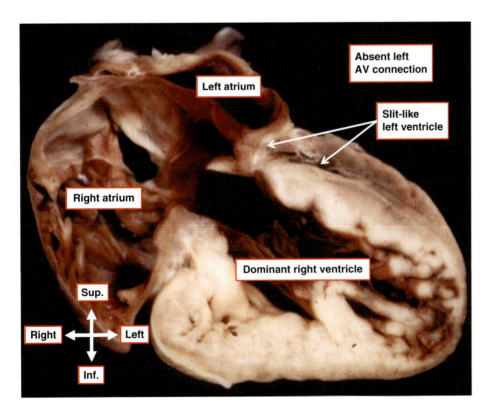

Figure 9.1.24 This heart with classical mitral atresia, from a patient with hypoplasia of the left heart, has again been sectioned to replicate the four-chamber echocardiographic view. There is absence of the left atrioventricular connection, albeit that a connection had been formed at some time during gestation (see Chapter 8.6).

period of evolution of the Fontan procedure to incorporate the incomplete right ventricle into the pulmonary circulation. At present, most surgeons have shifted to constructing total cavo-pulmonary connections, now mostly using external conduits. If the conduit is to be constructed within the right atrium, the architecture of its muscular walls, and the arterial supply, should be disturbed as little as possible. Preservation of the sinus node and its blood supply is particularly important, as atrial arrhythmia is a recognized life-threatening postoperative complication, particularly in the long term.

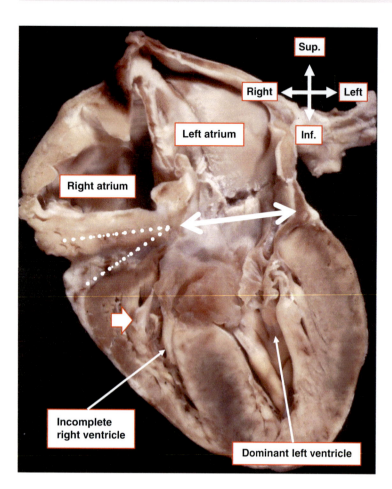

Figure 9.1.25 This heart, with absence of the right atrioventricular connection (white dotted lines), is sectioned to simulate the echocardiographic four-chamber view. The solitary atrioventricular junction (double-headed white arrow) is shared between the dominant left and the incomplete right ventricles because of straddling of the solitary atrioventricular valve (red-bordered arrow). This arrangement produces a uniatrial but biventricular connection.

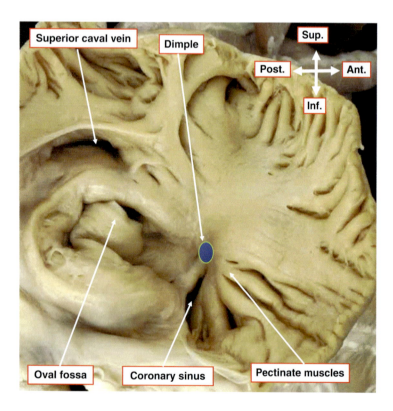

Figure 9.1.26 This view, of the opened right atrium seen in anatomical orientation from a specimen with tricuspid atresia, shows the muscular floor due to complete absence of the right atrioventricular connection. The site of the atrioventricular node has been superimposed in blue, and is closely related to the 'dimple'.

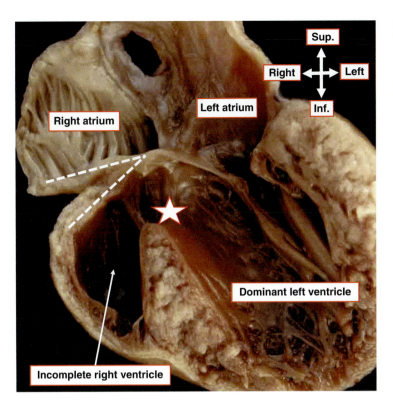

Figure 9.1.27 This specimen with classical tricuspid atresia due to absence of the right atrioventricular connection (white dotted lines), and concordant ventriculo-arterial connections, has been sectioned to simulate the echocardiographic four-chamber view. The hypoplastic ventricular septum separates the apical parts of the dominant left and incomplete right ventricles with a relatively large ventricular septal defect (star).

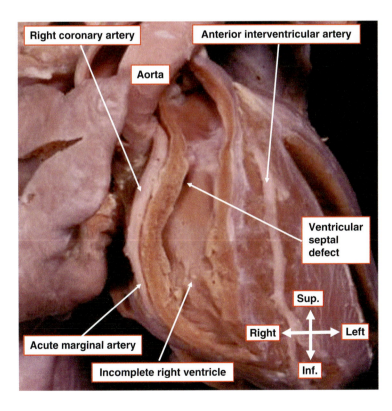

Figure 9.1.28 This dissection of a specimen with tricuspid atresia, again with concordant ventriculo-arterial connections, viewed in anatomical orientation, shows that the right delimiting coronary artery descends at the acute margin of the ventricular mass from the right coronary artery, rather than the crux. The other delimiting artery is the anterior interventricular artery. Note the antero-superior location of the incomplete right ventricle.

The rules for avoidance of these structures are as described above for double inlet ventricle. Whenever a well-formed Eustachian valve is encountered, it should be preserved. Such a valve can be incorporated in an internal baffle. Creation of such an internal baffle requires the surgeon to make a direct and wide connection between the right atrium and the pulmonary arteries. In such circumstances, the artery to the sinus node can be at risk as it traverses the interatrial groove. This potential complication is avoided when inserting an extracardiac conduit.

When the Fontan procedure is performed in hearts with discordant ventriculo-arterial connections, it may be necessary

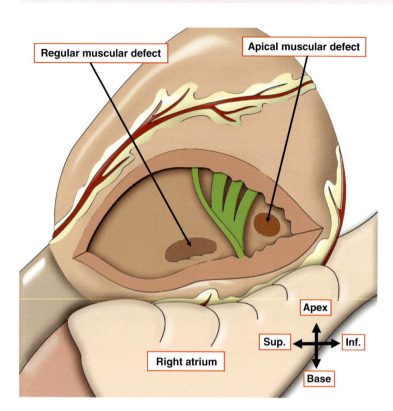

Figure 9.1.29 The cartoon, drawn in surgical orientation, shows the route of the axis of atrioventricular conduction tissue, shown in green, relative to the usual ventricular septal defect in tricuspid atresia, and to a defect opening between the apical trabecular component of the incomplete right ventricle and the dominant ventricle. In the latter situation, the axis is superior as opposed to inferior, and to the surgeon's left rather than right hand.

to resect the margins of the ventricular septal defect should it be restrictive. This must be done in a way that avoids the atrioventricular conduction axis on the left ventricular aspect of the septum. When seen from the right ventricle, this runs postero-inferior to the septal defect as in double inlet left ventricle. The rare exception is when the typical muscular ventricular septal defect is atretic, and an apical trabecular defect provides the interventricular communication (Figure 9.1.29).

Tricuspid atresia is not always the consequence of absence of the right atrioventricular connection. In rare circumstances, it may be produced because an imperforate valvar membrane is interposed between the right atrium and ventricle. This can be seen as part of pulmonary atresia with intact ventricular septum (Figure 9.1.30). This is another example of a functionally univentricular arrangement being found when the atrioventricular connections are biventricular. Similar arrangements are rarely found when there are concordant atrioventricular connections and a ventricular septal defect (Figure 9.1.31), or as part of Ebstein's malformation (Figure 9.1.32). We are unaware of any patient in whom the junction blocked by the imperforate membrane has been of sufficient size to permit resection of the valve, and replacement with a valvar prosthesis.

Operative treatment of mitral atresia is complicated because of its usual association with aortic atresia. This, of course, is one of the typical combinations producing hypoplasia of the left heart (see Chapter 8.6). Direct surgical correction involves reconstruction of the arterial pathways as an initial procedure, employing the Norwood protocol or one of its modifications. This is followed by a subsequent modified Fontan procedure. As we described in Chapter 8.6, the options in these procedures are dictated by the anatomy of the aortic pathways rather than the ventricular morphology, with the key features being the relations of the arterial duct and the size of the aortic root. In some patients having absence of the left atrioventricular valve, however, the aortic outflow tract is patent. 'Mitral atresia' may not be the best term for description of all these patients. This is because, in many, the morphology suggests that, had the left atrioventricular connection been formed, it would have been guarded by a morphologically tricuspid valve. The right atrium in this setting is connected to a morphologically left ventricle, with the incomplete right ventricle being anterior and left sided, usually with discordant ventriculoarterial connections (Figure 9.1.33). In this setting, there is no direct route for the pulmonary venous return to reach the dominant left ventricle. The blood must cross an atrial septal defect and traverse the right-sided atrioventricular valve. Initial survival in these cases, therefore, depends on the state of the atrial septum. Should the septum be restrictive, it will need to be enlarged. Some sort of modified Fontan procedure will then be the final option, usually a cavo-pulmonary connection. As with tricuspid atresia, left-sided atresia can be produced by an imperforate atrioventricular valve rather than being due to absence of the left atrioventricular connection. The imperforate valve can be found with biventricular (Figure 9.1.34) or double inlet (Figure 9.1.35) atrioventricular connections. Irrespective of the specific morphology, the only surgical option will be to create a functionally univentricular connection, the Fontan circulation being constructed following one of the options discussed above.

9.1 Functionally Univentricular Heart

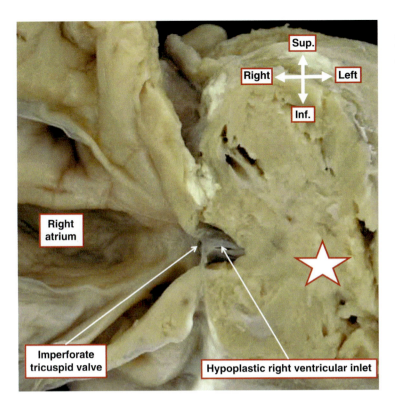

Figure 9.1.30 This specimen is sectioned across the right atrioventricular junction. There is pulmonary atresia with intact ventricular septum, with mural hypertrophy obliterating the apical (star) and outlet ventricular components. In addition, the tricuspid valve is imperforate. The atrioventricular connections are concordant.

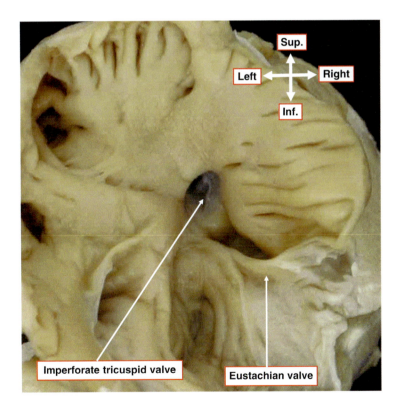

Figure 9.1.31 The right atrium in this specimen is viewed from above and behind, in anatomical orientation, to show the atrial aspect of an imperforate tricuspid valve. In this heart, the atrioventricular connections were again concordant (compare with Figure 9.1.30), and there was a ventricular septal defect.

References Cited

1. Fontan F, Baudet E. Surgical repair of tricuspid atresia. *Thorax* 1971; **26**: 240–248.
2. Norwood WI, Lang P, Hansen DD. Physiologic repair of aortic atresia – hypoplastic left heart syndrome. *NEJM* 1983; **308**: 23–26.
3. Jacobs ML, Anderson RH. Nomenclature of the functionally univentricular heart. *Cardiol Young* 2006; **16** (Suppl.1): 3–8.
4. Anderson RH, Macartney FJ, Tynan M, et al. Univentricular atrioventricular connection: the single ventricle trap unsprung. *Pediatr Cardiol* 1983; **4**: 273–280.

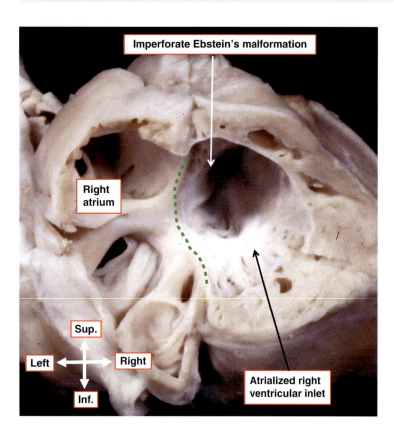

Figure 9.1.32 In this heart, with an imperforate tricuspid valve and concordant atrioventricular connections, the tricuspid valve itself is deformed by Ebstein's malformation. The dotted green line shows the location of the right atrioventricular junction.

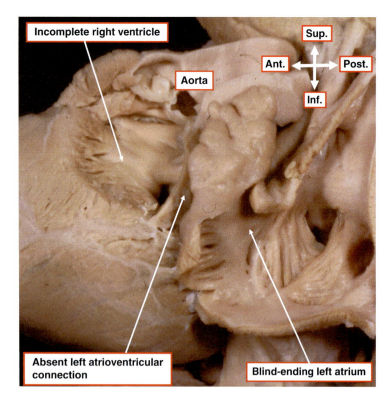

Figure 9.1.33 As shown by this specimen, shown in anatomical orientation viewed from the left, 'mitral atresia' is not always part of hypoplasia of the left heart. In this example, there is absence of the left atrioventricular connection, but the right atrium is connected to a dominant ventricle with left ventricular trabeculations (not seen). The incomplete right ventricle, supporting the aorta, is left sided and anterior. Had the left atrioventricular valve been formed, it would almost certainly of been of tricuspid morphology.

5. Anderson RH, Becker AE, Tynan M, et al. The univentricular atrioventricular connection: getting to the root of a thorny problem. *Am J Cardiol* 1984; **54**: 822–828.

6. Anderson RH, Ho SY. What is a ventricle? *Ann Thorac Surg* 1998; **66**: 616–620.

7. Kurosawa H, Imai Y, Fukuchi S, et al. Septation and Fontan repair of univentricular atrioventricular connection. *J Thorac Cardiovas Surg* 1990; **99**: 314–319.

8. Franklin RCG, Spiegelhalter DJ, Anderson RH, et al. Double-inlet

9.1 Functionally Univentricular Heart

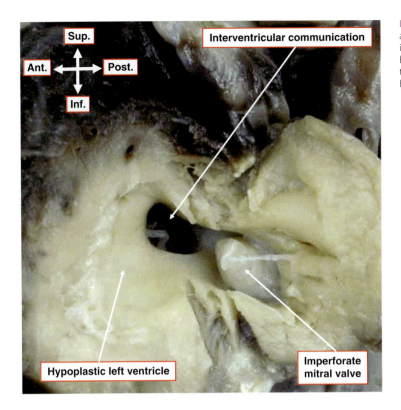

Figure 9.1.34 In this specimen, again seen in anatomical orientation and photographed from the left side, there is an imperforate mitral valve in the setting of concordant atrioventricular connections. Note the hypoplastic left ventricle and the interventricular communication, and the solitary cord and papillary muscle supporting the imperforate valve. Both arterial trunks arose from the morphologically right ventricle.

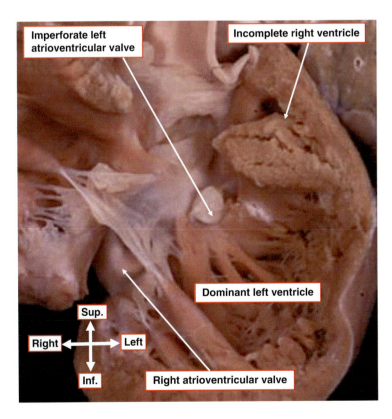

Figure 9.1.35 In this specimen, seen in anatomical orientation having opened the dominant left ventricle from the front, there is double inlet to the dominant ventricle, with the incomplete right ventricle in left-sided position, but with an imperforate left atrioventricular valve. The right atrioventricular valve is patent.

ventricle presenting in infancy. I. Survival without definitive repair. J Thorac Cardiovasc Surg 1991; **101**: 767–776.

9. Hosseinpour AR, Anderson RH, Ho SY. The anatomy of the septal perforating arteries in normal and congenitally malformed hearts. J Thorac Cardiovasc Surg 2001; **121**: 1046–1052.

10. Cheung HC, Lincoln C, Anderson RH, et al. Options for surgical repair in

hearts with univentricular atrioventricular connection and subaortic stenosis. *J Thorac Cardiovasc Surg* 1990; **100**: 672–681.

11. Abbott ME. Unique case of congenital malformation of the heart. Museum Notes. McGill University. 1992: pp. 522–525.

12. Fontan F, Kirklin JW, Fernandez G, et al. Outcome after a 'perfect' Fontan operation. *Circulation* 1990; **81**: 1520–1536.

13. de Leval MR, Kilner P, Gewillig M, Bull C. Total cavopulmonary connection: a logical alternative to atriopulmonary connection for complex Fontan operations. *J Thorac Cardiovasc Surg* 1988; **96**: 682–695.

14. Marcelletti C, Corno A, Giannico S, Marino B. Inferior vena cava-pulmonary artery extracardiac conduit: a new form of right heart bypass. *J Thorac Cardiovasc Surg* 1990; **100**: 228–232.

15. Anderson RH, Arnold R, Thaper MK, Jones RS, Hamilton DI. Cardiac specialized tissues in hearts with an apparently single ventricular chamber (double inlet left ventricle). *Am J Cardiol* 1974; **33**: 95–106.

16. Keeton BR, Macartney FJ, Hunter S, et al. Univentricular heart of right ventricular type with double or common inlet. *Circulation* 1979; **59**: 403–411.

17. Essed CE, Ho SY, Hunter S, Anderson RH. Atrioventricular conduction system in univentricular heart of right ventricular type with right-sided rudimentary chamber. *Thorax* 1980; **35**: 123–127.

18. Kiraly L, Hubay M, Cook AC, Ho SY, Anderson RH. Morphologic features of the uniatrial but biventricular atrioventricular connection. *J Thorac Cardiovasc Surg* 2007; **133**: 229–234.

19. Orie JD, Anderson C, Ettedgui J, Zuberbuhler JR, Anderson RH. Echocardiographic-morphologic correlations in tricuspid atresia. *J Am Coll Cardiol* 1995; **26**: 750–758.

Chapter 9.2
Discordant Ventriculo-Arterial Connections

Origin of the arterial trunks from morphologically inappropriate ventricles is usually described as 'transposition of the great arteries', and frequently abbreviated to 'TGA'.[1] In times gone by, individuals were sometimes described as having transposition of the organs, but this is now better described as the mirror-imaged arrangement. And we are unaware of any reported example of transposition of the great veins. We prefer, therefore, simply to describe the arrangement as transposition. The effects of such transposition are then conditioned by the atrioventricular connections. There are two major combinations, which we will address in this chapter. In the first combination, the discordant ventriculo-arterial connections exist in association with concordant atrioventricular connections.[1] This means that the systemic and pulmonary circulations are in parallel, rather than in series (Figure 9.2.1). In the second combination, discordant connections are found at both the atrioventricular and ventriculo-arterial junctions. This means that the two abnormal connections cancel each other out, such that, potentially, the circulations are congenitally corrected (Figure 9.2.2).[2] It is usually the case, however, that the haemodynamics in this second setting are disturbed by the presence of associated malformations.[3] As we described in Chapter 9.1, discordant ventriculo-arterial connections can be found in the setting of the functionally univentricular heart. They can also be found when in the setting of isomerism, when the atrioventricular connections are mixed, rather than being either concordant or discordant. When found with such mixed atrioventricular connections and left-handed ventricular topology, the combination can resemble closely the findings anticipated for congenitally corrected transposition. In the setting of isomerism, nonetheless, it is the anomalous venoatrial connections that dominate the picture. We will discuss these details in one of our final chapters. In this chapter, therefore, we will discuss the commonest form of transposition, and its congenitally corrected sibling. In the past, the most frequent variant was often described as being 'complete'. As was pointed out by Jaggers and his colleagues,[1] however, the arterial trunks are always completely 'transposed', in being placed across the septum,[4] whenever the ventriculo-arterial connections are discordant. 'Complete', in fact, was initially used to distinguish the discordant connections from double outlet right ventricle, in which it was argued that the transposition was 'partial', since the pulmonary trunk retained its connection with the right ventricle.[5] We agree that it is inappropriate to use 'complete' to describe the common variant. We will simply use the term 'transposition' as our own default option.

Transposition

It is now generally agreed that it is the combination of concordant atrioventricular with discordant ventriculo-arterial

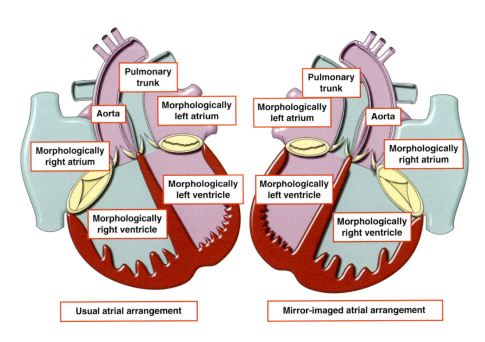

Figure 9.2.1 The drawing shows the segmental combinations of concordant atrioventricular and discordant ventriculo-arterial connections that produce the lesion usually described simply as transposition. The arrangement can exist in usual and mirror-imaged variants.

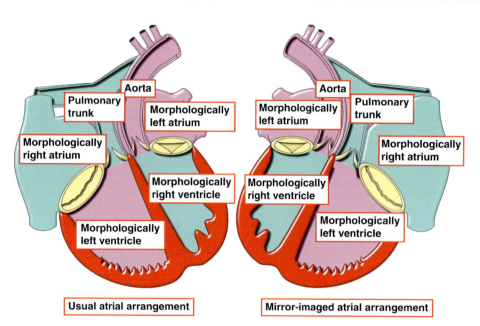

Figure 9.2.2 The drawing shows the segmental combinations of discordant atrioventricular and ventriculo-arterial connections that produce the lesion best described as congenitally corrected transposition. As with the commonest variant, the arrangement can be found in usual and mirror-imaged variants.

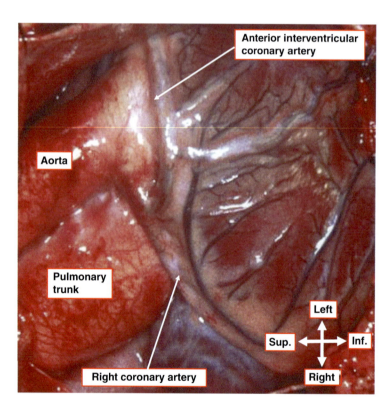

Figure 9.2.3 This surgical view, taken through a median sternotomy, shows a patient with transposition, defined on the basis of concordant atrioventricular and discordant ventriculo-arterial connections, in which the aorta is anterior and leftward relative to the pulmonary trunk. It would be a mistake to describe this arrangement as d-transposition. For those using segmental notation, it is properly described as exhibiting transposition {S,D,L}.

connections that produces the commonest variant of transposition.1,4 This has not always been the case. For quite some time, it was argued that 'transposition' described any situation in which the aorta was anterior to the pulmonary trunk.[6] This led to the confusing descriptions of 'double outlet right ventricle with transposition'. It is much easier to restrict the term to those with discordant ventriculo-arterial connections. This, however, does not solve all the current problems. It is still frequent to find the default option described as 'd-transposition', or 'd-TGA'. This is less than satisfactory, and totally illogical. In the first instance, this term fails to account accurately even for all patients having the usual atrial arrangement with concordant atrioventricular and discordant ventriculo-arterial connections. In a number of these patients, the aorta can be left sided, even when arising from the right-sided morphologically right ventricle (Figure 9.2.3). Nor does 'd-transposition' describe accurately the majority of patients with the combinations of mirror-imaged atrial arrangement, concordant atrioventricular, and discordant ventriculo-arterial connections. It is the rule for the aorta to be anterior and left-sided in this setting (Figure 9.2.4). All these patients are accurately described simply as having transposition. If the

9.2 Discordant Ventriculo-Arterial Connections

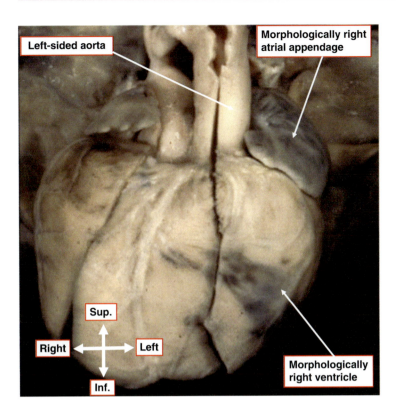

Figure 9.2.4 In this heart, again with concordant atrioventricular and discordant ventriculo-arterial connections, shown in anatomical orientation from the front, the aorta is left-sided relative to the pulmonary trunk. In this case, the heart is in the right chest, with the apex pointing to the right, in the setting of mirror-imaged atrial arrangement. The appropriate segmental notation is transposition {I.L.L}.

relationship of the aorta is to be emphasized, then this should be done by describing the full segmental set. Thus, the heart shown in Figure 9.2.3 is properly described as exhibiting transposition {S,D,L},[7] while the example shown in Figure 9.2.4 has transposition {I,L,L}.

From the surgical standpoint, two major subsets can be identified within the overall grouping of hearts with transposition. These are those without any major additional complicating lesions, usually described as simple transposition, and those with additional malformations sufficiently severe to complicate the clinical picture. The morphological aspects of the complicating lesions will be dealt with in turn, but the atrial anatomy is comparable within the whole group.

Nowadays, corrective surgical procedures are almost always performed at the arterial level. Operations designed to redirect venous blood at the atrial level should not be forgotten, however, particularly since these manoeuvres are an integral part of double switch procedures. When planning these operations, known as the Mustard and Senning options, it is the disposition of the cardiac nodes and their blood supply that is probably the most important factor. The presence of discordant ventriculo-arterial connections does not in any way affect the position of the sinus node, so the rules enunciated in Chapter 3 for avoidance of this node, and discussed in Chapter 9.1 in the setting of the Fontan procedure, are equally applicable in the setting of transposition. The entire terminal groove should be avoided, as should the crest of the atrial appendage, since the node can extend in horseshoe fashion across the crest, although it is usually in a lateral position. The nodal artery may enter the groove across the crest of the appendage, or after it has taken a retrocaval course. Of more importance is the course taken by the nodal artery as it ascends the interatrial groove. The artery frequently burrows into the atrial musculature, running across the superior border of the oval fossa, usually described as being the septum secundum (Figure 9.2.5). It is at risk in this position when incising the septum for either a Senning or Mustard procedure, or during a Blalock–Hanlon septostomy. A lateral course across the atrial appendage is also significant (Figure 9.2.6).

Other considerations remain significant when carrying out a venous switch procedure. Cannulation of the superior caval vein should be performed a good distance from the cavo-atrial junction, incising the right atrium well clear of the terminal groove. Traction, suction, or suturing should be avoided in the area of the superior border of the groove. If an incision is required across the terminal groove to widen the newly constructed pulmonary venous atrium in Mustard's operation, it can be made between the right pulmonary veins without fear of damaging the sinus node or its artery.

This discussion is also pertinent to the genesis of arrhythmias after Mustard's operation or the Senning procedure. It had been suggested, long since, that the arrhythmias are due to damage to purported specialized internodal pathways.[8] As we have explained in Chapter 3, there are no insulated tracts to be found within the atrial myocardium. Instead, the atrioventricular impulse is conducted from the sinus node through the thicker muscles of the right atrial wall and septum, with the anisotropic aggregation of the cardiomyocytes favouring preferential conduction (Figure 9.2.7). It is advantageous, therefore, to preserve at least one of these routes. If the terminal crest is to be divided to enlarge the new pulmonary venous atrium, this is a further reason to preserve the superior border of the oval fossa. These procedures, together with scrupulous

323

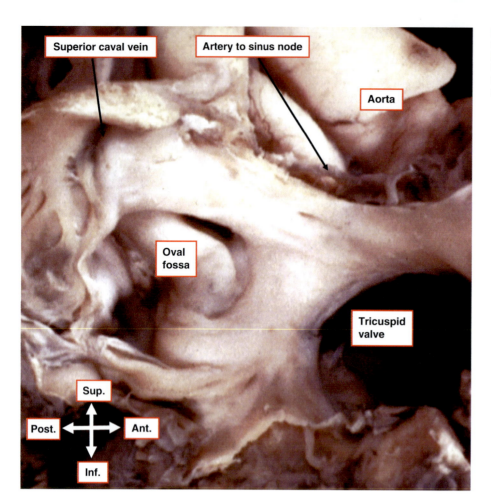

Figure 9.2.5 This dissection of a specimen of transposition seen in anatomical orientation from the right side shows the relationship of the artery to the sinus node, in this heart arising from the right coronary artery to the superior rim of the oval fossa.

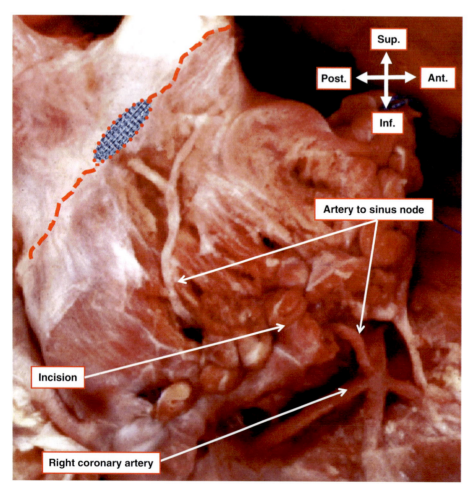

Figure 9.2.6 This anatomical specimen with transposition is photographed in anatomical orientation from the right side to show how the artery to the sinus node, arising laterally from the right coronary artery, with the site of the node shown by the textured oval, has been transected by a standard incision in the right atrial appendage.

9.2 Discordant Ventriculo-Arterial Connections

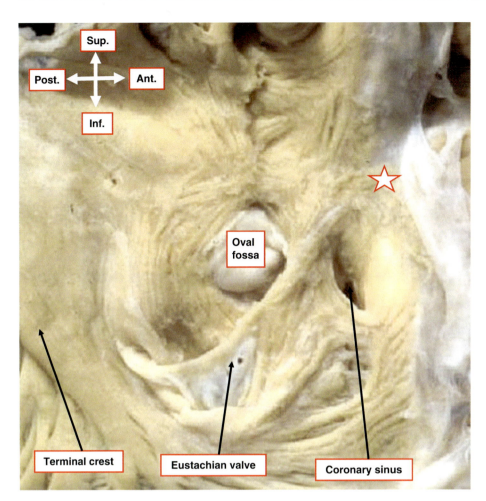

Figure 9.2.7 This dissection is made in a normal heart, oriented anatomically, by removing the endocardium from the inner surface of the right atrium. It shows the non-uniform anisotropic arrangement of the aggregated cardiomyocytes making up the atrial walls. There is preferential conduction along the major axis of muscle bundles such as the terminal crest, but no insulated tracts within the atrial musculature. The site of the atrioventricular node, at the apex of the triangle of Koch, is shown by the star.

avoidance of the sinus node and its blood supply, mean that arrhythmias can be considerably reduced, if not totally avoided, after atrial redirection procedures.[9] It is always important to avoid the atrioventricular node. The landmarks to this vital structure are the same as in the normal heart. Providing all surgery is performed outside the triangle of Koch, injury to the node will be avoided. The technique of cutting back the coronary sinus should be carefully considered. It is possible to perform this procedure without damaging the node and its zones of transitional cells, but the incision will undoubtedly cross one of the preferential routes of conduction. For this reason, it is safer to place the inferior suture line so as to avoid completely the triangle of Koch.

It is also important to place the interatrial baffles so as to minimize the risk of subsequent venous obstruction, either in the pulmonary or venous pathways. Although it was suggested that venous obstruction was less likely to complicate the Senning procedure, those who became skilled in Mustard's operation were able to achieve excellent results with a minimal incidence of late venous obstruction.[9] Almost certainly, therefore, it is the surgical technique which determines the likelihood of postoperative venous obstruction.

The major complicating lesions in transposition are the presence of a ventricular septal defect, along with obstruction of the left ventricular outflow tract. Often the two complications co-exist. Any other lesion can co-exist if anatomically possible. The anatomy of the additional lesions is then as described for the lesion found in isolation. It follows, therefore, that ventricular septal defects, when found in patients with transposition, can be just as variable as when found in isolation (Figure 9.2.8). The majority of defects open between the outlet components of the ventricular mass, but have their own peculiar characteristics. In such settings, typically with malalignment of the outlet septum, they can extend to become perimembranous when there is fibrous continuity between the leaflets of the tricuspid and mitral valves (Figure 9.2.9), or have a muscular postero-inferior rim (Figure 9.2.10). The distinguishing feature, as in tetralogy of Fallot, is whether or not the postero-caudal limb of the septo-marginal trabeculation, or septal band, fuses with the ventriculo-infundibular fold. If there is fusion (Figure 9.2.10), the resultant muscle bar will buttress the conduction axis, and there will be discontinuity between the leaflets of the tricuspid and mitral valves. If there is no fusion of the muscular bars, the defect will be perimembranous. The penetrating atrioventricular bundle will then be at risk in this area of fibrous continuity (Figure 9.2.9).

These defects have other features of surgical significance. The tension apparatus of the tricuspid valve tends to course over the defect, attaching itself to the outlet septum or to the

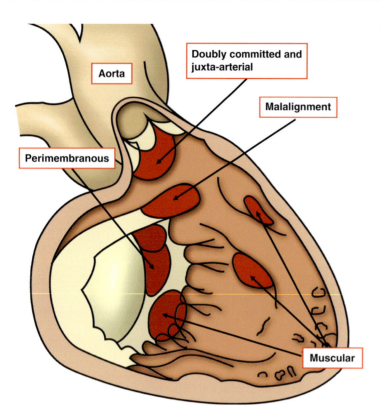

Figure 9.2.8 The drawing shows how the ventricular septal defect in hearts with transposition, as in the normal heart, can be perimembranous, muscular, or juxta-arterial. The drawing also emphasizes the potential for malalignment of the muscular outlet septum, a particular feature of the ventricular septal defect in the setting of transposition.

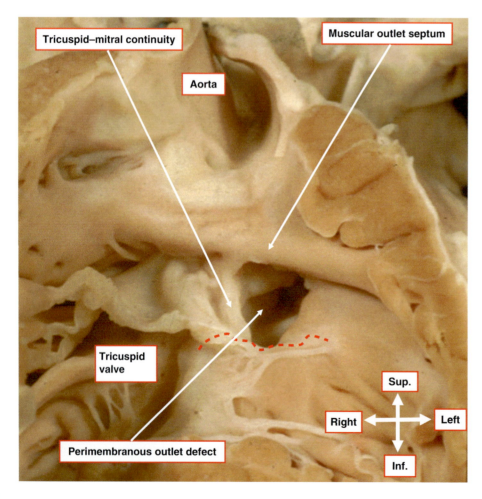

Figure 9.2.9 This view of a specimen with transposition, seen in anatomical orientation from the right ventricle, shows the right ventricular aspect of a perimembranous defect opening to the outlet of the right ventricle, with malalignment of the outlet septum. It is the fibrous continuity postero-inferiorly between the leaflets of the mitral and tricuspid valves that makes the defect perimembranous. The conduction axis is shown by the red dots.

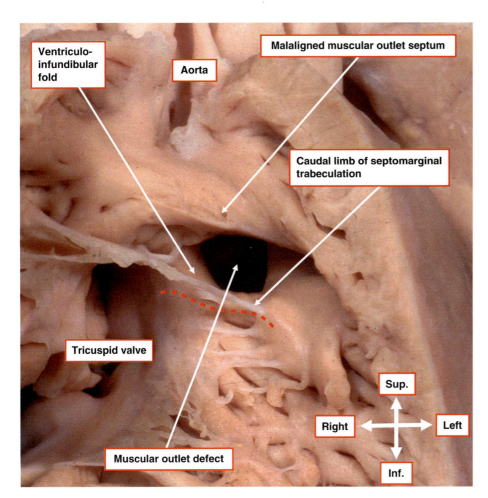

Figure 9.2.10 This specimen, again seen in anatomical orientation from the right side, again has a malalignment ventricular septal defect opening to the outlet of the right ventricle as in Figure 9.2.9, but this time with a muscular postero-inferior rim produced by continuity between the caudal limb of the septomarginal trabeculation and the ventriculo-infundibular fold. The muscular rim protects the conduction axis, shown by the red dotted line.

ventriculo-infundibular fold. This makes closure of the defect difficult without producing damage to the tricuspid valve, albeit that this is of less significance when the tricuspid valve is in the pulmonary circuit after an arterial switch. Of more significance is the divergence of the margins of the parietal and anterior heart walls. In hearts with concordant ventriculo-arterial connections, the anterior margin of a ventricular septal defect is usually well circumscribed. In the setting of transposition, the muscular outlet septum is frequently malaligned relative to the rest of the muscular ventricular septum as it inserts into the antero-cephalad wall of the right ventricular outflow tract. The defect, therefore, is more difficult to close at this anterior margin (Figures 9.2.9, 9.2.10).

Perimembranous defects can also open centrally to the right ventricle (Figure 9.2.11). They can also extend inferiorly when perimembranous, with the conduction axis similarly being deviated towards the crux of the heart. It is important to distinguish such perimembranous inlet defects from defects opening to the inlet of the right ventricle with exclusively muscular borders (Figure 9.2.12). The conduction axis will extend cranially relative to the muscular inlet defect, being to the left hand of the surgeon when viewed through the tricuspid valve. Muscular defects can also open centrally, while others open apically, often being multiple. Other defects opening to the ventricular inlet, which are also perimembranous, are the harbingers of straddling and overriding of the tricuspid valve (Figure 9.2.13).[10] The phenotypic feature is malalignment between the atrial and ventricular septal structures. Such defects should always be suspected when the right ventricle is hypoplastic. Straddling and overriding of the tricuspid valve increase markedly the risks of surgery, not least because of the abnormal disposition of the conduction tissues (Figures 9.2.13, 9.2.14). Outlet defects that are juxta-arterial, with the phenotypic feature of fibrous continuity between the leaflets of the arterial valves, but are the rarest variant. They can extend to become perimembranous (Figure 9.2.15).

The left ventricular outflow tract belongs to the ventricle. It follows, therefore, that subpulmonary obstruction in transposition (Figure 9.2.16) can be produced by any lesion which, in the normal heart, would produce subaortic obstruction. Valvar stenosis often accompanies the subvalvar abnormalities. Rarer lesions, such as anomalous insertion of the tension apparatus of the atrioventricular valve, are probably beyond surgical repair. Aneurysm of the membranous septum, or similar fibrous tissue tags (Figure 9.2.17), should be readily amenable to removal, although a subpulmonary fibrous shelf poses more problems, as it directly overlies the left bundle branch. The lesion also typically extends on to the pulmonary leaflet of the mitral valve, and can co-exist with a ventricular septal defect (Figure 9.2.18). The difficulties are compounded when the

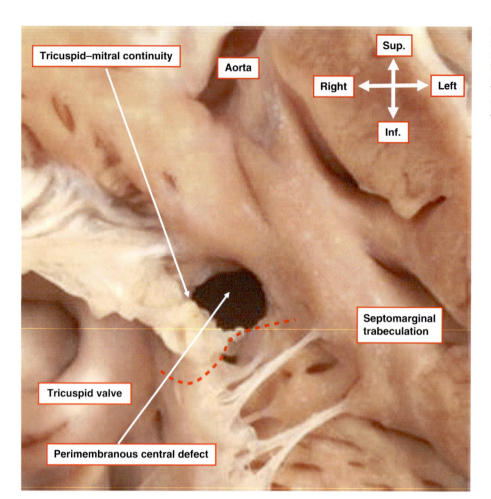

Figure 9.2.11 In this heart with transposition, seen in anatomical orientation from the right side, a perimembranous defect opens centrally to the right ventricle in the absence of malalignment of the muscular outlet septum. The conduction axis, shown by the red dots, relates directly to the postero-inferior rim of the defect.

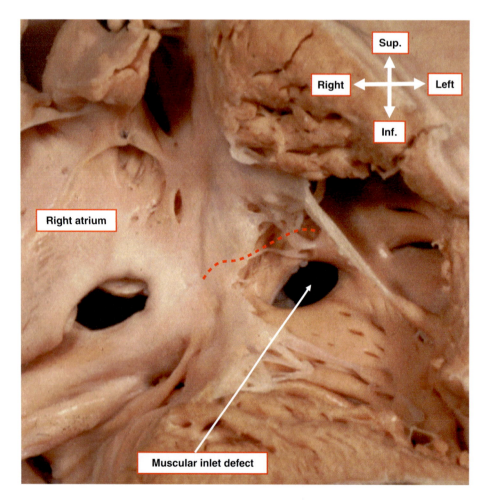

Figure 9.2.12 This heart, again with transposition, and photographed through the right atrioventricular junction, has a muscular defect opening to the inlet of the right ventricle. In this setting, the conduction axis, shown by the red dots, courses antero-superior relative to the defect.

9.2 Discordant Ventriculo-Arterial Connections

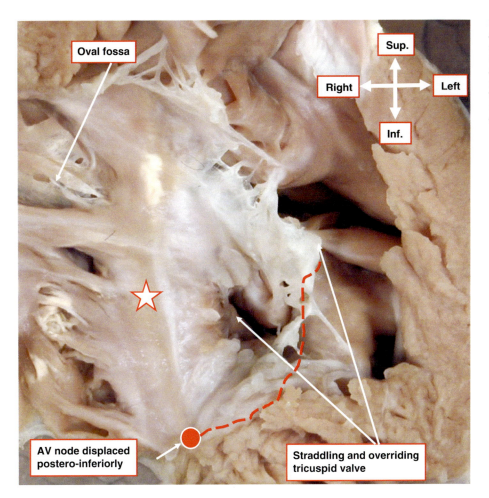

Figure 9.2.13 In this heart with transposition, again shown in anatomical orientation, there is straddling and overriding of the tricuspid valve. Because of the malalignment between the atrial and ventricular septums, the atrioventricular node (red circle) is no longer at the apex of the triangle of Koch (star), being deviated postero-inferiorly, as shown by the superimposed course of the conduction axis (red dashed line).

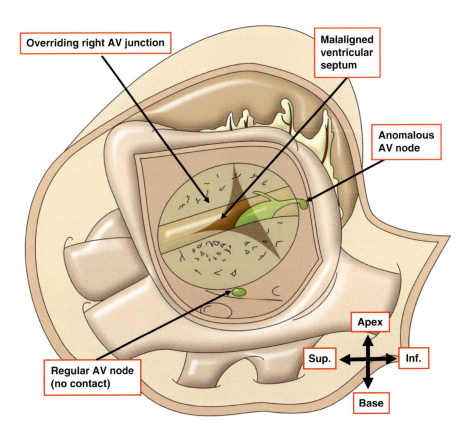

Figure 9.2.14 The cartoon, shown in surgical orientation, illustrates the location of the conduction axis in hearts with malalignment between the atrial and muscular ventricular septums as found when there is straddling and overriding of the tricuspid valve.

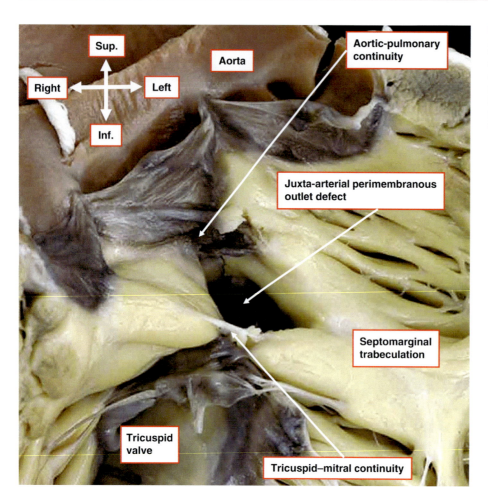

Figure 9.2.15 In this heart with transposition, seen in anatomical orientation from the front, the ventricular septal defect opening to the right ventricular outlet is juxta-arterial, with fibrous continuity between the leaflets of the aortic and pulmonary valves. The defect also extends to become perimembranous, with tricuspid-to-mitral fibrous continuity, reinforced with a membranous flap.

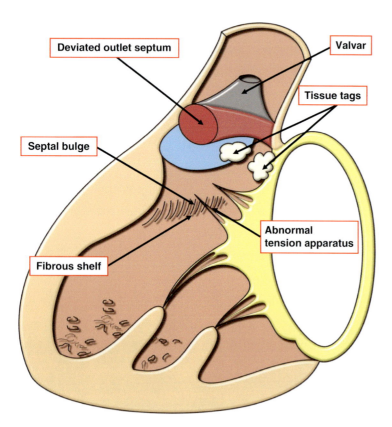

Figure 9.2.16 The drawing shows the lesions that can produce subpulmonary obstruction in the setting of transposition. Exactly the same lesions will produce subaortic obstruction in hearts with concordant ventriculo-arterial connections.

9.2 Discordant Ventriculo-Arterial Connections

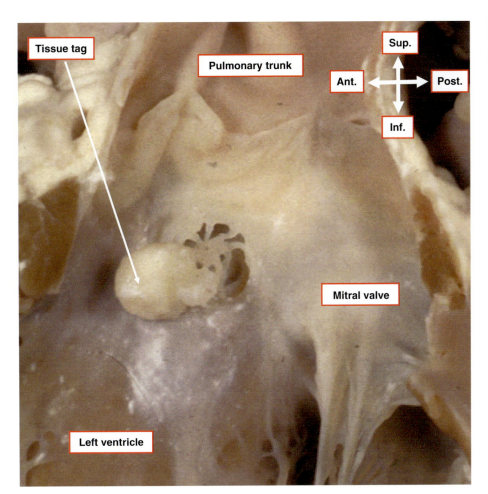

Figure 9.2.17 This view of the left ventricle from a specimen with transposition, seen in anatomical orientation from the left, shows a tissue tag from the septal leaflet of the tricuspid valve herniating through a perimembranous ventricular septal defect and producing subpulmonary obstruction.

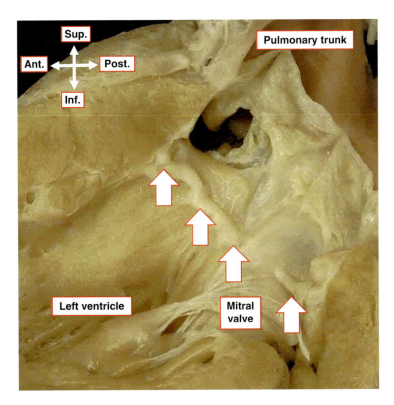

Figure 9.2.18 In this view of the left ventricular outflow tract of a specimen with transposition, seen in anatomical orientation, there is obstruction due to an extensive fibrous shelf that extends onto the leaflet of the mitral valve (red-bordered arrows).

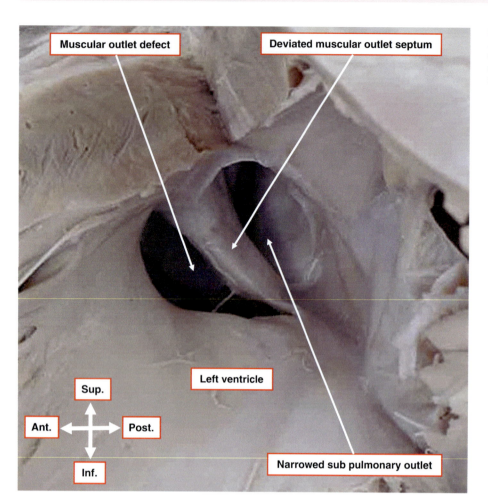

Figure 9.2.19 This specimen of transposition, seen from the left ventricle in anatomical orientation, has postero-caudal deviation of the outlet septum through a co-existing muscular outlet ventricular septal defect.

fibrous obstruction is more extensive, because then it can form a subvalvar tunnel. The other quadrants of the outflow tract are also vulnerable because of their proximity to the left coronary artery, or because they are formed by the pulmonary leaflet of the mitral valve. The safest area for resection is beneath the remnant of the left margin of the ventriculoinfundibular fold. When subpulmonary obstruction co-exists with a ventricular septal defect, there is frequently postero-caudal deviation of the outlet septum, which is then inserted in the left ventricle (Figure 9.2.19). This usually means that the aortic valve over-rides the septum. When the septal defect is substantial with this combination, the scene is set for an operative procedure such as the Rastelli or Nikaidoh operation.[11] When placing the aortic outlet into the left ventricle during these procedures, it is possible to resect safely the outlet septum, which never harbours conduction tissue. Such resection of the outlet septum is also part of the REV procedure, which is an acronym derived from 'reparation de l'etage ventriculaire'.[12] Nowadays, it is also possible to rotate the ventricular outflow tracts.[13] Should the co-existing septal defect be situated other than between the ventricular outlets, however, the chances of successfully transferring the aortic infundibulum into the left ventricle are considerably reduced.

Thus far, we have devoted attention exclusively to the segmental anatomy of transposition. There is further variation to be found in terms of arterial relationships and infundibular anatomy. These variations do not alter the intracardiac anatomy, and are of relatively minor surgical significance. For example, the aorta is usually anterior and to the right in transposition (Figure 9.2.20), but as already discussed, the aorta may be anterior and to the left. This is the rule when the atrial chambers are mirror imaged (Figure 9.2.4), but left sided and transposed aortas can also be encountered when there is usual atrial arrangement (Figure 9.2.3). In even rarer cases, the aorta can be posterior and to the right of the pulmonary trunk (Figure 9.2.21). This arrangement produces the paradoxical situation in which, although the arterial trunks are normally related, they remain discordantly connected. It was description of hearts of this type that spawned the polemic between those using connections as opposed to relations as the phenotypic feature of 'transposition'.[14] The different relationships, however, do not alter the basic anatomy. They do serve to show why it is inadvisable to use the term 'd-transposition' as a unifying terminology. It makes little sense to use this term for description of the patient in whom the aorta is left sided when there is usual atrial arrangement (Figure 9.2.3). There are, furthermore, some clues to associated lesions to be drawn from these unexpected arterial relationships. When the aorta is left sided with usual atrial arrangement,[7] any co-existing ventricular septal defect is frequently doubly committed and juxta-arterial. This arrangement is convenient for direct connection of the aorta to the left ventricle. When the aorta is posterior

9.2 Discordant Ventriculo-Arterial Connections

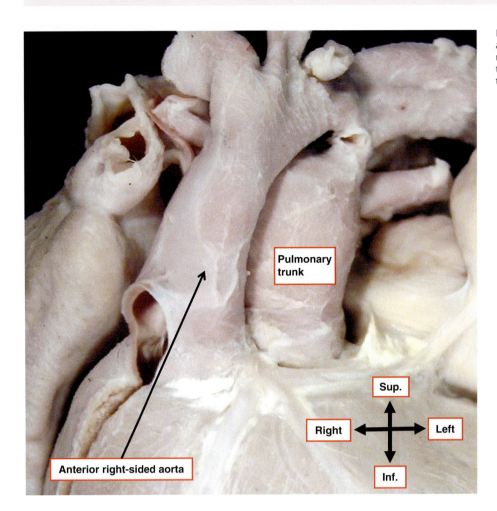

Figure 9.2.20 This heart is shown in anatomical orientation, demonstrating the usual relationship of the aorta in the setting of transposition, namely anterior and to the right of the pulmonary trunk.

and the arterial trunks are normally related, there is usually a subpulmonary infundibulum, with the leaflets of the aortic valve in fibrous continuity with the anterior leaflet of the mitral valve through the roof of a perimembranous septal defect.[15] This unusual anatomy can create difficulty both at initial diagnosis and at subsequent surgery. Variations in infundibular morphology in themselves are unlikely to give problems. The expected subaortic muscular infundibulum in the right ventricle is most frequently encountered along with fibrous continuity between the leaflets of the pulmonary and mitral valves in the left ventricle. Rarely, there may be a complete muscular infundibulum in both ventricles (Figure 9.2.22). Even more rarely, as described above, there may be a subpulmonary infundibulum with continuity between the leaflets of the aortic and mitral valves, particularly when the discordantly connected aorta is in posterior position.

The feature currently of greatest surgical importance in patients with transposition is the morphology of the coronary arteries. This is because of the universal acceptance of the arterial switch procedure as the surgical treatment of choice. This operation involves transecting the ascending aorta and pulmonary trunk, and reconnecting them to their morphologically appropriate ventricles. The significant morphological feature is that, with exceedingly rare exceptions, the coronary arteries arise from the aortic sinuses that are adjacent to the pulmonary trunk (Figure 9.2.23). When performing the arterial switch, therefore, the surgeon is required to transfer the origins of the coronary arteries across a relatively short distance (Figure 9.2.24). This holds true irrespective of the relationship of the aorta to the pulmonary trunk.

The variable relationships between the aorta and the pulmonary trunk, however, produce problems in naming the aortic sinuses and, hence, the origin of the coronary arteries. Truly formidable conventions are created if attempts are made to catalogue each and every pattern,[16] while use of simple alphabetic codes[17] is self-evidently procrustean. As suggested by the group from Leiden,[18] it is best to name the aortic sinuses as viewed from the stance of the observer standing in the non-adjacent sinus of the aorta and looking towards the pulmonary trunk (Figure 9.2.25). One sinus is then always to the observer's right hand. This is designated as sinus #1. The other sinus is to the left hand, and is called sinus #2. The three major coronary arteries can arise from either of these sinuses, giving only eight potential patterns of sinusal origin, including the arrangements in which both arteries arise from the same aortic sinus (Figure 9.2.26). All eight have now been seen in the setting of transposition.[19] Transfer of the arteries during the switch procedure can be compromised by an anomalous course of the coronary arteries themselves in relation to the vascular pedicle (Figure 9.2.27), albeit that such variations can be suitably accommodated by appropriate surgical technique.[20] Transfer can be particularly difficult, however, in the

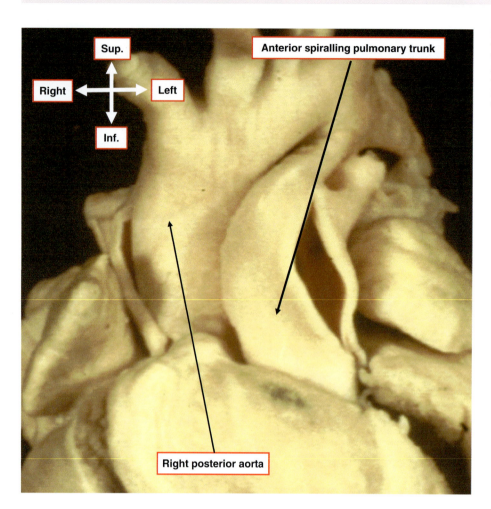

Figure 9.2.21 In this specimen of transposition, shown in anatomical orientation from the front, the aorta is positioned posteriorly and rightward position relative to the pulmonary trunk, with spiralling of the arterial trunks. This is normal relations of the arterial trunks, but still with discordant ventriculo-arterial connections.

exceedingly rare circumstance in which a coronary artery arises from the non-adjacent sinus.[21] This may require the use of a graft so as to connect the artery to the new aortic root.

It is the intramural course of the origin of the coronary artery across a valvar commissure (Figure 9.2.28), or through the aortic wall because of high origin (Figures 9.2.28, 9.2.29), which creates greater problems.[22] These can also now be resolved with appropriate surgical technique.[23] The origin of the artery to the sinus node can be very close to the origin of one coronary artery from an aortic sinus, or the sinus nodal artery can originate separately from the sinus. Also of note is mismatch between the commissures of the aortic and pulmonary valves (Figure 9.2.30).[24] Despite all these anatomical variations, surgeons now find it possible to perform the arterial switch procedure with remarkable success.

Congenitally Corrected Transposition

The combination of discordant atrioventricular and ventriculo-arterial connections (Figure 9.2.2) is well described as congenitally corrected transposition. When defined in this fashion, as with transposition itself (Figure 9.2.1)), the entity can exist with the atrial chambers in their usual arrangement (Figure 9.2.31), or in mirror-imaged position (Figures 9.2.32–9.2.34). It cannot exist when there is isomerism of the atrial appendages, since then the atrioventricular connections will be mixed, rather than discordant. Hearts with isomeric appendages, nonetheless, can have left-hand ventricular topology in association with discordant ventriculo-arterial connections (see Chapter 11).

The complexities of congenitally corrected transposition reflect the fact that, with usual atrial arrangement, there is malalignment between the inlet part of the muscular ventricular septum and the atrial septum. These two septal structures are in line at the crux but, when traced forward, they diverge markedly. This produces a gap, into which is wedged the subpulmonary outflow tract from the morphologically left ventricle (Figure 9.2.35). This abnormal feature accounts for perhaps the most important surgical aspect of congenitally corrected transposition, namely the unusual and unexpected disposition of the atrioventricular conduction tissues.[25] Because of the septal malalignment, it is not possible for the normal atrioventricular node, positioned at the apex of the triangle of Koch, to penetrate through the fibrous atrioventricular junction and make contact with the ventricular conduction tissues. Instead, it is an anomalous atrioventricular node, found in an antero-lateral position (Figure 9.2.36), which gives rise to the penetrating atrioventricular bundle. The bundle penetrates the insulating plane of the atrioventricular junction lateral to the area of fibrous continuity between the leaflets of the pulmonary and mitral valves. A long non-branching bundle then runs around the anterior quadrants of the

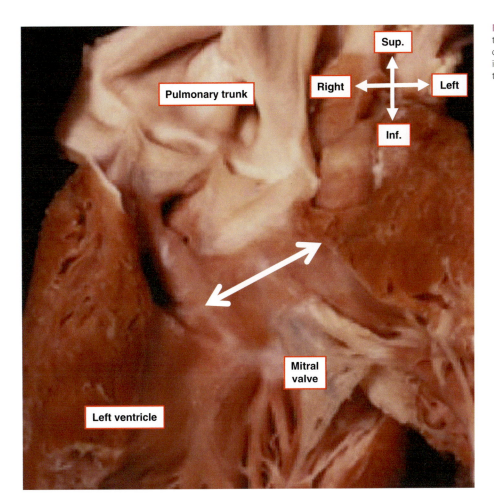

Figure 9.2.22 This heart, photographed through the left ventricle in anatomical orientation, shows a large subpulmonary infundibulum (double-headed arrow) separating the leaflets of the pulmonary and mitral valves.

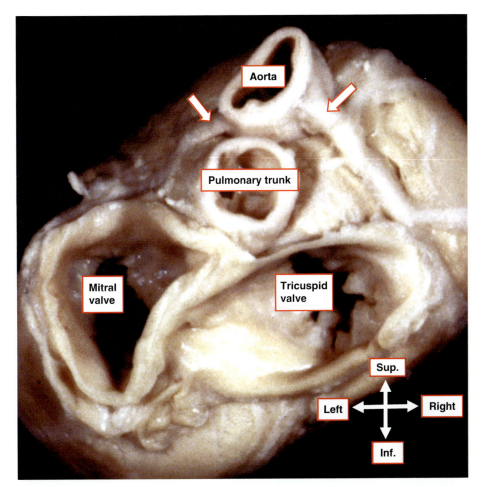

Figure 9.2.23 In this heart, the short axis is viewed from above in anatomical orientation, the atrial myocardium and the arterial trunks having been removed. The ventriculo-arterial connections are discordant. The dissection shows how the coronary arteries (red-bordered arrows) arise from the two aortic sinuses that are adjacent to the pulmonary trunk.

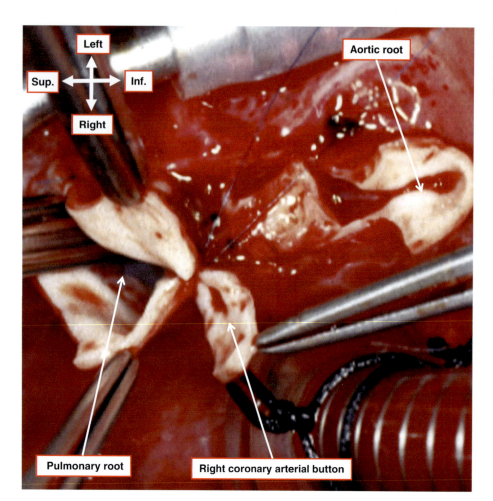

Figure 9.2.24 The picture, taken in the operating room, shows the short distance required to transfer a button supporting one of the coronary arteries from the old aortic to the old pulmonary root during the arterial switch procedure.

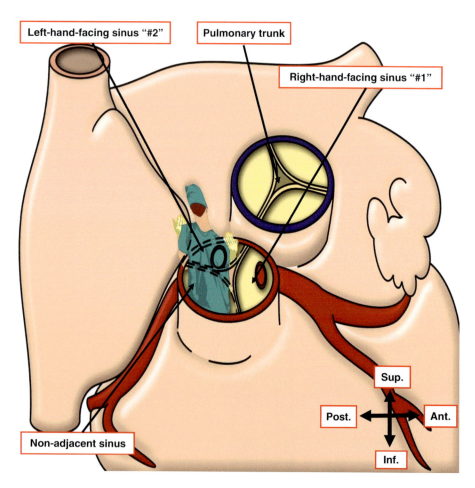

Figure 9.2.25 The cartoon shows how the two aortic sinuses that face the pulmonary trunk can always be described accurately as being to the surgeon's left hand or right hand, when standing in the non-adjacent sinus of the aorta and looking towards the pulmonary trunk, irrespective of the relationships of the arterial trunks. Conventionally, the sinus to the right hand is described as being #1, while that to the left hand is designated as being #2.

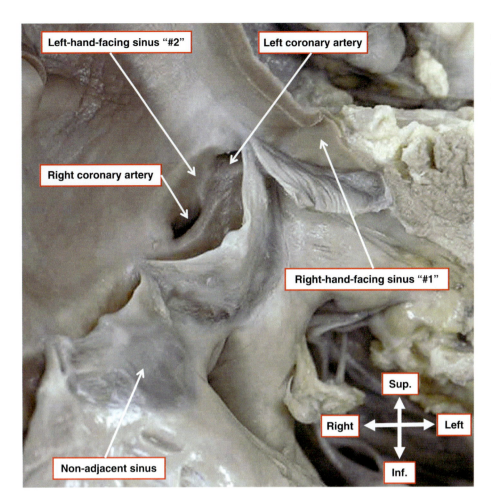

Figure 9.2.26 In this heart from a patient with transposition, the aortic root has been open and is viewed from the front. Both of the coronary arteries arise from the left-hand-facing sinus, or sinus #2. The main stem of the left coronary artery was noted to take an intramural course as it extended towards the left atrioventricular and interventricular grooves.

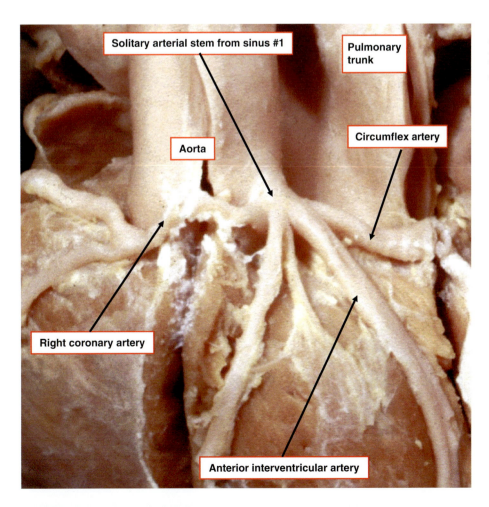

Figure 9.2.27 In this heart, photographed in anatomical orientation from the front, the right and the left coronary arteries arise from a solitary vessel, with the right coronary and the circumflex arteries then passing in front of the arterial pedicle.

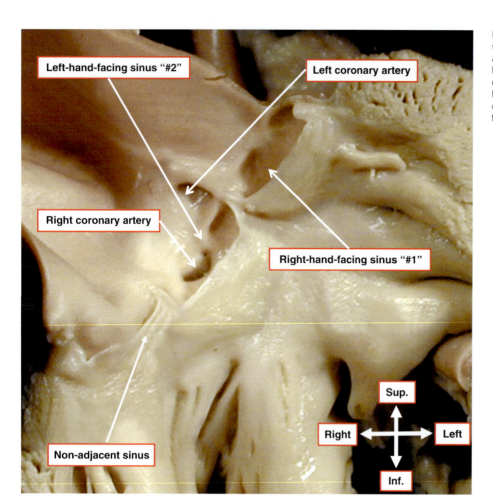

Figure 9.2.28 In this heart, as in the specimen shown in Figure 9.2.26, both coronary arteries arise within the left-hand-facing sinus. In this heart, the orifice of the main stem of the left coronary artery is above the sinutubular junction. Having exited from the aortic root, the artery courses between the arterial trunks in intramural fashion (see Figure 9.2.30).

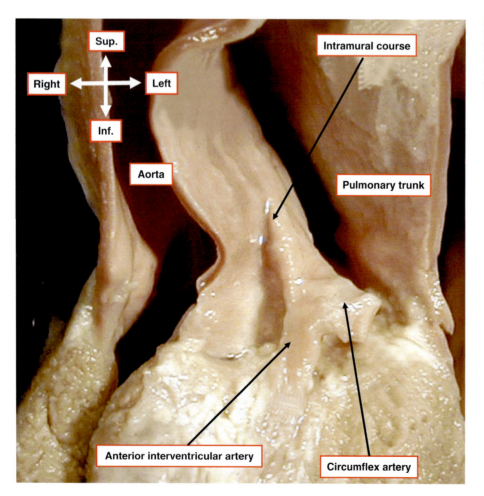

Figure 9.2.29 The heart shown in Figure 9.2.28 is photographed from the left side, showing how the main stem of the left coronary artery is embedded within the wall of the aorta as it runs towards the anterior surface of the heart, where it divides into its circumflex and anterior interventricular branches.

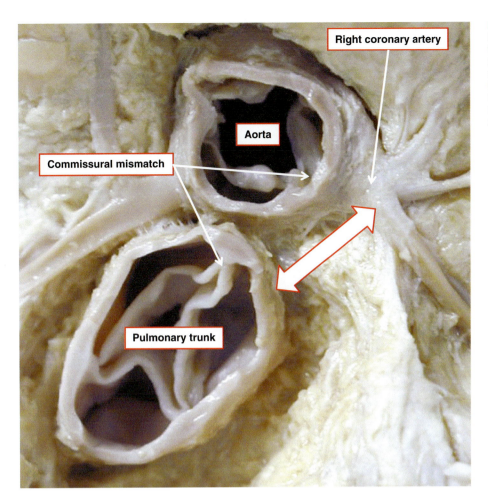

Figure 9.2.30 In this heart with transposition, in which the atrial myocardium and the arterial trunks have been removed, the heart being photographed from the atrial aspect, there is mismatch between the zones of apposition of the leaflets of the aortic and pulmonary valves. Because of this, the distance for transfer of the right coronary artery is increased (double-headed red-bordered arrow).

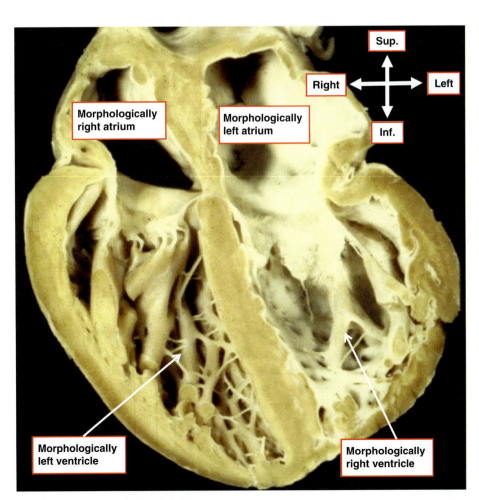

Figure 9.2.31 The heart with congenitally corrected transposition in the setting of usual atrial arrangement has been sectioned in four-chamber fashion to show the discordant atrioventricular connections.

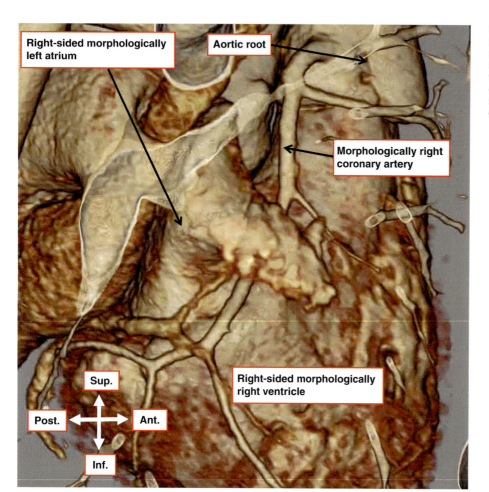

Figure 9.2.32 The computed tomographic angiogram, viewed from the right side, shows a right-sided morphologically left atrium that is connected to a right-sided morphologically right ventricle, which then supports the aorta. This is congenitally corrected transposition in the setting of mirror-imaged arrangement of the organs.

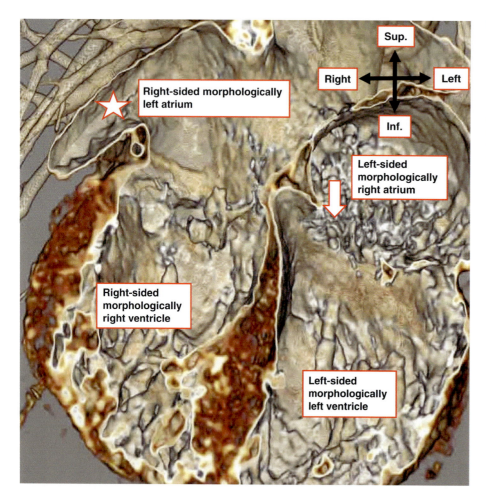

Figure 9.2.33 The image shows the four-chamber cut through the computed tomographic angiographic dataset shown in Figure 9.2.32. The narrow neck of the right-sided atrial appendage (star) shows that it has left morphology, while the other appendage has pectinate muscles extending to the crux (red-bordered white arrow), confirming the left-sided location of the morphologically right atrium. The nature of the apical trabeculations confirm that the atrial chambers are connected to inappropriate morphological ventricles.

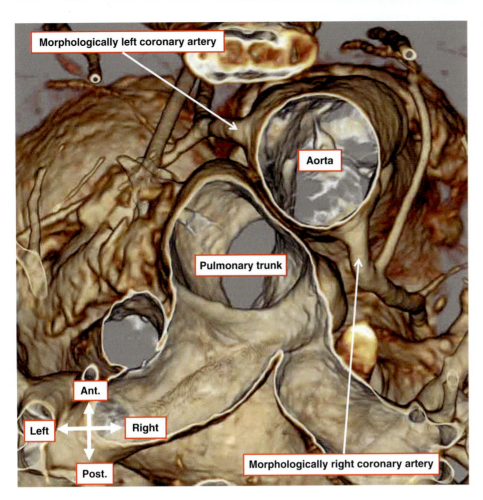

Figure 9.2.34 The short-axis cut through the dataset created from the computed tomographic angiograms shown in Figures 9.2.32 and 9.2.33 shows the right-sided and anterior location of the aorta relative to the pulmonary trunk. This shows that 'd-transposition' can also be congenitally corrected. The appropriate segmental notation is transposition {I,D,D}. Note the normal position of the coronary arteries because of the right-handed ventricular topology that is a feature of this segmental combination.

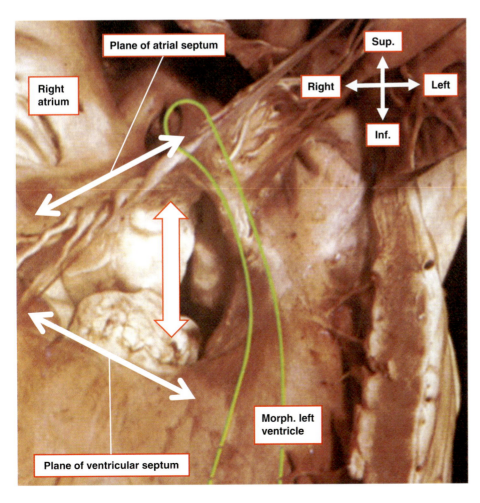

Figure 9.2.35 This specimen with congenitally corrected transposition, viewed in anatomical orientation from the morphologically left ventricle, shows the malalignment between the atrial and ventricular septal structures (white double-headed arrows), with the subpulmonary outflow tract wedged into this gap (red-bordered double-headed arrow). The site of the atrioventricular conduction axis has been superimposed in green.

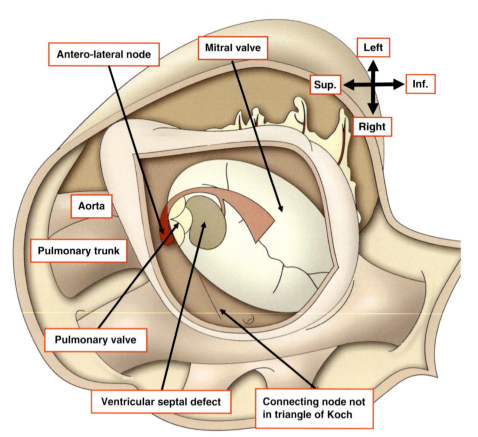

Figure 9.2.36 The drawing shows the view of the morphologically mitral valve in congenitally corrected transposition as seen by the surgeon working through a right atriotomy. The locations of the atrioventricular node and the conduction axis have been marked in red. There is a perimembranous ventricular septal defect.

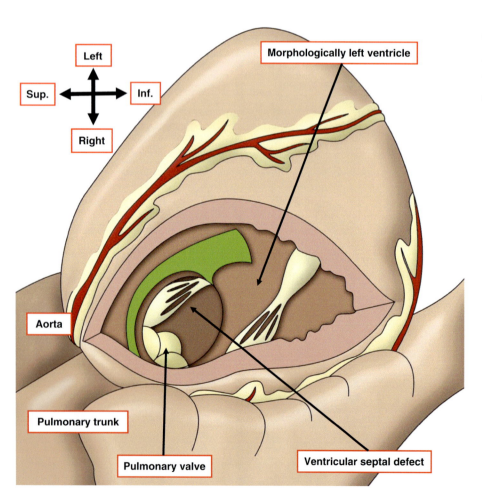

Figure 9.2.37 In this drawing, we show the view of a perimembranous ventricular septal defect in congenitally corrected transposition as would be seen by the surgeon working through a generous incision in the right-sided morphologically left ventricle. The course of the conduction axis has been marked in green.

9.2 Discordant Ventriculo-Arterial Connections

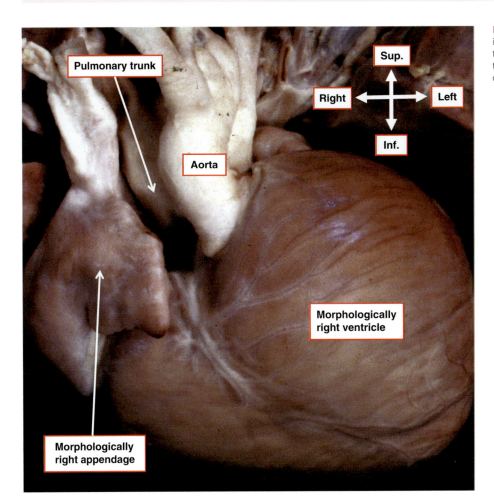

Figure 9.2.38 This specimen is photographed in anatomical orientation from the front, showing the usual left-sided location of the aorta relative to the pulmonary trunk in patients with congenitally corrected transposition.

subpulmonary outflow tract, crossing the characteristic anterior recess of the morphologically left ventricle, before descending onto the muscular ventricular septum (Figure 9.2.37). Having branched, the fan-like left branch is distributed in the right-sided morphologically left ventricle, while the cord-like right branch of the bundle penetrates the septum to reach the left-sided morphologically right ventricle. The discordantly connected aorta arises from this morphologically right ventricle, typically above a complete muscular infundibulum, and usually in a left-sided position (Figure 9.2.38). When congenitally corrected transposition is found in the mirror-imaged variant, however, it is the rule for the aorta to be located in anterior and right-sided position (Figure 9.2.34). This is why it is less than ideal to use d-transposition as an alternative term for regular transposition. When the right-sided aorta is found in the setting of congenitally corrected transposition, the correct segmental notation is transposition {I,D,D}.

When congenitally corrected transposition exists without any other anomaly, the circulation of the blood is normal. This situation is very much the exception. Usually, one or more of three associated lesions are found. These are a ventricular septal defect, pulmonary stenosis, or anomalies of the left-sided atrioventricular valve.[4] It is these associated lesions that require surgical treatment.

A ventricular septal defect is present in up to three-quarters of patients. As in the patient with concordant atrioventricular connections, it may be perimembranous, muscular, or juxta-arterial (Figure 9.2.39). Usually, it is of the perimembranous type. When viewed from the left ventricle, it usually seems to open between the ventricular inlets (Figure 9.2.40). As was emphasized by the group from Enfant Malades Hospital in Paris, nonetheless, when assessing the geography of ventricular septal defects, they should be viewed from the stance of the morphologically right ventricle.[26] When viewed from the morphologically left side, because of the wedged position of the pulmonary valve, the pulmonary trunk tends to override the defect (Figure 9.2.40). When seen from the right atrium, perimembranous defects are shielded by the superior end of the zone of apposition between the leaflets of the right-sided morphologically mitral valve (Figure 9.2.41). The abnormal position of the atrioventricular node and the non-branching atrioventricular bundle must be borne in mind when closing the defect. The atrioventricular bundle arises from the anomalous antero-lateral node, penetrates the area of pulmonary–mitral valvar continuity, and then runs around the subpulmonary outflow tract to descend on the antero-superior margin of the defect (Figure 9.2.42).

The safest way of closing the defect without damaging the conduction system is to place sutures from the left-sided morphologically right ventricular aspect (Figure 9.2.42).[27] Perimembranous defects can extend to become juxta-arterial. They are then roofed by the conjoined leaflets of the aortic and

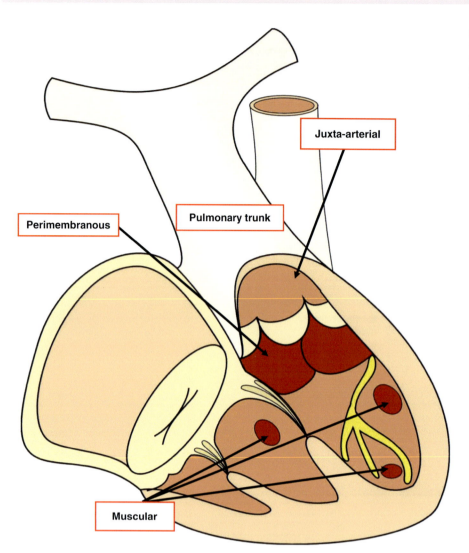

Figure 9.2.39 The cartoon shows that, in congenitally corrected transposition as in the otherwise normal heart, the ventricular septal defect can be perimembranous, muscular, or juxta-arterial. In congenitally corrected transposition, however, the conduction axis, shown in bright yellow, takes a grossly abnormal course relative to the defects.

pulmonary valves (Figure 9.2.43). When the defect is perimembranous and juxta-arterial, the conduction tissue remains in anterior position. In some patients, however, there can be a muscular inferior rim between the leaflets of the tricuspid and mitral valves. It is still likely that the conduction tissue remains in antero-superior position relative to the defect.

As with transposition, any of the lesions that produce obstruction of the left ventricular outflow tract will produce pulmonary stenosis when the transposition is congenitally corrected (Figure 9.2.44). Valvar stenosis in isolation is rare, but frequently co-exists with subvalvar obstructive lesions. Particularly significant in this respect are fibrous tissue tags (Figure 9.2.45). Fibrous diaphragmatic lesions (Figure 9.2.46), or muscular obstruction, are also encountered.[28] The overwhelming consideration in all of these types of stenosis is the presence of the non-branching bundle running around the anterior quadrants of the outflow tract. Apart from tissue tags, this relationship makes it very difficult to resect these various lesions. Placement of a conduit may be the safest means of avoiding postoperative heart block.

Ebstein's malformation is the lesion that most frequently afflicts the left-sided morphologically tricuspid valve, involving rotational displacement of the septal and mural leaflets (Figure 9.2.47). Only rarely is the inlet part of the ventricle dilated and thinned, as occurs so frequently in Ebstein's malformation with concordant atrioventricular connections. Should replacement of the valve become necessary, the location of the conduction tissues in the right-sided atrioventricular junction takes them out of the area of danger.

The other anomaly that affects the left valve, and that can also affect the right valve,[29] is straddling of its tension apparatus and overriding of the valvar orifice (Figure 9.2.48). These anomalies do not alter the origin of the conduction tissues from an antero-lateral node, but will markedly increase the risks of surgery. Indeed, in the presence of straddling atrioventricular valves, some may opt for functionally univentricular rather than biventricular surgical correction. Those who use biventricular correction have observed disappointing results subsequent to simple correction of the associated lesions, because these manoeuvres leave the morphologically right ventricle supporting the systemic circulation. Because of this, the trend is now to correct the patients using the so-called double switch procedure, combining atrial redirection with either an arterial switch[30] or use of an interventricular tunnel to the aorta, placing a conduit from the morphologically right

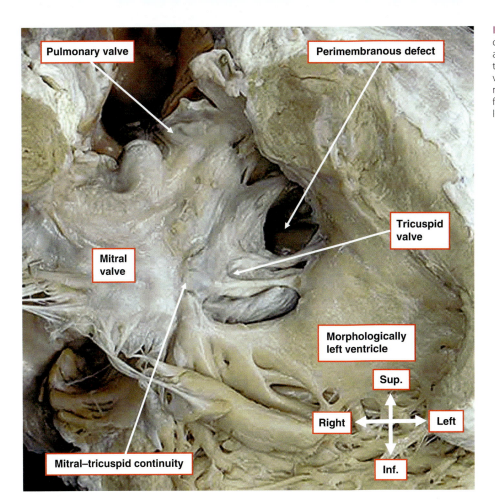

Figure 9.2.40 This view of a specimen with congenitally corrected transposition, shown in anatomical orientation from the front, illustrates the relationships of a perimembranous ventricular septal defect as seen from the morphologically left ventricle. Its phenotypic feature is the fibrous continuity between the leaflets of the mitral and tricuspid valves.

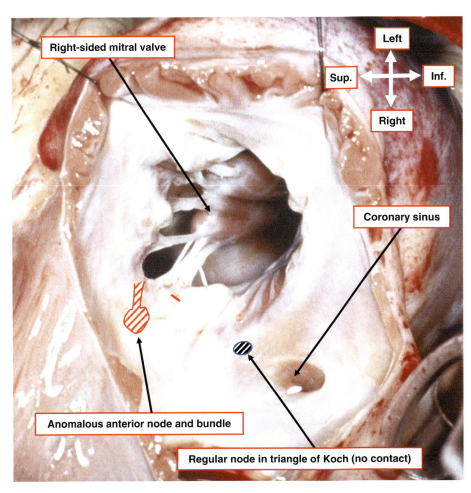

Figure 9.2.41 This view of a perimembranous inlet ventricular septal defect in congenitally corrected transposition taken in the operating room, as seen through the right-sided morphologically mitral valve, shows how the defect and the subpulmonary outflow tract are shielded behind the antero-septal commissure of the valve. The red cross-hatched area shows the location of the connecting atrioventricular node, with the non-connecting regular node shown by the blue cross-hatched oval. Reproduced by kind permission of Dr Jan Quaegebeur, Columbia University, New York.

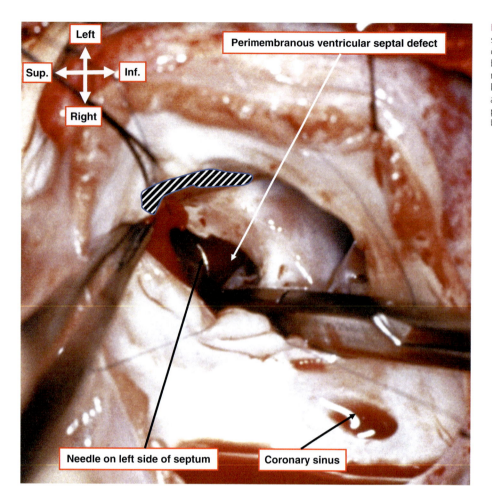

Figure 9.2.42 This further view of the patient shown in Figure 9.2.41 illustrates how the axis of conduction tissue (hatched area) can be avoided by placing sutures through the defect on its morphologically right ventricular aspect, which is left sided when, as in this patient, there was usual atrial arrangement. Reproduced by kind permission of Dr Jan Quaegebeur, Columbia University, New York.

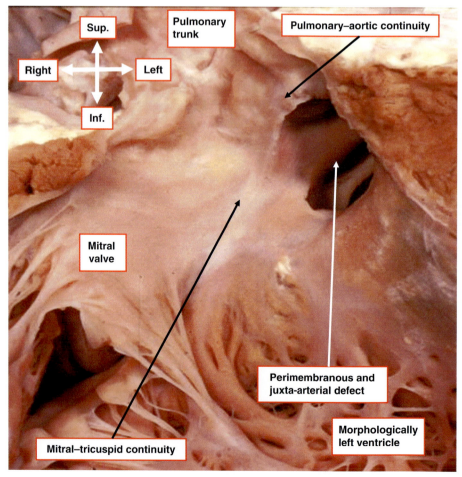

Figure 9.2.43 In this specimen, viewed in anatomical orientation, the perimembranous ventricular septal defect extends to become juxta-arterial, being roofed by fibrous continuity between the leaflets of the aortic and pulmonary valves.

9.2 Discordant Ventriculo-Arterial Connections

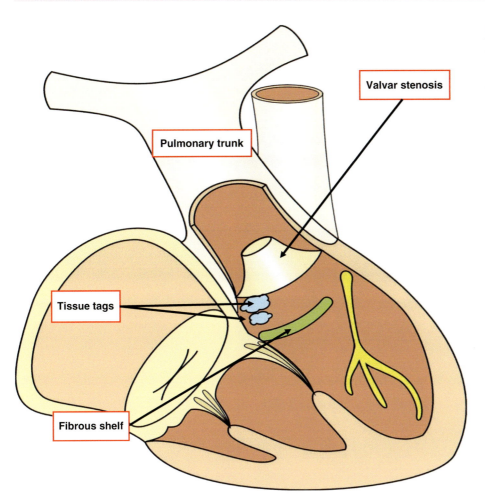

Figure 9.2.44 The drawing shows the lesions that can produce subpulmonary obstruction in the setting of congenitally corrected transposition. Note the anterior position of the conduction axis, shown in yellow. As with transposition, the same lesions produce subaortic obstruction in the setting of concordant ventriculo-arterial connections.

ventricle to the pulmonary atrium.[31] This also makes it possible to correct patients with co-existing pulmonary atresia.

Some patients with discordant atrioventricular connections will have ventriculo-arterial connections other than discordant ones. We will discuss the options for double outlet from the morphologically right ventricle in Chapter 9.3, but our emphasis there will be on patients with concordant atrioventricular connections. The variability to be described can also be found when the atrioventricular connections are discordant, but then the atrioventricular conduction axis will arise from an anterolateral atrioventricular node, as described for congenitally corrected transposition. In patients with discordant atrioventricular connections and double outlet right ventricle, nonetheless, it is also possible to find a sling of conduction tissue running along the crest of the muscular ventricular septum and joining anterior and regular atrioventricular nodes. This possibility should be borne in mind for all patients having discordant atrioventricular connections and double outlet from the morphologically right ventricle.

Some patients also have single outlet in association with discordant atrioventricular connections, most frequently because of pulmonary atresia (Figure 9.2.49). In this situation, there is typically a perimembranous ventricular septal defect. If the defect is large, then, as we have discussed, it is possible to achieve biventricular repair by channelling the morphologically left ventricle to the aorta, placing a conduit from the morphologically right ventricle to the pulmonary arteries, and performing an atrial redirection procedure.[31] The defect, however, is not always large enough to permit channelling of the morphologically left ventricle to the aorta (Figure 9.2.50). If restrictive, the decision must be made as to whether the defect can be enlarged, or whether the better option is to create the Fontan circulation. The antero-cephalad location of the atrioventricular conduction axis in the setting can make enlargement of the defect a daunting procedure (Figure 9.2.50). Exceedingly rarely, it is possible to find pulmonary atresia with an intact ventricular septum and an imperforate right-sided atrioventricular valve. When seen from the right atrium (Figure 9.2.51), the arrangement can be indistinguishable from pulmonary atresia with intact ventricular septum with concordant atrioventricular connections (see Chapter 8.5). The significant difference is that, unlike regular pulmonary atresia with intact ventricular septum, it is the morphologically right ventricle that must drive the systemic circulation when the atrioventricular connections are discordant (Figure 9.2.52). Aortic atresia, or common arterial trunk, can also rarely be found with discordant atrioventricular connections. A more important combination is that found

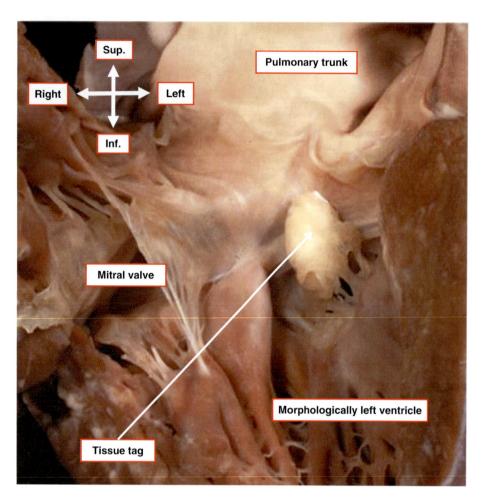

Figure 9.2.45 In this specimen, viewed in anatomical orientation through the morphologically left ventricle, a fibrous tissue tag derived from the septal leaflet of the left-sided morphologically tricuspid valve herniates into the subpulmonary outflow tract.

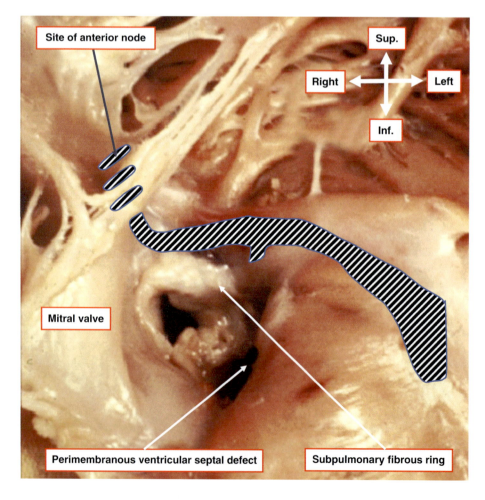

Figure 9.2.46 In this specimen, seen in anatomical orientation through the morphologically left ventricle, a fibrous shelf produces subpulmonary obstruction in presence of a perimembranous ventricular septal defect. The site of the axis of atrioventricular conduction tissue is shown by the hatched area.

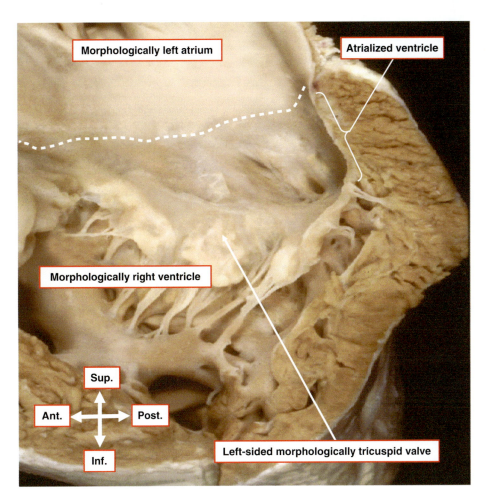

Figure 9.2.47 This specimen with congenitally corrected transposition, seen in anatomical orientation from the left side, shows Ebstein's malformation of the left-sided morphologically tricuspid valve. There is no thinning of the musculature of the inlet component of the morphologically right ventricle. The white dotted line shows the location of the atrioventricular junction.

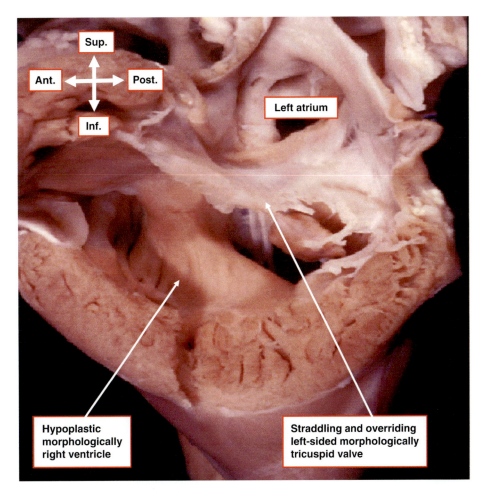

Figure 9.2.48 In this heart with congenitally corrected transposition, viewed in anatomical orientation from the left-sided morphologically right ventricle, there is straddling and overriding of the left-sided morphologically tricuspid valve. Note the hypoplastic nature of the morphologically right ventricle.

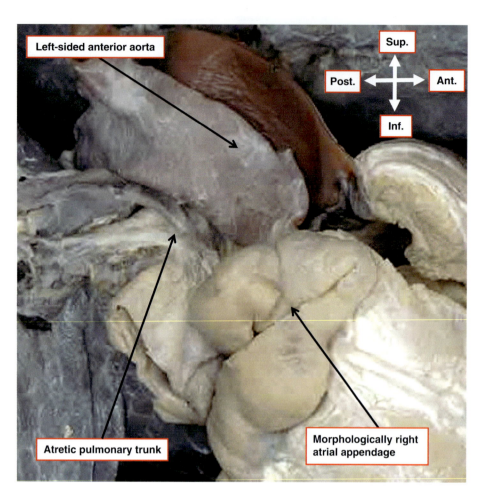

Figure 9.2.49 The image shows the base of the heart. The atretic pulmonary trunk is posterior and right-sided relative to the aorta. The pulmonary arteries were fed through a persistently patent arterial duct.

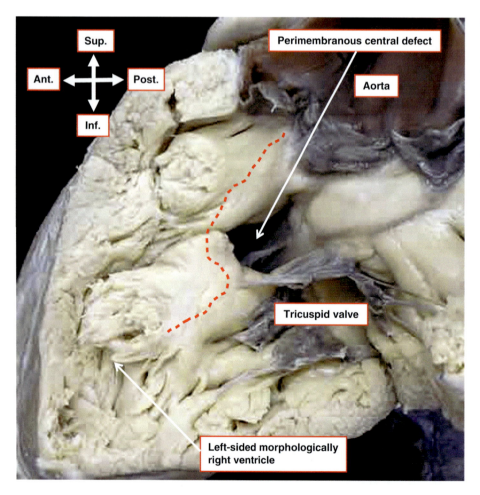

Figure 9.2.50 The image shows the left-sided ventricle from the heart illustrated in Figure 9.2.49. The atrioventricular connections are discordant, and the aorta is supported by the left-sided morphologically right ventricle. The perimembranous ventricular septal defect is restrictive. The dashed red line shows the course of the atrioventricular conduction axis, which is carried on the right side of the ventricular septum. Its antero-cephalad location relative to the defect would make enlargement difficult, if not impossible, to achieve without producing atrioventricular block if the decision was made to attempt biventricular repair by channelling the morphologically left ventricle to the aorta, and then performing an atrial redirection procedure.

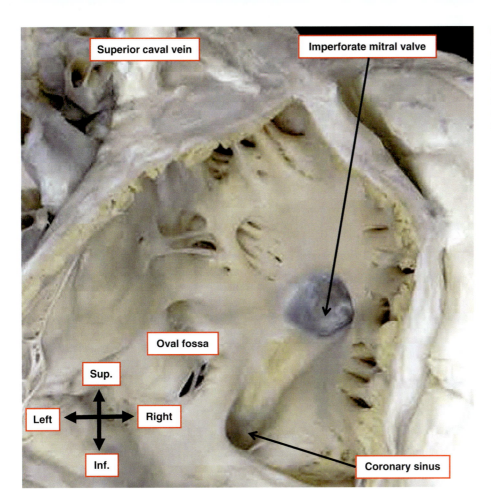

Figure 9.2.51 The morphologically right atrium is photographed from above and behind to reveal the presence of an imperforate atrioventricular valve. When viewed in isolation, it is not possible to distinguish the morphological nature of the valve. As shown in Figure 9.2.52, however, the atrioventricular connections were discordant, so the valvar membrane is morphologically mitral.

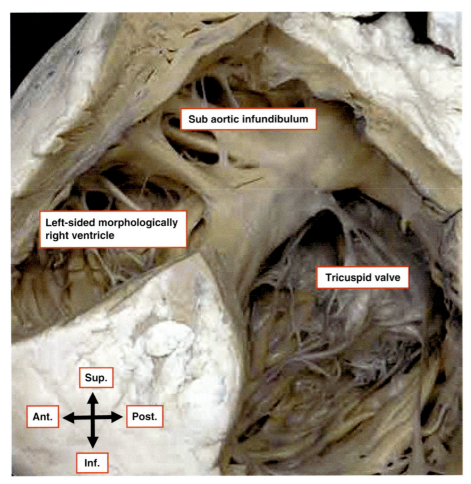

Figure 9.2.52 The image shows the left-sided ventricle in the heart shown also in Figure 9.2.51. The ventricle is coarsely trabeculated, and receives the morphologically tricuspid valve. The heart had pulmonary atresia with intact ventricular septum, but in the setting of discordant atrioventricular and ventriculo-arterial connections.

with concordant ventriculo-arterial connections. We will discuss this arrangement in greater detail in Chapter 9.5. The significant surgical feature is that the combination produces the ideal situation for employment of an atrial redirection procedure, since this restores the morphologically left ventricle to pumping the systemic circulation.

References Cited

1. Jaggers JJ, Cameron DE, Herlong JR, Ungerleider RM. Congenital Heart Surgery Nomenclature and Database Project: transposition of the great arteries. *Ann Thor Surg* 2000; **69**: 205–235.
2. Wilkinson JL, Cochrane AD, Karl TR. Congenital Heart Surgery Nomenclature and Database Project: corrected (discordant) transposition of the great arteries (and related malformations). *Ann Thor Surg* 2000; **69**: 236–248.
3. Van Praagh R. What is congenitally corrected transposition? *NEJM* 1970; **282**: 1097–1098.
4. Van Praagh R. Transposition of the great arteries II. Transposition clarified. *Am J Cardiol* 1971; **28**: 739–741.
5. Walters HL III, Mavroudis C, Tchervenkov CI, et al. Congenital heart surgery nomenclature and database project: double outlet right ventricle. *Ann Thor Surg* 2000; **69**: 249–263.
6. Van Mierop LHS. Transposition of the great arteries. Clarification or further confusion? Editorial. *Am J Cardiol* 1971; **28**: 735–738.
7. Houyel L, Van Praagh R, Lacour-Gayet F, et al. Transposition of the great arteries {S, D, L}: pathologic anatomy, diagnosis, and surgical management of a newly recognized complex. *J Thorac Cardiovasc Surg* 1995; **110**: 613–624.
8. Isaacson R, Titus JL, Merideth J, Feldt RH, McGoon DC. Apparent interruption of atrial conduction pathways after surgical repair of transposition of the great arteries. *Am J Cardiol* 1972; **30**: 533–535.
9. Ullal RR, Anderson RH, Lincoln C. Mustard's operation modified to avoid dysrhythmias and pulmonary and systemic venous obstruction. *J Thorac Cardiovasc Surg* 1979; **78**: 431–439.
10. Spicer DE, Anderson RH, Backer CL. Clarifying the surgical morphology of inlet ventricular septal defects. *Ann Thor Surg* 2013; **95**: 236–241.
11. Nikaidoh H. Nikaidoh procedure: a perspective. *Eur J Cardio-Thorac Surg* 2016; **50**: 1001–1005.
12. Lecompte Y. Reparation a l'etage ventriculaire – the REV procedure: technique and clinical results. *Cardiol Young* 1991; **1**: 63–70.
13. Prandstetter C, Tulzer A, Mair R, Sames-Dolzer E, Tulzer G. Effects of surgical en bloc rotation of the arterial trunk on the conduction system in children with transposition of the great arteries, ventricular septal defect and pulmonary stenosis. *Cardiol Young* 2016; **26**: 516–520.
14. Van Praagh R, Pérez-Treviño C, López-Cuellar M, et al. Transposition of the great arteries with posterior aorta, anterior pulmonary artery, subpulmonary conus and fibrous continuity between aortic and atrioventricular valves. *Am J Cardiol* 1971; **28**: 621–623.
15. Wilkinson JL, Arnold R, Anderson RH, Acerete F. 'Posterior' transposition reconsidered. *Br Heart J* 1975; **37**: 757–766.
16. Shaher RM, Puddu GC. Coronary arterial anatomy in complete transposition of the great arteries. *Am J Cardiol* 1966; **17**: 355–361.
17. Yacoub MH, Radley-Smith R. Anatomy of the coronary arteries in transposition of the great arteries and methods for their transfer in anatomical correction. *Thorax* 1978; **33**: 418–424.
18. Gittenberger-de-Groot AC, Sauer U, Oppenheimer-Dekker A, Quaegebeur J. Coronary arterial anatomy in transposition of the great arteries: a morphologic study. *Pediatr Cardiol* 1983; **4**: 15–24.
19. Michalak KW, Wernovsky G, Moll M, Anderson RH. The black swan: unique coronary arterial anatomy observed in a patient with transposition. *J Thorac Cardiovasc Surg* 2019; **158**: e107–109.
20. Lacour-Gayet F, Anderson RH. A uniform surgical technique for transfer of both simple and complex patterns of the coronary arteries during the arterial switch procedure. *Cardiol Young* 2005; **15** (Suppl.1): 93–101.
21. Konstantinov IE, Fricke TA, d'Udekem Y, Radford DJ. Translocation of a single coronary artery from the nonfacing sinus in the arterial switch operation: long-term patency of the interposition graft. *J Thorac Cardiovasc Surg* 2010; **140**: 1193–1194.
22. Gittenberger-de Groot AC, Sauer U, Quaegebeur J. Aortic intramural coronary artery in three hearts with transposition of the great arteries. *J Thorac Cardiovasc Surg* 1986; **91**: 566–571.
23. Asou T, Karl TR, Pawade A, Mee RB. Arterial switch: translocation of the intramural coronary artery. *Ann Thorac Surg* 1994; **57**: 461–465.
24. Massoudy P, Baltalarli A, de Leval MR, et al. Anatomic variability in coronary arterial distribution with regard to the arterial switch procedure. *Circulation* 2002; **106**: 1980–1984.
25. Anderson RH, Becker AE, Arnold R, Wilkinson JL. The conducting tissues in congenitally corrected transposition. *Circulation* 1974; **50**: 911–923.
26. Arribard N, Mostefa Kara M, Hascoët S, et al. Congenitally corrected transposition of the great arteries: is it really a transposition? An anatomical study of the right ventricular septal surface. *J Anat* 2020; **236**: 325–333.
27. De Leval M, Bastos P, Stark J, et al. Surgical technique to reduce the risks of heart block following closure of ventricular septal defect in atrioventricular discordance. *J Thorac Cardiovasc Surg* 1979; **78**: 515–526.
28. Anderson RH, Becker AE, Gerlis LM. The pulmonary outflow tract in classically corrected transposition. *J Thorac Cardiovasc Surg* 1975; **69**: 747–757.
29. Becker AE, Ho SY, Caruso G, Milo S, Anderson RH. Straddling right atrioventricular valves in atrioventricular discordance. *Circulation* 1980; **61**: 1133–1141.
30. Ilbawi MN, DeLeon SY, Backer CL, et al. An alternative approach to the surgical management for physiologically corrected transposition with ventricular septal defect and pulmonary stenosis or atresia. *J Thorac Cardiovasc Surg* 1990; **100**: 410–415.
31. Imai Y, Sawatori K, Hoshino S, et al. Ventricular function after anatomic repair in patients with atrioventricular discordance. *J Thorac Cardiovasc Surg* 1994; **107**: 1272–1283.

Chapter 9.3 Double Outlet Ventricle

As we discussed in Chapter 9.2, hearts with double outlet from the right ventricle were initially considered to represent a partial form of 'transposition', on the basis that only the aortic root had been transposed across the septum.[1] Hearts with double outlet from the left ventricle had initially been considered an embryological impossibility. The finding of a heart with both arterial trunks arising from the left ventricle when the ventricular septum was intact proved that the lesions do exist, albeit being very rare.[2] It is now accepted that hearts with double outlet ventricle constitute a specific type of ventriculo-arterial connection. As we will see, lesions with markedly varied morphology make up the group. The hearts within the group, however, have been the source of multiple controversies. For quite some time, it was argued that only hearts with bilateral infundibulums, or conuses, should be included as examples of double outlet right ventricle. The reason underscoring this definition was to distinguish between the hearts having a subaortic defect in the setting of double outlet and those with tetralogy of Fallot.[3] There are several reasons why this argument was fallacious. In the first instance, in the initial description offered by Fallot for the hearts now named in his honour, he included a case in which the aorta arose exclusively from the right ventricle.[4] Secondly, the argument for distinction between the lesions depended on hearts with tetralogy of Fallot having fibrous continuity between the leaflets of the aortic and mitral valves. Hearts with the phenotypic features of tetralogy of Fallot can be found not only with the aortic root largely supported by the morphologically right ventricle, but also with a subaortic infundibulum (Figure 9.3.1). Thirdly, using the criterion of bilateral infundibulums, or conuses, to

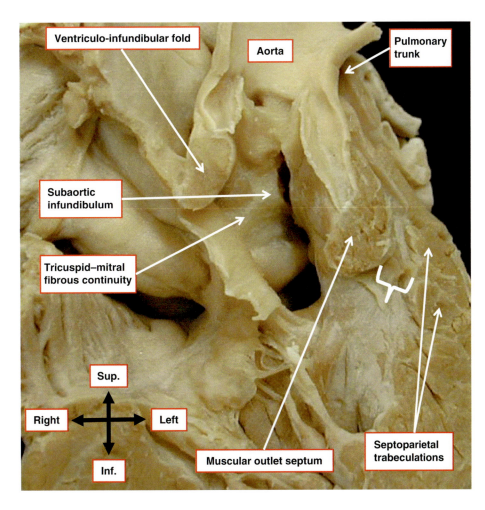

Figure 9.3.1 The heart illustrated has the phenotypic features of tetralogy of Fallot, namely the squeeze between the malaligned muscular outlet septum and the septoparietal trabeculations (bracket – see Chapter 8.5). There is also double outlet from the morphologically right ventricle and bilateral infundibulums. The specimen shows, first, that tetralogy of Fallot can co-exist with double outlet ventriculo-arterial connection, and, second, that not all examples of tetralogy of Fallot have fibrous continuity between the leaflets of the aortic and mitral valves.

define double outlet right ventricle abrogates the principle of the morphological method. As we have emphasized, this important principle states that one abnormal lesion should not be defined on the basis of another feature that is itself variable. The most important reason for discarding the notion that bilateral infundibulums are the phenotype of double outlet right ventricle, nonetheless, is that when autopsy archives are assessed to identify specimens with both arterial trunks arising from the right ventricle, almost half of those fulfilling this criterion have fibrous continuity between an arterial and an atrioventricular valve (Figure 9.3.2).[5]

Still further controversies have been related to the problems existing in arbitrating how to differentiate between those that have double outlet as opposed to concordant or discordant ventriculo-arterial connections. This reflects the fact that, when there is overriding of either the aortic and pulmonary roots, spectrums of malformation exist in the settings of tetralogy of Fallot, or transposition, respectively. For quite some time, it was argued that double outlet should be diagnosed only when nine-tenths of the overriding root arose from the same ventricle as supported the other arterial root. It is now accepted that it is better to define double outlet ventricle whenever more than half of the circumference of both arterial valves takes its origin from the same ventricle.[1] Until recently, however, arbitrating the support of the arterial roots had been far from easy. For those using echocardiography, for example, it was recognized that making designations on the basis of long-axis views could be misleading because of the motion of the heart during the cardiac cycle (Figure 9.3.3). Nowadays, with the advent of three-dimensional imaging techniques, it is possible to determine the precise extent of override. This is achieved by assessing the relationship of cord subtended by the crest of the ventricular septum to the circumference of the overriding arterial root (Figure 9.3.4). Using this approach, those with the greater part of both arterial trunks supported by the morphologically right ventricle can readily be identified (Figure 9.3.5).

Almost always, the hearts with double outlet ventricle exist in the setting of deficient ventricular septation. This creates another problem. When there are concordant or discordant ventriculo-arterial connections, the channel between the ventricles is appropriately described as a ventricular septal defect (Figure 9.3.6). This is harder to apply when both arterial trunks arise from the morphologically right ventricle. This is because, in this setting, the outlet part of the septum, of necessity, is exclusively a right ventricular structure. Hence, it is not interventricular. The channel between the ventricles, therefore, is the outlet for the morphologically left ventricle (Figure 9.3.7). In terms of development, it is the secondary, rather than the tertiary, interventricular communication (see Chapter 2). The channel cannot be closed during surgical correction, but instead must be tunnelled to one or the other of the ventricular

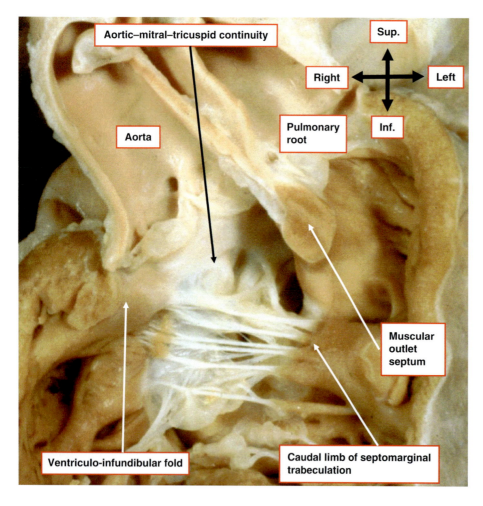

Figure 9.3.2 In this specimen, shown in anatomical orientation, the outlet septum is attached to the antero-cephalad limb of the septomarginal trabeculation so that the channel between the ventricles is subaortic. There is extensive fibrous continuity between the leaflets of the mitral and tricuspid valves, making the defect perimembranous, but there is also extensive continuity between the leaflets of the aortic and tricuspid valves, even though the aortic root is supported exclusively within the right ventricle. The specimen shows that hearts can have double outlet from the right ventricle without there being bilateral infundibulums.

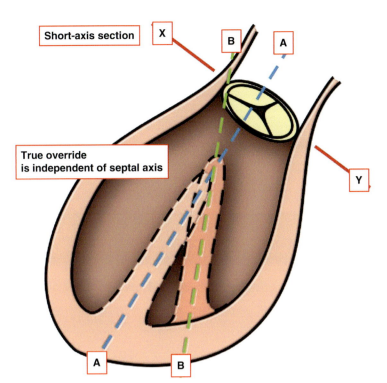

Figure 9.3.3 The cartoon shows how, when assessing the alignment of an overriding arterial root to the crest of the muscular septum, this can vary depending on the motion of the heart (lines A-A and B-B), meaning that the root could be considered to arise from either ventricle. This variable, however, does not come into play when the root is assigned according to the relationship of its short axis to the cord subtended by the crest of the ventricular septum (see Figure 9.3.4).

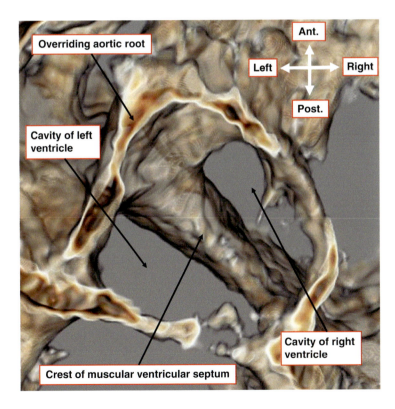

Figure 9.3.4 The image shows the short axis of the overriding aortic root as revealed by a computed tomographic scan from a patient with tetralogy of Fallot. When using such a three-dimensional technique, it is possible precisely to determine the portions of the overriding root committed to the morphologically right as opposed to the morphologically left ventricles.

outflow tracts. This creates problems for its description. If we return to the situation in tetralogy of Fallot, with overriding of the aortic root (Figure 9.3.8), there is a cone of space subtended beneath the circumference of the root and the crest of the muscular ventricular septum. Within this cone of space, it is possible to construct a geometric interventricular communication by continuing the long axis of the muscular ventricular septum. This space is not the area closed by the surgeon when undertaking repair. It is the right ventricular entrance to the cone of space that is closed by the surgeon. This is the area

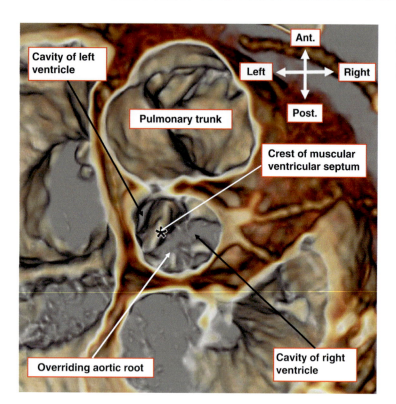

Figure 9.3.5 The image shows a similar view of the overriding aortic root as shown in Figure 9.3.4. In this instance, however, it is obvious that the greater part of the aortic root and all of the pulmonary root are supported above the cavity of the right ventricle. This is diagnostic for double outlet right ventricle.

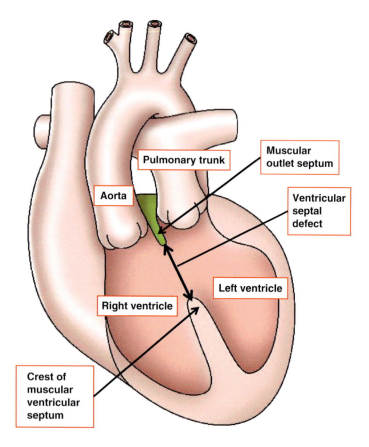

Figure 9.3.6 The cartoon illustrates the plane of space identified as the ventricular septal defect when there are concordant or discordant ventriculo-arterial connections. Both the apical muscular septum and the muscular outlet septum are interventricular structures in these settings.

usually defined as representing the 'ventricular septal defect' in the setting of tetralogy. The left ventricular entrance to the cone of space, of course, functions as the left ventricular outflow tract. It cannot be closed by the surgeon. When both arterial trunks arise from the right ventricle, the entirety of the cones of space subtended by both arterial roots are above the

9.3 Double Outlet Ventricle

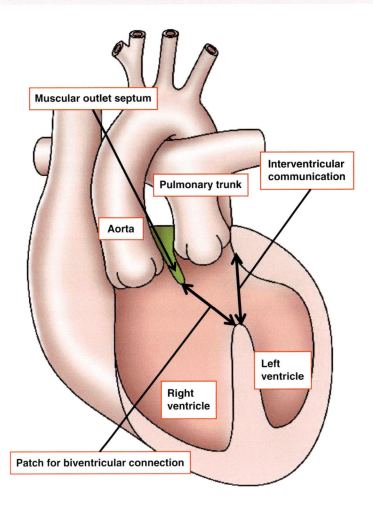

Figure 9.3.7 The cartoon, which should be compared with Figure 9.3.6, shows the arrangement of the channel between the ventricles when both arterial trunks are supported by the cavity of the right ventricle. The muscular outlet septum is no longer an interventricular structure. The interventricular communication is now the outlet for the morphologically left ventricle. Surgical repair involves constructing a tunnel within the cavity of the right ventricle.

cavity of the right ventricle (Figure 9.3.9). It is still the right ventricular entrance to the cone of space that is closed by the surgeon when tunnelling one or the other outflow tract into continuity with the left ventricle (Figure 9.3.10). And the left ventricular entrance to the cone of space remains the effective outlet for the left ventricle. By analogy with the arrangement in tetralogy of Fallot, therefore, it should still be the right ventricular entrance to the arterial root that is defined as the ventricular septal defect (compare Figures 9.3.8 and 9.3.9). In most instances, nonetheless, it is the left ventricular entrance to the arterial root that most investigators name as the 'ventricular septal defect'. This is illogical. For this reason, we prefer to name the channel between the ventricles when both arterial trunks arise from the right ventricle as the interventricular communication.[5]

It follows from these discussions that double outlet ventriculo-arterial connection is no more than an anatomical arrangement of the ventriculo-arterial junctions. Hearts unified by possession of this feature can exist with such a wide variety of configurations that the possible combinations seem almost limitless. The cases we will illustrate in this chapter will have both arteries arising from the morphologically right ventricle in the setting of concordant atrioventricular connections. The principles to be established, nonetheless, are equally applicable in the setting of the other atrioventricular connections, remembering that when the atrioventricular connections are discordant, or there is left-hand topology in the setting of isomerism, there is likely to be an anomalously located atrioventricular node, or even dual atrioventricular nodes.

As already emphasized, almost always there is a co-existing interventricular communication in the presence of double outlet.[6] It is then the anatomical relationship between the arterial roots and the defect in the ventricular septum that is of greatest importance to the surgeon. The relationship of the arterial trunks is another variable. In many patients, the aorta and the pulmonary trunk are related more-or-less normally. In this setting, the aortic valve is posterior and to the right of the pulmonary valve, and the pulmonary trunk spirals around the aorta as it extends towards its bifurcation (Figure 9.3.11). In most of the remaining patients, the arterial trunks arise from the base of the heart in parallel fashion, as anticipated when the ventriculo-arterial connections are discordant. For a good proportion of these, the arterial valves are side by side (Figure 9.3.12); otherwise, the aortic valve is anterior. In a few cases, the aorta is posteriorly located because the pulmonary trunk is enlarged. Almost always the aorta is to the right when the arterial trunks are parallel. In a small number of cases, the aorta can be left sided relative to the pulmonary trunk (Figure 9.3.13). Although the interventricular communication is most usually subaortic when the arterial trunks are spiralling, and subpulmonary when they extend into the mediastinum in parallel fashion, there is no direct correlation

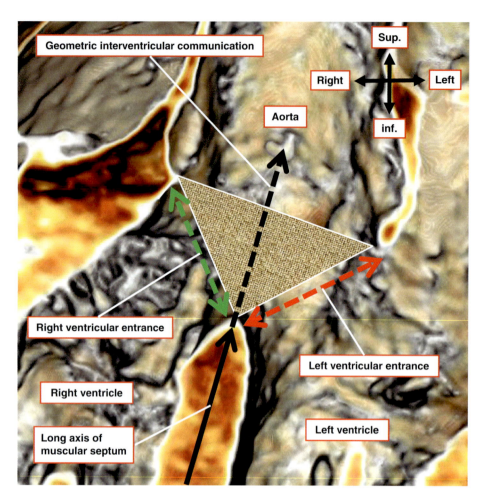

Figure 9.3.8 The image, from the same computed tomographic dataset with a patient with tetralogy of Fallot as used to create Figure 9.3.4, shows the cone of space subtended beneath the overriding aortic root relative to the crest of the muscular ventricular septum. The areas of interest are the geometric interventricular communication, and the right and left ventricular entrances to the cone of space. In tetralogy of Fallot, it is the right ventricular entrance that is closed by the surgeon, and which is usually nominated as the ventricular septal defect.

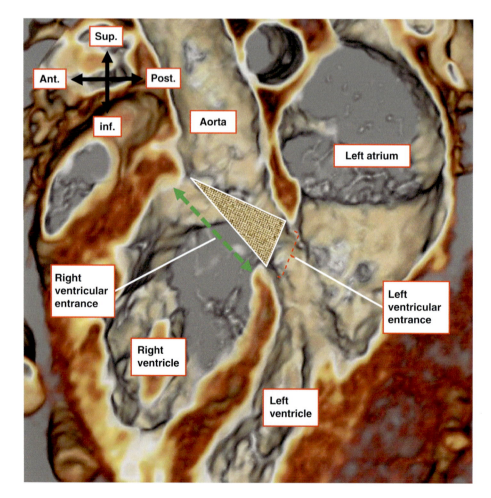

Figure 9.3.9 This image is from the computed tomographic dataset of the patient shown in Figure 9.3.5, with double outlet right ventricle. The left ventricular entrance to the cone of space is the outlet for the left ventricle. The surgeon will correct the lesion by closing the right ventricular entrance.

9.3 Double Outlet Ventricle

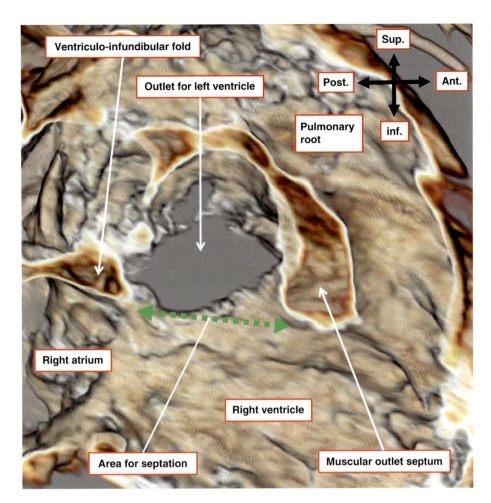

Figure 9.3.10 The image, again from the patient with double outlet right ventricle shown in Figures 9.3.9 and 9.3.5, shows that the area at the back of the overriding aortic root is the outlet for the left ventricle. The surgical correction will require the placement of a patch within the cavity of the right ventricle. The area closed will be analogous to the ventricular septal defect as nominated in the setting of tetralogy of Fallot (see Figure 9.3.8).

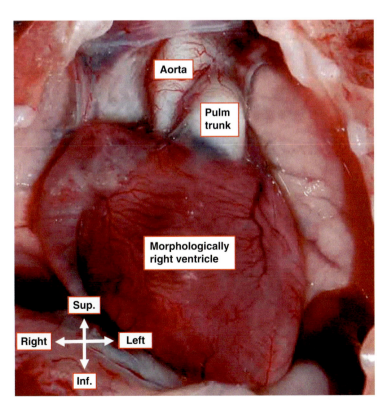

Figure 9.3.11 This specimen, shown in anatomical orientation from the front, has double outlet from the right ventricle with the interventricular communication in subaortic position. The great arterial trunks spiral in normal relationships as they leave the base of the heart.

359

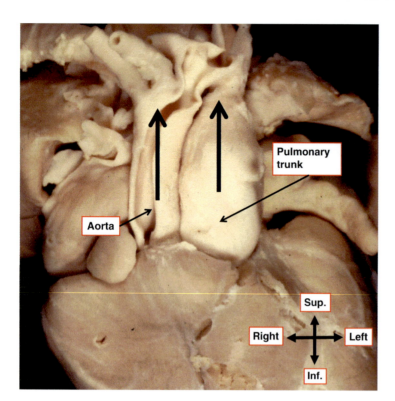

Figure 9.3.12 In this specimen, also seen in anatomical orientation from the front, and also with double outlet from the right ventricle, the interventricular communication was in subpulmonary position. The arterial trunks rise in parallel fashion (black arrows) as they exit from the base of the heart (compare with Figure 9.3.11).

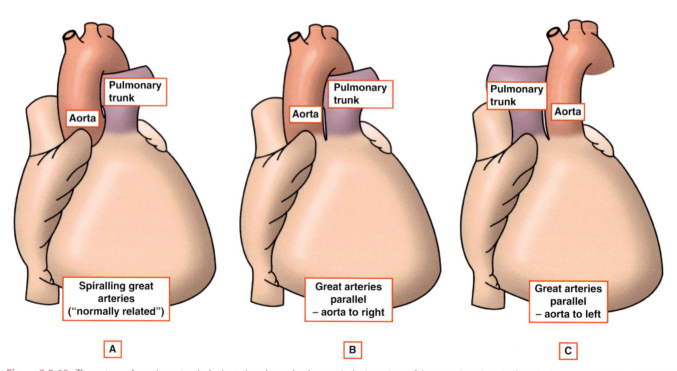

Figure 9.3.13 The cartoon, drawn in anatomical orientation, shows the three typical orientations of the arterial trunks to be found in hearts with double outlet right ventricle. The arrangements with spiralling and parallel arterial trunks with the aorta to the right have been shown in Figures 9.3.11 and 9.3.12. The rarest variant, shown in panel C, is for the arterial trunks to rise in parallel fashion, but with the aorta in left-sided position.

between these features. It is always necessary, therefore, to determine precisely the location of the interventricular communication relative to the arterial roots, and to establish whether it can safely be channelled to one or other arterial root in unobstructed fashion so as to achieve a biventricular surgical repair. A particular feature of the patients with left-sided and parallel aortas with concordant atrioventricular connections, nonetheless, is that the interventricular communication tends to be subaortic, making surgical repair that much easier.[7]

In the light of the above discussions, it is evident that the anatomy of the interventricular communication needs to be considered in two ways. The first feature of significance is its proximity to the great arteries.[6] The second feature concerns its own intrinsic morphology. When combining these two approaches, it must be remembered, again as already emphasized, that when there is double outlet from the right ventricle, the muscular ventricular septum itself separates only the inlet and apical trabecular components of the ventricles. The outlet septum, or its fibrous remnant, is found between the two outlets from the right ventricle, and does not form the roof of the interventricular communication (Figure 9.3.7). Except when non-committed, the interventricular communication is cradled between the limbs of the septomarginal trabeculation, or septal band. Its other borders vary depending on several features. The first is whether the caudal limb of the septomarginal trabeculation fuses with the ventriculo-infundibular fold. If it does, there is a muscular inferior rim to the defect. This then protects the conduction tissue axis as in tetralogy or transposition (Figure 9.3.14). If the caudal limb of the trabeculation does not fuse with the ventriculo-infundibular fold, there is continuity between the leaflets of the mitral and tricuspid valves, and the defect is perimembranous (Figure 9.3.15).

The second feature is the extent of the ventriculo-infundibular fold. It is the presence of well-formed folds bilaterally that produces bilateral muscular infundibulums. These are the so-called 'bilateral conuses', which were initially considered to be part and parcel of the definition of double outlet right ventricle. The significant surgical aspect of this feature is that the infundibulums move the arterial valves some distance away from the margins of the interventricular communication (Figure 9.3.15). Even in the setting of bilateral infundibulums, the interventricular communication can still be perimembranous, since there still can be continuity between the leaflets of the mitral and tricuspid valves (Figures 9.3.1, 9.3.15). When the ventriculo-infundibular fold is attenuated, the leaflets of one of the arterial valves are able to achieve fibrous continuity with an atrioventricular valve (Figure 9.3.2).

The final feature is the relationship of the outlet septum, which can be muscular or fibrous, to the other structures. When attached to the cranial limb of the septomarginal trabeculation, the defect is subaortic (Figures 9.3.1, 9.3.14, 9.3.15). When, in contrast, the outlet septum is attached to the ventriculo-infundibular fold, or to the caudal limb of the septomarginal trabeculation, the defect is placed beneath the left-sided great artery, which is almost always the pulmonary trunk (Figures 9.3.16, 9.3.17). When the outlet septum is attached to neither the cranial nor caudal limbs of the septomarginal trabeculation, the defect is doubly committed (Figure 9.3.18). If the outlet septum is fibrous, it is also juxta-arterial (Figure 9.3.19). When the outlet septum is fibrous, however, the defect can still be subaortic if the septum is attached to the cranial limb of the septomarginal trabeculation (Figure 9.3.20).

From this potential for variation, two groups of patients can be collected from those having double outlet from the right ventricle. The most frequent configuration is when the aortic valve is posterior and to the right of the pulmonary trunk (Figure 9.3.11), usually with the interventricular communication in subaortic position (Figures 9.3.14, 9.3.15). This arterial relationship can also be found with a juxta-arterial defect (Figure 9.3.19). The second group comprises hearts in which the aorta ascends parallel to the pulmonary trunk

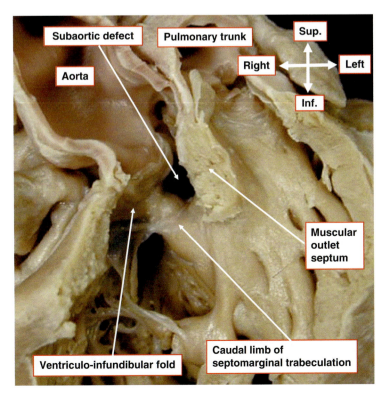

Figure 9.3.14 In this specimen, shown in anatomical orientation from the front, the interventricular communication, opening in subaortic position, is cradled within the limbs of the septomarginal trabeculation. The postero-caudal limb of the trabeculation fuses with the ventriculo-infundibular fold. The muscular buttress thus formed protects the atrioventricular conduction axis. There is fibrous continuity between the leaflets of the aortic and mitral valves in the roof of the interventricular communication, so that it is directly adjacent to the aortic root.

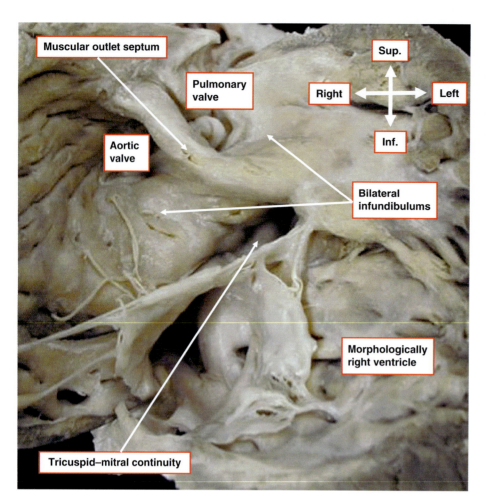

Figure 9.3.15 In this specimen with double outlet right ventricle, seen in anatomical orientation, there is an extensive subaortic infundibulum, along with a long subpulmonary infundibulum. The interventricular communication, however, is perimembranous because of the fibrous continuity between the leaflets of the tricuspid and mitral valves. The interventricular communication is relatively distant from the aortic valve because of the length of the subaortic infundibulum.

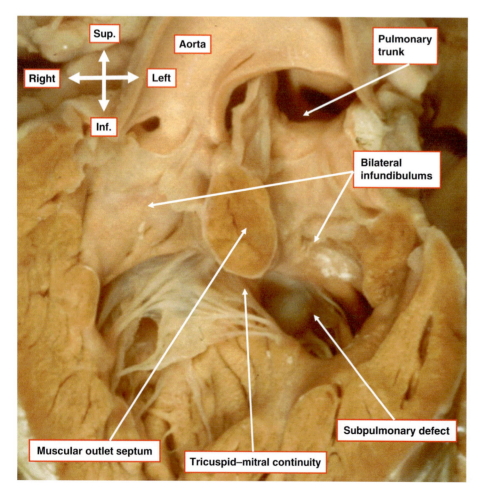

Figure 9.3.16 In this specimen, shown in anatomical orientation, the interventricular communication is positioned in subpulmonary location. This is the so-called Taussig–Bing malformation. Note the attachment of the muscular outlet septum to the midpoint of the ventriculo-infundibular fold, along with bilateral infundibulums. There is also tricuspid–mitral fibrous continuity, so the interventricular communication is perimembranous.

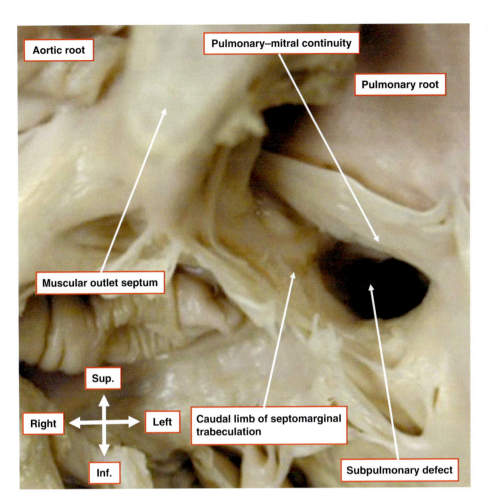

Figure 9.3.17 This specimen again is an example of the so-called Taussig–Bing malformation. In this heart, however, there is a muscular postero-inferior rim that protects the conduction axis, and fibrous continuity between the leaflets of the mitral and pulmonary valves.

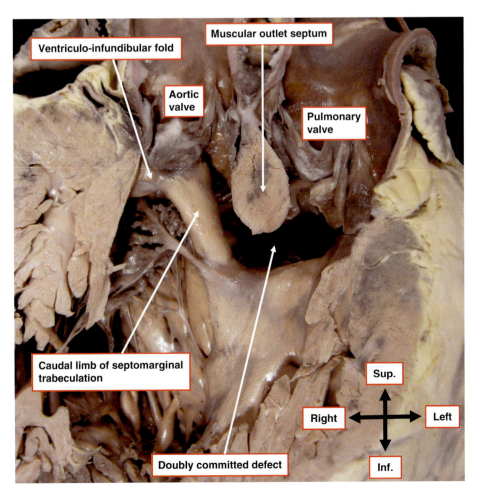

Figure 9.3.18 In this specimen, photographed by Professor Vera Aiello and reproduced with her permission, the muscular outlet septum is positioned at right angles to the crest of the muscular ventricular septum. This makes the defect doubly committed.

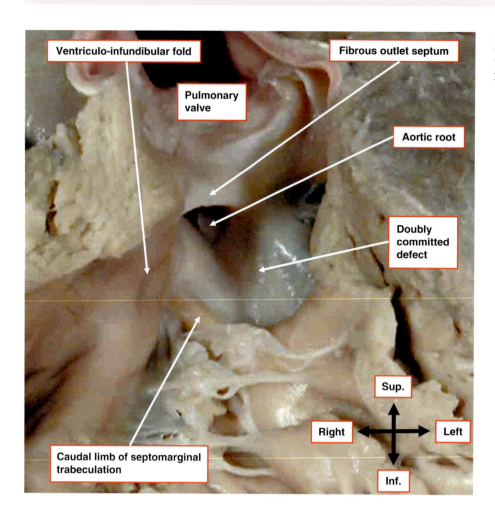

Figure 9.3.19 This specimen again has a doubly committed interventricular communication, but in this example with a fibrous rather than a muscular outlet septum. The defect is now also juxta-arterial.

(Figure 9.3.12), usually with its valve either in anterior or side-by-side position, and to the right relative to the pulmonary valve, and with the septal defect in perimembranous or muscular but subpulmonary position (Figures 9.3.16, 9.3.17). This is the so-called Taussig–Bing malformation.[8]

The surgeon should be particularly wary when the interventricular communication is non-committed.[9] Almost always, when it is subaortic, subpulmonary, or doubly committed, it is possible to place a patch within the right ventricle so as to channel the interventricular communication to one or other outflow tract, thus achieving biventricular circulations. This may not be possible if the defect is anatomically non-committed, or else if the interventricular communication is adjacent to an outflow tract, but the potentially corrective pathways are blocked by structures such as valvar tension apparatus (Figure 9.3.21). Anatomical non-commitment is most usually found when the interventricular communication is between the ventricular inlets (Figure 9.3.21), or is the ventricular component of an atrioventricular septal defect in patients with common atrioventricular junction (Figure 9.3.22). The surgeon may be able to overcome these impediments and still achieve biventricular repair.[10] In this situation, however, there may be arguments as to whether the defect was truly 'non-committed' (Figure 9.3.23). There is no question but that the defect is non-committed both anatomically and surgically when it is encased within the muscular septum and opens to the inlet of the right ventricle (Figure 9.3.24).

It is also important for the surgeon to identify any other abnormalities in the extremely heterogeneous group of malformations linked together because of a double outlet ventriculo-arterial connection. By far the most common set of anomalies relates to obstruction of the arterial outlets, such as infundibular stenosis, valvar stenosis, coarctation, or interruption of the aortic arch. The presence of subpulmonary infundibular stenosis is a particularly frequent finding when the septal defect is subaortic, often producing the morphology of tetralogy of Fallot, even in the setting of bilateral infundibulums (Figure 9.3.1). Coarctation and interrupted arch, together with straddling of the mitral valve, are frequent accompaniments of the Taussig–Bing variant.[8] Common atrioventricular valves also occur in a significant number of cases. Unusual coronary arterial anatomy, including the intramural arrangement, is found most frequently when the aorta is in anterior or side-by-side position. In this situation, special consideration is needed when performing either a right ventriculotomy or an arterial switch procedure.

Surgical and anatomical considerations for the potential corrective procedures relate to the particular combination of defects. It is possible, nonetheless, to establish some basic rules (Figure 9.3.25).[11] The outlet septum, almost always present, although it may be fibrous rather than muscular, serves as

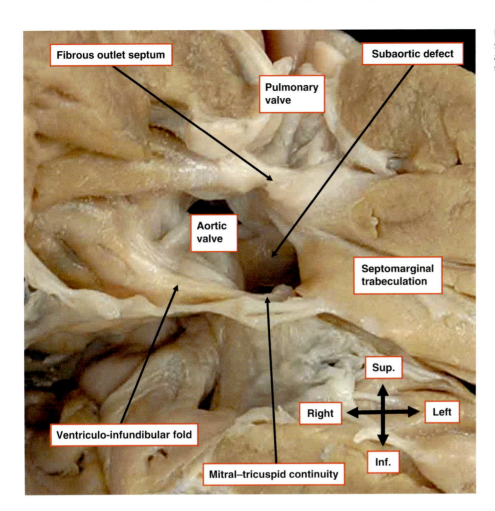

Figure 9.3.20 In this specimen, the outlet septum is fibrous rather than muscular. It is attached to the cranial limb of the septomarginal trabeculation, making the defect itself subaortic.

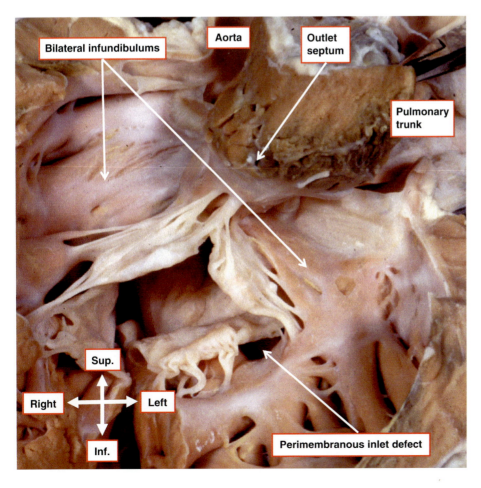

Figure 9.3.21 In this specimen, shown in anatomical orientation, the interventricular communication opens between the ventricular inlets, and is shielded by the septal leaflet of the tricuspid valve. This feature, coupled with the attachment of tendinous cords to the muscular outlet septum, makes the defect non-committed.

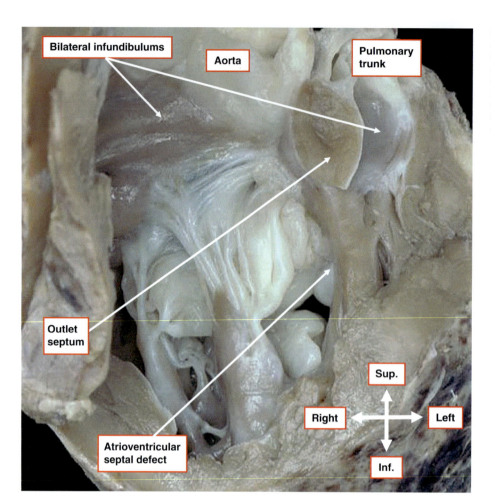

Figure 9.3.22 In this specimen with double outlet right ventricle and bilateral infundibulums, shown in anatomical orientation, there is a common atrioventricular junction guarded by a common atrioventricular valve. It is questionable whether the ventricular component of the atrioventricular septal defect could be channelled to the subpulmonary root. Anatomically, the defect is non-committed.

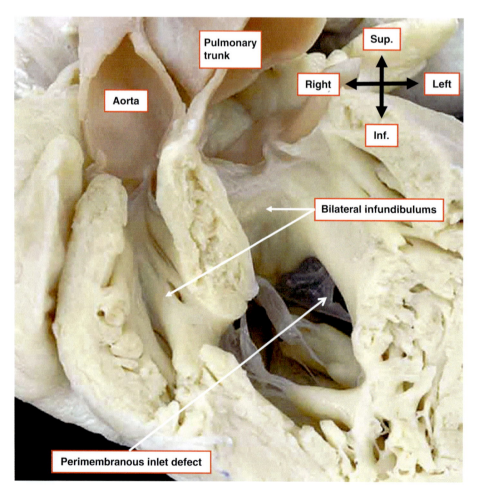

Figure 9.3.23 In this specimen with double outlet right ventricle and bilateral infundibulums, also seen in anatomical orientation, the interventricular communication is again between the ventricular inlets (compare with Figure 9.3.21). In this specimen, however, the inlet perimembranous defect could almost certainly be committed surgically to the subpulmonary outlet. In this instance, therefore, the defect might well be described as being subpulmonary rather than non-committed.

9.3 Double Outlet Ventricle

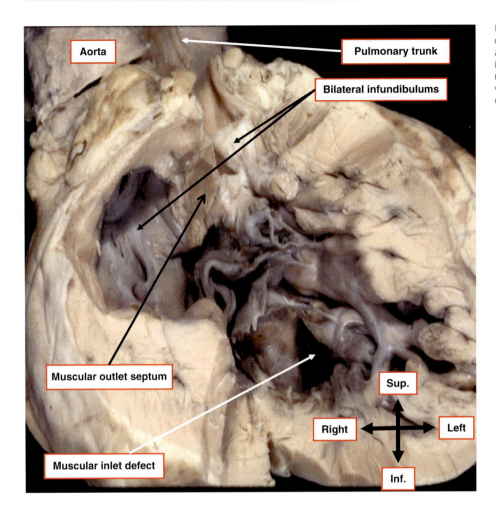

Figure 9.3.24 In this specimen with double outlet right ventricle and bilateral infundibulums, again shown in anatomical orientation, the interventricular communication is within the muscular septum and opens to the right ventricular inlet. This defect is unequivocally non-committed.

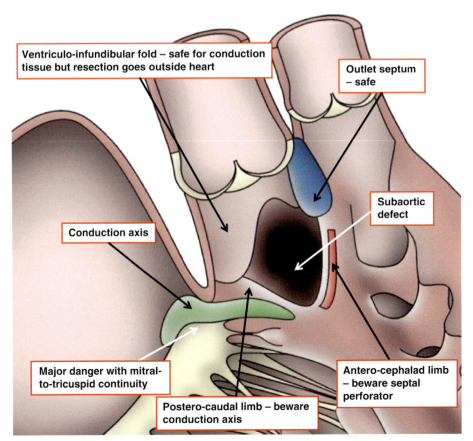

Figure 9.3.25 The drawing, illustrating double outlet right ventricle with subaortic interventricular communication, shows the major components of the outflow tracts, and illustrates the salient surgical features relating to each individual muscular component. The conduction axis is shown in green, and the first septal perforating artery as the red bar. The outlet septum is shown in blue. The 'limbs' are part of the septomarginal trabeculation.

a guide to the arterial valves and their relationships to each other, and to the interventricular communication. As described above, in cases with subaortic defects the outlet septum usually inserts into the antero-cephalad limb of the septomarginal trabeculation. With subpulmonary defects, it usually inserts into the ventriculo-infundibular fold, or into the inferior part of the muscular ventricular septum. The outlet septum is always devoid of any vital structure, so it can be resected, or used as a secure site for anchorage of sutures. In contrast, the ventriculo-infundibular fold is not a solid bar of muscle. Care must be taken to avoid extensive dissection or resection of this structure, since the right coronary artery lies within its fold.

Knowledge of the type of interventricular communication will, as in isolated ventricular septal defects, give accurate guidance to the disposition of the conduction tissue. Obstruction of the subpulmonary outflow tract requires the same attention to detail as when dealing with tetralogy of Fallot. Other cardiac anomalies will have to be dealt with in the context of the particular cardiac configuration present.

Double outlet from the left ventricle is very much rarer than double outlet right ventricle. It can present with similar variations in the position of the arterial trunks, and their relationship to the interventricular communication, as we have described for double outlet right ventricle. As with double outlet right ventricle, double outlet left ventricle can be found with any atrioventricular connections. The rules for the disposition of the conduction tissue will then change accordingly.

References Cited

1. Walters HL 3rd, Mavroudis C, Tchervenkov CI, et al. Congenital Heart Surgery Nomenclature and Database Project: double outlet right ventricle. *Ann Thorac Surg* 2000; **69**(Suppl.4): S249–263.

2. Paul MH, Muster AJ, Sinha SN, Cole RB, Van Praagh R. Double-outlet left ventricle with an intact ventricular septum: clinical and autopsy diagnosis and developmental implications. *Circulation* 1970; **41**: 129–139.

3. Baron MG. Radiologic notes in cardiology: angiographic differentiation between tetralogy of Fallot and double-outlet right ventricle relationship of the mitral and aortic valves. *Circulation* 1971; **43**: 451–545.

4. Fallot A. Contribution à l'anatomie pathologique de la maladie bleue (cyanose cardiaque). *Marseille Medicale* 1888; **25**: 77–93.

5. Ebadi A, Spicer DE, Backer CL, Fricker FJ, Anderson RH. Double-outlet right ventricle revisited. *J Thorac Cardiovasc Surg* 2017; **154**: 598–604.

6. Lev M, Bharati S, Meng CCL, et al. A concept of double-outlet right ventricle. *J Thorac Cardiovasc Surg* 1972; **64**: 271–281.

7. Lincoln C, Anderson R, Shinebourne EA, English TA, Wilkinson JL. Double outlet right ventricle with l-malposition of the aorta. *Br Heart J* 1975; **37**: 453–463.

8. Stellin G, Zuberbuhler JR, Anderson, RH, Siewers RD. The surgical anatomy of the Taussig-Bing malformation. *J Thorac Cardiovasc Surg* 1987; **93**: 560–569.

9. Stellin G, Ho SY, Anderson RH, Zuberbuhler JR, Siewers RD. The surgical anatomy of double-outlet right ventricle with concordant atrioventricular connection and non-committed ventricular septal defect. *J Thorac Cardiovasc Surg* 1991; **102**: 849–855.

10. Lacour-Gayet F, Haun C, Ntalakoura K, et al. Biventricular repair of double outlet right ventricle with non-committed ventricular septal defect (VSD) by VSD rerouting to the pulmonary artery and arterial switch. *Eur J Cardiothorac Surg* 2002; **21**: 1042–1048.

11. Hosseinpour A-R, Jones TJ, Barron DJ, Brawn WJ, Anderson RH. An appreciation of the structural variability in the components of the ventricular outlets in congenitally malformed hearts. *Eur J Cardio-thorac Surg* 2007; **31**: 888–893.

Chapter 9.4
Common Arterial Trunk

There is now general agreement that a common arterial trunk is one that supplies directly the systemic, pulmonary, and coronary arteries (Figure 9.4.1).[1] The phenotypic feature of the lesion is the commonality of the ventriculo-arterial junction, which is almost always guarded by a common arterial valve (Figure 9.4.2).[2] In this way, the anomaly is distinguished from the other types of ventriculo-arterial connection producing single outlet from the heart. These are a solitary aortic trunk with pulmonary atresia, a solitary pulmonary trunk with aortic atresia, and a solitary arterial trunk.[3] The presence of the common ventriculo-arterial junction serves to distinguish the entity from hearts with a large aortopulmonary window, which can effectively produce a common intrapericardial arterial component, but with separate aortic and pulmonary valves. While the difference between a common trunk and an aortopulmonary window is anatomical, the distinction between common and solitary arterial trunks is more semantic. We define an arterial trunk as being solitary, rather than common, when it is not possible to find any evidence of intrapericardial pulmonary arteries (Figure 9.4.3).[3] Such an approach resolves the controversy as to whether the pulmonary arteries, had they been present, would have arisen from the arterial trunk, or from the morphologically right ventricle. Had the pulmonary trunk been present but atretic, and arising from the arterial trunk itself, then the trunk would then have been common. Cases do exist in which an atretic intrapulmonary arterial trunk can be traced back to the arterial trunk exiting from the heart (Figure 9.4.4).[4] The intracardiac anatomy of hearts shown to have solitary trunks, however, with absence of the intrapericardial pulmonary arteries, is much more in keeping with the arrangement found when the atretic pulmonary arises from the right ventricle (Figure 9.4.5). In patients with a solitary trunk as thus defined, it is the arterial supply to the pulmonary circulation that is the key to surgical treatment. The trunk itself, to all intents and purposes, functions as the aorta. Patients with these arrangements, therefore, are best considered along with tetralogy with pulmonary atresia (see Chapter 8.5).

We describe the lesions to be discussed in this chapter as common arterial trunks. The lesions are still frequently described in terms of persistence of the 'truncus arteriosus'. As we discussed in Chapter 2, it was Kramer who introduced the terms 'truncus' and 'conus', arguing that use of these terms might clarify the development of the cardiac outflow tract.[5] In

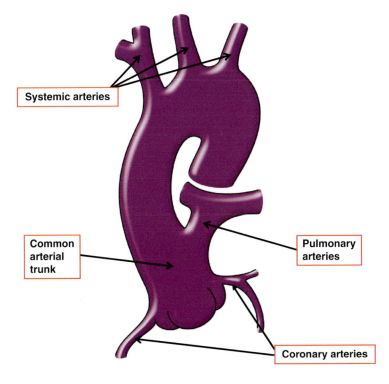

Figure 9.4.1 The drawing illustrates the essence of a common arterial trunk. It is a solitary trunk that leaves the base of the heart, and then supplies directly the systemic, pulmonary, and coronary arteries.

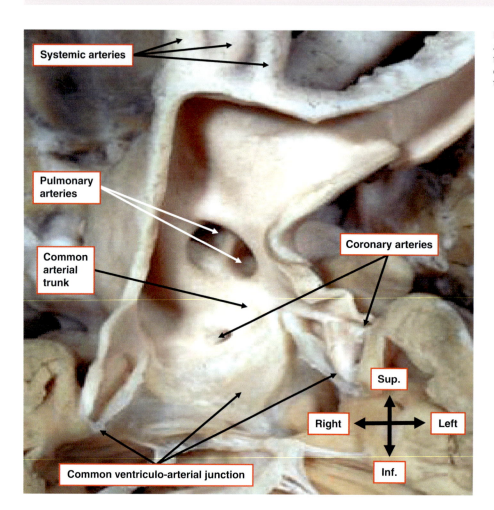

Figure 9.4.2 The specimen, photographed in anatomical orientation, shows the phenotypic feature of common arterial trunk to be the common ventriculo-arterial junction, guarded in this heart by a valve with three leaflets.

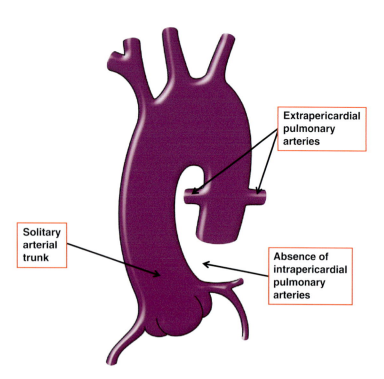

Figure 9.4.3 The drawing illustrates the potential dilemma in defining the nature of an arterial trunk in the absence of the intrapericardial pulmonary arteries. There is no way of knowing whether, had they existed, the pulmonary arteries would have originated directly from the heart or from the arterial trunk itself. The only logical way of describing the trunk in this setting is to nominate it as being solitary, even though, to all intents and purposed, it functions as an aorta.

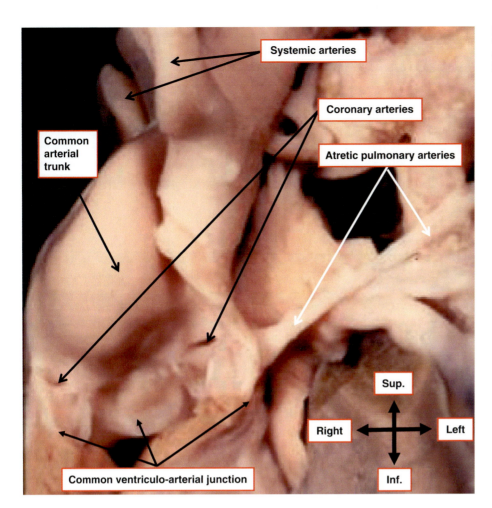

Figure 9.4.4 The specimen shows how, on very rare occasions, an atretic pulmonary trunk can arise from a common arterial trunk, in this instance with origin from a truncal valvar sinus.

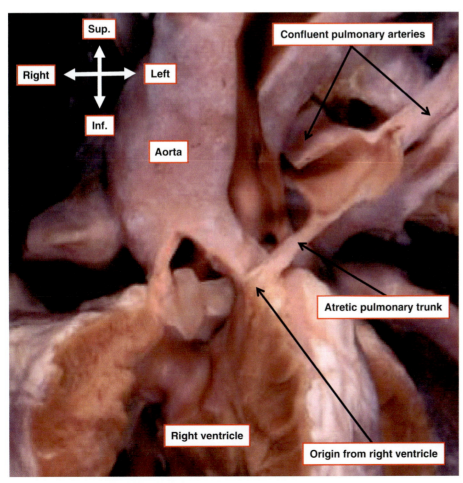

Figure 9.4.5 When the intrapericardial pulmonary trunk is atretic, it is usually the case that, as in this heart, it arises from the base of the right ventricle. The arterial trunk overriding the crest of the muscular ventricular septum is then correctly described as being aortic.

reality, the terms have produced confusion rather than clarity. There is no certainty as to which part of the outflow tract Kramer wished to define as the 'truncus'. And, as we have demonstrated, the developing intrapericardial outflow tract is much better described in terms of three components, these being the intrapericardial arterial trunks, the arterial roots, and the ventricular outflow tracts. Of these three parts, it is the commonality of the arterial roots that provides the phenotypic feature of the lesion (Figure 9.4.2). In this instance, a recapitulation of development is helpful in understanding the morphological variability to be found within hearts fitting this phenotypic pattern.[6]

When considering development, it is also helpful to draw analogies between the formation of the atrioventricular as opposed to the ventriculo-arterial junctions. So-called cushions are key to the normal septation and separation at both junctions. At the atrioventricular junctions, the cushions are formed superiorly and inferiorly within the atrioventricular canal. They separate, initially, an atrioventricular septal defect into its atrial and ventricular components. The atrial part is the primary atrial foramen. The ventricular part, subsequent to expansion of the atrioventricular canal, is the secondary interventricular foramen (Figure 9.4.6). At the ventriculo-arterial junction, the cushions are much more extensive. They differ, furthermore, from the cushions separating the atrioventricular canal in that they contain a contribution of cells derived from the neural crest. As at the atrioventricular junction, nonetheless, as they fuse, they separate the cavity of the outflow tract into a distal arterial part, which is the aortopulmonary foramen, and a proximal ventricular foramen. The ventricular channel is again the secondary interventricular communication (Figure 9.4.7).

With ongoing development, the cushions at both junctions remodel to form the leaflets of the valves that eventually guard the separate valvar orifices. In addition, the atrioventricular cushions contribute to providing atrioventricular insulation. They also produce the roof of the infero-septal recess, which supports the base of the atrial septum. The cushions within the outflow tract similarly have a dual purpose. The proximal parts of the cushions eventually muscularize. If development proceeds normally, these muscularized cushions form the free-standing subpulmonary infundibulum. Should ventricular septation be incomplete, the cushions form the outlet septum, which can be myocardial or fibrous depending on the extent of muscularization. Recognition of these features serves to show how several different lesions can be grouped together as either atrioventricular or ventriculo-arterial septal defects.[7] We have discussed the variants found in the setting of the atrioventricular septal defect in Chapter 8.3. It is an appreciation of the features of the ventriculo-arterial defect that permits understanding of the lesions unified because of the presence of a common ventriculo-arterial junction (Figure 9.4.8). As with the overriding arterial root in tetralogy of Fallot, a cone of space can be constructed between the circumference of the common truncal root and the

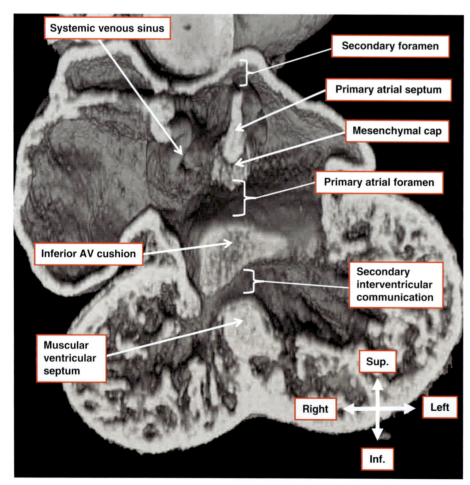

Figure 9.4.6 The section is from an episcopic dataset prepared from a mouse embryo sacrificed at embryonic day 11.5. The image shows how, subsequent to expansion of the atrioventricular canal, the atrioventricular cushions separate the primary atrial foramen from the secondary interventricular foramen.

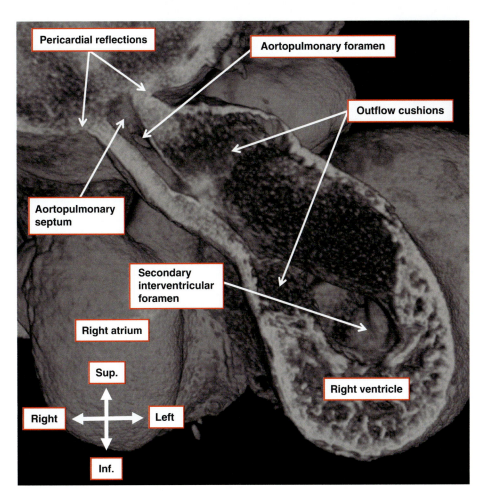

Figure 9.4.7 The section is again taken from a mouse embryo sacrificed at embryonic day 11.5. The image shows how the arrangement of the cushions formed in the outflow tract can be compared with the arrangement found at the atrioventricular junctions (Figure 9.4.6). In the outflow tract, the cushions are much more extensive, but they interpose between the aortopulmonary foramen and the secondary interventricular foramen. Comparison of these arrangements permits inferences to be drawn regarding the separation, in malformed hearts, of the atrioventricular and ventriculo-arterial septal defects.

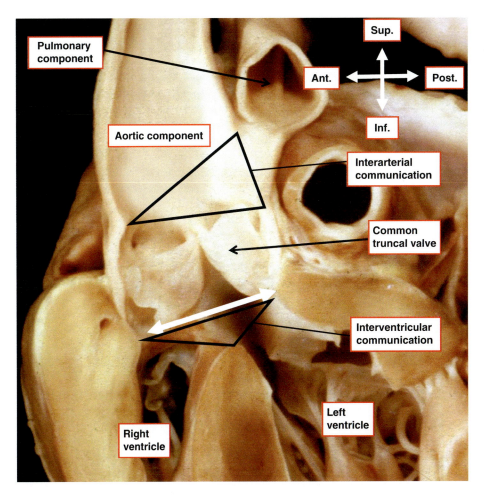

Figure 9.4.8 The image shows a long-axis section through the common ventriculo-arterial junction (double-headed white arrow) of a heart with a common arterial trunk. The triangles show the cones of space representing the arterial and ventricular components of the ventriculo-arterial septal defect.

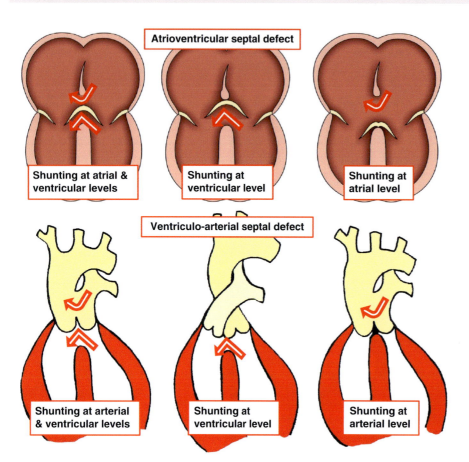

Figure 9.4.9 The drawings compare the phenotypic variability, depending on the relations between the cushions and the proximal and distal septal components, of the atrioventricular septal defect (upper panels) and the ventriculo-arterial septal defect (lower panels).

crest of the muscular ventricular septum. This is the interventricular communication, with right and left ventricular entrances as in tetralogy of Fallot (compare Figures 9.4.8 and 9.3.8). Depending on the extent of separation of the aortic and pulmonary components of the common trunk, a second cone of space can then be identified which represents the arterial component of the defect (Figure 9.4.8). It is the changes that take place between the cushions during their development that determine the morphological variability.

At both junctions, the commonest variants are found when the cushions fail to fuse, leaving a common valve guarding the respective junction (Figure 9.4.9 – left-hand panels). Although it was suggested that the common trunk reflected failure of growth of the pulmonary outflow tract,[8] Van Mierop and his colleagues produced strong evidence to show that the cause was, indeed, failure of fusion of the outflow cushions.[9] We have now confirmed those findings in two mouse models. In the first model, the *Tbx1* gene was knocked out. This is the gene responsible for 22q11 deletion, a syndrome associated with common arterial trunk. In all the hearts from these embryos, there was no fusion of the cushions within the middle and proximal parts of the outflow tract (Figure 9.4.10). When assessing the middle part of the outflow tract, some variants were found with unfused proximal cushions in the presence of paired intercalated valvar swellings (Figure 9.4.11 – upper panel). Others showed either absence or gross hypoplasia of one of the intercalated swellings (Figure 9.4.11 – lower panel). As we will show, these findings provide good explanations for the finding of common arterial valves with either four or three leaflets, and for leaflets of dissimilar size. In our second colony of mice, the activity of the Furin enzyme had been perturbed. We are unsure as to why perturbing this enzyme produced its specific effects, but many of the abnormal mice were found to have common ventriculo-arterial junctions. These mice differed from those with *Tbx1* knock-out in that there had been growth of the aortopulmonary septum. The distal outflow tract, therefore, was divided into aortic and pulmonary components. In some of the embryos, the separation by the aortopulmonary septum produced balanced aortic and pulmonary components (Figure 9.4.12). In other embryos, the distal outflow tract was separated in favour of the pulmonary component, which continued as the arterial duct, with interruption of the hypoplastic aortic component (Figure 9.4.13). These findings again serve to provide explanations for similar variants of common arterial trunk with common truncal valve in humans. In still other of the mice perturbed by perturbing the Furin enzyme, however, the common ventriculo-arterial junction had been divided into the aortic and pulmonary roots, with separate intrapericardial arterial trunks, but in the presence of a juxta-arterial interventricular communication (Figure 9.4.14). This lesion, of course, is equivalent to the juxta-arterial outlet ventricular septal defect (see Chapter 8.2). The variant can be compared with atrioventricular septal defects with exclusively ventricular shunting (Figure 9.4.9 – middle panels).

In the setting of the common atrioventricular junction, the lesion with exclusively ventricular shunting is the rarest variant. The second most frequent variant is found when the cushions have fused with each other to produce dual orifices within the junction, but also have fused with the crest of the

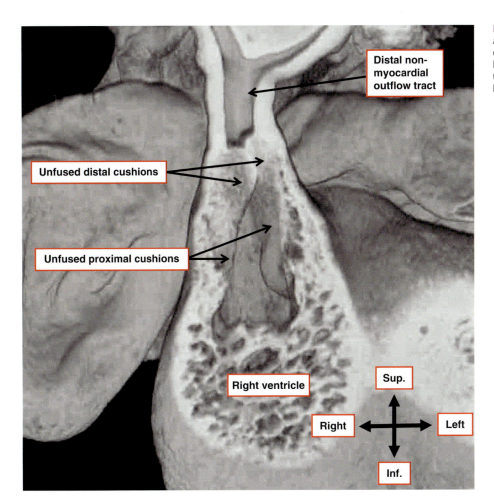

Figure 9.4.10 The images show a frontal long-axis section through a mouse embryo at embryonic day 12.5 in which the *Tbx1* gene has been knocked out. It shows a common arterial trunk, with lack of fusion of the outflow cushions both distally and proximally.

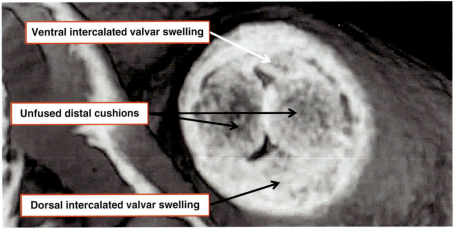

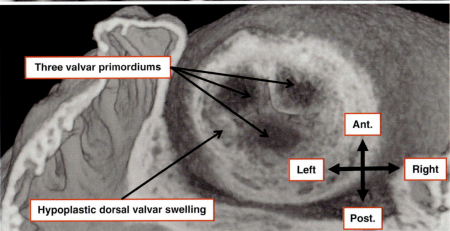

Figure 9.4.11 The images show short-axis sections through the distal outflow tracts of two mouse embryos at embryonic day 12.5 in which the *Tbx1* gene has been knocked out. The upper panel shows the arrangement that will produce a valve with four leaflets, whereas the lower panel shows the situation where the valve will either develop with three leaflets or with four leaflets, with one being grossly hypoplastic.

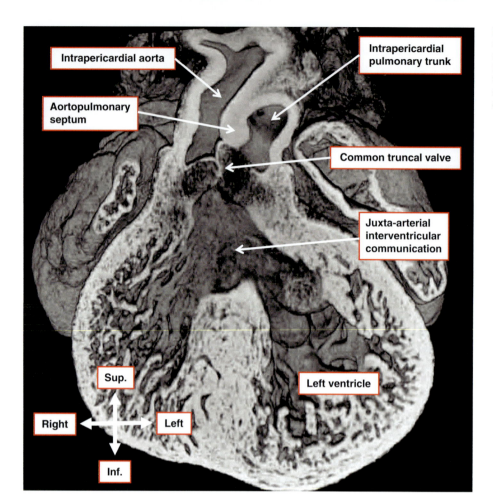

Figure 9.4.12 The image shows a frontal section through a mouse embryo at embryonic day 14.5 in which the Furin enzyme has been perturbed. There is a common arterial trunk with balanced aortic and pulmonary components due to growth of the aortopulmonary septum.

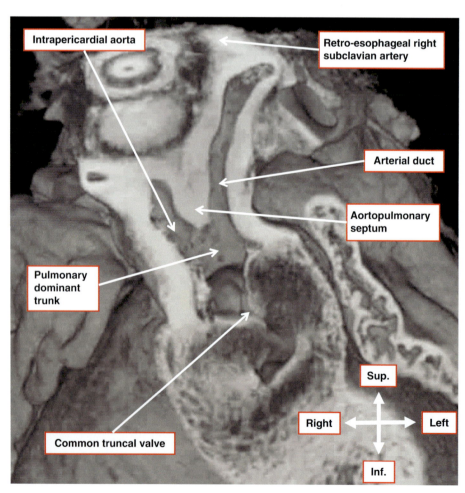

Figure 9.4.13 The image is another frontal section through a mouse embryo at embryonic day 14.5 in which the Furin enzyme has been perturbed. In this embryo, again with common arterial trunk, the aortopulmonary septum has developed so as to produce pulmonary dominance. The arterial duct feeds the descending aorta, and there is interruption of the aortic arch, with retro-esophageal origin of the right subclavian artery.

9.4 Common Arterial Trunk

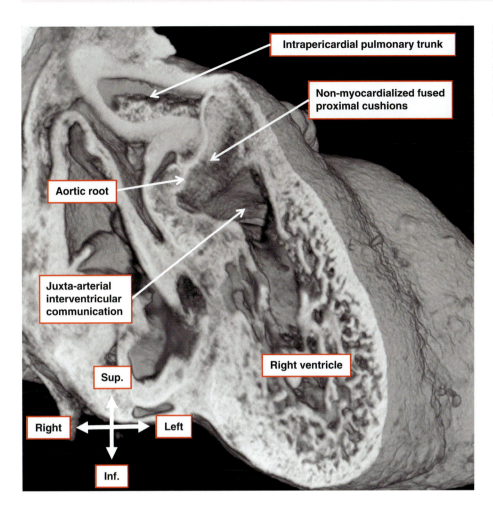

Figure 9.4.14 This is another mouse embryo at embryonic day 14.5 in which the Furin enzyme has been perturbed. In this heart, there is a common ventriculo-arterial junction, but with shunting only through the ventricular component of the ventriculo-arterial septal defect. The lesion presents as a juxta-arterial outlet ventricular septal defect.

muscular ventricular septum (Figure 9.4.9 – right-hand upper panel). This lesion, of course, is the so-called ostium primum defect. A comparable lesion is found at the level of the ventriculo-arterial junction. It represents the situation when the outflow cushions have fused with each other, but with the proximal cushions, rather than muscularizing, remaining fibrous and fusing with each other, and also to the crest of the muscular ventricular septum (Figure 9.4.9 – right-hand lower panel). This rare finding produces the arrangement in which a common arterial trunk exists with dual orifices in the common truncal valve, but with no shunting possible between the ventricles proximal to the level of the valvar leaflets (Figures 9.4.15–9.4.17). The lesion has also been encountered in the operating room,[10] as has the equally rare variant in which there are dual orifices within the truncal valve, but with the potential for shunting at both ventricular and arterial levels.[11]

The variants found with common ventriculo-arterial junction, but with either an exclusively arterial or exclusively ventricular communication, are rare. And, when the shunting is at the ventricular level, the lesions are usually classified as juxta-arterial ventricular septal defects. It is the lesions that have the potential for shunting at both arterial and ventricular levels that are most frequently described simply as common arterial trunks, or 'persistent truncus arteriosus'.[1–3] The anatomical features that underscore the options for, and success of, their surgical treatment are the connection of the trunk to the ventricular mass, the state of the truncal valve, the morphology of the interventricular communication, the presence of associated anomalies, and the arrangement of the intrapericardial systemic and pulmonary arterial channels. The lesions can be found with any atrial arrangement and any atrioventricular connection, but the majority have the usual atrial arrangement and concordant atrioventricular connections. The trunk itself usually overrides the crest of the muscular ventricular septum, being more-or-less equally committed to the right and left ventricles (Figure 9.4.8). Surgical repair involves patching the ventricular component of the defect such that the trunk is committed to the left ventricle. Separation of the pulmonary from the aortic component of the trunk, subsequent to closure of the initial origin of the pulmonary components, then permits the trunk itself to become the new aorta. On occasion, the trunk can arise predominantly (Figure 9.4.18) or exclusively (Figure 9.4.19) from the morphologically right ventricle. In this setting, the interventricular communication can be restrictive. Another problem with right ventricular origin is the association with an atrioventricular septal defect and a common atrioventricular junction (Figure 9.4.20).[12] This adds to the surgical complexity, since not only is the septal defect more distant from the arterial trunk, but also the left ventricular component of the common atrioventricular valve is trifoliate. The need to secure a competent left valve adds significantly to the problems of surgical repair. These problems do not

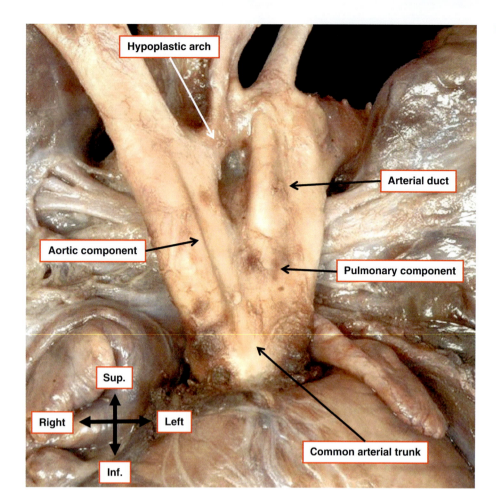

Figure 9.4.15 The image shows a heart with a balanced common arterial trunk, but with an arterial duct feeding the descending aorta and a hypoplastic transverse aortic arch.

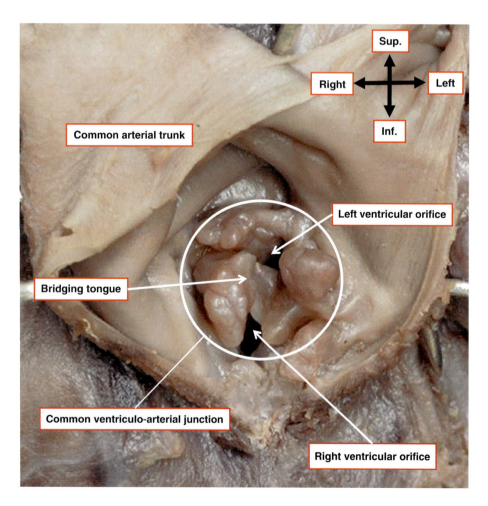

Figure 9.4.16 Opening the common arterial trunk of the heart shown in Figure 9.4.15 reveals dual orifice of the common truncal valve.

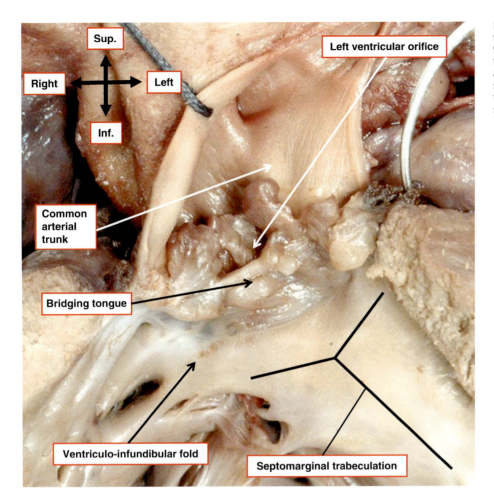

Figure 9.4.17 The right ventricular outflow tract of the heart shown in Figures 9.4.15 and 9.4.16 has been opened. The raphe that produces the dual orifice in the common truncal valve is attached to the crest of the muscular ventricular septum, so that shunting is possible only through the arterial component of the ventriculo-arterial septal defect.

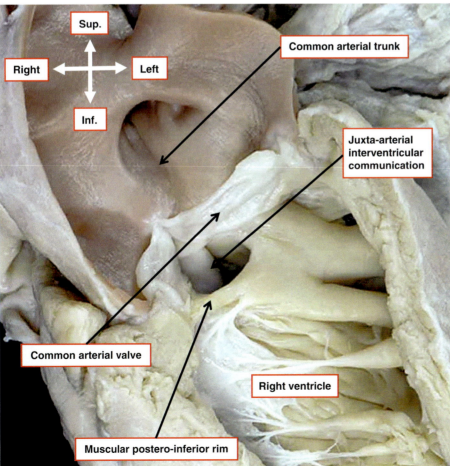

Figure 9.4.18 The heart is opened through the right ventricular outflow tract to show a common arterial trunk supported predominantly above the right ventricle. The interventricular communication has a muscular postero-inferior rim, with the pulmonary arteries arising from a confluent segment from the posterior aspect of the aortic dominant trunk.

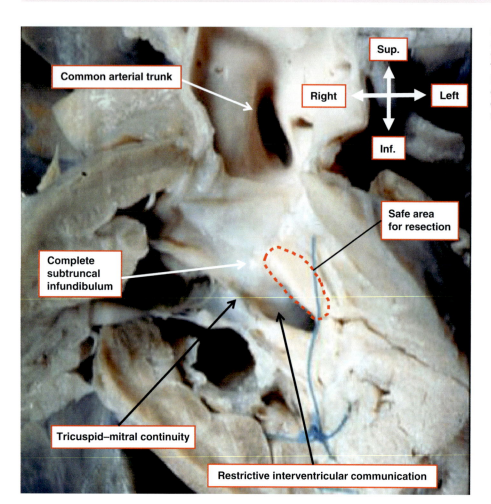

Figure 9.4.19 In this heart with common arterial trunk, seen in anatomical orientation, the trunk arises exclusively from the right ventricle. There is a completely muscular subtruncal infundibulum. The interventricular communication is restrictive. Should enlargement be attempted, then the safe area for resection is shown by the red dotted line.

occur when the trunk is committed predominantly or exclusively to the left ventricle (Figure 9.4.21). In this setting, it is an easy matter to close the ventricular component of the defect, leaving the new aorta in communication with the left ventricle.

In the majority of cases, the leaflets of the truncal valve are in fibrous continuity with those of the mitral valve. When the trunk arises exclusively from the right ventricle, nonetheless, it can be supported by a complete infundibulum (Figure 9.4.19). More usually, the interventricular communication is directly juxta-arterial and opens to the right ventricle between the limbs of the septomarginal trabeculation. There can then be fibrous continuity between the leaflets of the tricuspid, and mitral valves in the postero-inferior margin of the defect, making it perimembranous (Figure 9.4.22). As with all other perimembranous defects, the conduction axis is then at risk in the area of fibrous continuity between the atrioventricular valves. In most patients, however, the postero-caudal limb of the trabeculation fuses with the ventriculoinfundibular fold to provide the defect with a muscular postero-inferior rim (Figures 9.4.18, 9.4.23). The muscular structure thus formed then serves to buttress the axis of atrioventricular conduction tissue from potential surgical damage. Should it be deemed necessary to enlarge a restrictive interventricular communication, this can be achieved by resecting along its antero-superior margins (Figures 9.4.18, 9.4.19). Sometimes, a second muscular defect co-exists with the juxta-arterial defect. If present, such defects must be identified and closed.

Cases have been described in which the ventricular septum has been considered intact. In some instances, this was because the leaflets of the truncal valve closed on the septal crest during ventricular diastole, thus blocking the ventricular component of the ventriculo-arterial septal defect.[13] In this setting, the juxta-arterial defect is readily evident when the valvar leaflets open during diastole. It is possible to have a truly intact ventricular septum should the arterial trunk arise exclusively from the right ventricle, and there is spontaneous closure of a pre-existing interventricular communication. The latter cases are unlikely to come to surgical attention. As we have explained, it is also possible to find cases with a common ventriculo-arterial junction, but with exclusively arterial shunting. This occurs in the hearts with dual valvar orifices, with the bridging tongue attached to the crest of the muscular ventricular septum (Figures 9.4.15–9.4.17). When recognized, these cases can be corrected in surgically appropriate fashion.[10]

After surgical repair by closing both the ventricular and arterial components of the defect, the truncal valve becomes the aortic valve. Valvar incompetence or stenosis, if present, is therefore of considerable significance. This typically reflects dysplasia of the leaflets (Figure 9.4.24). The truncal valve itself usually has three leaflets (Figure 9.4.18). Quadrifoliate valves

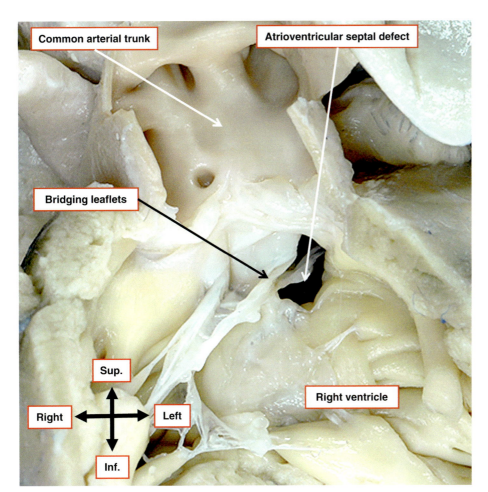

Figure 9.4.20 The heart, photographed from the front, the right ventricle having been opened, has a common arterial trunk supported exclusively by the right ventricle. The interventricular communication, however, is an atrioventricular septal defect. The bridging leaflets of the common atrioventricular valve are seen extending into the left ventricle. The left atrioventricular valve was trifoliate.

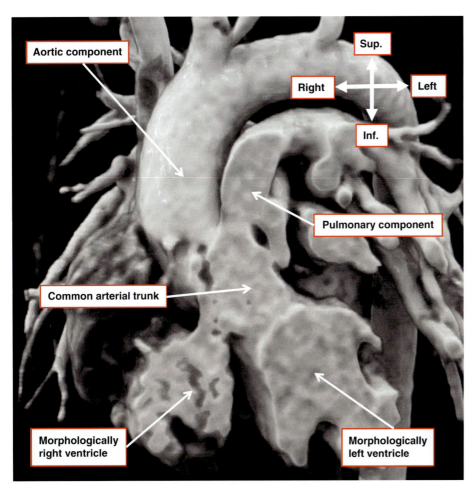

Figure 9.4.21 The frame in the frontal plane from a computed tomographic dataset shows a common arterial trunk with relatively balanced aortic and pulmonary components, with the trunk arising exclusively from the left ventricle. The image was prepared by Dr Niraj Pandey, from All India Institute of Medical Studies, and is reproduced with his permission.

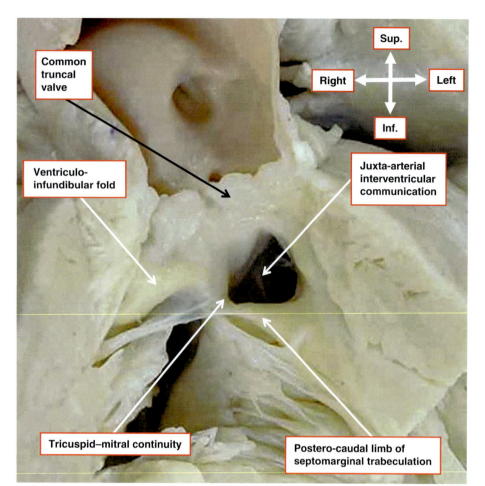

Figure 9.4.22 This heart with a common arterial trunk, again viewed in anatomical orientation, has an interventricular communication which is perimembranous, with fibrous continuity between the leaflets of the mitral and tricuspid valves because the ventriculo-infundibular fold stops short of the caudal limb of the septomarginal trabeculation. The atrioventricular conduction axis is at risk in the postero-inferior rim of the defect.

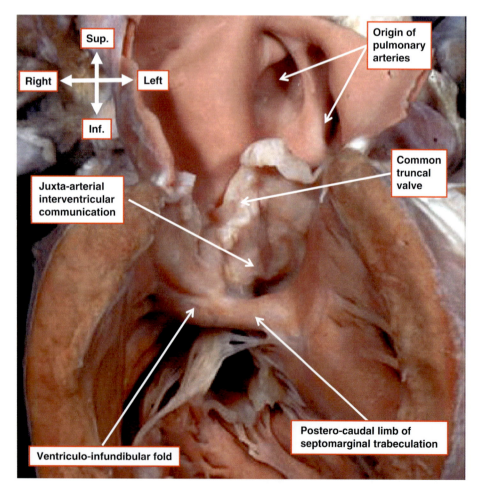

Figure 9.4.23 This heart, shown in anatomical orientation as seen from the right ventricle, has a common arterial trunk overriding an interventricular communication with a muscular postero-inferior rim formed by fusion of the ventriculo-infundibular fold with the postero-caudal limb of the septomarginal trabeculation. The muscular rim protects the atrioventricular conduction axis. There is fibrous continuity between the leaflets of the truncal and mitral valves in the roof of the left ventricle.

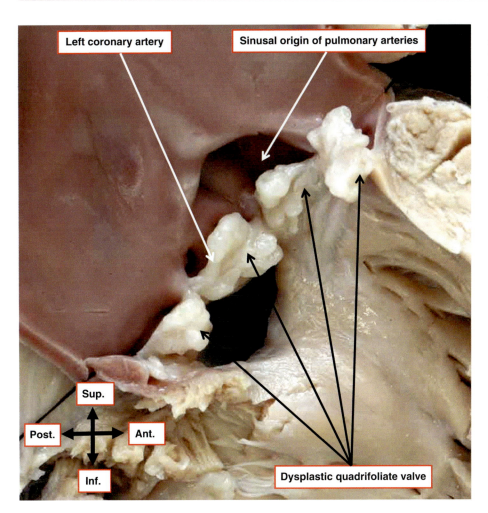

Figure 9.4.24 In this heart, the common arterial trunk has been opened from the right side and is shown in anatomical orientation. The pulmonary arteries arise from within a truncal valvar sinus. Note the origin of the left coronary artery from within the same sinus. The truncal valve is dysplastic and has four leaflets.

are also relatively frequent, although the leaflets are often of unequal size (Figures 9.4.25, 9.4.26). In such circumstances, the surgeon may choose to convert the valve into a trifoliate pattern.[14] Valves with two leaflets are also found. The different patterns are now well explained on the basis of the arrangement of the major outflow cushions, along with hypoplasia or absence of the intercalated valvar swellings (Figure 9.4.11).

The greatest variation of surgical significance is the arrangement of the intrapericardial arterial pathways. Conventionally, two classifications have commonly been used to account for the morphological variations. Both are procrustean, and both use numeric categorizations. The seminal study of Collett and Edwards, which also established the phenotypic feature of the lesion,[1] was exclusively based on the mode of origin of the pulmonary arteries. The possibilities initially described were for the arteries to arise from a short confluent channel (Figure 9.4.18), to arise separately and directly from the left posterior aspect of the trunk (Figure 9.4.27), or to arise separately from either side of the trunk (Figure 9.4.28). The initial classification also included a fourth category, but those fitting in this grouping are better described as having solitary rather than common trunks (Figure 9.4.3). These lesions are now recognized as representing examples of tetralogy with pulmonary atresia, with pulmonary arterial supply via systemic-to-pulmonary collateral arteries, although very rarely the pulmonary arteries can arise extrapericardially from the underside of the aortic arch.[15,16]

The second classification was proposed by Van Praagh and Van Praagh.[8] They initially divided the cases into groups with or without an interventricular communication, with those having no ventricular defects classified as Group B. As we have discussed, it is exceedingly rare to find patients having common ventriculo-arterial junction with exclusively arterial shunting, and it is not clear whether the examples included in the classification of Van Praagh and Van Praagh matched this phenotype. It is their first group, which they designated as Group A, that is of most significance. They also described four subtypes, grouping together the first two categorizations of Collett and Edwards to make their own first type, and retaining the third group of Collett and Edwards as their second type. The importance of their approach was that it highlighted cases with obstruction of the systemic circulation, which they established as their fourth group. They also emphasized the possibility for separate origin of discontinuous pulmonary arteries, with one fed by a persistently patent arterial duct, which could then become ligamentous, with these examples making up their third group. They also noted that the overall group could be divided into those with aortic as opposed to pulmonary dominance within the trunk itself.[8] It is this notion of aortic as opposed to pulmonary dominance that simplifies categorization and description.[2] It is relatively rare for

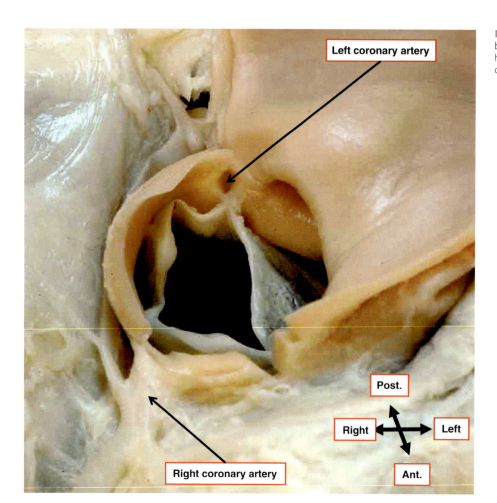

Figure 9.4.25 The common arterial trunk has been windowed from the front. The truncal valve has three leaflets. Note the high origin of the left coronary artery.

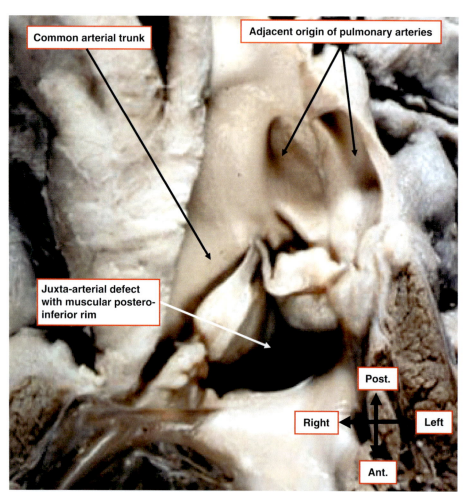

Figure 9.4.26 In this example of common arterial trunk, opened through the right ventricle from the front, the pulmonary arteries take origin in adjacent fashion from the leftward and posterior part of an aortic dominant trunk. The interventricular communication has a muscular postero-inferior rim. The truncal valve has four leaflets.

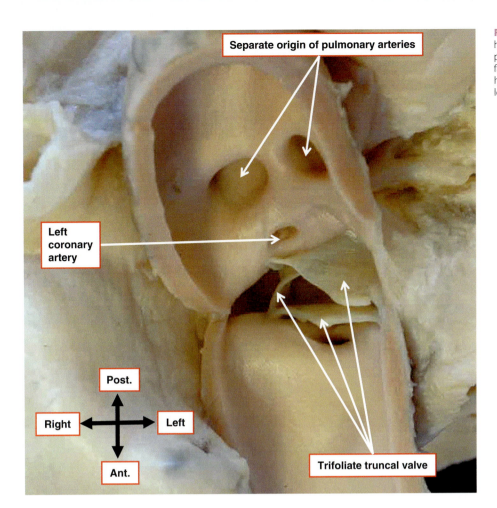

Figure 9.4.27 In this heart, the common trunk has been windowed to show origin of the pulmonary arteries in separate but adjacent fashion from the posterior wall. The truncal valve has three leaflets. There is again high origin of the left coronary artery.

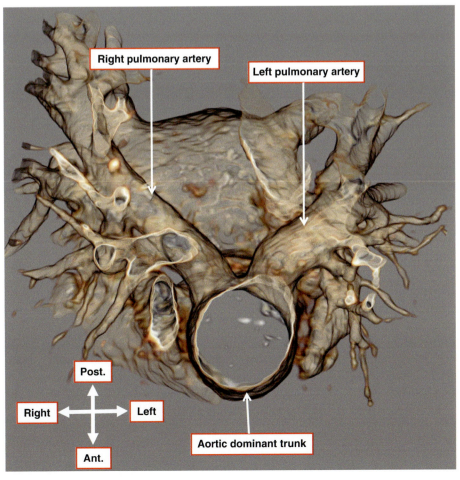

Figure 9.4.28 This computed tomographic angiogram, viewed from above, shows right and left pulmonary arteries arising separately from either side of a common arterial trunk with aortic dominance.

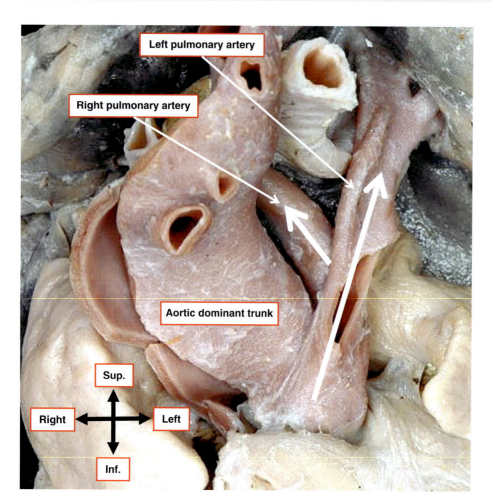

Figure 9.4.29 In this example of common arterial trunk with aortic dominance, photographed from the front, the pulmonary arteries are crossed, and take their origin from the anterior wall of the trunk.

the intrapericardial common trunk to divide into aortic and pulmonary components of comparable dimensions (Figure 9.4.21). In most instances, it is the aortic component of the trunk that is dominant. The pulmonary arteries then usually arise adjacent to one another from the leftward posterior component of the trunk (Figure 9.4.2). If there is a confluent pulmonary component, it is usually very short. The pulmonary arteries, however, can arise more anteriorly, and are then typically crossed at their origins (Figures 9.4.29, 9.4.30). With the increasing availability of three-dimensional techniques for imaging, it is becoming evident that the pulmonary arteries can arise within a truncal valvar sinus (Figures 9.4.31, 9.4.32).[17,18] None of these patterns compromises connection of the pulmonary component to the right ventricle during complete repair. The less common pulmonary dominant trunk is found when the aortic component of the trunk is hypoplastic, in association with either coarctation or interruption of the aortic arch (Figures 9.4.33, 9.4.34). In this arrangement, in which the pulmonary arteries arise from the sides of the trunk, the pulmonary dominant trunk continues through a persistently patent arterial duct to feed the descending aorta.[2] The pulmonary arteries can still be crossed even when there is pulmonary dominance (Figure 9.4.35). The cases with pulmonary dominance produce greater problems for surgical correction. Apart from these cases, or when the pulmonary arteries are discontinuous, with one fed via an arterial duct, it is rare to find persistence of the arterial duct. On occasion, it is also possible to encounter still rarer patterns that justify description as variants of common arterial trunk. Such an example is that case described quite some time ago by Rubay and colleagues, in which the pulmonary arteries arose extrapericardially from the underside of the aortic arch.[15] Another example has been described recently, with an explanation offered as to why the case justifies description as a common arterial trunk,[16] although a case can be made for considering the trunk as being a solitary entity.

The surgeon should always take care to identify the origins of the coronary arteries.[19] When the truncal valve has four sinuses, then the arteries typically arise from the right- and left-sided sinuses. There is less uniformity when, as is most frequently the case, the truncal root has three sinuses. It is unusual, nonetheless, for coronary arteries to arise from the anterior sinus.[20] Solitary coronary arteries, however, are frequent. When there are two coronary arteries, then the left coronary artery often takes an origin above the sinutubular junction (Figures 9.4.25, 9.4.27). On occasion, the origin can be very high, with transmural passage through the truncal wall (Figure 9.4.36). The left coronary artery can also be closely related to the origin of the pulmonary arteries, particularly when the pulmonary arteries themselves take a sinusal origin (Figure 9.4.31). In all these settings, the coronary arteries are at risk if unrecognized when the surgeon separates the pulmonary arteries from the common trunk during complete surgical repair.

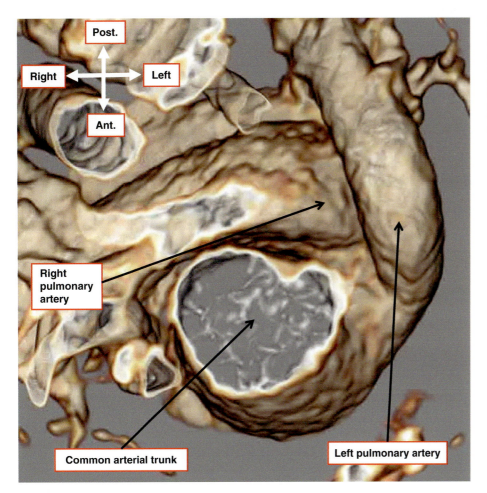

Figure 9.4.30 This computed tomographic angiogram, viewed from above, shows how, in the setting of common arterial trunks, the pulmonary arteries usually arise adjacent to one another from the leftward and posterior component of the trunk. Note the crossing of the left pulmonary artery over the origin of the right pulmonary artery. Such crossing is exaggerated when the pulmonary arteries take a more anterior origin (see Figure 9.4.29).

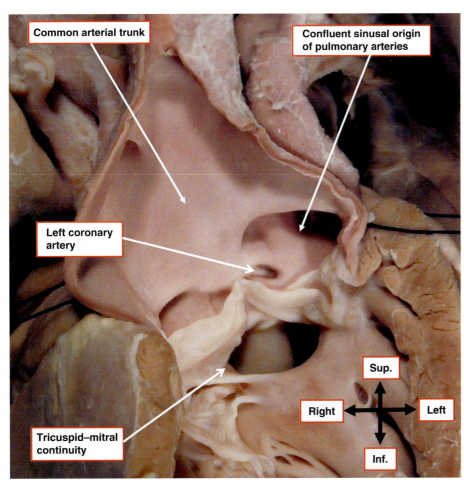

Figure 9.4.31 In this example of common arterial trunk with aortic dominance, the pulmonary arteries take origin from a small confluent component which itself is confluent with the truncal valvar sinus. The interventricular communication is perimembranous, since there is fibrous continuity between the leaflets of the mitral and tricuspid valves, with the continuity reinforced by a membranous flap.

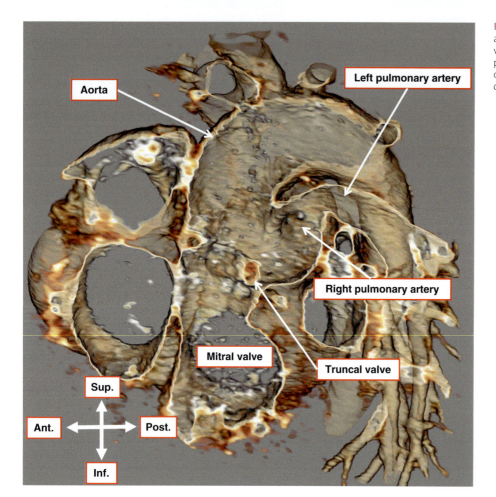

Figure 9.4.32 In this computed tomographic angiogram, cropped in a plane revealing the left ventricular inflow and outflow, the right and left pulmonary arteries arise from a small confluent component within the truncal valvar sinus. The common trunk is aortic dominant.

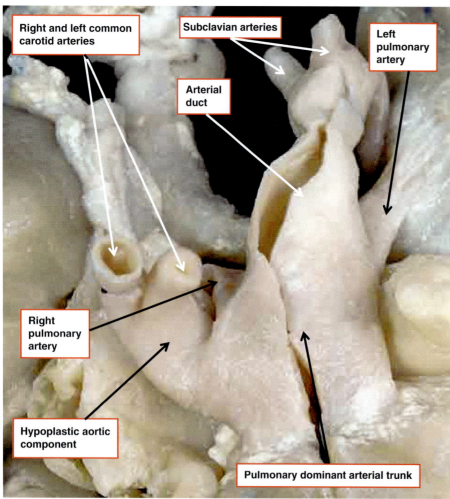

Figure 9.4.33 In this heart, the pulmonary component of the common arterial trunk is dominant. It gives rise to the arterial duct, and to the right and left pulmonary arteries, the latter arising from the sides of the pulmonary component. The aortic component of the trunk is grossly hypoplastic, supplying the right common carotid artery, but is then interrupted beyond the origin of the left common carotid artery. There is retro-esophageal origin of the right subclavian artery, which arises from the descending aorta along with the left subclavian artery, the descending aorta itself being fed by the arterial duct.

9.4 Common Arterial Trunk

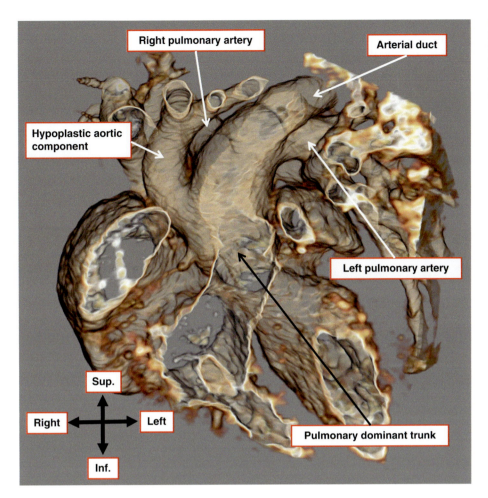

Figure 9.4.34 The computed tomographic angiogram, reconstructed and seen from the front, shows another example of a pulmonary dominant common arterial trunk. In this patient, the aortic arch was interrupted at the isthmus. The arterial duct remains patent and supplies the descending aorta.

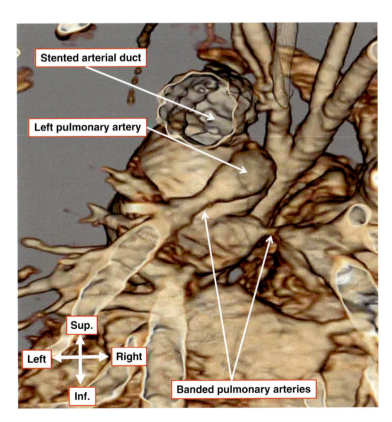

Figure 9.4.35 This computed tomographic angiogram, reconstructed and viewed from behind, is another example of a pulmonary dominant common arterial trunk. It shows crossing of the pulmonary arteries as they arise from the posterior aspect of the common trunk. Note that the right and left pulmonary arteries have been banded. The arterial duct, which feeds the descending aorta in the setting of the interrupted aortic arch, has been stented.

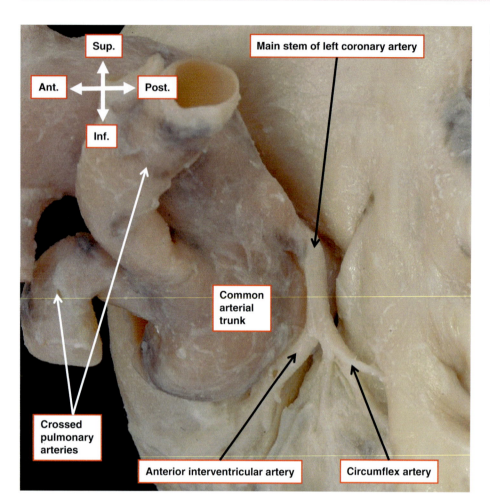

Figure 9.4.36 The common arterial trunk is photographed from the left side to show a very high origin of the left coronary artery, which extends in intramural fashion as it exits the aortic dominant component of the trunk (compare with Figure 9.4.27). Note the crossed origin of the right and left pulmonary arteries.

References Cited

1. Collett RW, Edwards JE. Persistent truncus arteriosus. A classification according to anatomic types. *Surg Clin North Am* 1949; **29**: 1245–1270.

2. Russell HM, Jacobs ML, Anderson RH, et al. A simplified categorization for common arterial trunk. *J Thorac Cardiovasc Surg* 2011; **141**: 645–653.

3. Anderson RH, Thiene G. Categorization and description of hearts with common arterial trunk. *Eur J Cardio-thoracic Surg* 1989; **3**: 481–487.

4. Schofield DE, Anderson RH. Common arterial trunk with pulmonary atresia. *Int J Cardiol* 1988; **20**: 290–294.

5. Kramer TC. The partitioning of the truncus and conus and the formation of the membranous portion of the interventricular septum in the human heart. *Am J Anat* 1942; **71**: 343–370.

6. Anderson RH, Mohun TJ, Spicer DE, et al. Myths and realities relating to development of the arterial valves. *J Cardiovasc Devel Dis* 2014; **1**: 177–200.

7. Spicer DE, Steffensen TS. A rare presentation of common arterial trunk with intact ventricular septum. *J Cardiovasc Devel Dis* 2020; **7**: 43.

8. Van Praagh R, Van Praagh S. The anatomy of common aorticopulmonary trunk (truncus arteriosus communis) and its embryologic implications: a study of 57 necropsy cases. *Am J Cardiol* 1965; **16**: 406–425.

9. Van Mierop LHS, Patterson DF, Schnarr WR. Pathogenesis of persistent truncus arteriosus in light of observations made in a dog embryo with the anomaly. *Am J Cardiol* 1978; **41**: 755–762.

10. Garg P, Mishra A, Shah R, Parmar D, Anderson RH. Neonatal repair of common arterial trunk with intact ventricular septum. *World J Pediatr Congenit Heart Surg* 2015; **6**: 93–97.

11. Tsang VT, Kang N, Sullivan I, Marek J, Anderson RH. Ventriculoarterial septal defect with separate aortic and pulmonary valves, but common ventriculoarterial junction. *J Thorac Cardiovasc Surg* 2008; **135**: 222–223.

12. Adachi I, Ho SY, Bartelings MM, et al. Common arterial trunk with atrioventricular septal defect: new observations pertinent to repair. *Ann Thorac Surg* 2009; **87**: 1495–1499.

13. Carr I, Bharati S, Kusnoor VS, Lev M. Truncus arteriosus communis with intact ventricular septum. *Br Heart J* 1979; **42**: 97–102.

14. Backer CL. Techniques for repairing the aortic and truncal valves. *Cardiol Young* 2005; **15** (Suppl.1): 125–131.

15. Rubay JE, Macartney FJ, Anderson RH. A rare variant of common arterial trunk. *Br Heart J* 1987; **57**: 202–204.

16. Sekelyk RI, Yusifli IB, Kozhokar DM, et al. Surgical repair of a rare variant of common arterial trunk, with considerations of its significance for morphogenesis. *World J Ped Card Surg* 2023; **14**: 446–450.

17. Adachi I, Uemura H, McCarthy KP, Seale A, Ho SY. Relationship between orifices of pulmonary and coronary arteries in common arterial trunk. *Eur J Cardiothorac Surg* 2009; **35**: 594–599.

18. Gupta SK, Aggarwal A., Shaw M, et al. Clarifying the anatomy of common arterial trunk: a clinical study of 70 patients. *Eur Heart J-Cardiovasc Imag* 2020; **21**, 914–922.

19. Suzuki A, Ho SY, Anderson RH, Deanfield JE. Coronary arterial and sinusal anatomy in hearts with a common arterial trunk. *Ann Thorac Surg* 1989; **48**: 792–797.

20. Bogers AJ, Bartelings MM, Bokenkamp R, et al. Common arterial trunk, uncommon coronary arterial anatomy. *J Thorac Cardiovasc Surg* 1993; **106**; 1133–1137.

Chapter 9.5
Concordant Ventriculo-Arterial Connections with Parallel Arterial Trunks

The hearts to be discussed in this chapter do not necessarily have abnormal segmental combinations, since if the atrioventricular connections, along with the ventriculo-arterial connections, are concordant, then the segmental junctions will be normal, despite the unexpected relationships of the arterial trunks. It is also the case that patients with the arrangements to be discussed are exceedingly rare. Although rare, however, the combinations have been the source of much discussion and controversy. Indeed, for quite some time the possibility that the aorta could arise anteriorly from the morphologically left ventricle, and extend into the mediastinum in parallel fashion relative to the pulmonary trunk, was considered an embryological impossibility.[1] There is no question now, however, that such hearts do exist. It is also the case that the unusual arrangement at the ventriculo-arterial junctions can be found with any atrial arrangement, and with any possible atrioventricular connection. It is for this reason that we have allocated the hearts their own specific chapter.

It is also the case that, in the past, the lesions have been described using some of the most arcane of terminologies, including such spectacular phrases as isolated ventricular inversion,[2] and anatomically corrected malposition.[3] The feature that unifies the combinations is the feature emphasized above. Although the arterial trunks arise from the morphologically appropriate ventricles, usually with the aorta in anterior position, they extend towards the mediastinum in parallel rather than spiralling fashion.[4,5] On occasion, although still extending in parallel fashion relative to the pulmonary trunk, the aortic root can be found in rightward and posterior location. A right-sided and posterior origin of the aorta, of course, is found in the normal heart. But in the normal heart, the right-sided aorta takes its origin from the left-sided morphologically left ventricle (Figure 9.5.1). In the situation described by some as 'isolated ventricular inversion', the right-sided aorta takes origin from the morphologically left ventricle also located in right-sided position, with the ventricular mass showing left-handed topology. In this setting, there is fibrous continuity between the leaflets of the aortic and mitral valves, but unlike the situation in the normal heart, the mitral valve in the arrangement alleged to show 'isolated ventricular inversion' is itself right sided (Figure 9.5.2). Under no circumstances can such an arrangement be considered to represent 'normal

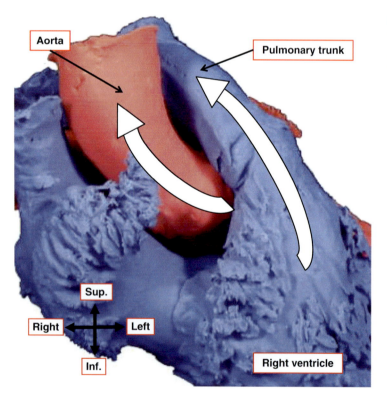

Figure 9.5.1 The base of a cast of the normal heart, with the right side cast in blue, and the left side in red, is photographed to show the normal spiralling of the arterial trunks, with the pulmonary trunk extending in counter-clockwise fashion around the aortic root (large white arrows).

9.5 Concordant Ventriculo-Arterial Connections with Parallel Arterial Trunks

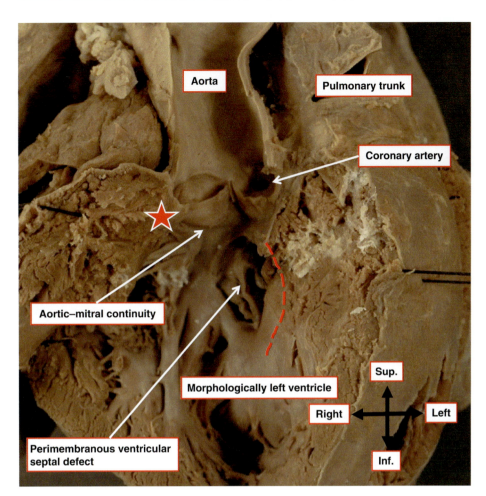

Figure 9.5.2 The morphologically left ventricle in this heart is connected in discordant fashion to the right atrium, but gives rise to the aorta. Because of the discordant atrioventricular connections, the atrioventricular node is anomalously located in anterior position (red star with white borders), and the conduction axis (dashed red line) descends in cranial fashion relative to the perimembranous ventricular septal defect.

relations' of the arterial trunks. The features of the abnormal heart do no more than focus attention on the issues we discussed in Chapter 7, namely the need to assess connections, relationships, and infundibular morphology as discrete and separate features of the ventriculo-arterial junctions.[6] When assessing the relationship of the arterial trunks, furthermore, this must be determined according to the topology of the ventricular mass, not on the basis of atrial arrangement.

There are also problems with the use of the term 'malposition'. The word was introduced because, when the lesions having a concordantly connected aorta arising anteriorly were first described, they were considered to represent 'anatomically corrected transposition'.[7] As we discussed when considering the hearts having discordant ventriculo-arterial connections, this approach reflected the fact that, initially, all lesions having the aorta positioned anterior to the pulmonary trunk were considered to represent 'transposition'. The finding of the aorta arising posteriorly from the morphologically left ventricle in discordant fashion identified the problems produced by those using this approach.[8] Those defining the anterior aorta as being 'transposed', however, mounted a strong defence of their position.[9] Nowadays, nonetheless, it has become accepted that continuing to use the anterior position of the aorta as the criterion for 'transposition' is less than satisfactory, since it continues to permit the confusing nomination of 'double outlet right ventricle with transposition'. The introduction of 'malposition', however, has not resolved the problem. As already indicated, those favouring the use of 'isolated ventricular inversion' argue that the right-sided aortic root, arising from the right-sided morphologically left ventricle, and in fibrous continuity with the right-sided mitral valve, is 'normally related'. The root, however, is just as malposed in this location as when arising in similar position, but with its leaflets separated from those of the mitral valve by a completely muscular infundibulum (Figure 9.5.3).

To clarify the situation, the 'normal relations' of the arterial roots are found when the right-sided and posterior aortic root arises from the left-sided morphologically left ventricle, with fibrous continuity present between the leaflets of the aortic and left-sided aortic valves. This is found in the setting of right-handed ventricular topology (Figure 9.5.1). In the setting of left-handed topology, the mirror-imaged normal arrangement is found when the aortic root is left-sided and posterior, arising from the right-sided morphologically left ventricle. This combination is found in the mirror-imaged, but otherwise normal, heart (Figure 9.5.4).

We are now able not only to provide a rational explanation for the grouping of the lesions on the basis of the parallel nature of the arterial trunks, distinguishing them from those with spiralling arterial trunks. We can also offer an explanation

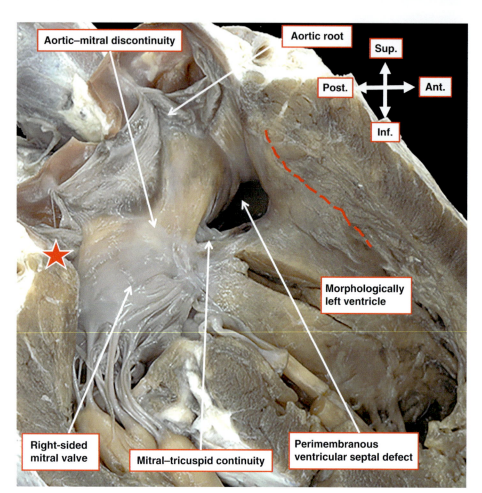

Figure 9.5.3 The left-sided morphologically left ventricle is photographed in another heart with usual atrial arrangement and discordant atrioventricular connections. Again, the left ventricle supports the aorta, as in the heart shown in Figure 9.5.2, but in this heart above a complete muscular infundibulum. The pulmonary trunk exits the heart parallel to the aorta, and arises from the morphologically right ventricle (see Figure 9.5.17). The conduction axis again descends cranial to the perimembranous ventricular septal defect.

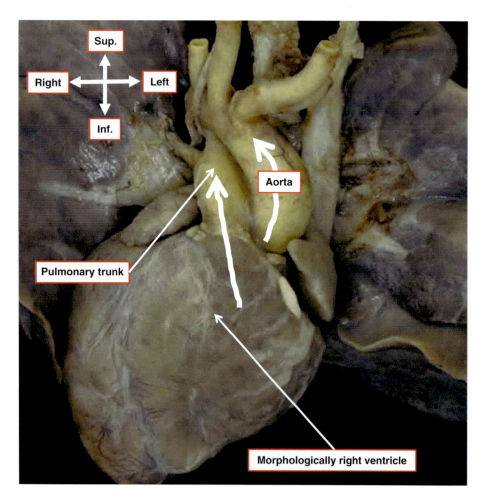

Figure 9.5.4 This heart is from a normal individual with mirror-imaged arrangement of all the organs. The ventricular mass shows left-handed topology, and the pulmonary trunk spirals in mirror-imaged fashion relative to the aortic root as it extends into the mediastinum (thick white arrows).

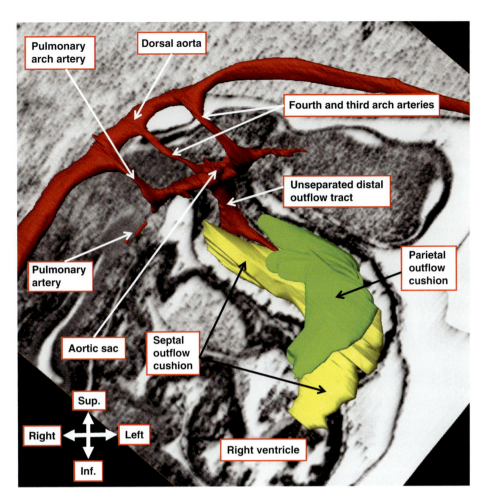

Figure 9.5.5 The reconstruction shows the developing outflow tract and pharyngeal arch arteries of a developing mouse embryo sacrificed during embryonic day 11.5. The outflow cushions are spiralling through the part of the outflow tract that has retained its myocardial walls; however, the distal part of the outflow tract already has non-myocardial walls, but has yet to be separated into its aortic and pulmonary components. The reconstruction was made by Dr Simon Bamforth, from Newcastle University, and is reproduced with his permission.

of the abnormal development producing the unusual segmental combinations. As we showed in Chapter 2, during normal development it is the manner of separation of the channels within the outflow tract that serves to unite the cavity of the right ventricle with the pulmonary arteries, which arise from the arteries of the ultimate pharyngeal arch. The feature that ensures this appropriate channelling of the ventricular outflow tracts is the spiral nature of the cushions that separate the outflow tract into its aortic and pulmonary components. When selecting the illustrations for Chapter 2, we chose, as far as possible, to use images of developing human hearts. The changes are seen equally well in the developing mouse heart. At embryonic day 11.5 in the murine model, the distal part of the outflow tract has still to be separated into aortic and pulmonary channels (Figure 9.5.5). The image shows well also the relationship between the arteries of the pharyngeal arches and the aortic sac. It is the growth of the dorsal wall of the aortic sac into the unseparated distal part of the outflow tract, which has non-myocardial walls, which separates the sac into its aortic and pulmonary components. The protrusion from the dorsal wall produces the aortopulmonary septum (Figure 9.5.6). The parts of the outflow tract that have retained their myocardial walls are not separated by the aortopulmonary septum. Instead, they are divided into the aortic and pulmonary channels by fusion of the major outflow cushions. As can be seen in Figure 9.5.5, these cushions spiral around one another as they extend from proximal to distal within the outflow tract of the right ventricle. At the stage at which the distal parts of the cushions fuse with each other, and also with the leading edge of the aortopulmonary septum, the proximal parts of the cushions have yet to fuse (Figure 9.5.7). The flow into the aortic root at this stage is through the secondary interventricular foramen (Figure 9.5.8). The fusion of the proximal parts of the cushions builds a shelf in the roof of the right ventricle, in this way committing the aortic root to the left ventricle (Figure 9.5.9). As is also shown in Figure 9.5.9, at the stage at which the cavity of the aortic root is brought into continuity with the cavity of the left ventricle, the aortic root remains supported above the cavity of the right ventricle. It is only after the closure of the tertiary interventricular foramen, which is the persisting part of the primary foramen between the aortic root and the right ventricle, that remodelling of the aortic root brings it predominantly above the cavity of the left ventricle. After the closure of the embryonic communication, furthermore, and hence after the completion of ventricular septation, the aortic leaflets retain a completely muscular infundibulum (Figure 9.5.10). Further remodelling subsequent to the closure of the interventricular communication, therefore, is required to produce the area of mitral-to-aortic continuity which is the feature of the normal heart.

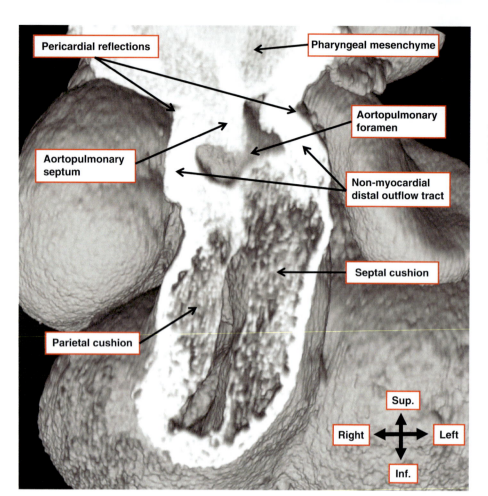

Figure 9.5.6 The frontal section is from an episcopic dataset prepared from a mouse embryo sacrificed a little later during embryonic day 11.5 when compared with the reconstruction shown in Figure 9.5.5. The image shows how the aortopulmonary septum is protruding into the distal outflow tract, separating it into the aortic and pulmonary components. The major outflow cushions have yet to fuse, but will separate the part of the outflow tract that has retained its myocardial walls.

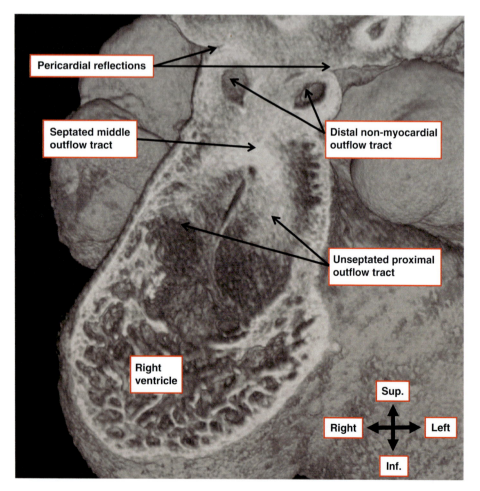

Figure 9.5.7 The image shows another frontal section from a developing mouse embryo, this time sacrificed early during embryonic day 12.5. The aortopulmonary septum has fused with the distal outflow cushions, themselves also by now fused. The proximal parts of the cushions, however, have yet to fuse.

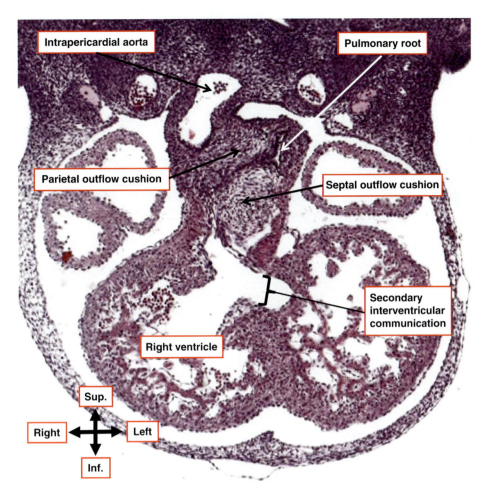

Figure 9.5.8 The histological section, stained using the trichrome technique, is from a mouse embryo at the same stage of development as the example shown in Figure 9.5.7. The major cushions are sectioned as they spiral at the level of the developing arterial roots (compare with Figure 9.5.11). Both arterial roots are supported by the right ventricle, with the secondary interventricular foramen providing the outflow tract for the left ventricle.

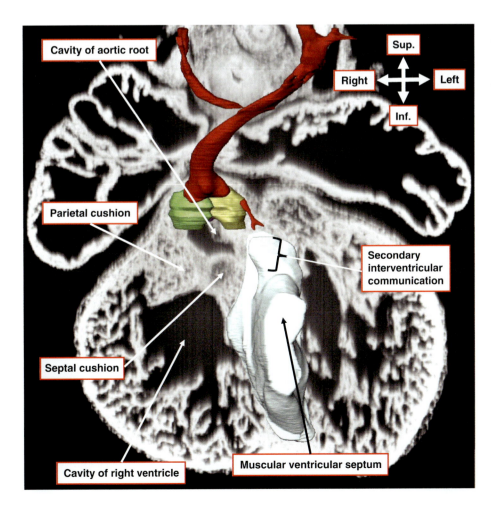

Figure 9.5.9 The frontal section is taken from an episcopic dataset prepared from a mouse embryo sacrificed at embryonic day 13.5. The proximal outflow cushions have now fused to build the shelf in the roof of the right ventricle that commits the aortic root through the secondary interventricular foramen to the cavity of the left ventricle. The reconstruction was made by Dr Simon Bamforth, from Newcastle University, and is reproduced with his permission.

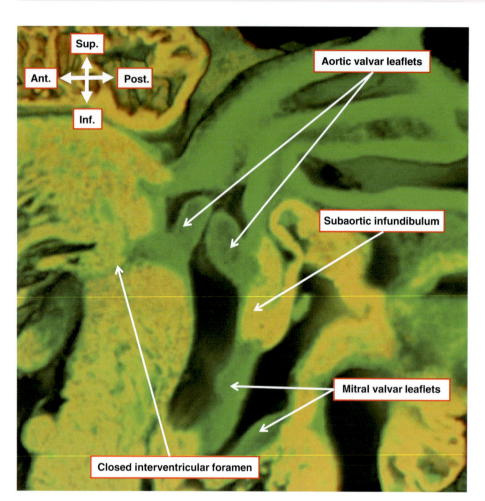

Figure 9.5.10 The image is from an episcopic dataset prepared from a mouse embryo sacrificed at embryonic day 14.5, and programmed to show the myocardium as yellow. At this stage, subsequent to closure of the embryonic interventricular foramen, the left ventricle retains a completely muscular subaortic infundibulum.

All of these mechanisms of normal development are pertinent to the understanding of hearts with concordant ventriculo-arterial connections, but parallel arterial trunks. A parallel arrangement of the arterial trunks, of course, is seen most frequently when the ventriculo-arterial connections are discordant, in other words, transposition. It is now established that the reason the trunks are attached to morphologically inappropriate ventricles is because the outflow cushions fuse in straight rather than spiralling fashion (Figure 9.5.11). This then permits the arterial root adjacent to the ventricular septum, which is the pulmonary root, to be transferred to the left ventricle subsequent to the formation of the shelf in the roof of the right ventricle. The images illustrating the process of normal development also serve to demonstrate the independence of the separation of the channels derived from the aortic sac as opposed to those formed within the outflow tract. The anatomical findings permit the inference to be made that the manner of fusion between the aortopulmonary septum and the distal margins of the outflow cushions is comparable in normal development and in the arrangement producing discordant ventriculo-arterial connections (Figure 9.5.12 – columns A and B). Should the outflow cushions fuse in straight rather than spiralling fashion, as is the case to produce discordant ventriculo-arterial connections, but the aortopulmonary septum then fuses with the distal end of the major outflow cushion in reversed fashion, then the ventriculo-arterial connections would be concordant, but with parallel arterial trunks (Figure 9.5.12 – column C). In this arrangement, it would again be the aortic root that is transferred to the left ventricle, but in an anterior as opposed to its usual posterior position. All the evidence now available from hearts and patients described with concordant ventriculo-arterial connections, but in the setting of parallel arterial trunks,[5] is in keeping with these proposed mechanisms of normal as opposed to abnormal development.

In most of the hearts described with parallel arterial trunks with concordant ventriculo-arterial connections, the atrioventricular connections have been concordant, and with usual atrial arrangement. In this combination, the aorta arises from the ventricular mass in left-sided and anterior position (Figure 9.5.13). As in the example shown in Figure 9.5.13, the arrangement is frequently accompanied by left-sided juxtaposition of the atrial appendages.[10] The leaflets of the aortic valve are supported anteriorly within the left ventricle by a complete muscular infundibulum (Figure 9.5.14). Ventricular septation is usually deficient, and as shown in Figure 9.5.14, the ventricular septal defect can be perimembranous when there is fibrous continuity postero-inferiorly between the leaflets of the mitral and tricuspid valves. In this arrangement, as is always the case for perimembranous defects, the conduction axis is at risk in the postero-inferior margin of the defect. In other hearts of this type, nonetheless, the defect can have a muscular postero-inferior rim, which then protects the conduction axis (Figure 9.5.15). In all these hearts, the

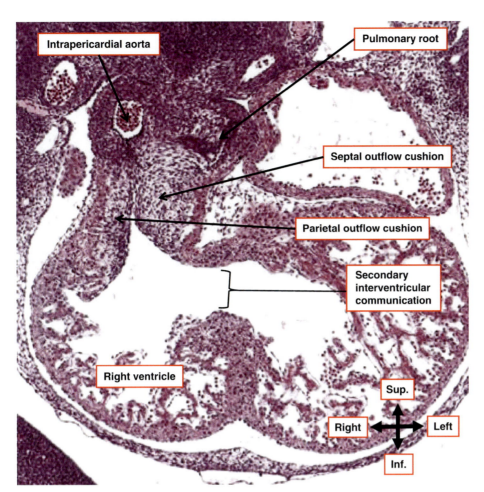

Figure 9.5.11 The histological section is from a mouse embryo sacrificed at embryonic day 12.5 in which the *Pitx2* gene has been knocked out. All of these embryos either develop discordant ventriculo-arterial connections, or double outlet right ventricle with subpulmonary interventricular foramen. The key difference with the normal arrangement at this stage (see Figure 9.5.8) is that the outflow cushions are fusing in straight, rather than spiralling, fashion.

ventricular septal defect opens to the outlet of the right ventricle beneath the anteriorly positioned aortic root (Figure 9.5.16). This feature points to the spectrum that likely existed during development between this variant of concordant ventriculo-arterial connections and the rare variant of double outlet right ventricle with left-sided aorta and subaortic interventricular communication.[11]

Although found most frequently with concordant atrioventricular connections, the concordant ventriculo-arterial connections with parallel trunks can be found with any atrioventricular connection. Tricuspid atresia, due to absence of the right atrioventricular connection, is one of the more frequent alternative connections.[12] The combination can also be found in the setting of isomerism, when the atrioventricular connections are mixed, as opposed to being concordant or discordant.[13] The variant of most surgical importance, however, is the combination with discordant atrioventricular connections (Figures 9.5.2, 9.5.3). It is this arrangement that has, in the past, been described as 'isolated ventricular inversion', or when seen with mirror-imaged atrial arrangement, 'isolated ventricular non-inversion'. As we have explained, there is no justification for using this terminology, which depends on the finding of fibrous continuity between the leaflets of the aortic and mitral valves (Figure 9.5.2). As we have also shown, the combination can be found in almost identical fashion when there is a muscular subaortic infundibulum (Figure 9.5.3). The latter lesion would be dubbed 'anatomically corrected nomenclature'. The physiological features are identical, in that the combination of discordant and concordant connections at the atrioventricular and ventriculo-arterial junctions produces the hemodynamic picture of transposition.[14] With this combination, it is the morphologically left ventricle that is already supporting the aortic root (Figures 9.5.2, 9.5.3), and the morphologically right ventricle that supports the pulmonary trunk (Figure 9.5.17). As with the variants with concordant atrioventricular connections, there is usually a ventricular septal defect, which opens to the outlet of the right ventricle between the limbs of septomarginal trabeculation (Figure 9.5.17). The defect is usually perimembranous (Figures 9.5.2, 9.5.3), but can have a muscular postero-inferior rim. The significant point in this setting, however, is that, because of the discordant atrioventricular connections, and the associated malalignment between the atrial and ventricular septums because of the interposing aortic outflow tract, the conduction axis will take origin from an anomalous atrioventricular node, and extend cranially relative to the defect, descending the septum along its cranial rim (Figures 9.5.2, 9.5.3). From the surgical stance, the other significant point is that the lesion can be corrected both anatomically and physiologically by performing an atrial switch, taking care, of course, to deal with all associated malformations.[14]

The concordant ventriculo-arterial connections in the setting of parallel arterial trunks can also be found when there is double inlet to a dominant left ventricle (Figures 9.5.18,

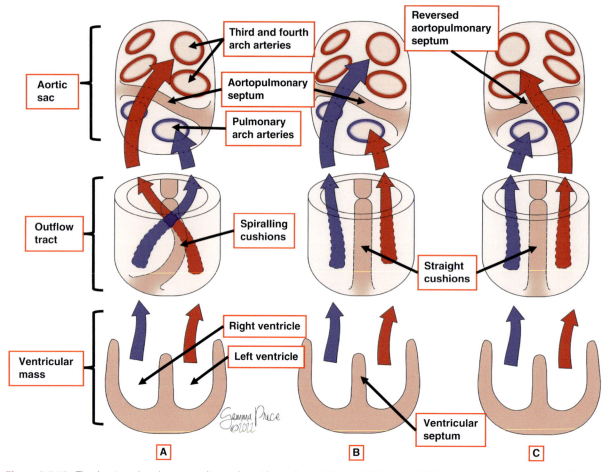

Figure 9.5.12 The drawings show how, according to the evidence shown in Figures 9.5.5 through 9.5.11, a concept can be put forward to explain the difference between the normal arrangement (column A), the arrangement with discordant ventriculo-arterial connections (column B), and the combination of concordant ventriculo-arterial connections, but with parallel rather than spiralling arterial trunks.

9.5.19). This combination, in the past, has again been described as 'isolated ventricular inversion',[15] but without any good reason. It produces a variant of the so-called Holmes heart, in which the arterial trunks spiral when double inlet left ventricle is associated with concordant ventriculo-arterial connections (Figure 9.5.20). The hemodynamics, however, are identical between the lesions having spiralling as opposed to parallel arterial trunks. The optimal surgical approach when the trunks are parallel (Figure 9.5.18) is likely to be conversion to the Fontan procedure.

As discussed above, when the atrioventricular connections are discordant in the setting of concordant ventriculo-arterial connections with parallel arterial trunks, the ideal surgical repair is an atrial redirection procedure, since this operation restores the morphologically left ventricle to its systemic role. This operation will also be the procedure of choice in those situations where the arterial trunks spiral in normal fashion as they extend into the mediastinum, but again in the setting of discordant rather than concordant ventriculo-arterial connections. The understanding of this combination, however, is clouded by the finding that the majority of the cases described thus far with spiralling arterial trunks have been associated with left isomerism, rather than usual or mirror-imaged atrial arrangement.[14] In the report of Laux and colleagues,[16] for example, five of their six cases had left isomerism. The three cases reported by Sharma and colleagues,[17] nonetheless, all were described with usual atrial arrangement and discordant ventriculo-arterial connections, with mirror-imaged spiralling of the trunks as they extended from a ventricular mass with left-handed topology. Sporadic cases are also described of discordant atrioventricular and concordant ventriculo-arterial connections, with spiralling arterial trunks, when there is mirror-imaged atrial arrangement, with one case described with an intact ventricular septum.[18]

It is the finding of spiralling but concordantly connected arterial trunks in the setting of left isomerism that requires particular surgical attention. The feature of hearts with isomeric atrial appendages, of course, is the grossly abnormal venoatrial connections. Despite the essential anatomical abnormalities that are produced when both appendages have the same morphology, the particular connections can produce quasi-usual drainage when all the systemic veins connect to the right-sided atrium, and all the pulmonary veins to the left-sided atrium (Figure 9.5.21). If connected in opposite fashion, the result would be quasi-mirror-imaged drainage. If, in the setting of the quasi-usual drainage, there were biventricular

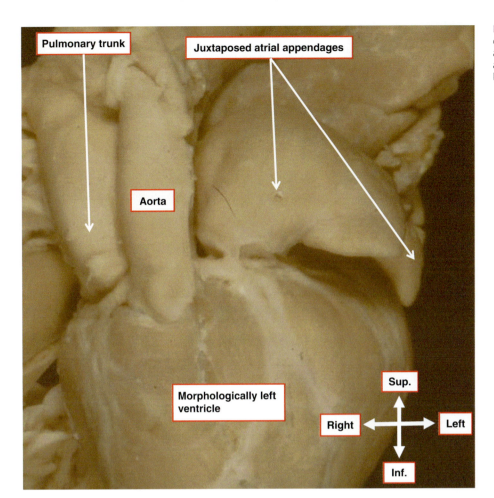

Figure 9.5.13 This heart is from a patient with concordant atrioventricular and ventriculo-arterial connections. The aorta is left sided and anterior relative to the pulmonary trunk. There is left-sided juxtaposition of the atrial appendages.

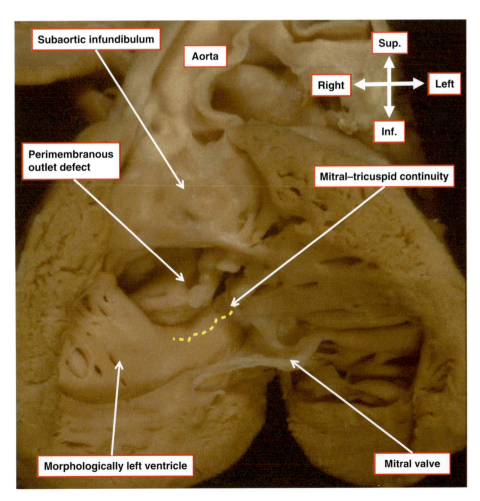

Figure 9.5.14 The left side of the heart shown in Figure 9.5.13 is shown, opened from its left side. The morphologically left atrium is connected to the morphologically left ventricle with right-handed ventricular topology. The aorta arises from the left ventricle, with its valvar leaflets supported by an extensive muscular infundibulum. There is also a large perimembranous ventricular septal defect. The atrioventricular conduction axis is postero-inferiorly positioned relative to the defect (yellow dotted line), but is at risk in the fibrous postero-inferior margin.

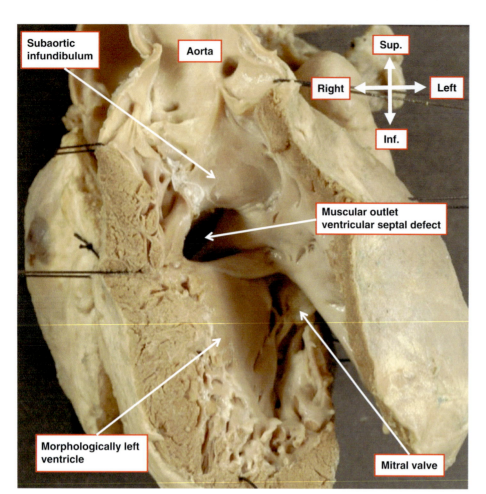

Figure 9.5.15 The left side of another heart is shown with concordant ventriculo-arterial connections and parallel arterial trunks. As with the heart shown in Figure 9.5.14, there is a large subaortic infundibulum, but in this heart, the defect has a muscular postero-inferior rim, which will protect the atrioventricular conduction axis. Note the glued together halves of the muscular outlet septum forming the roof of the defect.

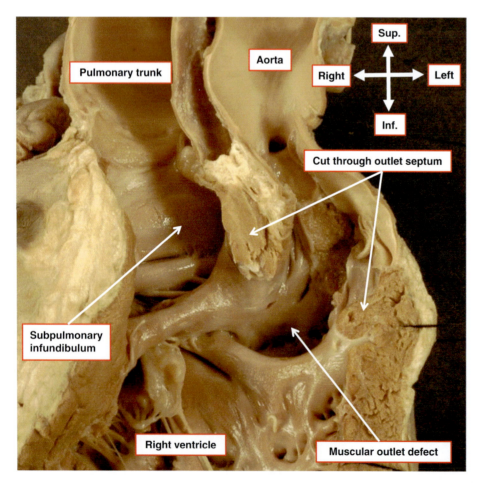

Figure 9.5.16 This image shows the right side of the heart photographed in Figure 9.5.15, but with the outlet septum divided across its middle. The aortic root opens to the right ventricle through the muscular outlet defect. There is also a completely muscular subpulmonary infundibulum.

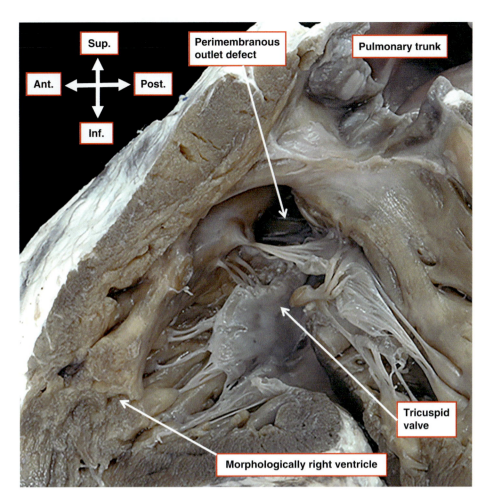

Figure 9.5.17 The left-sided morphologically right ventricle is shown from the heart also illustrated in Figure 9.5.3. The atrioventricular connections are discordant, but the pulmonary trunk arises from the right ventricle because of the concordant ventriculo-arterial connections. The combination with discordant atrioventricular connections produces the haemodynamics of transposition. Correction with an atrial redirection procedure will restore the morphologically left ventricle to a systemic role.

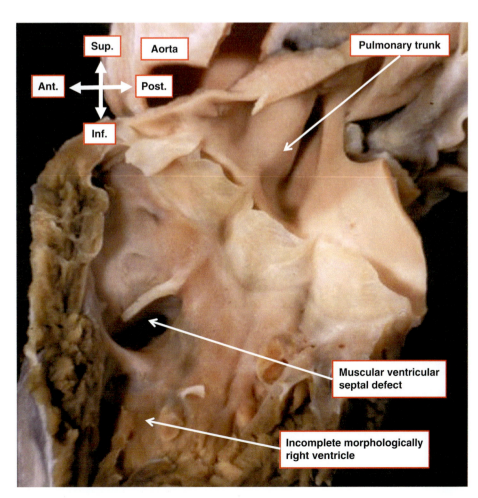

Figure 9.5.18 The heart exhibits double inlet left ventricle, with an incomplete right ventricle and concordant ventriculo-arterial connections. In this specimen, the incomplete right ventricle is left sided, and the pulmonary trunk arises in parallel fashion. This is an example of concordant ventriculo-arterial connections with parallel arterial trunks in the setting of double inlet ventricle.

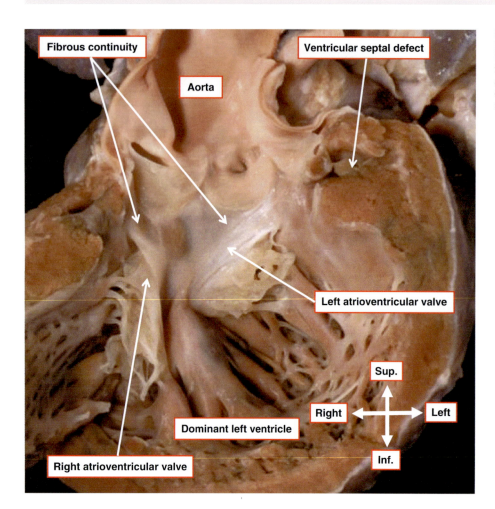

Figure 9.5.19 The image shows the dominant left ventricle from the heart shown in Figure 9.5.18. The leaflets of the aortic valve are in fibrous continuity with the leaflets of both of the atrioventricular valves. The ventricular septal defect is seen providing the outlet for the left-sided incomplete right ventricle.

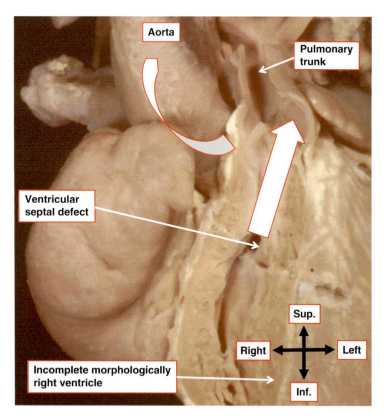

Figure 9.5.20 The image shows the anterior view of the incomplete right ventricle more usually found when double inlet left ventricle is combined with concordant ventriculo-arterial connections. This is the lesion known as the Holmes heart. The arterial trunks spiral in normal fashion (twisted white arrow with red borders), with the pulmonary trunk extending in counter-clockwise fashion relative to the aortic root (straight white arrow with red borders).

9.5 Concordant Ventriculo-Arterial Connections with Parallel Arterial Trunks

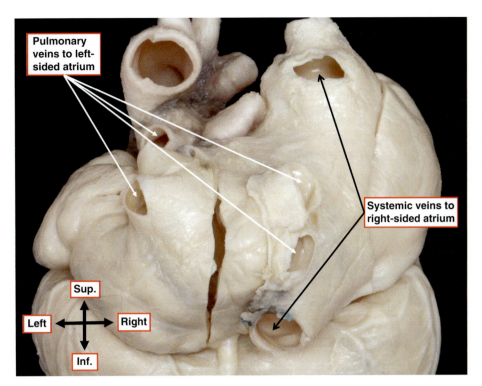

Figure 9.5.21 The heart, which has isomeric left atrial appendages, is photographed from behind to show all the systemic veins connecting to the right-sided atrium, and all the pulmonary veins connected to the left-sided atrium. If this quasi-usual venous drainage was found in a heart as shown in Figure 9.5.22, which as left-handed ventricular topology, then there would be transposition physiology with concordantly connected and mirror-imaged spiralling arterial trunks. In this heart, however, the aorta is discordantly connected to the morphologically right ventricle, which has right-handed topology, so the ventriculo-arterial connections are discordant.

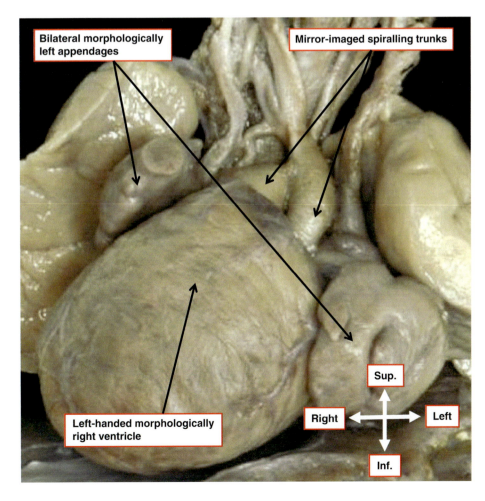

Figure 9.5.22 This heart again has isomeric left atrial appendages. There is left-handed ventricular topology, with concordant ventriculo-arterial connections and mirror-imaged spiralling arterial trunks. If the venoatrial connections had been as shown in Figure 9.5.21, then this heart would have exhibited transposition physiology despite the presence of concordant ventriculo-arterial connections and spiralling arterial trunks.

atrioventricular connections with left-handed ventricular topology, then the arrangement with mirror-imaged spiralling arterial trunks (Figure 9.5.22) would replicate the arrangement described for discordant atrioventricular connections with usual atrial arrangement.[17] It is very likely that, in the arrangements with left isomerism, the atrioventricular conduction would continue to arise from an anomalous anterior atrioventricular node.[19] The sinus node, however, would be anticipated to be grossly abnormal. Indeed, in many instances it is not possible to identify the sinus node when there are isomeric left atrial appendages. All of these considerations point to the need to distinguish between patients having lateralized as opposed to isomeric atrial appendages when these rare segmental combinations are encountered.

Taken together, the hearts with concordant ventriculo-arterial connections but parallel arterial trunks,[5] along with those producing transposition despite the presence of concordant ventriculo-arterial connections,[14] are exemplary in serving to demonstrate the importance of analysing separately the arterial relationships and infundibular morphology as opposed to the origin of the arterial trunks from the ventricular mass.

References Cited

1. Van Mierop LHS, Wiglesworth FW. Pathogenesis of transposition complexes. II. Anomalies due to faulty transfer of the posterior great artery. *Am J Cardiol* 1963; **12**:226–232.

2. Van Praagh R, Van Praagh S. Isolated ventricular inversion: a consideration of the morphogenesis, definition and diagnosis of nontransposed and transposed great arteries. *Am J Cardiol* 1966; **17**: 395–406.

3. Van Praagh R, Durnin RE, Jockin H, et al. Anatomically corrected malposition of the great arteries (S, D, L). *Circulation*. 1975; **51**: 20–31.

4. Bernasconi A, Cavalle-Garrido T, Perrin DG, Anderson RH. What is anatomically corrected malposition? *Cardiol Young* 2007; **17**: 26–34.

5. Cavalle-Garrido T, Bernasconi A, Perrin D, Anderson RH. Hearts with concordant ventriculoarterial connections but parallel arterial trunks. *Heart* 2007; **93**: 100–106.

6. Macartney FJ, Shinebourne EA, Anderson RH. Connexions, relations, discordance and distortions. *Br Heart J* 1976; **38**: 323–326.

7. Van Praagh R, Van Praagh S. Anatomically corrected transposition of the great arteries. *Br Heart J* 1967; **29**: 112.

8. Van Praagh R, Pérez-Treviño C, López-Cuellar M, et al. Transposition of the great arteries with posterior aorta, anterior pulmonary artery, subpulmonary conus and fibrous continuity between aortic and atrioventricular valves. *Am J Cardiol* 1971; **28**: 621–631.

9. Van Mierop LH. Transposition of the great arteries. I. Clarification or further confusion? *Am J Cardiol* 1971; **28**: 735–738.

10. Freedom RM, Harrington DP. Anatomically corrected malposition of the great arteries. Report of 2 cases, one with congenital asplenia; frequent association with juxtaposition of atrial appendages. *Br Heart J* 1974; **36**: 20–26.

11. Lincoln C, Anderson R, Shinebourne EA, English TA, Wilkinson JL. Double outlet right ventricle with 1-malposition of the aorta. *Br Heart J* 1975; **37**: 453–463.

12. Anderson RH, Becker A, Losekoot TG, Gerlis LM. Anatomically corrected malposition of great arteries. *Br Heart J* 1975; **37**: 993–1013.

13. Salazar J, López C, Felipe J, et al. Anatomically corrected malposition of the great arteries in situs ambiguous with polysplenia. *Ped Cardiol* 1985; **6**: 53–55.

14. Chowdhury UK, Anderson RH, Spicer DE, et al. Transposition physiology in the setting of concordant ventriculo-arterial connections. *J Card Surg* 202; **37**: 2823–2834.

15. Freedom RM, Nanton M, Dische MR. Isolated ventricular inversion with double inlet left ventricle. *Eur J Cardiol* 1977; **5**: 63–86.

16. Laux D, Houyel L, Bajolle F, et al. Problems in the diagnosis of discordant atrioventricular with concordant ventriculo-arterial connections: anatomical considerations, surgical management, and long-term outcome. *Cardiol Young* 2016; **26**: 127–138.

17. Sharma R, Marwah A, Shah S, Maheshwari S. Isolated atrioventricular discordance: surgical experience. *Ann Thorac Surg* 2008; **85**: 1403–1406.

18. Santoro G, Masiello P, Farina R, et al. Isolated atrial inversion in situs inversus: a rare anatomic arrangement. *Ann Thorac Surg* 1995; **59**: 1019–1021.

19. Smith A, Ho SY, Anderson RH, et al. The diverse cardiac morphology seen in hearts with isomerism of the atrial appendages with reference to the disposition of the specialised conduction system. *Cardiol Young* 2006; **16**: 437–454.

Chapter 10.1

Abnormalities of the Great Vessels

Anomalous Systemic Venous Connections

Abnormal systemic venous connections are usually of little surgical significance, since their clinical consequences are limited, although in the severest form, totally anomalous connection, the changes can be profound. Fortunately, totally anomalous systemic venous connection is very rare. The less severe variants are more likely to be encountered as the surgeon pursues a more complex associated intracardiac anomaly, such as the sinus venosus interatrial communication. The anomalous connections in general are of most significance in the setting of isomeric atrial appendages, which we discuss in Chapter 11, emphasizing how so-called visceral heterotaxy is best considered in terms of right versus left isomerism. In this chapter, we consider the features of the anomalous systemic venous connections in their own right. They may be grouped into the categories of absence or abnormal drainage of the right caval veins, persistence or abnormal drainage of the left caval vein, abnormal hepatic venous connections, and totally anomalous systemic venous connections. Abnormalities of the coronary sinus usually fall into one of these groups, although unroofing, which produces an interatrial communication through the right atrial orifice of the sinus, has been discussed in Chapter 8.1.

Abnormalities of the Right Superior Caval Vein

One of the features of the majority of patients with superior sinus venosus interatrial communications is overriding of the superior rim of the oval fossa by the orifice of the superior caval vein. The situation can be compared with overriding of the crest of the ventricular septum by the aortic root in the setting of tetralogy of Fallot.[1] In some of these arrangements, the superior caval vein can drain exclusively to the cavity of the morphologically left atrium, with no obvious sign of the sinus venosus defect (Figure 10.1.1). Apart from such associations with the superior sinus venosus defect, anomalies of the right

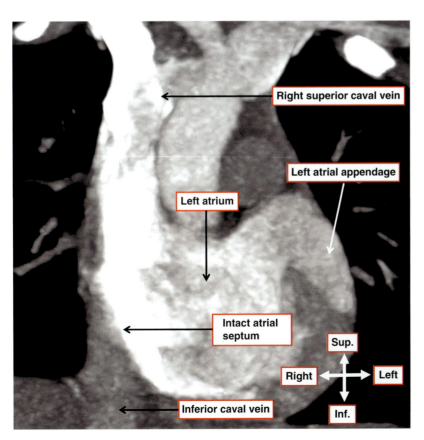

Figure 10.1.1 This coronal reconstruction from a computed tomographic angiographic dataset shows the right superior caval vein draining exclusively to the left atrium, with the inferior caval vein connected to the right atrium. The atrial septum is intact.

superior caval vein are rare. The vein may be diminished in size. Alternatively, it may be completely absent when the venous return from the head, neck and arms passes through a persistent left superior caval vein to the right atrium by way of the coronary sinus (Figures 10.1.2–10.1.4) or, rarely, directly into the morphologically left atrium (Figure 10.1.5). Only this last situation requires surgical intervention. The other conditions, if encountered during an open-heart operation, would require some adjustment from the usual technique used for cannulation. Though there is no definite evidence to this effect, we would not expect these abnormalities to affect the location of the sinus node.

Abnormalities of the Inferior Caval Vein

The inferior caval vein has been described to connect directly to the morphologically left atrium,[2] producing right-to-left shunting. When found, this is usually because a persistent Eustachian valve directs flow from the right atrium through the oval fossa (Figure 10.1.6). Such right-to-left shunting can also be an iatrogenic phenomenon, occasionally observed when low-lying atrial septal defects are improperly closed (see Chapter 8.1). Flow from the vein can also be directed towards the left atrium when there is an inferior sinus venosus defect. As with the superior caval vein, it is possible to envisage this arrangement with the inferior caval vein draining exclusively into the left atrium.

The more frequent anomaly involving the inferior caval vein is interruption of its terminal segment, with return of the venous blood from the lower body through the azygos or hemiazygos venous systems (Figures 10.1.7, 10.1.8).[3] The malformation is seen most frequently with isomerism of the left atrial appendages.[4] The hepatic veins then usually drain independently into the right-sided or left-sided atrium, although there can be a confluent suprahepatic channel, as is usually the

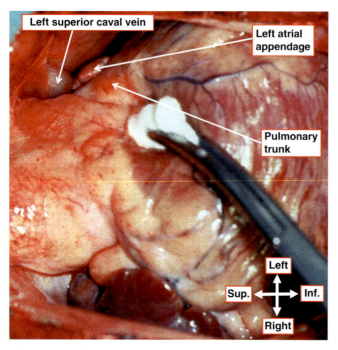

Figure 10.1.2 This operative view through a median sternotomy shows a left superior caval vein entering the pericardial cavity between the left atrial appendage and the pulmonary trunk.

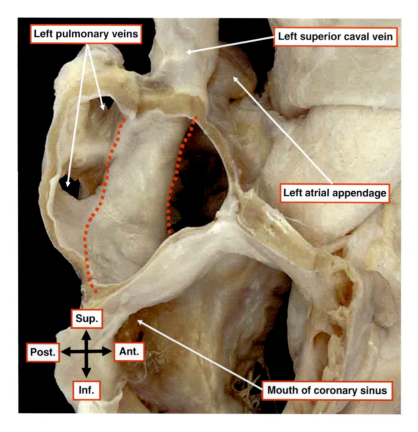

Figure 10.1.3 The heart is photographed from above in anatomical orientation, the domes of both atrial chambers having been removed. A persistent left superior caval vein enters the left atrioventricular groove between the left appendage and the left pulmonary veins, with its course through the groove marked by the red dotted lines. It enters the right atrium through the enlarged coronary sinus (see Figure 10.1.10). As it passes through the left atrioventricular groove, it potentially obstructs pulmonary venous flow to the mitral valvar vestibule.

10.1 Anomalous Systemic Venous Connections

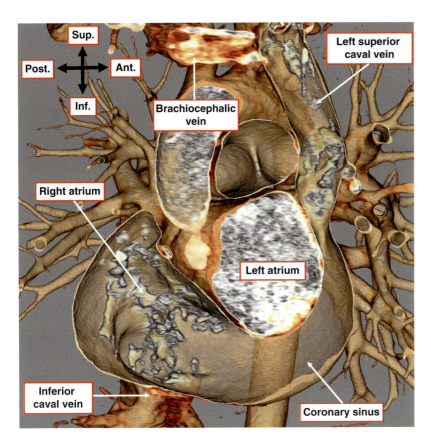

Figure 10.1.4 This computed tomographic angiogram, viewed in a frontal projection, shows absence of the right superior caval vein with the brachiocephalic vein diverting flow to the persistent left superior caval vein, which connects to the coronary sinus. The inferior caval vein connects normally to the right atrium.

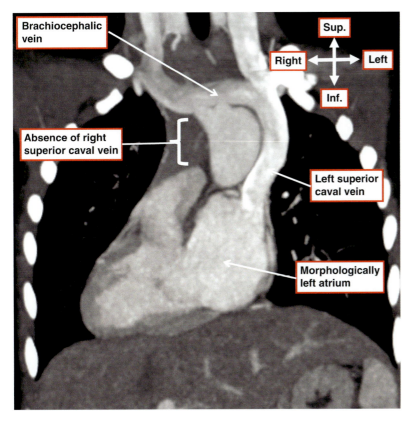

Figure 10.1.5 The computed tomographic angiogram, taken in frontal projection in a patient with a right-sided heart, also shows absence of the right superior caval vein with the brachiocephalic vein diverting flow to the persistent left superior caval vein. In this case, the left superior caval vein connects to the roof of the morphologically left atrium. The image was provided by Dr Madan Madali, from the Royal Hospital in Muscat, Oman, and is reproduced with his permission.

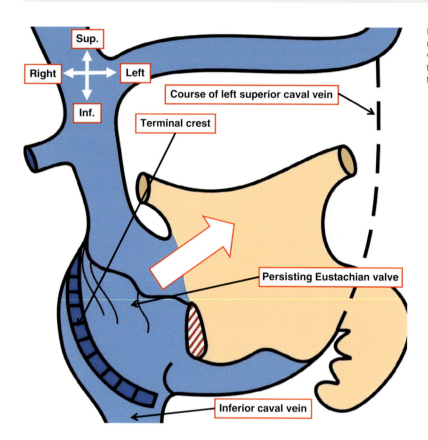

Figure 10.1.6 The cartoon shows the most frequent mechanism by which the venous return through the inferior caval vein drains to the left atrium. It is deflected across a defect within the oval fossa (red-bordered white arrow) due to persistence of the Eustachian valve.

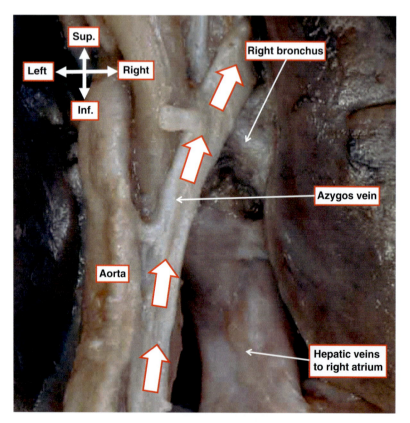

Figure 10.1.7 The heart is photographed from behind, showing the venous return from the abdomen returned to the heart through the azygos system of veins (white arrows with red borders). The inferior caval vein is interrupted below the diaphragm, and returns only the blood received through the hepatic veins.

10.1 Anomalous Systemic Venous Connections

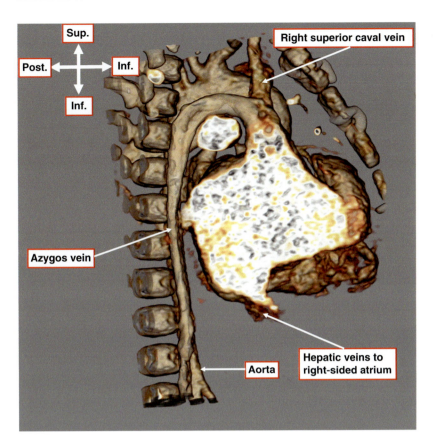

Figure 10.1.8 This computed tomographic angiogram, viewed from the right, shows a dilated azygous vein draining into a right superior caval vein. The aorta can be seen in the background running parallel to the azygous vein. Hepatic veins are seen draining into the right-sided atrium.

case when interruption and azygos continuation is found with usual or mirror-imaged atrial chambers (Figure 10.1.9).

Persistence of the Left Superior Caval Vein

Persistence of the left superior caval vein is the commonest malformation involving the caval veins (Figures 10.1.2, 10.1.3). In about three-fifths of reported cases,[5] the persisting left vein is joined to the right superior caval vein by a brachiocephalic vein. When arranged in this fashion, the left caval vein can simply be clamped or ligated, so as to avoid flooding the field when the heart is opened. If connections with the right vein are not apparent, a trial period of occlusion will usually indicate whether venous hypertension will give problems. A left superior caval vein is found not infrequently in patients with cyanotic heart disease, being reported in up to one-fifth of patients with tetralogy of Fallot, and one-twelfth of patients with Eisenmenger's syndrome.[6] The channel can also empty directly into the left atrium, as in the constellation described as unroofing of the coronary sinus (see Chapter 8.1), and as shown in Figure 10.1.5, when the vein drains the systemic venous return from the arms and head in absence of the right superior caval vein. Much more frequently, the vein persists as an isolated venous channel, which usually receives the hemiazygos vein before penetrating the pericardium and passing between the left atrial appendage and the left pulmonary veins. It then connects as the coronary sinus, traversing the inferior left atrioventricular groove to empty into the right atrium through a larger than normal orifice (Figure 10.1.10). In such hearts, the Thebesian valve is often attenuated or absent. There are also reports of the persistent vein obstructing flow from the pulmonary veins towards the atrial vestibule.[7] It is certainly the case that the venous channel can bulge into the cavity of the left atrium (Figure 10.1.3). The persistent left superior caval vein can also drain the coronary sinus blood into the brachiocephalic vein when an intact Thebesian valve produces atresia of the mouth of the sinus (Figures 10.1.11, 10.1.12).

Totally Anomalous Systemic Venous Connection

This rare variant is found when the entirety of the systemic venous sinus, along with the pulmonary venous sinus, is connected to the morphologically left atrium (Figures 10.1.13–10.1.16). It should be distinguished from the arrangement in which the systemic veins connect to the left-sided atrial chamber in the setting of left isomerism, although the physiological consequences are the same.[8]

Levoatrial Cardinal Vein

Another anomaly that, although rare, warrants consideration is the levoatrial cardinal vein.[9,10] In reality, the channel is neither levo, nor atrial, and arguably not cardinal. This term, nonetheless, is usually used to describe a collateral channel connecting the left atrium to the systemic venous system. It is typically found with associated lesions such as mitral atresia, where it can function as the major route for pulmonary venous return (Figures 10.1.17, 10.1.18). Then, although the pulmonary veins are normally

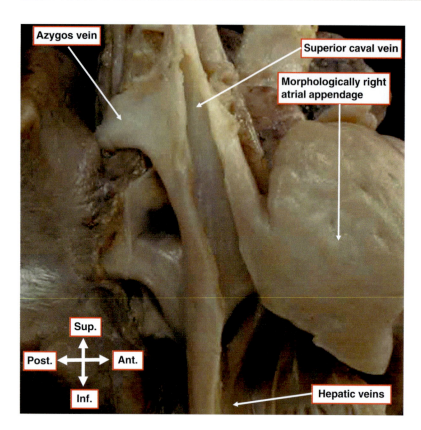

Figure 10.1.9 This heart, photographed from the right side in anatomical orientation, shows the termination of the azygos vein, which is returning the blood from below the diaphragm to the superior caval vein in the setting of interruption of the inferior caval vein (see Figure 10.1.7). Note the presence of the morphologically right appendage, indicating usual atrial arrangement.

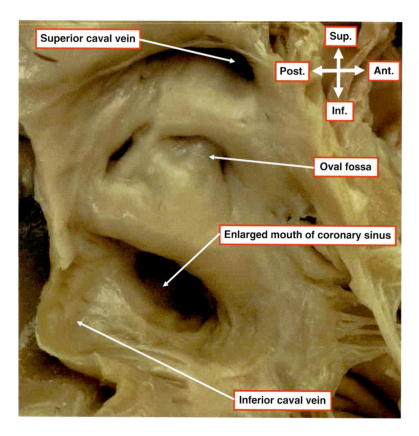

Figure 10.1.10 This photograph, again in anatomical orientation, shows the enlarged orifice of the coronary sinus within the right atrium of a heart with a persistent left superior caval vein. This is not the same heart as is shown in Figure 10.1.3.

connected to the morphologically left atrium, the pattern of venous return is comparable to the 'snowman' types of anomalous pulmonary venous connection. The collateral venous channel, however, is now increasingly becoming recognized in absence of any left-sided obstructive lesions.[11]

10.1 Anomalous Systemic Venous Connections

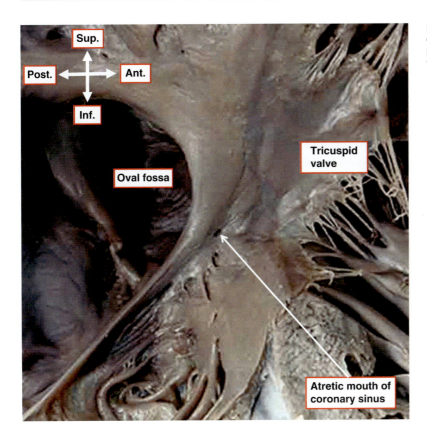

Figure 10.1.11 In this heart, there is atresia of the mouth of the coronary sinus. The coronary venous blood is directed through a persistent left superior caval vein to the brachiocephalic vein, and thence to the right superior caval vein (see Figure 10.1.12).

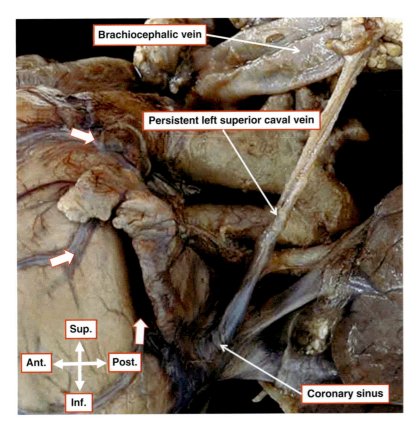

Figure 10.1.12 The heart shown in Figure 10.1.11 is photographed here from behind to show the persistent left superior caval vein, which drains the coronary veins (white arrows with red borders), themselves connected to the obstructed coronary sinus (see Figure 10.1.11), to the left brachiocephalic vein, and thence to the superior caval vein.

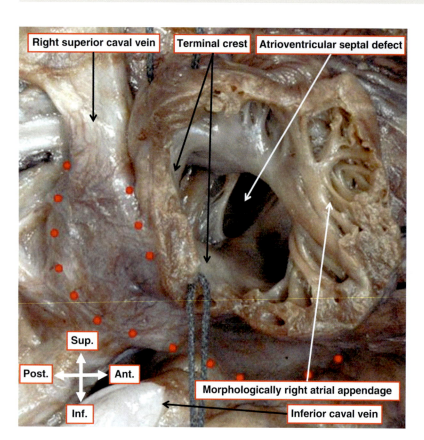

Figure 10.1.13 The heart is photographed from the right side, showing the right superior caval vein taking an anomalous course (dotted red lines) to the left side of the terminal crest and the atrial septum, and connecting to the morphologically left atrium (see Figure 10.1.14). Note the presence of the atrioventricular septal defect, along with an oval fossa defect.

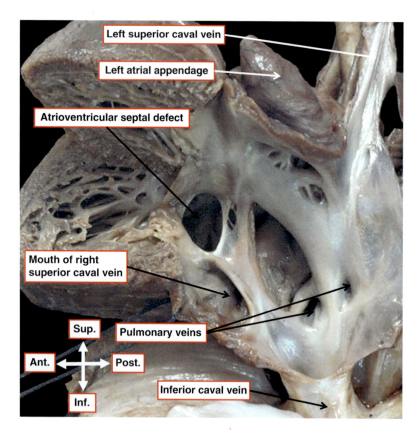

Figure 10.1.14 The left side of the heart shown in Figure 10.1.13 is photographed to show that not only does the right superior caval vein connect to the morphologically left atrium, but so do the inferior caval vein and the left superior caval vein, along with all the pulmonary veins. This is totally anomalous systemic venous connection.

10.1 Anomalous Systemic Venous Connections

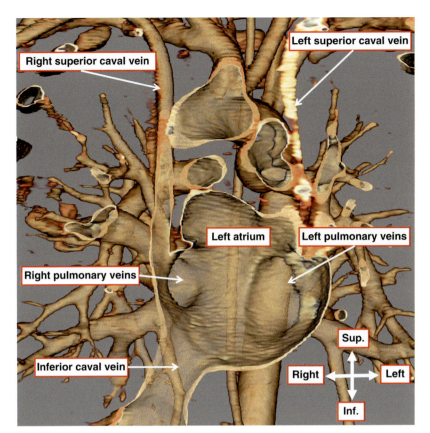

Figure 10.1.15 This computed tomographic angiogram, viewed from the front, was performed in a patient with totally anomalous systemic venous connection. The right and left superior caval veins, along with the inferior caval vein, are seen draining into the morphological left atrium. The right and left pulmonary veins can be seen draining into the left atrium as well.

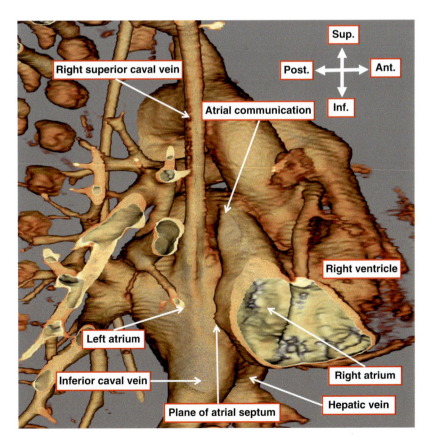

Figure 10.1.16 This is the same computed tomographic angiogram as was seen in 10.1.15, now viewed from the right. A small right atrium is seen. The only source of systemic blood flow into the right atrium is via a superior atrial septal defect. The right superior caval vein, inferior caval vein, and a hepatic vein are seen draining into the morphological left atrium.

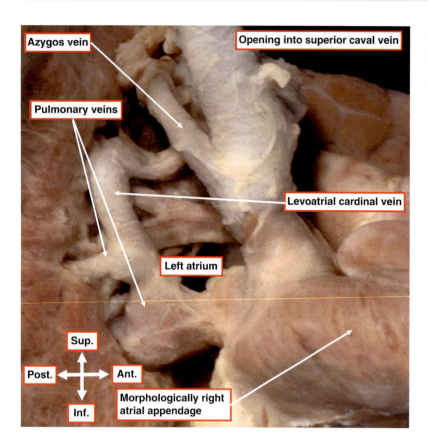

Figure 10.1.17 This specimen, from a patient with hypoplasia of the left heart, photographed in anatomical orientation, shows the course of the so-called levoatrial cardinal vein. The pulmonary veins connect in normal fashion to the left atrium, but the anomalous vein drains the atrial contents to the superior caval vein.

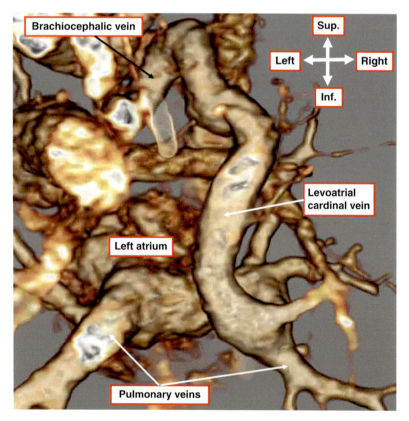

Figure 10.1.18 The reconstructed dataset prepared from a computed tomographic angiogram shows a levoatrial cardinal vein extending from the right lower pulmonary vein and taking a tortuous course before draining into the brachiocephalic vein. The patient had co-existing mitral atresia and an intact atrial septum.

References Cited

1. Relan J, Gupta SK, Rajagopal R, et al. Clarifying the anatomy of the superior sinus venosus defect. *Heart* 2022; **108**: 689–694.
2. Anderson RC, Heilig W, Novick R, Jarvis C. Anomalous inferior vena cava with azygos drainage: so-called absence of the inferior vena cava. *Am Heart J* 1955; **49**: 318–322.
3. Moller JH, Nakib A, Anderson RC, Edwards JE. Congenital cardiac disease associated with polysplenia: a developmental complex of bilateral 'left-sidedness'. *Circulation* 1967; **36**: 789–799.
4. Venables AW. Isolated drainage of the inferior vena cava to the left atrium. *Br Heart J* 1963; **25**: 545–548.
5. Winter FS. Persistent left superior vena cava: survey of world literature and report of 30 additional cases. *Angiology* 1954; **5**: 90–132.
6. Bankl H. *Congenital Malformations of the Heart and Great Vessels*. Baltimore – Munich: Urban and Schwarzenberg; 1977: p. 194.
7. Agnoletti G, Annechino F, Preda L, Borghi A. Persistence of the left superior caval vein: can it potentiate obstructive lesions of the left ventricle? *Cardiol Young* 1999; **9**: 285–290.
8. Madali MM, Al Kindi HN, Kandachar PS, et al. Identifying anomalies of systemic venous drainage. *World J Ped Card Surg* 2023; **14**: 490–496.
9. Edwards JE, DuShane JW. Thoracic venous anomalies. 1. Vascular connection between the left atrium and the left innominate vein (levoatriocardinal vein) associated with mitral atresia and premature closure of the foramen ovale (case 1). 11. Pulmonary veins draining wholly to the ductus arteriosus (case 2). *Arch Pathol* 1950; **49**: 517–537.
10. Pinto CAM, Ho SY, Redington A, Shinebourne EA, Anderson RH. Morphological features of the levoatriocardinal (or pulmonary-to-systemic collateral) vein. *Pediatr Pathol* 1993; **13**: 751–761.
11. Pandey NN, Spicer DE, Anderson RH. Is it really a levoatrial cardinal vein? *J Card Surg* 2022; **37**: 3754–3759.

Chapter 10.2
Anomalous Pulmonary Venous Connections

Very rarely, the pulmonary veins may be totally atretic at their atrial junction.[1] This is unlikely to be a surgically remedial situation. On other occasions, the pulmonary veins can be stenotic, either in segmental fashion (Figure 10.2.1), or with hour-glass stenosis at the venoatrial junction, with dilation of the pulmonary veins themselves (Figure 10.2.2).[2] Such pulmonary venous stenosis, which can be congenital or acquired subsequent to surgical correction of anomalously connected veins, creates great problems in subsequent surgical repair.[3] Attempts have been made to provide a so-called sutureless repair, which in essence means opening the stenotic veins and reinforcing them with the adjacent pericardium.[4] The procedure does, of course, require the use of sutures. Even this approach frequently proves less than perfect. It remains the case that pulmonary venous stenosis carries a relatively poor prognosis.

Fortunately, the surgical repair of anomalously connected pulmonary veins is now a much more successful undertaking. The pulmonary venous system can be connected anomalously in total or partial fashion. The anomalously connected veins must, of course, be distinguished from those that drain anomalously despite their normal connections. We have discussed this latter apparent paradox in the setting of the so-called levoatrial cardinal vein (see Chapter 10.1). The arrangement can also be produced by fenestrations of the walls of the coronary sinus (see Chapter 8.5). The pulmonary veins are anomalously connected when they are joined to a site, or sites, other than the morphologically left atrium. There is a plethora of possibilities for such abnormal connections.[5] Totally anomalous connection is found when all of the pulmonary veins connect to a site other than the left atrium (Figure 10.2.3 – panel A). Should it be that all the veins from one lung connect to a site other than the left atrium, the arrangement can be described as unilateral totally anomalous pulmonary venous connection (Figure 10.2.3 – panel B). When only one of the pulmonary veins is anomalously connected, then this is usually described simply as partially anomalous connection (Figure 10.2.3 – panel C).

In all of these combinations, it is then equally important to specify the site of the anomalous connection, or connections.

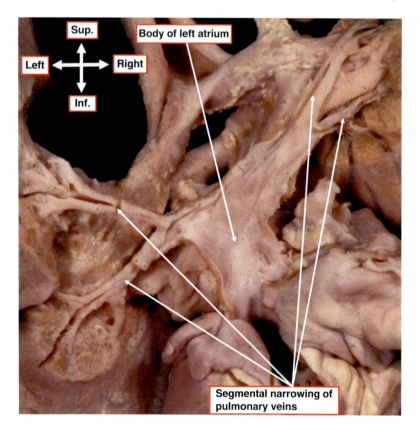

Figure 10.2.1 The heart is photographed from behind to show congenital segmental stenosis of all four pulmonary veins.

10.2 Anomalous Pulmonary Venous Connections

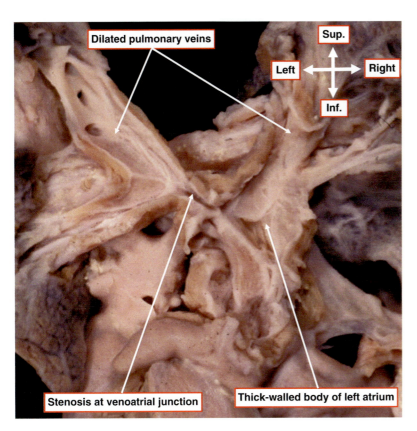

Figure 10.2.2 There is severe congenital pulmonary venous stenosis in this specimen, photographed from behind as was the heart shown in Figure 10.2.1. In this example, however, the stenosis is at the venoatrial junction, with dilation of the individual pulmonary veins and is due to fibromuscular thickening of the walls of the pulmonary veins themselves.

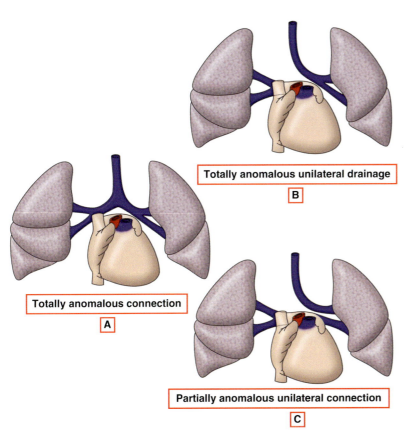

Figure 10.2.3 The drawing, in anatomical orientation, shows how anomalous connection of the pulmonary veins can be well accounted for by describing the connection of the veins from each lung as separate entities, and then describing partially as opposed to totally anomalous drainage on each side. The site of anomalous connection needs to be specified separately (see Figure 10.2.4).

This is conventionally described as being supradiaphragmatic or infradiaphragmatic (Figure 10.2.4). Supradiaphragmatic drainage can further be subdivided into supracardiac and cardiac patterns. Supracardiac connection may be to a right or left superior caval vein, the brachiocephalic vein, or even the azygos vein. Connection to the brachiocephalic vein is most

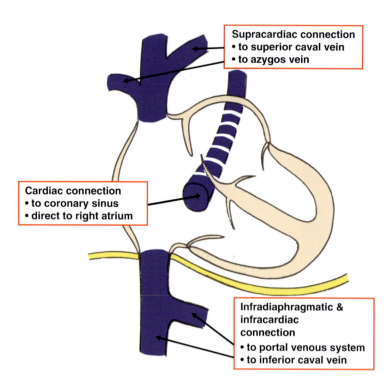

Figure 10.2.4 This drawing, in anatomical orientation, shows the potential sites for anomalous connection of the pulmonary veins.

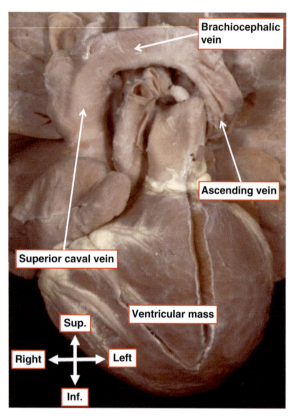

Figure 10.2.5 This heart, photographed from the front in anatomical orientation, has totally anomalous pulmonary venous connection to the superior caval vein. With this arrangement, the heart forms the body of the 'snowman' seen in the chest radiograph, with the anomalous vein forming the head of the snowman as it courses to drain to the superior caval vein via the brachiocephalic vein.

frequent. The combination of drainage via a left-sided vertical vein, and thence via the brachiocephalic vein to the superior caval vein (Figures 10.2.5, 10.2.6), produces the typical snowman configuration as seen on chest radiography. The venous pathways can be obstructed when the vertical vein crosses in front of the left bronchus, but obstruction is more usually produced when the venous channel is caught in a vice between the left pulmonary artery and the left bronchus (Figure 10.2.7). When the route of drainage involves the azygos vein, then the left pulmonary veins tend to join together before crossing vertically beneath the heart, then ascending in the right paravertebral gutter where they receive the right pulmonary veins, before draining to the superior caval vein via the azygos vein (Figure 10.2.8). Bizarre patterns are frequently found with this type of connection, for example when the right-sided veins cross to the left, join with the left-sided veins, and make their connection to the azygos vein adjacent to the diaphragm.[6]

Direct connection to the right atrium is typically through the coronary sinus (Figure 10.2.9). Totally anomalous connection to the right atrium, other than through the coronary sinus, is most usually found in the setting of isomerism of the right atrial appendages (Figure 10.2.10). The pulmonary veins, even when they return to the heart, are always connected in anatomically anomalous fashion when both of the atrial appendages are of right morphology.

Infradiaphragmatic connection is usually total except when there is partially right-sided connection to the inferior caval vein. This latter arrangement is the so-called scimitar syndrome, a name taken from its likeness to a Turkish sword when seen in the chest radiograph.[7] In the usual infradiaphragmatic connection, the common channel connecting both lungs lies outside

10.2 Anomalous Pulmonary Venous Connections

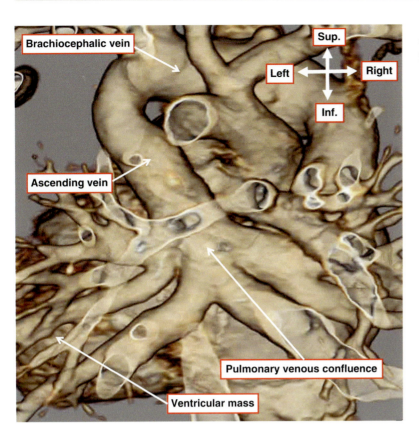

Figure 10.2.6 The reconstructed dataset prepared from a computed tomographic angiogram shows supracardiac totally anomalous pulmonary venous drainage as viewed from behind. The brachiocephalic vein drains to the superior caval vein.

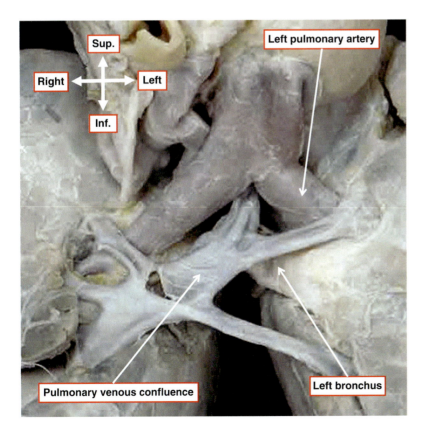

Figure 10.2.7 In this specimen, from a patient with totally anomalous pulmonary venous connection, the mediastinum is photographed from the front having reflected the heart from its pericardial cradle. The pathway from the pulmonary venous confluence is obstructed in a bronchopulmonary vice.

the pericardium posterior to the left atrium (Figure 10.2.11). A descending vein drains through the diaphragm as a single channel to enter the portal vein or the venous duct (Figures 10.2.12, 10.2.13). The return from the lungs becomes obstructed as it passes through the diaphragm, or subsequent to closure of the venous duct. Occasionally, the channel breaks up into a series of

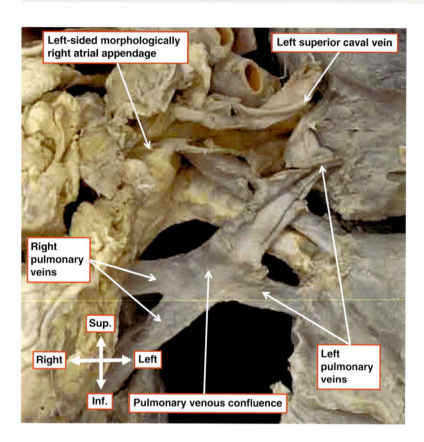

Figure 10.2.8 This heart is from a patient with mirror-imaged arrangement of all the organs, including the heart. Note the left-sided position of the morphologically right atrial appendage. The heart has again been reflected from its pericardial cradle, and the photograph taken from the front. The pulmonary veins drain anomalously to the left-sided superior caval vein, with the collecting channel passing below the heart and ascending within the left-sided paravertebral gutter.

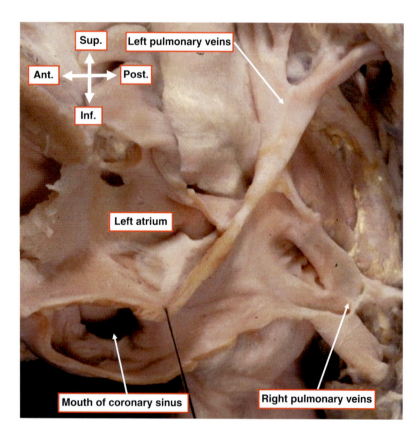

Figure 10.2.9 This specimen, viewed from the left side in anatomical orientation, has anomalous connection of all four pulmonary veins to the coronary sinus, which drains to the right atrium.

branches which connect to the gastric veins (Figure 10.2.14). It is very rare to find infradiaphragmatic connection directly to the inferior caval vein. Totally anomalous pulmonary venous connection can also drain to mixed sites. There are multiple potential patterns.[8] In the image shown in Figure 10.2.15, the upper left pulmonary vein drains in supracardiac fashion via the

10.2 Anomalous Pulmonary Venous Connections

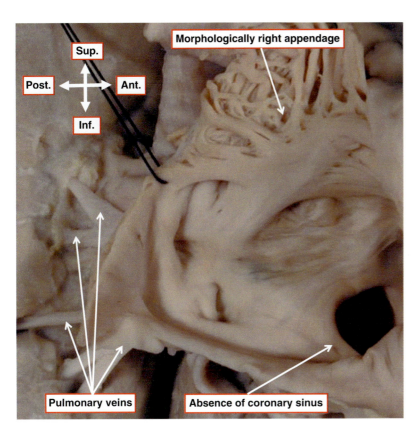

Figure 10.2.10 In this heart, all pulmonary veins are connected directly to the right atrium, the lowermost vein through two tributaries. There was isomerism of the right atrial appendages. Note the absence of the coronary sinus.

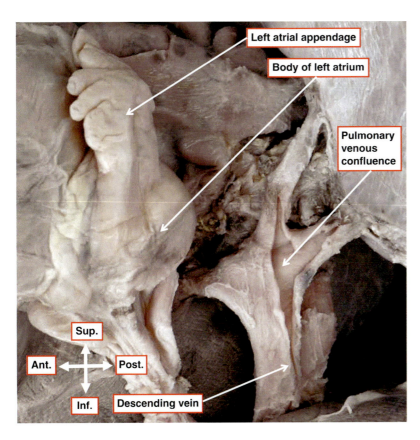

Figure 10.2.11 This specimen, viewed from the left side in anatomical orientation, has anomalous connection of all pulmonary veins to a descending channel that passes through the diaphragm to join the portal venous circulation.

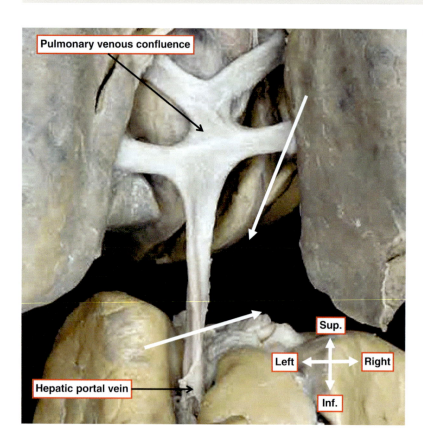

Figure 10.2.12 In this specimen, from a patient with totally anomalous pulmonary venous connection, the mediastinum is viewed from behind. The descending pulmonary venous channel passes through the diaphragm and empties into the hepatic portal vein.

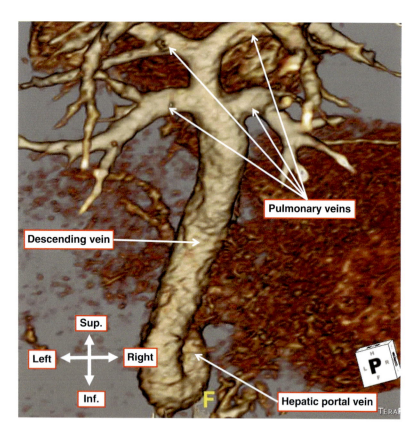

Figure 10.2.13 The reconstructed dataset prepared from a computed tomographic angiogram shows infracardiac and infradiaphragmatic totally anomalous pulmonary venous pulmonary drainage as viewed from behind. The descending vein drains to the hepatic portal venous system. Orientation cube, lower right: P, posterior; H, head, F, feet, A, anterior.

10.2 Anomalous Pulmonary Venous Connections

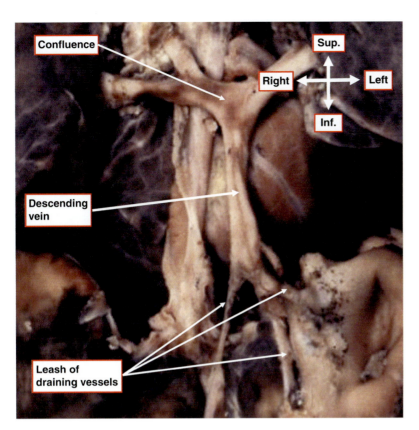

Figure 10.2.14 In this specimen, from a patient with totally anomalous pulmonary venous connection, the heart has been reflected from its pericardial cradle. The descending channel passes through the diaphragm and fragments into a leash of small veins that join the gastric veins.

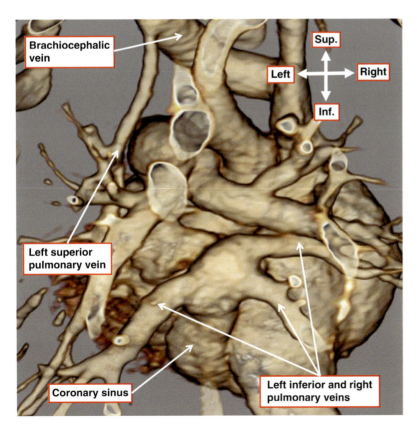

Figure 10.2.15 The reconstructed dataset prepared from a computed tomographic angiogram shows mixed totally anomalous pulmonary venous pulmonary drainage as viewed from behind. The left superior pulmonary vein drains to the brachiocephalic vein, and thence to the superior caval vein, while the left inferior and the right pulmonary veins connect to the coronary sinus.

brachiocephalic vein to the superior caval vein, while the remaining veins drain to the coronary sinus. Any combination should be anticipated.

The salient anatomical features relating to surgical repair of the anomalous connections include the type of abnormal connection, the site of anomalous connection, and the proximity of the anomalous veins to the left atrium. As pointed out in Chapter 8.1, interatrial communications in the mouth of the caval veins, the so-called sinus venosus defects, are always accompanied by anomalous connection of the right pulmonary veins, either to the superior or inferior caval vein. The need to safeguard the sinus node and its blood supply has already been emphasized.

Other sites of connection, or potential sites of anastomosis, often require construction of an extensive atrial junction to guard postoperatively against pulmonary venous obstruction. The appropriate landmarks must be borne in mind. Two types of anomalous connections pose particular problems. The first is when the anomalous venous return is by way of the coronary sinus (Figures 10.2.9, 10.2.15). We initially thought that the myocardium between the coronary sinus and the left atrium was common to both structures. We now know that the sinus has its own myocardial wall, separate from that of the left atrium.[9] It is possible, nonetheless, to incise both walls so as to unroof the sinus. At the same time, the orifice of the coronary sinus can be made confluent with the atrial septal defect, which is typically within the oval fossa. It is important to remove enough of the walls to ensure that the patch placed across the orifice of the coronary sinus and oval fossa does not produce obstruction at the site of the incised sinus septum. Ideally, the incised walls of atrium and coronary sinus should also be repaired, since the incisions create a route to the inferior atrioventricular groove. Thus far, however, we are unaware of any reports of tamponade following such procedures. The surgeon should be aware, nonetheless, that a potential opening is created to the extracardiac spaces. When incising the coronary sinus, it is also important to avoid the atrioventricular node at the apex of the triangle of Koch.

The second problematic type of connection is the infradiaphragmatic variant. The extrapericardial common pulmonary venous trunk can be farther from the posterior left atrial wall than might be expected (Figure 10.2.11). Because of this, the anastomosis constructed between the trunk and left atrium is vulnerable to obstruction, particularly at its lateral extreme. This may become evident only when bypass is discontinued and the heart fills with blood.

References Cited

1. Lucas RV Jr, Woolfrey BF, Anderson RC, Lester RG, Edwards JE. Atresia of the common pulmonary vein. *Pediatr* 1962; **29**: 729–739.

2. Fong LV, Anderson RH, Park SC, Zuberbuhler JR. Morphologic features of stenosis of the pulmonary veins. *Am J Cardiol* 1988; **62**: 1136–1138.

3. Seale AN, Webber SA, Uemura H, et al. Pulmonary vein stenosis: the UK, Ireland and Sweden collaborative study. *Heart* 2009; **95**: 1944–1949.

4. Yun TJ, Coles JG, Konstantinov IE, et al. Conventional and sutureless techniques for management of the pulmonary veins: evolution of indications from postrepair pulmonary vein stenosis to primary pulmonary vein anomalies. *J Thoracic Cardiovasc Surg* 2005; **129**: 167–174.

5. DeLisle G, Ando M, Calder AL, et al. Total anomalous pulmonary venous connection: report of 93 autopsied cases with emphasis on diagnostic and surgical considerations. *Am Heart J* 1976; **91**: 99–122.

6. Gupta SK, Gulati GS, Juneja R, Devagourou V. Total anomalous pulmonary venous connection with descending vertical vein: unusual drainage to azygos vein. *Ann Ped Card* 2012; **5**: 188–190.

7. Neill CA, Ferencz C, Sabiston DC, Sheldon H. The familial occurrence of hypoplastic right lung with systemic arterial supply and venous drainage 'scimitar syndrome'. *Bull Johns Hopkins Hosp* 1960; **107**: 1–15.

8. Chowdhury UK, Airan B, Malhotra A, et al. Mixed total anomalous pulmonary venous connection: anatomic variations, surgical approach, techniques, and results. *J Thoracic Cardiovasc Surg* 2008; **135**: 106–116.

9. Chauvin M, Shah DC, Haisseguerre M, Marcellin L, Brechenmacher, C. The anatomic basis of connections between the coronary sinus musculature and the left atrium in humans. *Circulation* 2000; **101**: 647–652.

Chapter 10.3
Obstructive Abnormalities of the Extrapericardial Systemic Pathways

The obstructive congenital anomalies of the extrapericardial thoracic aorta and its branches that are of interest to the surgeon are aortic coarctation, and its relationship to the spectrum of partial to complete interruption of the aortic arch.

Aortic Coarctation

Coarctation is a congenitally-derived discrete shelf-like (Figure 10.3.1) or waist-like (Figure 10.3.2) lesion within the aorta, which causes obstruction to the flow of blood. It is most often found adjacent to the opening of the persistently patent arterial duct (Figure 10.3.3), or the arterial ligament if the duct has closed. It can occur proximally, or more distally, and even in the abdominal aorta. The latter, which can be congenital and often referred to as 'middle or mid-aortic syndrome', is likely to be of different aetiology and is out of the scope of this book. In the thoracic segment, coarctation is usually accompanied by some degree of tubular hypoplasia of the aortic arch, but is anatomically independent of the hypoplasia. It can co-exist with other lesions that diminish left-sided flow, but coarctation can, and does, occur independently. Tubular hypoplasia, when involving the isthmic segment of the aortic arch, can then be considered as part of a spectrum leading to atresia or interruption of the aortic arch.

Much has been made of the role of ductal tissue in the aetiology of coarctation. Although there was a time when some doubted its significance, the evidence supporting its inclusion in the coarctation shelf (Figure 10.3.1) is now unequivocal.[1-3] The surgeon, therefore, needs to be aware of the importance of removing all the ductal tissue during repair. The significance of the duct itself devolves upon its patency. If the duct is patent, typically there is an associated congenital anomaly that promotes increased flow of blood through the pulmonary trunk, and diverts blood away from the proximal aorta. In these circumstances, the associated anomaly tends to dominate the picture, and will determine the most appropriate surgical therapy. On the other hand,

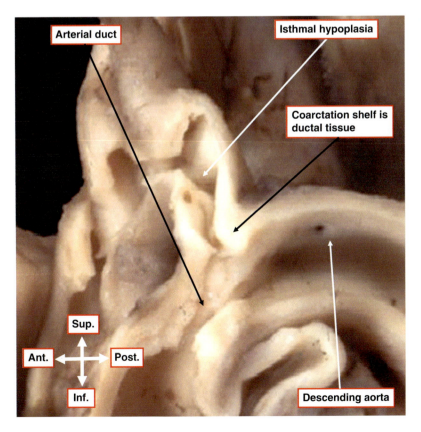

Figure 10.3.1 This specimen, viewed in anatomical orientation, shows the ductal tissue that forms the shelf lesion of aortic coarctation. Note the co-existing hypoplasia of the aortic isthmus.

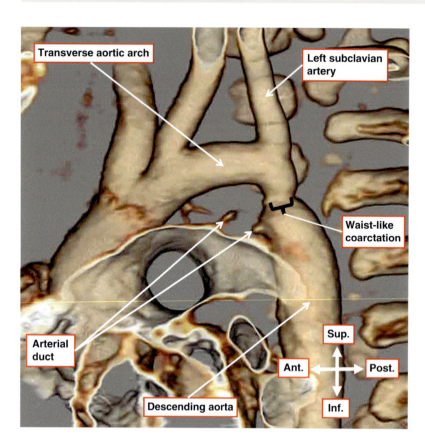

Figure 10.3.2 The reconstructed dataset prepared from a computed tomographic angiogram shows a waist-like constriction between the aortic isthmus and the descending aorta. In this patient, the arterial duct has closed.

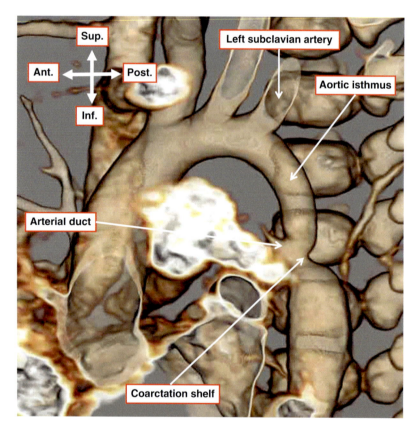

Figure 10.3.3 The reconstructed dataset prepared from a computed tomographic angiogram shows a coarctation lesion in juxtaductal position with a persistently patent arterial duct. In this patient, there is considerable length to the aortic isthmus (compare with Figure 10.3.2).

coarctation with a closed duct is very likely to be an isolated lesion (Figure 10.3.4), except for the occasional association with a bifoliate aortic valve.[4]

The chief concerns of the surgeon relate to the specific anatomy of the coarctation. The nature of the collateral circulation is of particular significance. With well-developed collateral arteries (Figure 10.3.4) there is little danger of cross-clamping the aorta during repair. If the collateral arteries are less well developed (Figure 10.3.5), however, clamping the aorta may have several deleterious consequences. These include strain on the left ventricle due to proximal hypertension, which may also induce a cerebrovascular accident

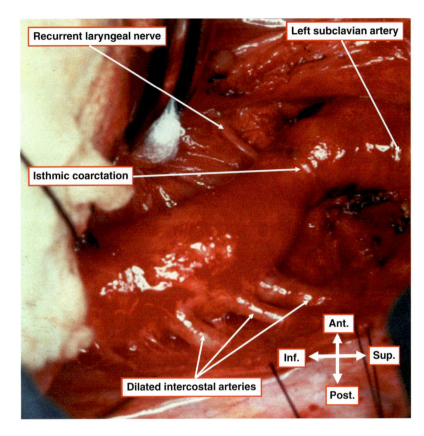

Figure 10.3.4 This operative view, through a left thoracotomy, shows aortic coarctation with enlarged intercostal arteries, part of a well-developed collateral circulation.

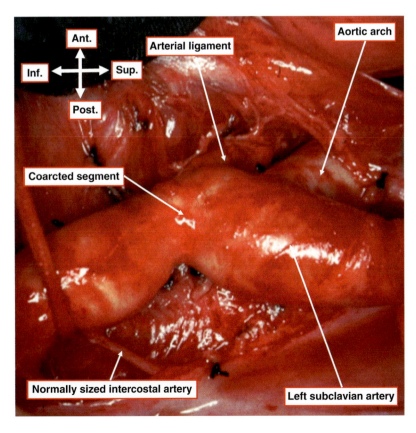

Figure 10.3.5 In this operative view through a left thoracotomy, again from a patient with aortic coarctation (compare with Figure 10.3.4), the collateral circulation is not well developed.

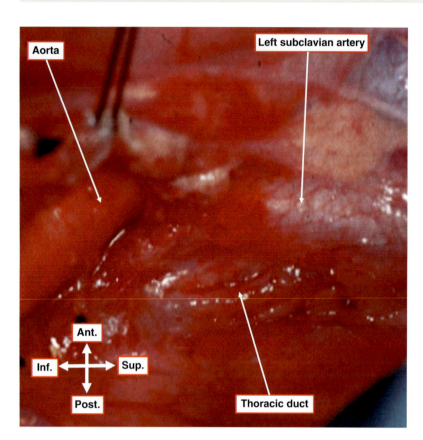

Figure 10.3.6 This view, through a left lateral thoracotomy, shows the thoracic duct as it passes from the area of coarctation behind the left subclavian artery.

secondary to rupture of a berry aneurysm. There may be distal aortic hypotension, at pressures of less than 50 millimetres of mercury, which endangers the splanchnic and spinal vascular beds. Irrespective of the nature of the collateral arteries, the spinal circulation is best preserved by interrupting none, or as few as possible, of the intercostal vessels. Temporary occlusion of the intercostal vessels adjacent to the operative field seems to be a reasonable compromise in this difficult situation.

Other noteworthy features include the position of the thoracic duct (Figure 10.3.6), and the occasional presence of an anomalous artery (Figure 10.3.7), sometimes referred to as Abbott's artery. When present, this artery arises from the postero-medial aspect of the proximal descending aorta. The surgeon needs to be aware of the existence of this anomalous vessel. If not properly managed, its presence can lead to substantial bleeding during the repair.[5]

Interruption of the Aortic Arch

Discontinuity of the aorta, as opposed to coarctation, has been variously referred to as absence, atresia, or interruption of the arch. Included in this group are those cases with a fibrous cord or bridge of tissue (Figure 10.3.8), as well as those with a gap, or absolute discontinuity, at some point in the arch (Figures 10.3.9, 10.3.10). Interruption can occur at one of three positions. When found at the isthmus (Figure 10.3.11), the variant is usually dubbed Type A, and is flow related. The interruption can also be found between the left common carotid and subclavian arteries, so-called Type B, with this variant commonly having a genetic background (Figure 10.3.12). The rarest variant is interruption between the common carotid arteries (Figure 10.3.13). The lesions typically are found in the setting of a unilateral left aortic arch but, rarely, a right arch can be similarly affected.[6] Since patients with discontinuity of the aorta are unlikely to survive without surgical treatment, they are a particular challenge to the clinician. The associated cardiovascular malformations are of critical importance, for they affect the operative outcome as much as does interrupted arch itself. Almost always there is a patent connection to the distal aorta through the duct (Figure 10.3.10). A proximal septal defect is also the rule. This is most frequently a ventricular septal defect but, occasionally, an aortopulmonary window is found. The ventricular septal defect is typically associated with posterior and leftward displacement of the outlet septum, resulting in subaortic stenosis. Although the outlet septum is usually muscular (Figure 10.3.14), it can be no more than a fibrous shelf, or raphe between the leaflets of the arterial valves (Figure 10.3.15), when the defect itself is juxta-arterial. Any type of defect, nonetheless, can be found. Abnormal ventriculo-arterial connections are not unusual, and present their own particular problems for operative reconstruction.[7] Of particular note is the so-called Taussig–Bing malformation, which is a spectrum between transposition and double outlet right ventricle with subpulmonary defect. A particularly problematic surgical combination can be found with this lesion when a restrictive subaortic defect, associated with either severe coarctation or interruption, is accompanied by straddling of the mitral valve (Figure 10.3.16).[8] The other

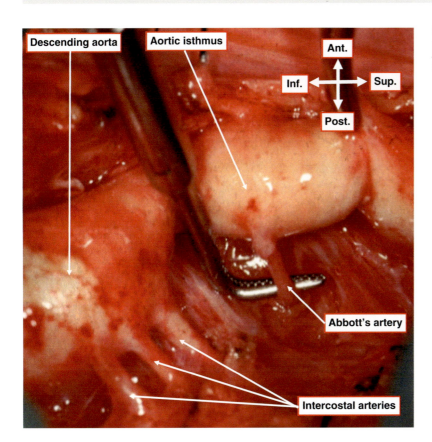

Figure 10.3.7 As seen through a left thoracotomy, the proximal descending aorta and distal arch have been rotated anteriorly. The large collateral vessel referred to as Abbott's artery is seen arising proximally to the area of coarctation.

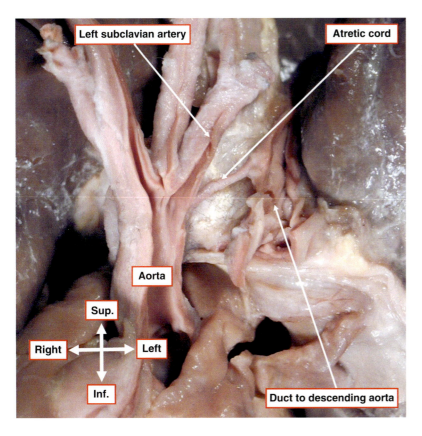

Figure 10.3.8 This specimen, photographed in anatomical orientation, has atresia of the isthmus, with a thin fibrous cord running from the site of effective interruption at the left subclavian artery to the distal descending aorta, which is fed through the arterial duct.

combination of note is a restrictive ventricular septal defect in the setting of a dominant left ventricle and an incomplete right ventricle with discordant ventriculo-arterial connections (Figure 10.3.17).

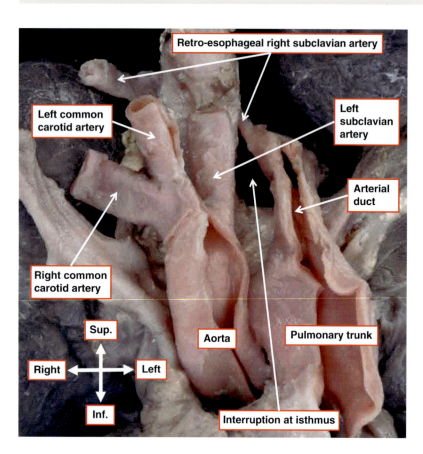

Figure 10.3.9 In this specimen, shown in anatomical orientation as photographed from the front, the aortic arch is interrupted at the isthmus, with retro-esophageal origin of the right subclavian artery. The descending aorta is fed from the pulmonary trunk via the arterial duct.

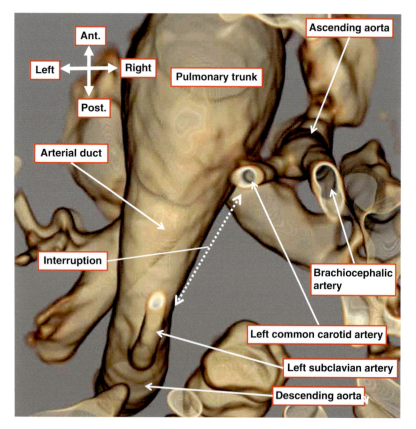

Figure 10.3.10 The reconstructed dataset prepared from a computed tomographic angiogram shows interruption of the aortic arch (white dotted double-headed arrow) in between the left common carotid artery and the left subclavian artery. The hypoplastic ascending aorta also supplies the brachiocephalic artery.

10.3 Obstructive Abnormalities of the Extrapericardial Systemic Pathways

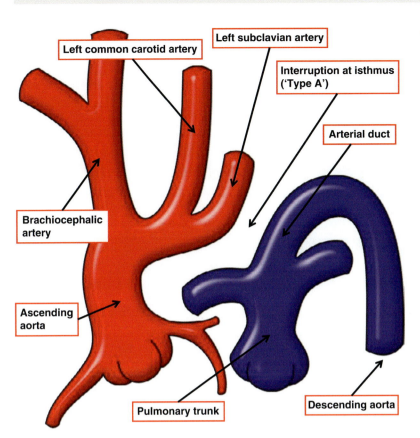

Figure 10.3.11 The drawing shows interruption at the aortic isthmus, so-called Type A interruption.

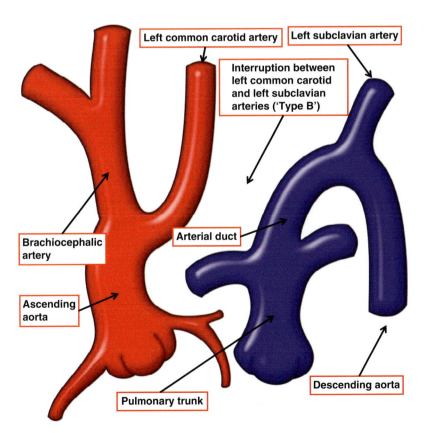

Figure 10.3.12 This drawing shows interruption between the left common carotid and left subclavian arteries, which is described as Type B interruption.

A less lethal, but fairly frequently associated, arterial abnormality is aberrant origin of a retro-esophageal right subclavian artery from the distal aorta (Figure 10.3.9). Since the arch is interrupted, symptoms of a vascular ring are unlikely unless a ring is created while reconstructing the arch. Conversely, if the aberrant artery is brought

433

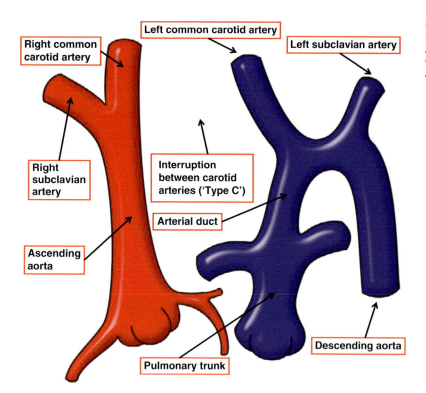

Figure 10.3.13 The drawing shows the rarest type of interruption, so-called Type C, which is between the carotid arteries. This should not be confused with Type B interruption, when there is retro-esophageal origin of the right subclavian artery.

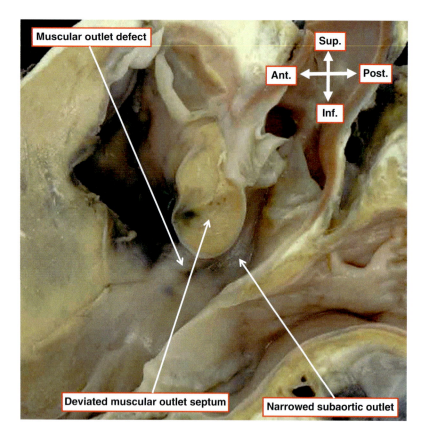

Figure 10.3.14 This view of a specimen sectioned to replicate the parasternal echocardiographic cut, in the setting of interruption of the aortic arch, seen in anatomical orientation, shows posterior deviation of the muscular outlet septum into the left ventricle, with obstruction of the subaortic outflow tract. The outlet ventricular septal defect has a muscular postero-inferior rim.

forward, it can be useful in repairing the aorta. This emphasizes the importance of defining clearly the nature and effect of associated abnormalities. Successful anatomical correction is as dependent on appropriate management of these accompanying lesions as it is on establishing aortic continuity.

10.3 Obstructive Abnormalities of the Extrapericardial Systemic Pathways

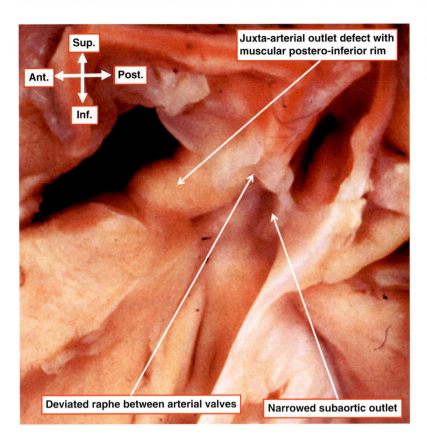

Figure 10.3.15 In this specimen, sectioned as for the specimen shown in Figure 10.3.14, there is a fibrous raphe between the leaflets of the arterial valves, which is deviated in posterior fashion. As with the heart with a muscular outlet septum, there is again obstruction to the subaortic outlet.

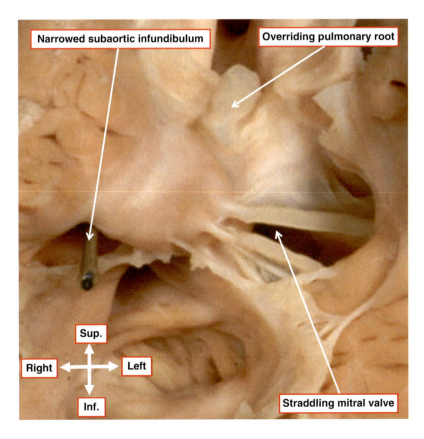

Figure 10.3.16 This image, photographed from the front, shows the problematic combination of a restrictive subaortic infundibulum and straddling of the mitral valve as seen in the setting of the Taussig–Bing malformation.

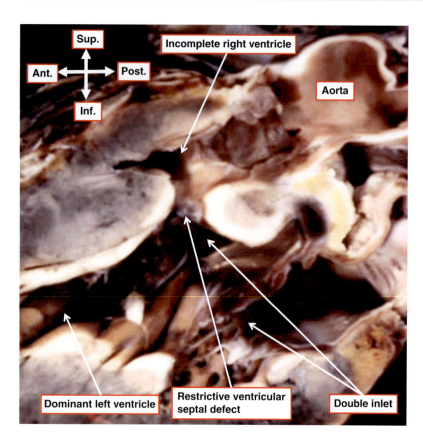

Figure 10.3.17 The image shows another problematic combination for the surgeon, namely a restrictive ventricular septal defect when there is a dominant right ventricle, an incomplete right ventricle, and discordant ventriculo-arterial connections. In this specimen, there is double inlet left ventricle.

References Cited

1. Brom AG. Narrowing of the aortic isthmus and enlargement of the mind. *J Thorac Cardiovasc Surg* 1965; **50**: 166–180.
2. Ho SY, Anderson RH. Coarctation, tubular hypoplasia and the ductus arteriosus: a histological study of 35 specimens. *Br Heart J* 1979; **41**: 268–274.
3. Elzenga NJ, Gittenberger-de-Groot AC. Localised coarctation of the aorta. An age dependent spectrum. *Br Heart J* 1983; **49**: 317–323.
4. Becker AE, Becker MJ, Edwards JE. Anomalies associated with coarctation of the aorta. Particular reference to infancy. *Circulation* 1970; **41**: 1067–1075.
5. Lerberg DB. Abbott's artery. *Ann Thorac Surg* 1982; **33**: 415–416.
6. Pierpont MEM, Zollikofer CL, Moller JH, Edwards JE. Interruption of the aortic arch with right descending aorta. *Pediatr Cardiol* 1982; **2**: 153–159.
7. Ho SY, Wilcox BR, Anderson RH, Lincoln JCR. Interrupted aortic arch-anatomical features of surgical significance. *Thorac Cardiovasc Surg* 1983; **31**: 199–205.
8. Muster AJ, Bharati S, Aziz KU, et al. Taussig-Bing anomaly with straddling mitral valve. *J Thorac Cardiovasc Surg* 1979; **77**: 832–842.

Chapter 10.4

Vascular Rings

Understanding vascular rings requires an appreciation of the abnormal regression of part of a double aortic arch. Since, during their development, the arch arteries are initially bilaterally symmetrical, it follows that knowledge of development is an aid to understanding the morphology of these anomalies. The understanding, however, needs to be based on the current knowledge, since confusion is produced if emphasis is placed on traditional accounts. These accounts are usually based on the initial diagram allegedly accredited to Rathke.[1] Rathke's initial diagram, however, had but five arches depicted. It was the modification produced by Boas[2] that introduced the supposed fifth set of arteries, now usually depicted in vestigial fashion. As we showed in Chapter 2, however, there are never six sets of arteries formed during human development. Nor is there any evidence to support such a situation during development of any mammal.[3] The arteries percolate through the pharyngeal arches, which themselves are delimited by pouches extending from the gut. There are four such pouches formed during development, with the first four sets of arteries positioned cranial to these pouches. When first seen, arteries are associated with the first two pouches (Figure 10.4.1). These arteries are themselves evanescent, persisting only as parts of the mandibular and hyoid arteries. To all intents and purposes, the first two sets have disappeared by the time the arteries develop, which will become the definitive extrapericardial vessels. These definitive arteries occupy the third and fourth arches. The arteries of the ultimate arches occupy the pharyngeal mesenchyme caudal to the fourth pouch (Figure 10.4.2). In human development, therefore, there are five sets of arch arteries. The ultimate arch arteries, which will give rise to the right and left pulmonary arteries, are the fifth set. Confusion would be produced, however, if we sought to describe these arteries as belonging to the 'fifth arch'. This, of course, is because of the significant literature currently devoted to interpretation of congenital lesions on the basis of persistence of arteries of the non-existent evanescent fifth set of the sixth pairs of arteries as shown in the traditional Rathke diagram as modified by Boas.[4] One of us has contributed significantly to

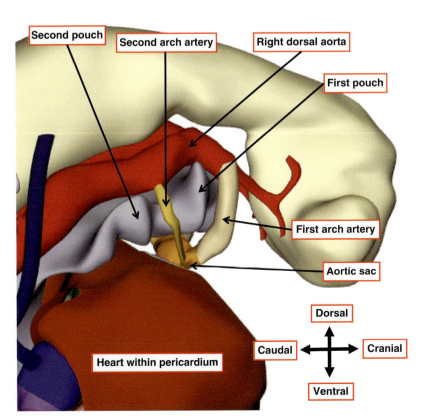

Figure 10.4.1 The image shows the reconstruction of the developing arteries of the pharyngeal arches in a human embryo at Carnegie stage 12, when the embryo is around 30 days subsequent to fertilization. Only the first two arches are formed at this stage.

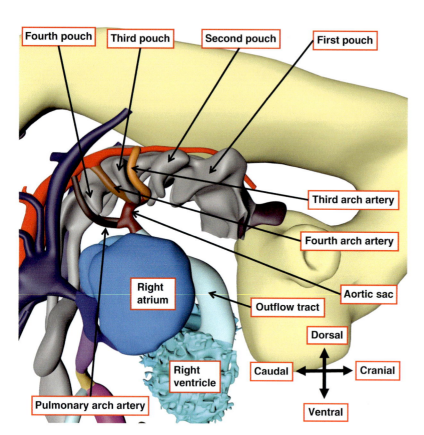

Figure 10.4.2 This image, comparable to the one shown in Figure 10.4.1, is from a human embryo at Carnegie stage 14, which is around four days later. The arteries of the first two arches have essentially attenuated, with arteries now formed in the caudal two arches, with an additional artery formed caudal to the fourth pharyngeal pouch. This ultimate artery will provide the origin for the right and left pulmonary arteries, with the left arch artery becoming the arterial duct (see Figure 10.4.5).

this literature.[5] Indeed, at one stage we harboured the belief that we had discovered an evanescent fifth arch artery (Figure 10.4.3).[6] We now realize that such interpretations were incorrect. If there have never been six pharyngeal arches, then it is obviously not possible to find persistence of a set of arteries that have never existed. The reputed 'arteries of the fifth arch', in all instances, can be better explained either on the basis of persistence of collateral channels, or remodelling of the aortic sac.[7,8] To avoid any semantic problems relating to the enigmatic presumed arteries of the fifth arch, therefore, we describe the ultimate arch as being pulmonary. As already indicated, it is the arteries of these arches which give rise to the right and left pulmonary arteries, with the left ultimate arch artery itself becoming the arterial duct.

It is the derivatives of the arteries of the third, fourth, and pulmonary arches that are seen in the postnatal heart. The significant feature of these arteries relative to vascular rings is that, initially, they are bilaterally symmetrical (Figure 10.4.4). They arise from the aortic sac, with the arteries of the third and fourth arches on each side arising from its cranial horns. The arteries of the pulmonary arches arise in similarly symmetrical fashion from the caudal part of the sac. Also of significance are the seventh cervical intersegmental arteries, which will eventually become the subclavian arteries. At the initial stage of development, these arteries arise caudal to the union of the two dorsal aortas (Figure 10.4.4). Significant remodelling of these vessels occurs as the heart itself moves caudally with ongoing development.

The essence of normal development is then the regression of the larger part of the right-sided structures, leaving a left aortic arch, a left-sided descending aorta, and a left-sided arterial duct (Figure 10.4.5). Subsequent to the remodelling, the initial right cranial horn of the aortic sac has become the brachiocephalic artery, while the left cranial horn remodels to become the initial segment of the transverse aortic arch. It is failure of the normal regression of the right-sided components that leaves the double arch, thus forming a ring around the trachea and the esophagus. Incomplete regression of a hypothetical perfect double arch is then the basis of the concept established by Edwards and his colleagues to explain the many and varied arterial patterns that encircle the tracheo-esophageal pedicle.[9] The hypothetical arch has a midline anterior aorta, which divides to produce bilateral arches, which in turn join posteriorly to form a midline descending aorta. Common carotid and subclavian arteries arise cranially from each of the arches in the hypothetical system, while an arterial duct connects each arch caudally to its companion pulmonary artery (Figure 10.4.6). Persistent patency of both sides of the hypothetical arch provides a pattern that encircles the tracheo-esophageal pedicle (Figure 10.4.7). The variant with all components present of the hypothetical model are exceedingly rare, with to the best of our knowledge only a solitary case thus far described.[10] Cases are more frequent with all the cranial components present, and with one of the arterial ducts present either as a patent channel, or more usually as an arterial ligament (Figure 10.4.8). Inappropriate interruption, or atresia with a fibrous remnant, at any part of the ring can then account for all the described abnormal variations. In this regard, Stewart and colleagues[9] provided an exhaustive list of the potential malformations, which they catalogued in complex alphanumeric fashion. Our preference is to opt for descriptive analysis, rather than alphanumeric notation.[8]

10.4 Vascular Rings

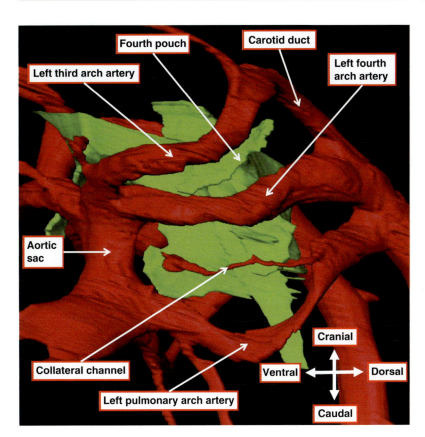

Figure 10.4.3 The image shows the reconstructed left-sided arch arteries from a human embryo at Carnegie stage 15. We initially interpreted the findings to suggest presence of a persistent 'fifth arch artery'. Since we now know that six arches are never formed, we believe the finding is better considered to represent a collateral channel. The reconstruction was made by Dr Simon Bamforth, from Newcastle University, and is reproduced with his permission.

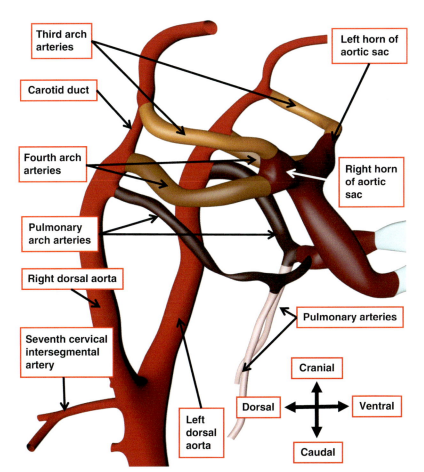

Figure 10.4.4 The image shows a reconstruction of the stage of remodelling of the initially bilaterally symmetrical arteries of the caudal three pharyngeal arches at Carnegie stage 16, when the embryo is around 36 days subsequent to fertilization. The right-sided vessels are beginning to diminish in size when compared with the left-sided components. Note, however, the caudal location of the seventh cervical intersegmental artery, which will become the subclavian artery.

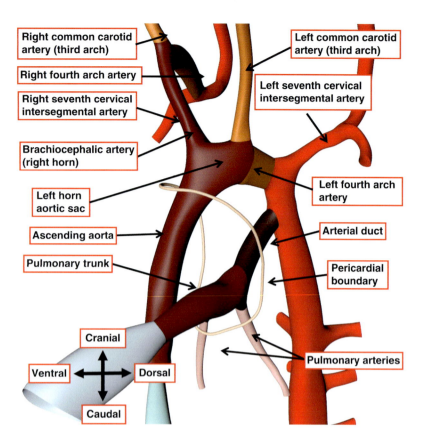

Figure 10.4.5 The image shows a view of the arch system in a human embryo at Carnegie stage 20, representing around 49 days of development. The remodelling is essentially complete, with persistence of the left-sided components. Note that the left subclavian artery has crossed the union of the arterial duct with the descending aorta creating the aortic isthmus.

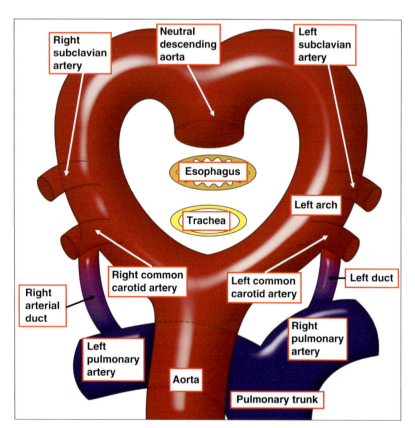

Figure 10.4.6 The drawing shows the perfect hypothetical double arch, with right and left arches, and with a subclavian and common carotid arising cranially, and arterial duct arising caudally, from each arch. The descending aorta is in the midline, or in a 'neutral' position.

10.4 Vascular Rings

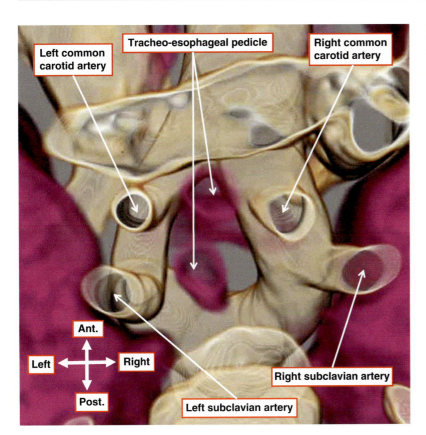

Figure 10.4.7 This computed tomographic angiogram, viewed from above, shows a double aortic arch, with persistence of both the right- and left-sided aortic arches. The common carotid and subclavian arteries originate in symmetrical fashion from the superior surface of the arches.

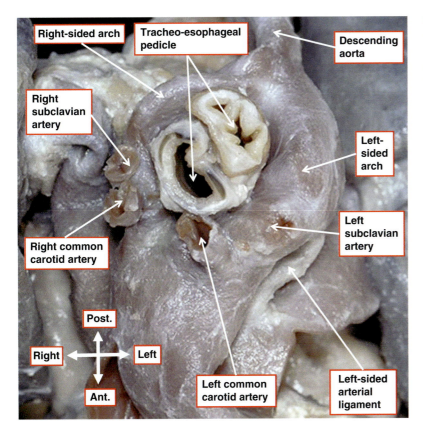

Figure 10.4.8 The specimen shows a double arch, with persistence of both the right- and left-sided aortic arches, with origin of the common carotid and subclavian arteries in symmetrical fashion from the superior surface of the arches. In this example, there is a ligamentous left-sided arterial duct, and the left-sided arch is dominant. The arrangement produces obvious compression of the tracheo-esophageal pedicle.

An example of interruption of part of the hypothetical double arch is shown in Figure 10.4.9. The lesion illustrated is an aberrant right subclavian artery extending in retro-esophageal fashion, having arisen from a left-sided aortic arch (Figure 10.4.10). The persisting part of the right-sided dorsal arch, which feeds the subclavian artery, is known as the diverticulum of Kommerell.

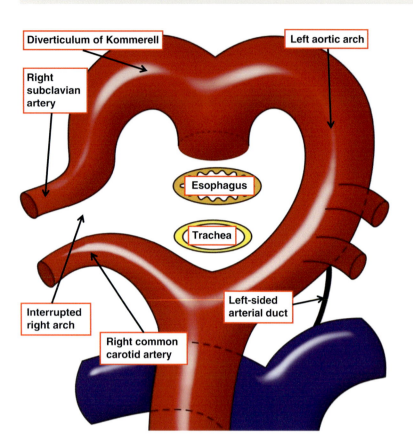

Figure 10.4.9 The drawing shows how aberrant retro-esophageal origin of the right subclavian artery from a left aortic arch is explained on the basis of the hypothetical double arch. The proximal portion of the right arch is known as the diverticulum of Kommerell. The initial segment of the hypothetical right arch is interrupted between the right common carotid and right subclavian arteries. The duct, in left-sided position, is shown as being ligamentous.

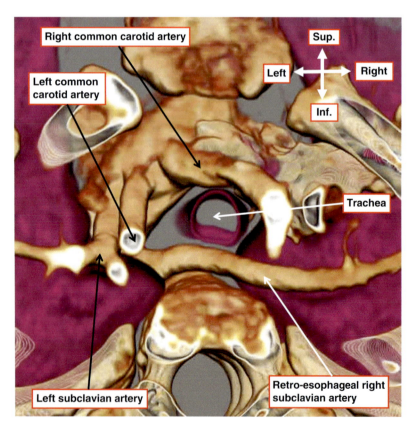

Figure 10.4.10 This computed tomographic angiogram, viewed from above, shows a retro-esophageal right subclavian artery arising from a left-sided aortic arch as depicted in the drawing of Figure 10.4.9. The trachea is seen in the reconstruction, but not the esophagus. The arterial duct is not seen in this reconstruction, but was left sided. This patient did not have a complete vascular ring.

The mere presence of a retro-esophageal subclavian artery, however, does not imply the presence of symptomatic esophageal compression, which is the usual problem produced by the vascular ring. Persistence of the arterial duct as a patent channel in the setting of a retro-esophageal subclavian artery is able to complete the ring, as shown in Figure 10.4.11 in the setting of a right aortic arch. The duct, of course, can itself become ligamentous, and persist as a fibrous cord (Figure 10.4.12). Compression is not always present in this setting. Even when the duct is patent, tracheo-esophageal compression may not be obvious in the operating room until the duct is divided, and its ends are allowed to spring apart (Figures 10.4.13, 10.4.14). There is another caveat that

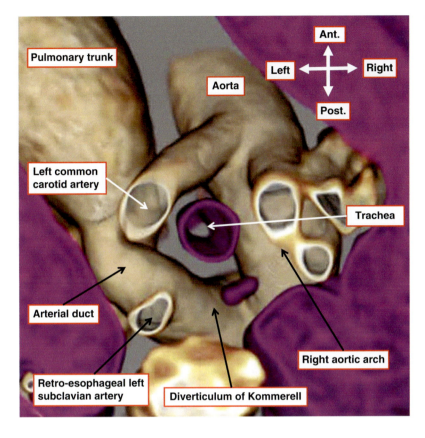

Figure 10.4.11 The image from this computed tomographic angiogram is the mirror-image of the arrangement shown in Figure 10.4.10. There is retro-esophageal origin of the left subclavian artery from a right-sided aortic arch, with the dorsal part of the left arch persisting as the diverticulum of Kommerell. In this instance, however, the diverticulum of Kommerell continues as the left-sided arterial duct, creating a vascular ring. The trachea is seen in the reconstruction, but not the esophagus. The potentially complete double arch is divided between the left subclavian and left common carotid arteries.

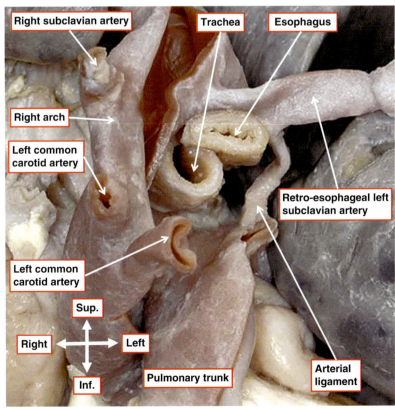

Figure 10.4.12 The specimen is comparable to the image shown in Figure 10.4.11. There is a potential double aortic arch that is interrupted between the left common carotid artery and the left subclavian artery, with the subclavian artery arising in retro-esophageal fashion from the right-sided aortic arch. Despite the incomplete nature of the hypothetical double arch, the presence of the arterial ligament, running from the left subclavian artery to the left pulmonary artery, produces a vascular ring around the tracheo-esophageal pedicle.

should be remembered by the operating surgeon. Not only can the duct persist as a fibrous remnant, but so can the seemingly interrupted segment of the double arch. In the setting shown for the retro-esophageal subclavian artery arising from the right arch, the compression will be much greater when both components of the hypothetical perfect double arch exist as fibrous cords

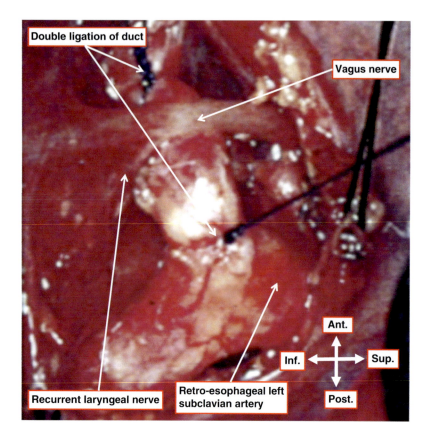

Figure 10.4.13 This operative view, taken through a left thoracotomy, shows an arterial duct that arises from an aberrant left subclavian artery, itself coursing in retro-esophageal position from a right aortic arch. As was shown in the previous two figures, this arrangement produces a vascular ring, which was found to be symptomatic in this patient. The duct has been doubly ligated prior to its division. Note the size and location of the vagus nerve and its recurrent laryngeal branch.

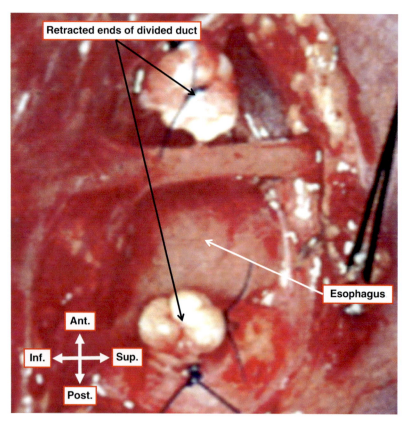

Figure 10.4.14 After division of the duct in the patient shown in Figure 10.4.13, the ends of the arch have sprung apart to free the esophagus. The appearance subsequent to the surgical procedure shows the initial effect of the compression produced by the vascular ring.

(Figure 10.4.15). The same situation can be found when the diverticulum of Kommerell itself exist with dual fibrous cords (Figure 10.4.16).

A right-sided aortic arch can also exist aside from its association with vascular rings. The arch is right sided when it crosses over the main stem of the right-sided bronchus. It may then connect to the descending aorta on either the right or left side of the vertebral column. Such a right-sided aortic arch is considered abnormal with the usual atrial arrangement, but is to be expected in patients with the mirror-imaged arrangement. In

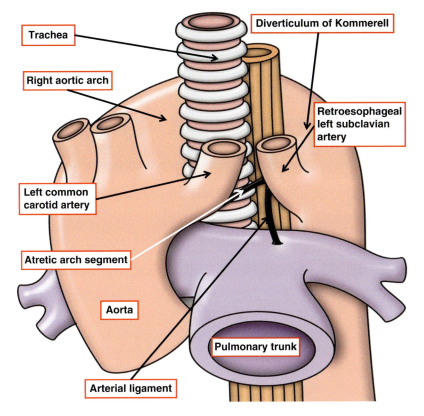

Figure 10.4.15 The drawing shows how, in the setting of retro-esophageal origin of the left subclavian artery from a right aortic arch, there is the potential for two fibrous cords to join the subclavian artery to both the left common carotid artery and the left pulmonary artery. Both cords may persist to produce compressive symptoms.

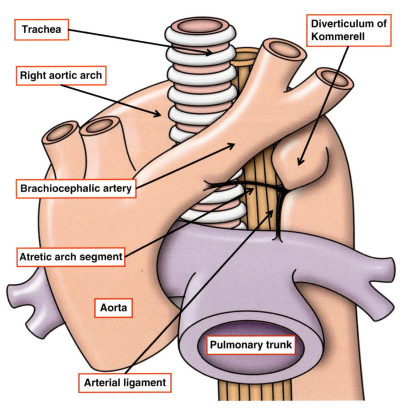

Figure 10.4.16 The potential for persistence of dual compressing fibrous remnants should also be suspected when the diverticulum of Kommerell persists as a ductal diverticulum in the setting of a right aortic arch with mirror-imaged branching.

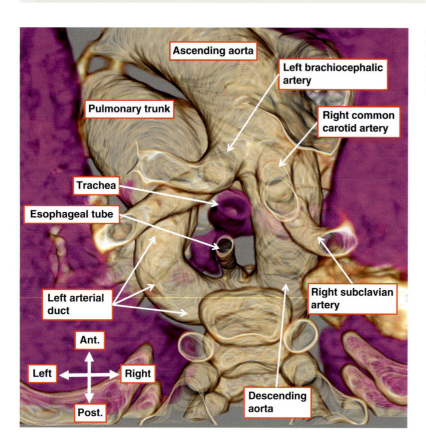

Figure 10.4.17 This computed tomographic angiogram, viewed from above, shows a right aortic arch with mirror-imaged branching. A left-sided arterial duct is seen connecting the left pulmonary artery to the descending aorta, creating a vascular ring encircling the trachea and esophagus. There is a feeding tube in the esophagus.

either case, it may or may not produce clinical problems. Its chief surgical significance lies in its association with about one-quarter of cases of tetralogy of Fallot, and approximately half of all patients with common arterial trunks. Patients with a right aortic arch usually have a mirror-imaged arrangement of the brachiocephalic arteries. This can be significant when contemplating construction of a subclavian-to-pulmonary arterial shunt. With mirror-imaged branching, the first branch of the aorta beyond the coronary arteries is the brachiocephalic trunk, which then gives rise to the left subclavian and common carotid arteries. Under such circumstances, the surgeon may elect to perform a left-sided anastomosis so as to avoid kinking of the right subclavian artery as it is turned down into the mediastinum. In patients with a right aortic arch and mirror-imaged branching, the duct usually remains a left-sided structure connecting the brachiocephalic trunk to the left pulmonary artery. The left-sided duct, nonetheless, can occasionally connect the left pulmonary artery to the aortic isthmus, creating a vascular ring (Figure 10.4.17).

The hypothetical double arch also provides a rational explanation for isolation of the brachiocephalic arteries. In these anomalies, which can involve either the brachiocephalic artery itself or the common carotid or subclavian arteries, and which can be associated with either the usual left-sided aortic arch or a right aortic arch, the isolated artery arises from one or other of the pulmonary arteries via a persistently patent arterial duct. In the example shown in Figure 10.4.18, there is persistence of both the right-sided and left-sided arterial ducts. The aortic arch is interrupted between the left common carotid and left subclavian arteries, with the isolated right subclavian artery arising via a right-sided arterial duct from the right pulmonary artery. Figure 10.4.19 is another example, seen in the context of an intact right aortic arch. The right-sided and left-sided arterial ducts are persistently patent, with an isolated left subclavian arising from the left-sided arterial duct.

References Cited

1. Rathke H. Über die Entwickelung der Arterien, welche bei den Säugethieren von den Bogen der Aorta ausgehen. *Arch Anat* 1843; **16**: 270–302.
2. Boas JEV. Über die Arterienbogen der Wirbelthiere. Briefliche Mittheilung an den Herausgeber. *Morph Jahrb* 1887; **13**: 115–118.
3. Graham A, Poopalasundaram S, Shone V, Kiecker C. A reappraisal and revision of the numbering of the pharyngeal arches. *J Anat* 2019; **235**: 1019–1023.
4. Van Praagh R, Van Praagh S. Persistent fifth arterial arch in man: congenital double-lumen aortic arch. *Am J Cardiol* 1969; **24**: 279–285.
5. Gerlis LM, Ho SY, Anderson RH, Da Costa P. Persistent 5th aortic arch – a great pretender: three new covert cases. *Int J Cardiol* 1989; **23**: 239–247.
6. Bamforth SD, Chaudhry B, Bennett M, et al. Clarification of the identity of the mammalian fifth pharyngeal arch artery. *Clin Anat* 2013; **26**: 173–182.
7. Anderson RH, Bamforth SD, Gupta SK. How best to describe the pharyngeal arch arteries when the fifth arch does not exist? *Cardiol Young* 2020; **30**: 1708–1710.
8. Anderson RH, Bamforth SD. Morphogenesis of the mammalian aortic

10.4 Vascular Rings

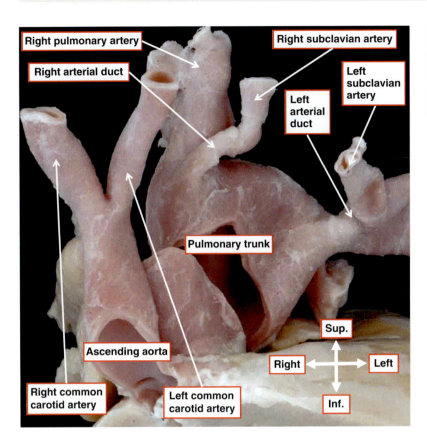

Figure 10.4.18 The specimen shows interruption of the aortic arch between the right common carotid and left subclavian arteries. The ascending aorta, however, gives rise only to the right subclavian and right common carotid arteries. The left common carotid artery is isolated, arising from the right pulmonary artery via the right-sided arterial duct. The descending aorta and the left subclavian artery are fed by the left-sided arterial duct.

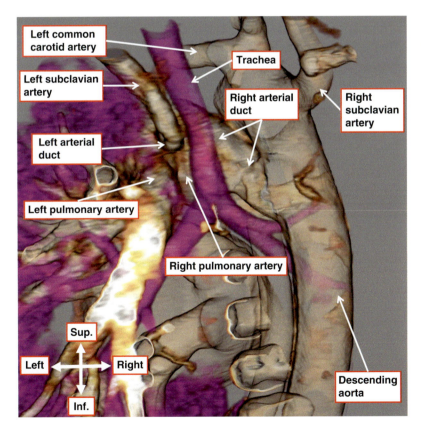

Figure 10.4.19 This computed tomographic angiogram, viewed from behind, shows a right aortic arch with a patent right-sided arterial duct. An isolated left subclavian artery is seen arising from the left pulmonary artery via a left-sided arterial duct.

arch arteries. *Front Cell Dev Biol* 2022 **10**; 892900.

9. Stewart JR, Kincaid OW, Edwards JE. *An Atlas of Vascular Rings and Related Malformations of the Aortic Arch System.* Springfield: Charles C. Thomas; 1964.

10. Shirali GS, Geva T, Ott DA, Bricker JT. Double aortic arch and bilateral patent ducti arteriosi associated with transposition of the great arteries: missing clinical link in an embryologic theory. *Am Heart J* 1994; **127**: 451–453.

Chapter 10.5
Pulmonary Arterial and Ductal Anomalies

By far the most common malformation of the pulmonary arteries, excluding atresia or stenosis, is for either the right or left pulmonary artery to have an aortic origin. Most frequently, the anomalous artery arises via an arterial duct. Although seen in the presence of pulmonary atresia, usually with the other lung supplied by major systemic-to-pulmonary collateral arteries (Figure 10.5.1), it can be found with the other pulmonary artery connected to the patent pulmonary trunk.[1] In this arrangement, the duct will often close with time. There will then be apparent unilateral absence of that pulmonary artery that was initially fed through the duct. This is common in tetralogy of Fallot or double outlet right ventricle, but about half of the patients thus afflicted have otherwise normal hearts. In our experience, it is rare to find true absence of the hilar pulmonary artery.

Less frequently, the anomalous pulmonary artery, usually the right, can arise directly from the ascending aorta (Figures 10.5.2, 10.5.3). This is sometimes termed a hemitruncus, but we do not recommend use of this term, because almost always there are two normally formed arterial roots (Figure 10.5.2). Rarely, the right pulmonary artery may take an unusually high origin from the right side of the ascending portion of a common arterial trunk. Even in this setting, the descriptive title of 'common trunk with anomalous origin of the right pulmonary artery' is preferable to 'hemitruncus'.

When the anomalously connected pulmonary artery arises directly from the aorta, surgical repair consists simply of detachment from the aorta and reattachment to the pulmonary trunk. This is somewhat more difficult in the presence of a common trunk, but the same basic principle is followed for repair. When the anomalous pulmonary artery is fed through a duct, or connected by a ligament, it will arise from the aortic arch or a brachiocephalic artery. Care must then be taken during surgical reconstruction to ensure that ductal tissue is not incorporated with the anastomosis, since it may subsequently constrict and produce stenosis at the site of repair. In cases with unilateral absence of a pulmonary artery, it is usual to find pulmonary hypertension and pulmonary hypertensive

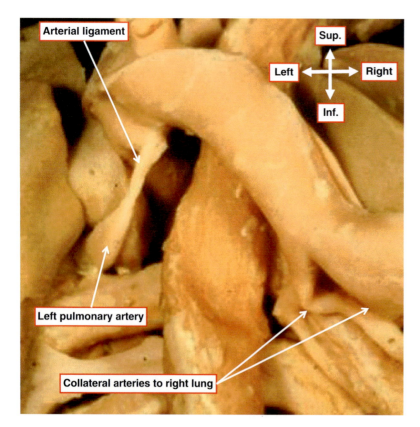

Figure 10.5.1 In this specimen, photographed from behind, the left pulmonary artery was initially fed from a left-sided duct, which has become ligamentous. The right lung is fed through systemic-to-pulmonary collateral arteries.

10.5 Pulmonary Arterial and Ductal Anomalies

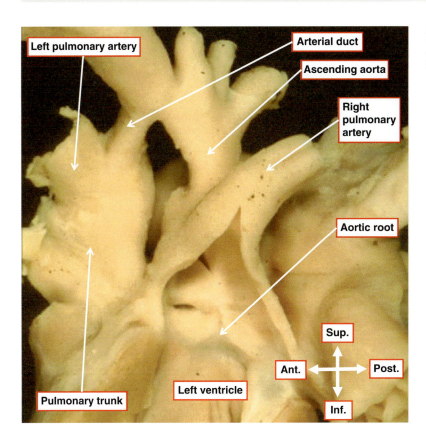

Figure 10.5.2 This specimen, viewed from the left side the left ventricle having been opened, shows anomalous origin of the right pulmonary artery from the ascending intrapericardial aorta. Note the separate arterial roots.

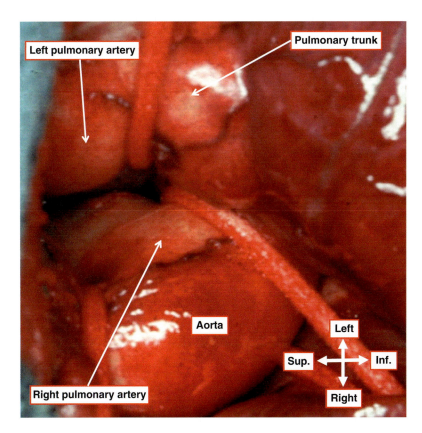

Figure 10.5.3 In this operative view, taken through a median sternotomy, the right pulmonary artery is seen arising directly from the aorta. This should not be described as hemitruncus, since there are separate aortic and pulmonary pathways, the pulmonary trunk continuing as the left pulmonary artery.

vascular disease in the normally connected lung, probably because of its being disproportionately small and having to receive the entire right ventricular output.[2]

In a much rarer anomaly, the left pulmonary artery arises from the right pulmonary artery. The abnormal left pulmonary artery originates within the right chest (Figures 10.5.3, 10.5.4),

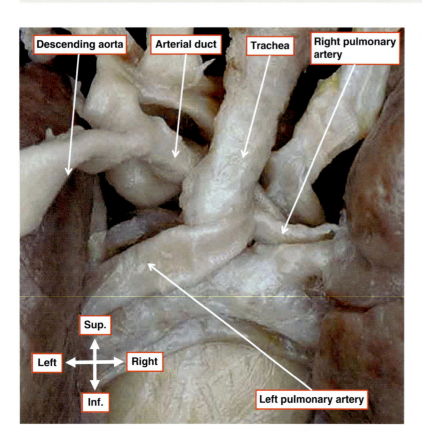

Figure 10.5.4 This specimen is photographed from behind. The left pulmonary artery arises from the right pulmonary artery. It then extends between the trachea and the esophagus, which has been removed, producing the pulmonary arterial sling (see Figure 10.5.6).

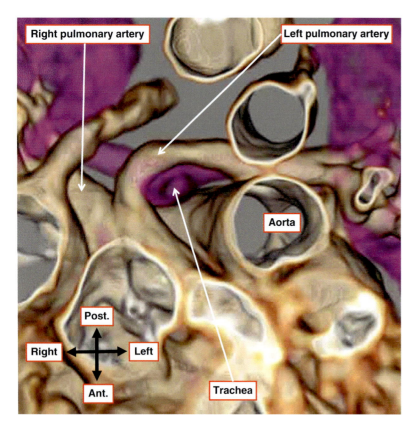

Figure 10.5.5 This computed tomographic dataset shows origin of the left pulmonary artery from the right pulmonary artery. It extends between the trachea and the esophagus, producing the pulmonary arterial sling (see Figure 10.5.6).

and passes between the trachea and esophagus to the left pulmonary hilum, creating a pulmonary arterial sling (Figures 10.5.5, 10.5.6).[3] This may result in repeated respiratory problems due to the frequent accompaniment of complete tracheal rings. This may require division and transplantation of the offending artery. As discussed above,

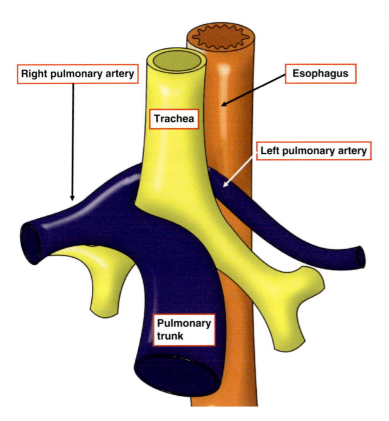

Figure 10.5.6 The drawing shows the arrangement known as the pulmonary arterial sling, as illustrated in Figures 10.5.4 and 10.5.5.

the right pulmonary artery may arise anomalously from the aorta or brachiocephalic artery, but an abnormal right pulmonary vessel arising from the left pulmonary artery has not, to our knowledge, been reported. The reason for this is not clear.

In the rare occurrence of agenesis of the right lung, displacement of the heart into the right chest may create a ring-like disposition which can obstruct the left bronchus. The displaced heart, pulling on the left pulmonary artery, draws the ligament and descending aorta across the left bronchus, compressing the bronchus against the spinal column. Division of the ligament, and grafting of the aorta, may be necessary to allow the pulmonary trunk and aorta to spring apart and 'unroof' the constricting circle.[4–6]

Persistence of the Arterial Duct and Aortopulmonary Window

Persistence of the arterial duct (Figure 10.5.7) occupies a special place in the study of cardiovascular disease, since it was the first congenital malformation to be cured by operative intervention.[7] Though the duct can now safely be closed by techniques of interventional catheterization,[8,9] its interruption remains a paradigm of the best of surgical science. The anatomy is almost always predictable, and the operative results uniformly excellent.

Because the arterial system develops with bilateral symmetry, a persistent duct may be either right or left sided, although the latter is overwhelmingly more common. Because the duct can persist on either side, or bilaterally, then as discussed above, it may be important as part of a vascular ring, or providing the origin of an isolated brachiocephalic artery (see Figure 10.4.17). Persistent patency may also play an important physiological role when it accompanies other complex congenital cardiovascular anomalies, such as interruption of the aortic arch, aortic or pulmonary valvar atresia, or discordant ventriculo-arterial connections. In this chapter, we confine our discussion to the primary congenital condition of isolated left-sided persistently patent arterial duct.

Although it is possible to approach the patent duct anteriorly, and sometimes necessary to use this route (Figure 10.5.7), the normal operative approach is through a left lateral thoracotomy (Figure 10.5.8). The duct arises from the postero-superior aspect of the junction of the pulmonary trunk and left pulmonary artery (Figure 10.5.9). It courses posteriorly and slightly leftward to join the junction of the aortic arch and descending aorta just distal to, and opposite, the origin of the left subclavian artery. Its pulmonary end is covered by a fold of pericardium, and its aortic end by parietal pleura. It may be confused with the aortic isthmus, particularly in the infant, and it is possible to identify the left pulmonary artery as a patent duct. Even under the best conditions, these other structures may be mistakenly ligated in place of the duct. The caveats of this procedure have been elegantly reviewed.[10] Approached laterally, the best anatomical guide to the duct is the vagus nerve and its recurrent laryngeal branch. The vagus nerve passes along the subclavian artery, crossing over the aortic arch before heading in a posterior direction to disappear behind the hilum. Just at the level of the duct, it gives off the recurrent nerve (Figure 10.5.8), which then curves beneath the

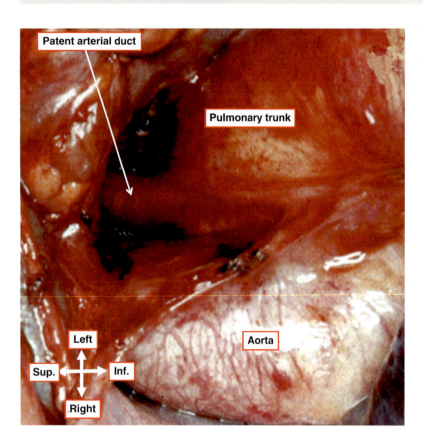

Figure 10.5.7 This operative view through a median sternotomy shows the origin of a persistently patent arterial duct from the distal extent of the pulmonary trunk.

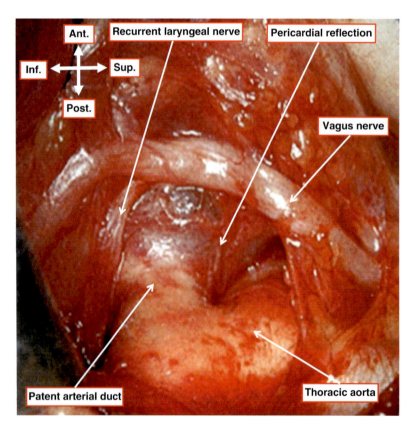

Figure 10.5.8 In this operative view, a persistently patent arterial duct is seen through a left thoracotomy (compare with Figure 10.5.7). Note the location of the vagus nerve and its recurrent laryngeal branch.

inferomedial wall of the duct before ascending along the postero-medial aspect of the aorta into the groove between the trachea and esophagus.

Access to the duct may be achieved by incising the mediastinal parietal pleura, either between the phrenic and vagus nerves or, more posteriorly, over the aorta

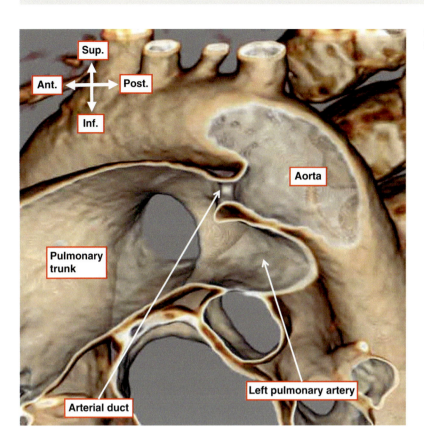

Figure 10.5.9 The reconstructed computed tomographic angiogram shows a persistently patent arterial duct.

itself. With either approach, the recurrent nerve must be visualized to guard against direct trauma or injury by traction. The fold of pericardium extending over the pulmonary end of the duct may be lifted away by sharp dissection. The postero-medial wall of the duct is firmly attached by another more fibrous fold to the bronchus. It is this firm fibrous fold that prevents easy circumscription of the duct with a right-angle clamp. To minimize the risk of tearing the wall of the duct, this tissue must be divided by sharp dissection. This can be done through a superior approach over the aortic end of the duct, or by freeing the aorta and retracting it medially. In the latter instance, small but potentially troublesome bronchial vessels may be encountered, arising from the posterior wall of the aorta. Another anatomical note of caution involves the thoracic duct and its tributaries in the area of the origin of the subclavian artery. Division of any of these major lymph vessels is liable to lead to chylothorax and its attendant difficulties. Should the lymphatic trunks be inadvertently divided, they must be ligated to avoid chylothorax. The duct in an infant or small child can measure from one to fifteen millimetres in length and diameter. Rarely, it can be aneurysmally dilated (Figure 10.5.10).[11] These may be aneurysms of a truly patent duct, or may simply be a dilated ductal diverticulum with a closed pulmonary end. In general, the short and fat duct should be cross-clamped, divided, and oversewn to minimize the chances of incomplete ligation or tearing of the vessel wall. For the longer thin duct, a triple ligation technique has proved to be safe and effective.[12]

The persistently patent arterial duct must be distinguished from an aortopulmonary window. The distinguishing feature is that the window is intrapericardial, whereas the duct is always outside the pericardial cavity. Clinical presentation of the window is often similar to that of a common arterial trunk. The anatomical distinction lies in the mode of ventriculo-arterial connection. The phenotypic feature of the common trunk is its common and solitary arterial root. Aortopulmonary window, in contrast, is always associated with separate aortic and pulmonary roots (Figure 10.5.11). Though the ventricular septum is usually intact, this defect is frequently associated with additional congenital cardiovascular anomalies.[13]

The defect itself is usually located in the right lateral wall of the pulmonary trunk anterior and opposite to the origin of the right pulmonary artery, which frequently overrides the window, or arises directly from the aorta (Figure 10.5.12). This means that its opening into the left side of the ascending aorta is just distal to the sinutubular junction. The window can also be associated with the origin of one of the coronary arteries from pulmonary trunk.[14] The defect itself can take the form of a well-demarcated short tubular channel, or present as an extensive fenestration. Surgical repair is best accomplished through an incision in the ascending aorta using standard cardiopulmonary bypass techniques. As a general rule, closed methods are not advisable, not even for the more tubular defects. When the window supplies a vital part of the circulation, it cannot be closed without providing an alternate source of blood for the dependent segment of the circulation.

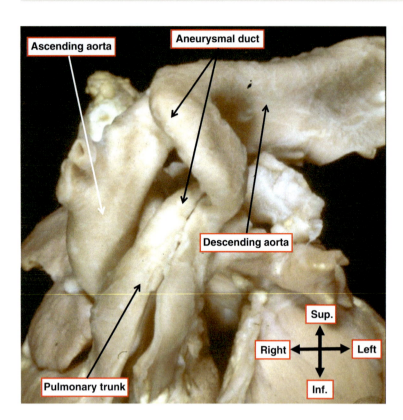

Figure 10.5.10 The heart is photographed in anatomical orientation from the front. The arterial duct is patent, elongated, and aneurysmal.

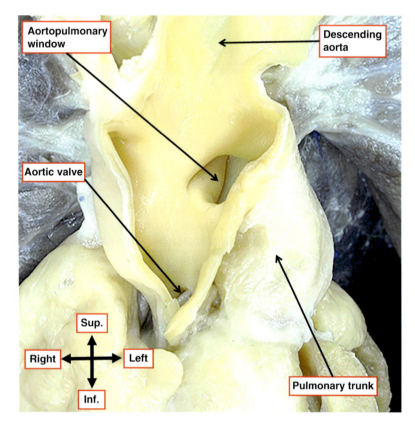

Figure 10.5.11 This specimen, shown in anatomical orientation having opened the aorta, shows an aortopulmonary window. Note the presence of the separate arterial trunks and valves proximal to the defect.

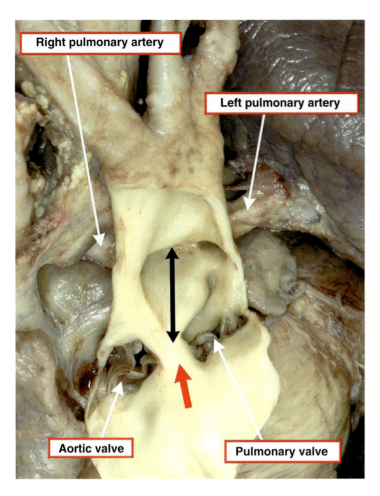

Figure 10.5.12 This specimen also has a large aortopulmonary window, with the right pulmonary artery directly adjacent to the aorta. The anterior wall of the arterial trunks has been removed to show the discrete and separate arterial roots. In this heart, the window (double headed black arrow) has significant length. Note also the separate walls of the arterial trunks proximal to the window (red arrow).

References Cited

1. Loomba RS, Aiello S, Tretter JT, et al. Left pulmonary artery from the ascending aorta: a case report and review of published cases. *J Cardiovasc Dev Dis* 2020; **8**: 1.

2. Pool PE, Vogel JHK, Blount SG Jr. Congenital unilateral absence of a pulmonary artery. The importance of flow in pulmonary hypertension. *Am J Cardiol* 1962; **10**: 706–732.

3. Contro S, Miller RA, White H, Potts WJ. Bronchial obstruction due to pulmonary artery anomalies. I. Vascular sling. *Circulation* 1958; **17**: 418–423.

4. Maier HC, Gould WJ. Agenesis of the lung with vascular compression of the tracheobronchial tree. *J Pediatr* 1953; **43**: 38–42.

5. Harrison MR, Hendren WH. Agenesis of the lung complicated by vascular compression and bronchomalacia. *J Pediatr Surg* 1975; **10**: 813–817.

6. Harrison MR, Heldt GP, Brasch RC, de Lorimier AA, Gregory GA. Resection of distal tracheal stenosis in a baby with agenesis of the lung. *J Pediatr Surg* 1980; **15**: 938–943.

7. Gross RE. Surgical management of patent ductus arteriosus with summary of four surgically treated cases. *Ann Surg* 1939; **110**: 321–356.

8. Ali Kahn MA, Al Yousef S, Mullins CE, Sawyer W. Experiences with 205 procedures of transcatheter closure of ductus arteriosus in 182 patients, with special reference to residual shunts and long term follow-up. *J Thorac Cardiovasc Surg* 1992; **104**: 1721–1727.

9. Lloyd TR, Fedderly R, Mendelsohn AM, Sandhu SK, Beekman RH. Transcatheter occlusion of patent ductus arteriosus with Gianturco coils. *Circulation* 1993; **88** (part 1): 1414–1420.

10. Pontius RG, Danielson GK, Noonan JA, Judson JP. Illusions leading to surgical closure of the distal left pulmonary artery instead of the ductus arteriosus. *J Thorac Cardiovasc Surg* 1981; **82**: 107–113.

11. Mendel V, Luhmer J, Oelert H. Aneurysma des Ductus arteriosus bei einem Neugeborenen. *Herz* 1980; **5**: 320–323.

12. Wilcox BR, Peters RM. The surgery of patent ductus arteriosus: a clinical report of 14 years' experience without an operative death. *Ann Thorac Surg* 1967; **3**: 126–131.

13. Faulkner SL, Oldham RR, Atwood GF, Graham T P. Aortopulmonary window, ventricular septal defect and membranous pulmonary atresia with a diagnosis of truncus arteriosus. *Chest* 1974; **65**: 351–353.

14. Anderson RH, Cook A, Brown NA, et al. Development of the outflow tracts with reference to aortopulmonary windows and aortoventricular tunnels. *Cardiol Young* 2010; **20**(Suppl.3): 92–99.

Chapter 10.6
Anomalies of the Coronary Arteries and Aortoventricular Tunnels

Congenital malformations of the coronary arteries in otherwise normally structured hearts have, traditionally, been categorized as major or minor. This approach was rooted in the belief that the so-called major anomalies were those that produced symptomatology, whereas the minor lesions were thought to be of no clinical relevance.[1] The potential danger of such a classification became evident when it was realized that some lesions categorized as minor within this concept could be a cause of sudden cardiac death.[2] Because of this discrepancy between presumed anatomical and revealed clinical significance, it now seems preferable to account for these malformations on a descriptive basis. Within such a descriptive categorization, the anomalies can be grouped into those with anomalous origin of the coronary arteries from the arterial roots, those with anomalous course of the epicardial coronary arteries, those with anomalous communications between the coronary arteries and other structures within the heart, or combinations of such findings.

Anomalous Origin of the Coronary Arteries

The coronary arteries can arise anomalously either from the pulmonary trunk or, rarely, from the right or left pulmonary artery. They can also take an anomalous origin from the aorta itself. Anomalous origin from the pulmonary trunk is often described as the Bland–White–Garland syndrome (Figures 10.6.1–10.6.3). Patients usually present in infancy with ischaemia of the left ventricle (Figure 10.6.4). If there is well-developed collateral circulation, presentation can be markedly delayed, some cases not presenting until childhood or even adolescence. The clinical problems are produced by the extent of ischaemia of the left ventricular myocardium, which can be extreme. It is important to re-attach the artery to the aorta as soon as the diagnosis is made. In most instances, the artery arises from the left sinus of the pulmonary trunk, to the right hand of the observer standing, figuratively speaking, in the non-adjacent sinus.[3] It is relatively easy to transfer the arterial origin, together with a button of pulmonary sinus, back to the left-hand adjacent sinus of the aorta. It is rare nowadays to

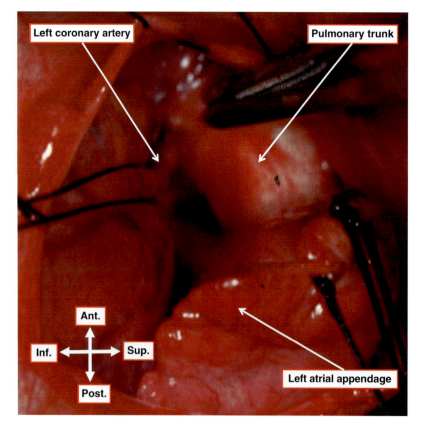

Figure 10.6.1 This view through a left lateral thoracotomy shows a silk ligature encircling a left coronary artery that is arising from the pulmonary trunk.

10.6 Anomalies of the Coronary Arteries and Aortoventricular Tunnels

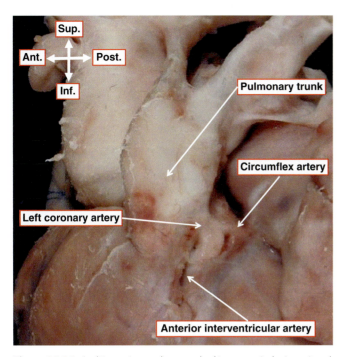

Figure 10.6.2 In this specimen, photographed in anatomical orientation, the main stem of the left coronary artery takes origin from the pulmonary trunk, arising from one of the sinuses adjacent to the aorta. It then divides into the circumflex and anterior interventricular arteries.

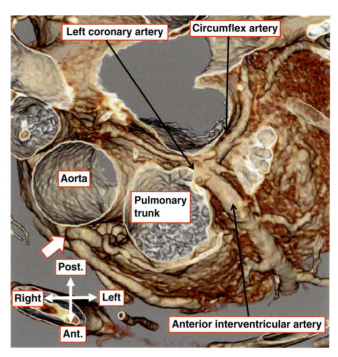

Figure 10.6.3 The reconstructed computed tomographic angiogram shows anomalous origin of the left coronary artery from the pulmonary trunk. The right coronary artery (red-bordered arrow) is dilated.

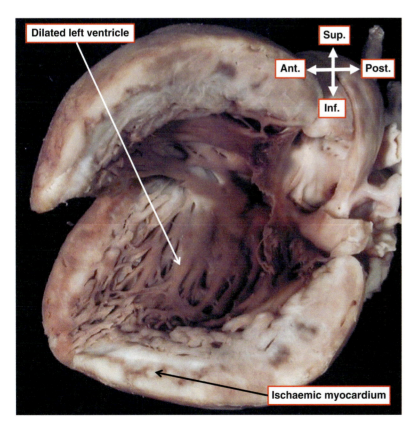

Figure 10.6.4 In this anatomical specimen, photographed in anatomical orientation, the left ventricle is dilated secondary to anomalous origin of the left coronary artery from the pulmonary trunk, while the ventricular myocardium is obviously ischaemic.

create an aortopulmonary tunnel in order to reconnect the artery to the aorta.[4] The pattern that may create problems in transfer is when the artery arises from a branch of the pulmonary trunk rather than the trunk itself. Other patterns, such as anomalous origin of the right coronary artery from the pulmonary trunk, do not produce the same degree of symptomatology, and often do not come to the attention of the surgeon. If encountered, an anomalous right coronary artery can readily be transferred back to the aortic root.

We have already discussed the significance of anomalous origin of one coronary artery from the aorta itself in Chapter 5. As we showed, the coronary arteries usually arise from the two aortic sinuses that are adjacent to the pulmonary trunk. In the normal heart, the left coronary artery arises from the left-hand-facing sinus, while the right coronary artery arises from the right-hand-facing sinus. Accessory orifices supplying either the infundibular artery, the artery to the sinus node, or an artery supplying the walls of the arterial trunks are by no means uncommon. These accessory branches should not be interpreted as representing anomalies. The circumflex and anterior interventricular branches of the left coronary artery can also rarely take separate origins from the left-hand-facing sinus in an otherwise normal heart. Usually, the arteries arise within the coronary aortic sinuses, but origin at the sinutubular junction, or just above it, should not be considered abnormal. High origin, however, or an oblique origin and course of a coronary artery through the wall, particularly when crossing the peripheral end of a zone of apposition between the valvar leaflets, usually described as the valvar commissure, should be considered anomalous, as should origin of either coronary artery from an inappropriate sinus or, as occurs very rarely, from the non-adjacent aortic sinus.[5] The origin from an inappropriate sinus is of greatest importance, since this is now well established to be a harbinger of sudden cardiac death.[6] As we showed in Chapter 5, either coronary artery can arise from an inappropriate sinus. The artery then courses between the arterial trunks, typically crossing the valvar commissure. This is described as an intramural arrangement (Figure 10.6.5). Surgical unroofing is not difficult, but whether such relief is always necessary has still to be determined.

The finding of a single coronary artery also represents anomalous origin from the aortic root. This can be found in two patterns. In the first, all three coronary arteries arise from the same aortic sinus, with either one, two, or three orifices within the sinus. Usually, it is the right-hand sinus that gives origin to the coronary arteries. There is then an associated anomalous epicardial course of the branches of the left coronary artery as they reach the anticipated locations. As discussed in Chapter 5, this can involve the anterior interventricular branch tracking between the aorta and the pulmonary trunk, with the potential for its constriction. Alternatively, the main stem of the left coronary artery can run across the subpulmonary infundibulum, tracking towards the left atrial appendage before dividing into the circumflex and anterior interventricular arteries (Figure 10.6.6). The solitary coronary artery can also arise from the left aortic sinus, and the right coronary artery can then course between the aortic root and the subpulmonary infundibulum to reach the right atrioventricular groove (Figure 10.6.7). Yet another pattern is for the right coronary artery to take its normal origin from the right-hand-facing sinus, but then to continue beyond the crux as the circumflex artery, and to terminate at the obtuse margin as the anterior interventricular artery (see Chapter 5). This pattern probably has no

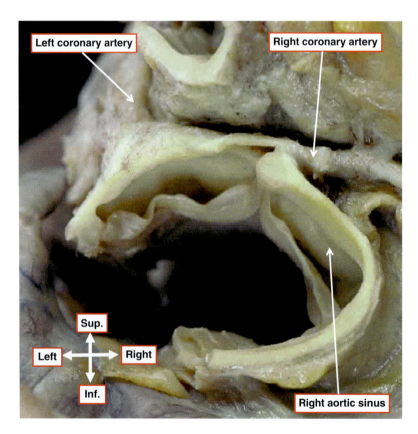

Figure 10.6.5 The tubular aorta has been removed from the aortic root, showing origin of the right coronary artery from the left coronary aortic sinus, with intramural coursing across the commissure, which is the peripheral attachment of the valvar leaflets at the sinutubular junction.

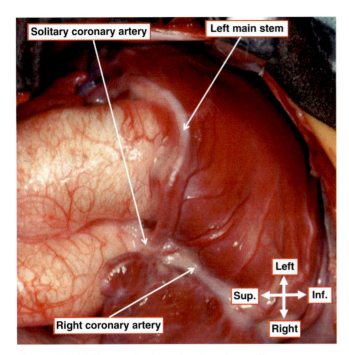

Figure 10.6.6 This operative view, taken through a median sternotomy, shows a heart in which all the coronary arteries arise from a solitary coronary artery, which takes origin from the right-hand adjacent aortic sinus. The main stem, which divides beneath the left appendage to become the circumflex and anterior interventricular arteries, crosses the origin of the pulmonary trunk from the right ventricle.

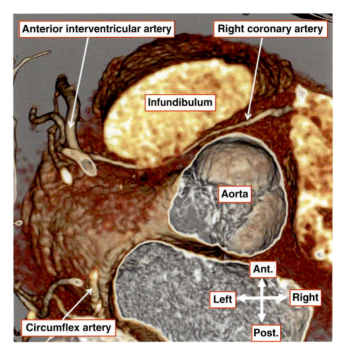

Figure 10.6.7 This computed tomographic dataset shows the origin of the right coronary artery from the anterior interventricular artery, with subsequent coursing between the subpulmonary infundibulum and the aortic root. There was a solitary coronary artery arising from the left coronary aortic sinus. Note the narrowed profile of the right coronary artery.

clinical significance. In addition to anomalous origin, congenital malformations can also afflict normally attached arteries, producing the effect of anomalous origin. Particularly important in this respect is congenital atresia of the main stem of the left coronary artery (Figure 10.6.8). This can be another substrate for sudden death in an adolescent or young adult.[7] Unfortunately, this anomaly is unlikely to be diagnosed prior to the event, when it could readily be treated by surgical manoeuvres.

Anomalous Epicardial Course of the Coronary Arteries

Although an anomalous epicardial course can be found in otherwise normally structured hearts, it is seen more frequently in hearts that are themselves malformed, such as those with discordant ventriculo-arterial connections or common arterial trunk. The clinical significance of these anomalies has yet to be fully determined. Some are found as chance observations at autopsy, such as the origin of the circumflex coronary artery from the right coronary artery, with passage through the transverse sinus to reach the left atrioventricular groove (Figure 10.6.9). Others may be of significance for sudden death, such as the passage between the aorta and the pulmonary trunk as discussed in Chapter 5. In this respect, muscular bridging of the epicardial coronary arteries (Figure 10.6.10) may also be of relevance, although the significance of this finding has still to be established.

Anomalous Communications of the Coronary Arteries

Fistulous communications between the coronary arteries and the ventricles are seen most frequently when atresia of an outflow tract is seen in the setting of an intact ventricular septum, notably in pulmonary atresia with intact ventricular septum (see Chapter 8.5). Such communications can also be found in otherwise normally structured hearts, and the anomalous artery can be joined to any other cardiac structure. The right coronary artery is most frequently involved, and it may connect to the right atrium (Figures 10.6.11, 10.6.12), the superior caval vein, the coronary sinus, the right ventricle, the pulmonary trunk, a pulmonary vein, or the left ventricle (Figure 10.6.13). The fistulas can also take origin from the left coronary artery. The communication itself can be a large solitary orifice, or a complex worm-like aneurysmal cavity. When the communication is simple and large, shunting across it can be considerable and the artery itself can be markedly dilated. Steals can also result, with consequent ischaemia in the area of myocardium from which the steal has occurred.

Aortoventricular Tunnels

The tunnels are rare lesions. The anatomical arrangement is not difficult to understand, since the essence of the lesions is to bypass the hinge of an aortic valvar leaflet (Figure 10.6.14). Typically, the tunnels extend between the aorta

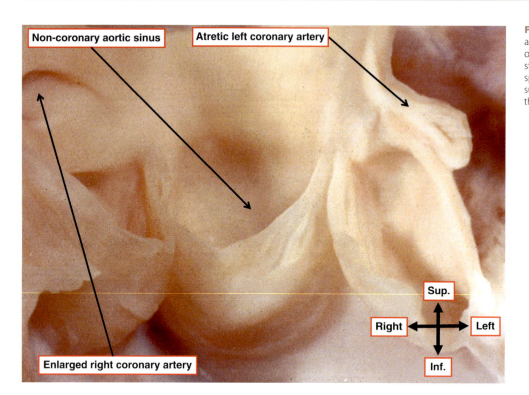

Figure 10.6.8 This view of the opened aortic root, photographed in anatomical orientation, shows atresia of the main stem of the left coronary artery. The specimen came from an adult who died suddenly. Note the enlarged orifice of the right coronary artery.

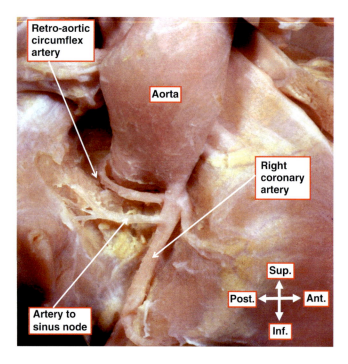

Figure 10.6.9 This infant heart is photographed in anatomical orientation. The circumflex coronary artery arises from the right coronary artery, and passes through the transverse sinus, behind the aorta, to reach the left atrioventricular groove.

and the left ventricle, although tunnels can also communicate with the right ventricle (Figure 10.6.15). It is the ones communicating with the left ventricle that are most frequent.[8,9] The anomalous channel, coursing from the left ventricle at the base of the interleaflet triangle between the two coronary aortic sinuses, then extends through the tissue plane that separates the aortic and pulmonary roots. It enters the aortic root above the sinutubular junction. The base of the tunnel is supported by the ventricular myocardium, while its roof is made up of arterial wall.

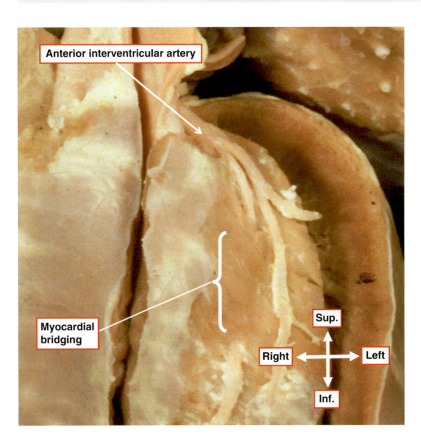

Figure 10.6.10 In this heart, photographed from the front in anatomical orientation, there is extensive myocardial bridging across the anterior interventricular artery.

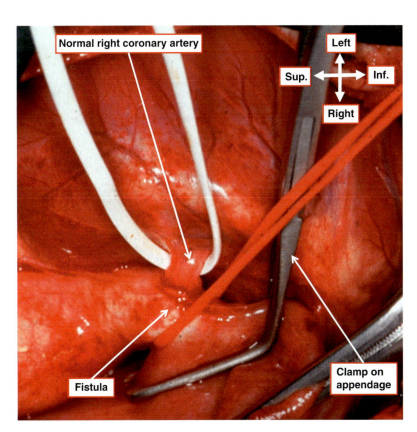

Figure 10.6.11 This operative view, taken through a median sternotomy, with the right atrial appendage retracted, shows a fistula running from the right coronary artery to the base of the appendage. The white loop is placed around the normal distal segment of the right coronary artery, while the red loop encircles the fistula itself.

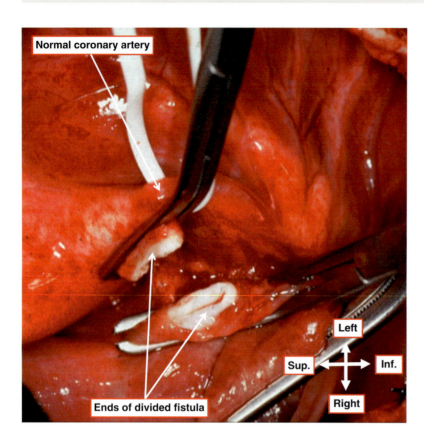

Figure 10.6.12 The broad fistula shown in Figure 10.6.11 has been divided.

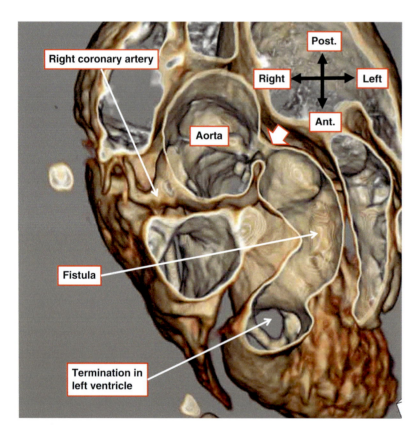

Figure 10.6.13 The reconstructed computed tomographic angiogram shows a fistula taking origin from the left coronary artery (red-bordered arrow) and terminating in the left ventricle.

10.6 Anomalies of the Coronary Arteries and Aortoventricular Tunnels

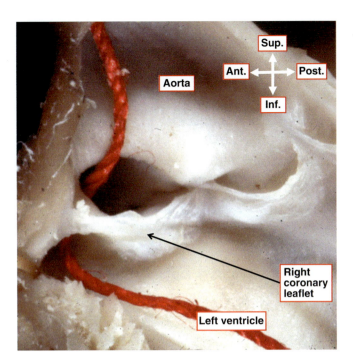

Figure 10.6.14 The aortic root has been opened and photographed from the front. The red cord is passing through an aorto–left ventricular tunnel, which bypasses the hinge of the right coronary aortic valvar leaflet.

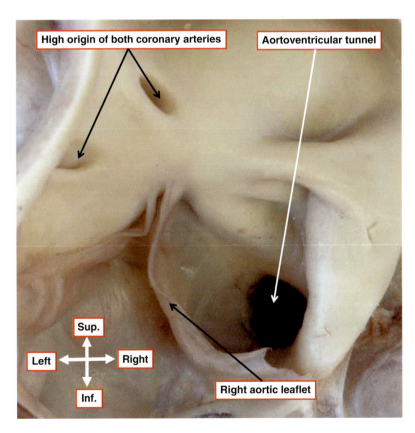

Figure 10.6.15 The aortic root has been opened and is photographed from behind. The aortic end of a tunnel is seen that courses through the supraventricular crest and opens into the right ventricular infundibulum. Note the high origin of the coronary arteries.

References Cited

1. Ogden JA. Congenital anomalies of the coronary arteries. *Am J Cardiol* 1970; **25**: 474–479.

2. Becker AE. Variations of the main coronary arteries. In AE Becker, T Losekoot, C Marcelletti, RH Anderson, eds., *Paediatric Cardiology*. 3rd ed. Edinburgh: Churchill Livingstone; 1983: pp. 263–277.

3. Smith A, Arnold R, Anderson RH, et al. Anomalous origin of the left coronary artery from the pulmonary trunk. Anatomic findings in relation to pathophysiology and surgical repair. *J Thorac Cardiovasc Surg* 1989; **98**: 16–24.

4. Takeuchi S, Imamura H, Katsumoto K, et al. New surgical method for repair of anomalous left coronary artery from the pulmonary artery. *J Thorac Cardiovasc Surg* 1979; **78**: 7–11.

5. Ishikawa T, Otsuka T, Suzuki T. Anomalous origin of the left main coronary artery from the non-coronary sinus of Valsalva. (Letter) *Pediatr Cardiol* 1990; **11**: 173–174.

6. Kragel AH, Roberts WC. Anomalous origin of either right or left main coronary artery from the aorta with subsequent coursing between aorta and pulmonary trunk: analysis of 32 necropsy cases. *Am J Cardiol* 1988; **62**: 771–777.

7. Debich DE, Williams KE, Anderson RH. Congenital atresia of the orifice of the left coronary artery and its main stem. *Int J Cardiol* 1989; **22**: 398–404.

8. McKay R, Anderson RH, Cook AC. The aorto-ventricular tunnels. *Cardiol Young* 2002; **12**: 563–580.

9. Protopapas EM, Anderson RH, Backer CL, et al. Surgical management of aorto-ventricular tunnel. A multicenter study. *Semin Thorac Cardiovasc Surg* 2020; **32**: 271–279.

Chapter 11

Positional Anomalies of the Heart

The surgical problems posed by cardiac malformations may be considerably increased when the heart itself is in an abnormal position. This is, in part, due to the unusual anatomical perspective presented to the surgeon because of the malposition, and also to the abnormal locations of the cardiac chambers, which may necessitate approaches other than those already discussed. Cardiac malposition in itself, nonetheless, does not constitute a diagnosis. Any normal or abnormal segmental combination can be found in a heart which itself is abnormally located. The heart may be normal, despite its abnormal location, but extremely complex anomalies are frequently present. Consequently, the very presence of an abnormal cardiac position emphasizes the need for a full and detailed segmental analysis of the heart. All the rules enunciated in Chapter 7 apply should the heart not be in its anticipated position. In this chapter, we confine ourselves to a description of abnormally positioned hearts, giving a more detailed discussion for specific types of malposition. We conclude with a review of the surgical significance of isomerism of the atrial appendages, which is generally agreed to be one of the major harbingers of abnormal cardiac position. We emphasize the need to segregate these lesions into the subsets of right as opposed to left isomerism, since the prognosis is markedly different for the two variants.

The Abnormally Positioned Heart

Account should be taken not only of an abnormal position of the heart within the chest, but also the direction of its apex. These are independent features. In the normal individual, the heart is positioned with its apex to the left, and with two-thirds of its bulk to the left of the midline. Mirror-imaged atrial arrangement is usually accompanied by mirror-imaged cardiac arrangement. The expected arrangement is then for the cardiac apex to point to the right, with the greater part of the cardiac mass in the right hemithorax (Figure 11.1). In the setting of isomerism of the atrial appendages, there is no norm. Thus, for all patients with isomerism, and equally for those with the usual or mirror-imaged atrial arrangements and abnormally positioned hearts, it is necessary to have a system that permits simple and straightforward description of the abnormal cardiac position. In the past, formidable conventions have been constructed, using terms such as dextrocardia, dextroposition, dextrorotation, or arcane variants such as pivotal dextrocardia.[1] In practice, the only requirement is for a system that accounts in independent fashion for the two major features, namely the position of the cardiac mass relative to the silhouette of the chest, and the direction of the cardiac apex. In the past, we have the situation in which the heart is in the right chest, with the apex pointing to the right (Figure 11.1) as 'dextrocardia'. But what happens on the rare occasion when the heart is in the right chest, but its apex is pointing to the left? This situation is readily, and unambiguously, described as the heart located in the right chest, with its apex pointing to the left. Those who wish to give nominative definitions to the arrangement are free so to do, but the descriptive approach is entirely adequate, and much less liable to misconstruction. Thus, the heart can be described as being mostly in the left chest, mostly in the right chest, or symmetrical. The apical orientation can be to the left, to the right, or to the midline.

Exteriorization of the Heart

The description given above does not account for the most severe cardiac malposition, namely exteriorization of the heart, or ectopia cordis. It has been said that the heart can protrude from the thoracic cavity in cervical, thoracic, thoracoabdominal, or abdominal positions. A previous review[2] questioned the existence of the cervical and abdominal variants, arguing that all cases can be described as thoracic or thoracoabdominal. In the thoracic type, which is the most common, there is a sternal defect and absence of the parietal pericardium. The heart protrudes directly from the thorax.[3] There is usually an associated omphalocele, and the thoracic cavity is small.

In the thoracoabdominal type, the sternal defect is usually confluent with deficiencies of the abdominal wall and diaphragm, so the heart and various abdominal organs are displaced into an omphalocele. A variant of this abnormality is seen in patients with Cantrell's syndrome.[4] These patients have a cleft lower sternum. The heart is beneath the skin in the upper epigastrium, and is associated with an omphalocele (Figure 11.2). When the skin was opened in the patient shown in Figure 11.2, the heart was seen to occupy a position in the midline (Figure 11.3), extending towards the omphalocele through a diaphragmatic defect. These patients frequently have complex intracardiac defects, often including a diverticulum of the left ventricle.

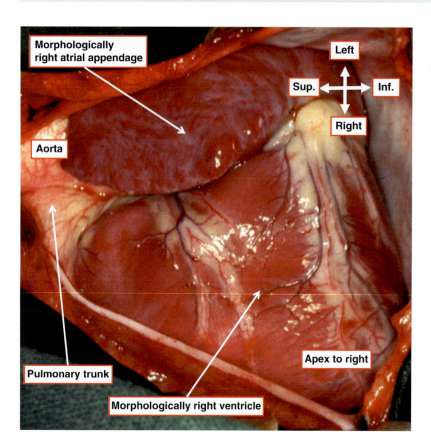

Figure 11.1 This operative view through a median sternotomy shows a patient with mirror-imaged arrangement of the organs. The heart is mostly in the right chest, with the apex pointing to the right.

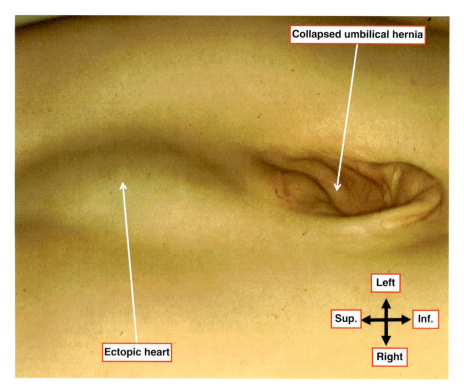

Figure 11.2 This picture, taken from the right side of the epigastrium with the patient supine, shows the heart bulging through the skin because of a cleft in the lower sternum and diastasis of the rectus muscles. An associated abdominal hernia is collapsed.

Right-Sided Heart

Our descriptive system provides no information as to whether the abnormal location of the heart is the result of congenital malformation. The heart may be in the right chest secondary to a pulmonary defect, left diaphragmatic hernia, or because of gross enlargement of its right-sided chambers. In each case, the problems of surgical access are similar. Indeed, there is no reason why, in a patient with a lesion such as congenitally

11 Positional Anomalies of the Heart

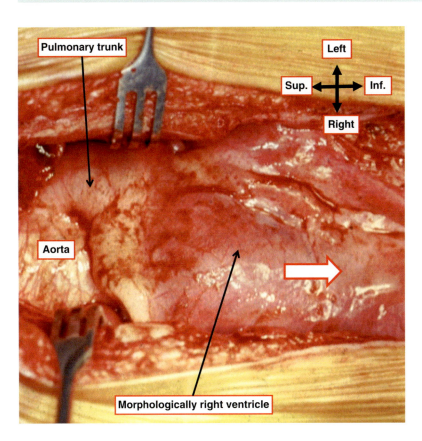

Figure 11.3 The skin and upper sternum have been opened in the patient shown in Figure 11.2, revealing the heart to be positioned in the midline, with the apex pointing to the middle of the chest (white arrow with red borders).

corrected transposition, the heart should not be positioned in the right chest because of pulmonary problems, diaphragmatic hernia, or right-sided hypertrophy.

There are certain lesions, nonetheless, that spring to mind when the heart is located in the right chest with usual atrial arrangement, or when the heart is left sided in patients with mirror-imaged atrial chambers. The most notable of these is, indeed, congenitally corrected transposition. The feature of this lesion is that the ventricles are not in their expected positions. In all patients with abnormally positioned hearts, therefore, it is essential that the surgeon establish the locations of the chambers within the abnormally located organ so that the operation can be planned appropriately.

Twisted Atrioventricular Connections and Supero-Inferior Ventricles

With the sophistication of modern diagnostic techniques, it is unlikely that the surgeon will be presented with a patient having an abnormally located heart without a full preoperative diagnosis. Particular arrangements of the cardiac chambers can still give major difficulties in diagnosis, notably the arrangements in which the ventricular mass is twisted around its long axis, producing the so-called criss-cross heart, or tilted to produce supero-inferior ventricles. In these anomalies, the ventricular relationships, or very rarely the ventricular topology, are not as anticipated for the given atrioventricular connections.[5] In a patient with congenitally corrected transposition and twisted atrioventricular connections, the morphologically right ventricle will usually be predominantly right sided, rather than in its anticipated left-sided position.[6] As emphasized, this is because of rotation of the apex of the ventricular mass with respect to its base around its long axis (Figure 11.4 – upper right-hand panel). The distribution of the coronary arteries is of considerable help in determining the position of the ventricles. In congenitally corrected transposition with usual atrial arrangement, the anterior interventricular coronary artery arises from the right-sided morphologically left coronary artery. Thus, in a heart which at first sight appears to represent simple transposition, finding the anterior interventricular artery arising from the right-sided coronary artery should alert the surgeon to the possible diagnosis of discordant atrioventricular connections and congenitally corrected transposition. The criss-cross arrangement, better described as twisted atrioventricular connections,[7] can also be found in the setting of concordant atrioventricular connections, and then twisting will usually bring the morphologically right ventricle to the left side (Figures 11.5–11.7). When the atrioventricular connections are twisted so as to produce the criss-crossing arrangement, then usually there is an additional superior–inferior relationship of the atrioventricular valves and ventricles (Figure 11.5). This is a consequence of the cardiac mass being rotated as well as tilted (Figure 11.4 – lower panels). Again, the interventricular coronary arteries are useful because they indicate the plane of the ventricular septum, serving as excellent guides to the position of the ventricular cavities. The distribution of the conduction tissue in these bizarre hearts, however, is governed by the connections between the chambers, and not by their position. These hearts are often further complicated by the presence of

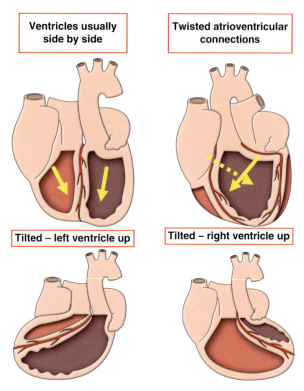

Figure 11.4 The drawing, in anatomical orientation, illustrates the rotational abnormality around the long axis that produces the so-called criss-cross abnormality (right-hand upper panel) in the setting of congenitally corrected transposition (left-hand upper panel). Subsequent to rotation (right-hand panel), the morphologically right ventricle occupies a right-sided position, although still connected discordantly to the morphologically left atrium. The arrows in the left-hand and right-hand upper panels show the consequence of the rotation to produce the twisted atrioventricular valves. The lower panels show the consequence of tilting, to produce supero-inferior ventricles.

straddling and overriding atrioventricular valves. These abnormal relationships can be found with any combination of atrioventricular and ventriculo-arterial connections. Even in these rare situations, the topological arrangement of the ventricular mass is usually as anticipated for the atrioventricular connections. Thus, when there is rotation of the ventricular mass sufficient to produce crossing of the atrioventricular connections, this does not disturb the intrinsic relationships of the two ventricles.[7] In exceedingly rare circumstances, however, not only do the ventricles occupy unusual positions, but the topology is not as expected for the existing atrioventricular connections. Thus, when usual atrial arrangement co-exists with concordant atrioventricular connections, the ventricular topology is usually right handed (Figures 11.5, 11.7). On occasion, nonetheless, the right atrium can be joined to a morphologically right ventricle which shows left-hand ventricular topology, with the right ventricle being additionally left sided (Figure 11.8). This situation is one of the rare occasions when it is necessary to describe ventricular topology in addition to accounting for the atrioventricular connections.[5]

Hearts with Isomeric Atrial Appendages

The problems occurring in hearts with isomeric atrial appendages have already been mentioned. Hearts with this arrangement are not only found in unusual positions, but are almost always associated with an abnormal arrangement of the thoracoabdominal organs, hence the popular rubric of visceral heterotaxy. Many continue to classify these patients in terms of 'asplenia' and 'polysplenia'.[8] It is of greater value for the surgeon to base any system of categorization on the morphology of the

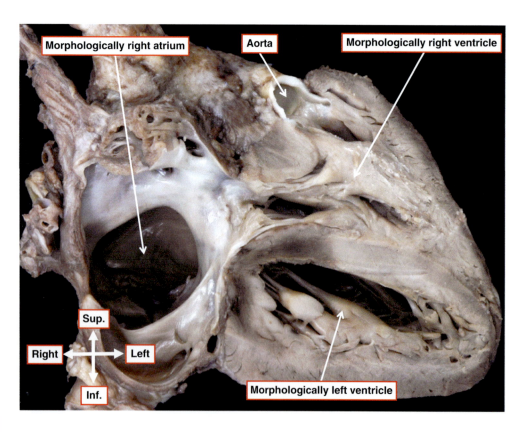

Figure 11.5 In this heart, the atrioventricular connections are concordant, and the ventriculo-arterial connections are discordant. Twisting of the ventricular mass, however, has moved the morphologically right ventricle, along with the aorta, into a left-sided position relative to the morphologically left ventricle and the pulmonary trunk. The ventricular topology, however, despite the twisting, remains right handed.

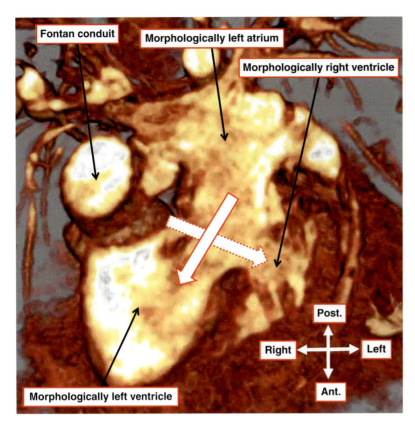

Figure 11.6 The reconstructed three-dimensional magnetic resonance image, shown in cross section, illustrates the twisted atrioventricular connections (arrows – the one with dotted borders is situated posteriorly) that produce the criss-cross heart. In this patient, as in the heart shown in Figure 11.5, there are concordant atrioventricular connections, so the twisting of the ventricular mass places the morphologically right ventricle in left-sided position relative to the morphologically left ventricle. As shown in Figure 11.7, both arterial trunks arose from the morphologically right ventricle.

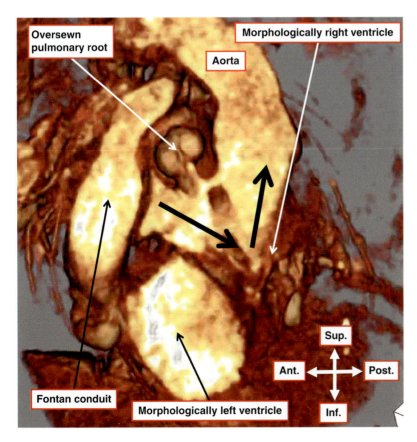

Figure 11.7 The reconstructed three-dimensional magnetic resonance image is from the patient shown in Figure 11.6, but viewed from the right side. The morphologically right ventricle is superiorly located relative to the morphologically left ventricle, but as shown by the thick black arrows, it retains its right-hand topology despite being left sided. Both arterial trunks arise from the right ventricle, with the aorta in left-sided position. The pulmonary trunk has been divided and oversewn, and a conduit placed from the inferior caval vein to the pulmonary arteries so as to create the Fontan circulation.

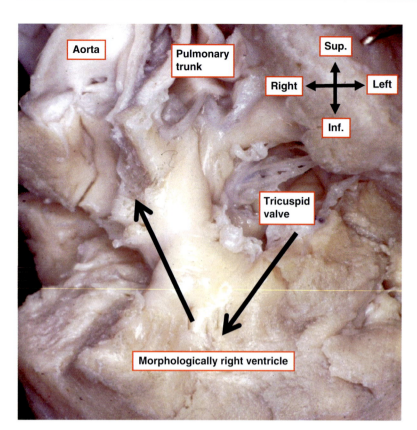

Figure 11.8 In the heart shown in Figure 11.7, the right ventricle with double outlet showed right-hand topology despite the twisted atrioventricular connections. In this image, the morphologically right ventricle exhibits left-hand topology (black arrows), again with double outlet from the ventricle. The atrioventricular valve, however, is morphologically tricuspid. It connects the morphologically right ventricle to the usually positioned right atrium. Despite the left-hand topology, the atrioventricular connections in this heart are concordant. This is a very rare example of segmental disharmony.[5]

atrial appendages.[9] Splenic morphology does not always correspond to the atrial anatomy, itself based on the extent of the pectinate muscles relative to the atrial vestibules. There is a greater correspondence between the anatomy of the appendages as thus determined and what is expected of the 'splenic syndromes' than between these syndromes and splenic morphology.[10,11] More important, it is of little consequence to the cardiac surgeon, at the time of operation, whether his or her patient has one spleen, multiple spleens, or no spleen at all. Determining the morphology of the appendages brings attention directly to the heart, enabling the surgeon working in the operating room to make immediately the diagnosis of isomerism, even if this had not been predicted by the preoperative studies.

The surgeon can readily distinguish the appendages as being either morphologically right or left (Figure 11.9). The surgeon should always confirm whether or not the patient possesses lateralized atrial appendages. The finding of isomeric left (Figure 11.10) or right (Figure 11.11) appendages should immediately alert the surgeon to potential problems over and above those anticipated in the patient with usual or mirror-imaged atrial arrangement. It is now also possible to distinguish directly the presence of isomeric atrial appendages using computed tomography (Figures 11.12–11.15), along with revealing the arrangement of the bronchial tree and the abdominal organs. There should be no problem, therefore, in distinguishing those patients having isomeric right as opposed to isomeric left appendages. In hearts from patients with isomeric right appendages (Figures 11.16–11.18), it is the rule to find complex intracardiac anomalies, usually with absence of the spleen. The pulmonary veins will be connected in totally anomalous fashion even when they are joined to the heart (Figure 11.19). Almost always there are major anomalies of systemic venous drainage. A common atrioventricular valve is usually present (Figures 11.16–11.18), often with double inlet ventricle (Figure 11.19). Pulmonary stenosis or atresia is frequently found with the aorta arising from the right ventricle, and there are bilateral sinus nodes.[12–14] Increasing operative experience now shows that even the most complex combinations can now be treated surgically.[15]

Although isomerism of the morphologically right appendages is almost always accompanied by severe intracardiac malformations, this is not necessarily the case when there are isomeric left appendages (Figures 11.20, 11.21). Thus, the surgeon is more likely to be confronted with an undiagnosed case in the setting of left isomerism. It then becomes important to know that the sinus node is in an anomalous position. It is usually hypoplastic. If it can be found, it will be located close to the atrioventricular junction.[12–14] Interruption of the inferior caval vein, with return through the azygos venous system, is a frequent accompaniment. In the more severely affected cases, there may be a common atrioventricular valve.[15,16] Pulmonary stenosis or atresia is not usually a feature, nor is the presence of univentricular atrioventricular connection, but there is frequently aortic coarctation.

Whatever the types of isomerism, when there is a common atrioventricular valve and each atrium is connected to its own ventricle, it is frequent to find a left-hand pattern of ventricular topology. In this setting, the patient may well have been diagnosed as having congenitally corrected transposition. The presence of isomeric appendages, however, makes it highly

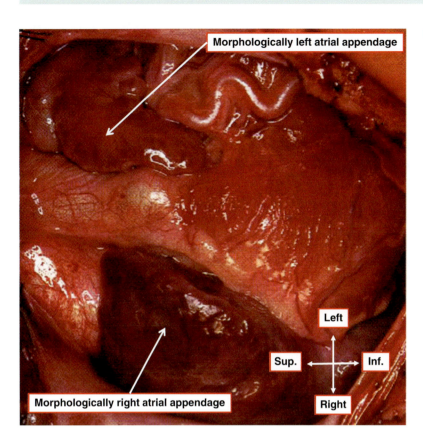

Figure 11.9 This operative view, taken through a median sternotomy, shows the different morphology of the morphologically right as opposed to the morphologically left atrial appendages in a patient with usual atrial arrangement.

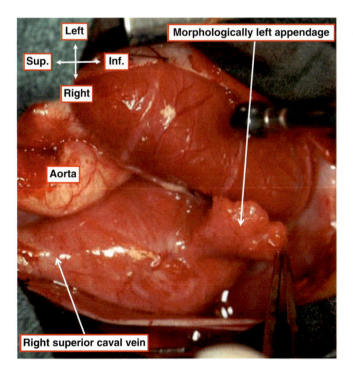

Figure 11.10 This operative view, taken through a median sternotomy, shows that the appendage on the right side of the heart has left morphology. In this patient, the left-sided appendage was also morphologically left, so the patient had isomerism of the morphologically left atrial appendages.

likely that there will be a sling of ventricular conduction tissue joining dual atrioventricular nodes (Figure 11.22).[12] This places the entire edge of the ventricular septum at risk should surgical correction be attempted. When isomerism of the appendages is found with biventricular atrioventricular connections and a right-hand pattern of ventricular topology, the atrioventricular conduction axis should be expected in its usual posterior position (Figure 11.23). This entire discussion emphasizes the significance of full sequential segmental analysis of any patient presented for cardiac surgery.

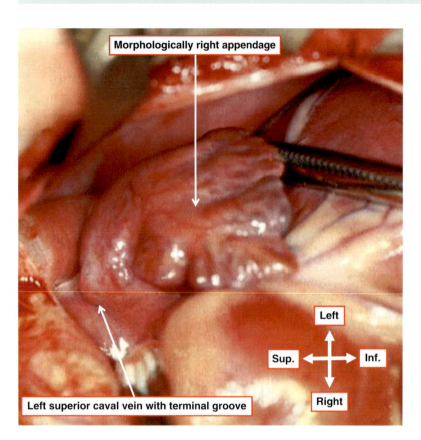

Figure 11.11 In this patient, the left-sided atrial appendage is broad based, with a wide junction to the body of the atrium. Note that the left-sided superior caval vein joins to the atrial roof, and that there is a left-sided terminal groove. The right-sided appendage was also of right morphology. The patient has isomerism of the right atrial appendages.

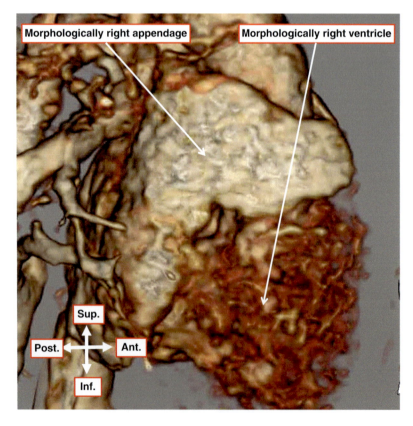

Figure 11.12 The reconstructed computed tomographic angiogram shows a patient with a right-sided morphologically right atrial appendage, the right-sided atrium joining to a morphologically right ventricle.

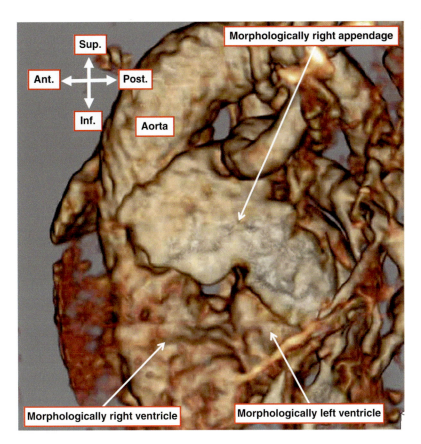

Figure 11.13 The image shows the left side of the heart reconstructed in Figure 11.12. The left-sided atrial appendage also has a broad base, and is morphologically right. The patient has isomerism of the morphologically right appendage. Note the incomplete left ventricle in postero-inferior position. The aorta arises from the dominant right ventricle.

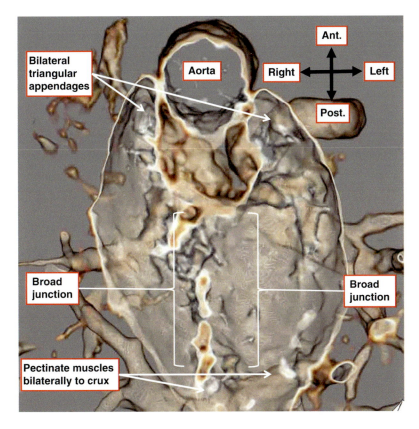

Figure 11.14 The cross-sectional image is from the same dataset as shown in Figures 11.12 and 11.13. Both appendages are broad based, with pectinate muscles extending to the crux (see also Figure 11.18). There is obvious isomerism of the right atrial appendages (compare with Figure 11.15).

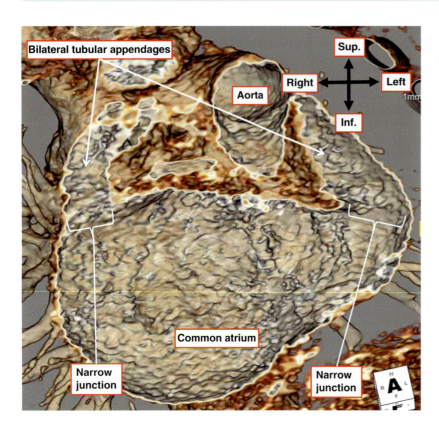

Figure 11.15 The computed tomogram in this patient, seen from the front, shows the presence of two tubular appendages with narrow necks. This patient has isomerism of the morphologically left atrial appendages (compare with Figure 11.14). Orientation cube, lower right: A, anterior; H, head; L, left; F, foot; R, right.

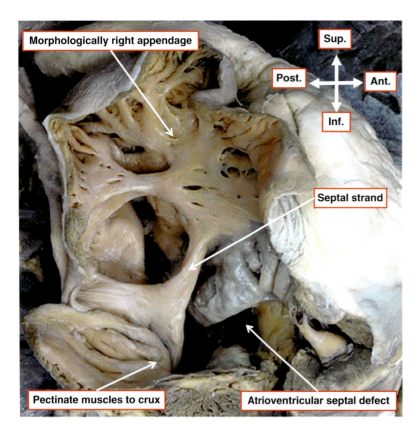

Figure 11.16 The heart has been opened through the right atrioventricular junction close to the crux, and the parietal wall spread upwards. The pectinate muscles encircle the right-sided vestibule, indicating that the right-sided appendage is morphologically right. Note the common atrioventricular valve, and absence of the coronary sinus.

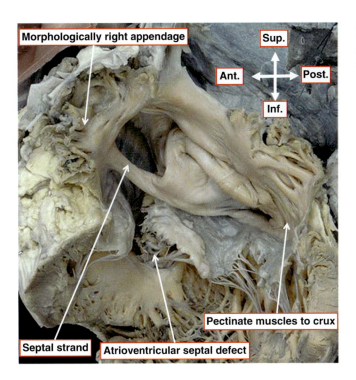

Figure 11.17 The left side of the heart shown in Figure 11.16 has been opened through an incision close to the crux. The pectinate muscles also encircle the left-sided vestibule, showing that there are morphologically right atrial appendages bilaterally. Note the common atrioventricular valve.

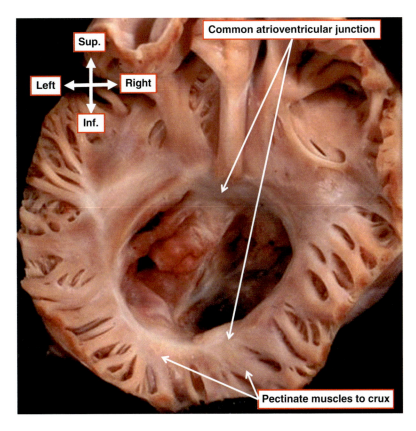

Figure 11.18 In this heart, the atrial chambers have been disconnected from the atrioventricular junctions inferiorly, and tilted superiorly. The pectinate muscles encircle the entirety of the common atrioventricular junction, indicating the presence of isomeric right atrial appendages. The common junction is guarded by a valve with separate right and left atrioventricular valvar orifices.

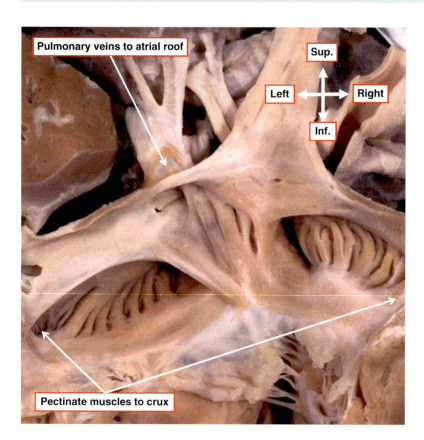

Figure 11.19 In this heart from a patient with isomeric right atrial appendages, the pulmonary veins drain in anatomically anomalous fashion to the atrial roof, even though returning directly to the heart. Note that the common atrioventricular valve is connected exclusively to a dominant left ventricle, indicating the presence of double inlet connection.

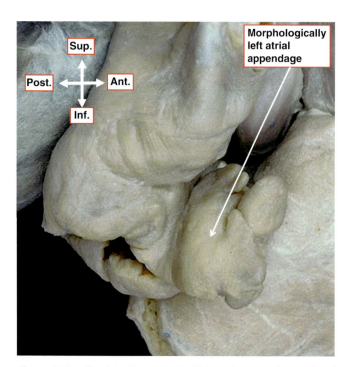

Figure 11.20 The right-sided atrium in this heart has a morphologically left appendage.

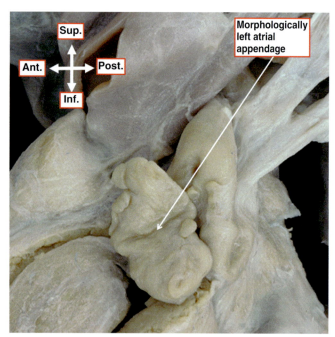

Figure 11.21 The image shows the opposite side of the heart illustrated in Figure 11.20. The left-sided appendage is also of left morphology.

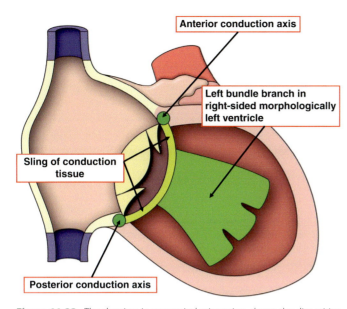
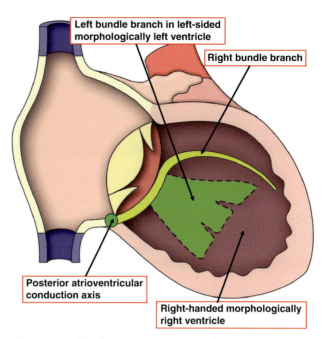

Figure 11.22 The drawing, in anatomical orientation, shows the disposition of the axis of atrioventricular conduction tissue in hearts with isomerism of the atrial appendages, biventricular atrioventricular connections, and a common atrioventricular valve. When there is left-handed topology, the ventricular conduction tissues are frequently connected by both posterior and anterior atrioventricular bundles, producing a sling of conduction tissue along the crest of the muscular ventricular septum.

Figure 11.23 The drawing, again in anatomical orientation, shows the disposition of the axis of atrioventricular conduction tissue in hearts with isomerism of the atrial appendages, biventricular atrioventricular connections, and a common atrioventricular valve when there is right-handed ventricular topology. The ventricular conduction axis arises from a posterior atrioventricular node.

References Cited

1. Wilkinson JL, Acerete F. Terminological pitfalls in congenital heart disease. Reappraisal of some confusing terms, with an account of a simplified system of basic nomenclature. *Br Heart J* 1973; **35**: 1166–1177.
2. Van Praagh R, Weinberg PM, Matsuoka R, Van Praagh S. Malpositions of the heart. In FH Adams, GC Emmanouilides, eds., *Moss's Heart Disease in Infants, Children and Adolescents*. 3rd ed. Baltimore: Williams & Wilkins; 1983: pp. 422–458.
3. Byron F. Ectopia cordis. Report of a case with attempted operative correction. *J Thorac Surg* 1948; **17**: 717–722.
4. Cantrell JR, Haller JA, Ravitch MM. A syndrome of congenital defects involving the abdominal wall, sternum, diaphragm, pericardium and heart. *Surg Gynecol Obstet* 1958; **107**: 602–614.
5. Anderson RH, Smith A, Wilkinson JL. Disharmony between atrioventricular connections and segmental combinations – usual variants of 'criss-cross' hearts. *J Am Coll Cardiol* 1987; **10**: 1274–1277.
6. Symons JC, Shinebourne EA, Joseph MC, et al. Criss-cross heart with congenitally corrected transposition: report of a case with d-transposed aorta and ventricular preexcitation. *Eur J Cardiol* 1977; **5**: 493–505.
7. Seo J-W, Yoo S-J, Ho SY, Lee HJ, Anderson RH. Further morphological observations on hearts with twisted atrioventricular connections (criss-cross hearts). *Cardiovasc Pathol* 1992; **1**: 211–217.
8. Stanger P, Rudolph AM, Edwards JE. Cardiac malpositions: an overview based on study of sixty-five necropsy specimens. *Circulation* 1977; **56**: 159–172.
9. Loomba RS, Hlavacek AM, Spicer DE, Anderson RH. Isomerism or heterotaxy: which term leads to better understanding? *Cardiol Young* 2015; **25**: 1037–1043.
10. Uemura H, Ho SY, Devine WA, Kilpatrick LL, Anderson RH. Atrial appendages and venoatrial connections in hearts with patients with visceral heterotaxy. *Ann Thorac Surg* 1995; **60**: 561–569.
11. Uemura H, Ho SY, Devine WA, Anderson RH. Analysis of visceral heterotaxy according to splenic status, appendage morphology, or both. *Am J Cardiol* 1995; **76**: 846–849.
12. Smith A, Ho SY, Anderson RH, et al. The diverse cardiac morphology seen in hearts with isomerism of the atrial appendages with reference to the disposition of the specialized conduction system. *Cardiol Young* 2006; **16**: 437–454.
13. Dickinson DF, Wilkinson JL, Anderson KR, et al. The cardiac conduction system in situs ambiguus. *Circulation* 1979; **59**: 879–885.
14. Ho SY, Seo J-W, Brown NA, et al. Morphology of the sinus node in human and mouse hearts with isomerism of the atrial appendages. *Br Heart J* 1995; **74**: 437–442.
15. Chowdhury UK, Anderson RH, Spicer DE, et al. Surgical management of hearts with isomeric atrial appendages. *J Card Surg* 2022; **37**: 1340–1352.
16. Uemura H, Anderson RH, Ho SY, et al. Left ventricular structures in atrioventricular septal defect associated with isomerism of the atrial appendages compared with similar features with usual atrial arrangement. *J Thorac Cardiovasc Surg* 1995; **110**: 445–452.

Index

Abbott's artery, 430, *431*
abnormal systemic venous connections, 407
absent pulmonary valve syndrome, *280*
aggregated cardiomyocytes, *325*
alternative therapy, 252
anomalous pulmonary venous drainage
　supracardiac totally, *421*
ansa subclavia, 9
anterior interventricular coronary artery, 263
anterior papillary muscle, 177
antero-cephalad limb, 170
aorta, the, 70–73
　ascending aortic trunk, 71
　coarctation of, 245
　coronary arteries and, 113
　posterior, 332
　proximal descending, *431*
aortic arch, 438
　double, 437, *441*, *443*
　interrupted at the isthmus, *432*
　interruption, *433*
　interruption of, *447*
　interruption of the, 430–434, *432*, *434*
　left-sided, *442*
　right, *445*, *447*
　right-sided, *443*, *445*
　tubular hypoplasia of the, *427*
　Type A interruption, *433*
　Type B interruption, *433*
　Type C interruption, *434*
　with mirror-imaged branching of the right, *446*
aortic atresia, 316, 347
　with mitral stenosis, 284
aortic coarctation, 286, 427, *429*, *431*
　role of ductal tissue and, 427
　shelf lesion of, *427*
　with enlarged intercostal arteries, *429*
aortic insufficiency, 252
aortic isthmus
　interruption at the, *432*, *433*
aortic leaflet, 91
aortic regurgitation, 241
aortic root, *460*
　location of, 392

aortic sinuses
　pulmonary trunk and, *336*
aortic stenosis
　patients with, 246
aortic valve insufficiency, 252
aortic valve, the, 100–105
aortopulmonary foramen, 29
　closure of, 29
aortopulmonary septum, 28, *31*
aortopulmonary window, 451, *454*, *455*
aorto-ventricular tunnels, 459
　anomalies of the, 456
apposition, zone of, *103*
arch
　double, *441*
　hypothetical double, *440*
arch arteries, 437
arrhythmia, 138
arrhythmia surgery
　congenital heart disease and, 148–149
arterial channel, 6
arterial duct, 444, 452, 454
　operative intervention, 451
　patent, 453
　persistence of the, 451, *455*
arterial duct, patent, *452*
arterial ligament, 6
arterial trunk
　common, *369*, *370*, *382*
　with absent intrapericardial pulmonary arteries, *370*
arterial trunks, 117, 169, 170, 332, 333, 369, 392–393, 458, *469*
　common, *380*, *446*
　double outlet ventricle and, *353*
　fibrous walls of, 98
　intrapericardial, 27, 33, 372, 374
　morphologically right ventricle and, 354
　morphology of the, *169*
　normal spiraling of the, *392*
　parallel, 398–406, *402*
　relationship of the, *357*, *360*
　relationships of the, 169
　right ventricle and, 354, 356
　solitary, 369
arterial trunks, 114

arterial valvar morphology, 169
arterial valvar sinuses
　lesions in, 147
arterial valves, 170
　abnormalities of the, 239
　arrangement of, 95–99
　morphology of, 169
asplenia, 468
atresia, 438, 470
atrial appendage, *157*
atrial appendages, 41, *157*
　isomerism of the morphologically left, *474*
　isomerism of the right, *472*, *473*
　morphologically left, *471*
　morphologically right, *471*
　right, 71
　right-sided morphologically right, *472*
atrial chambers
　appearance of the, 13
atrial depolarization, 34
atrial fibrillation
　interventional therapy and, 146
　treatments of, 149
atrial flutter, 144
atrial foramen, 13
atrial septal defects, *133*, 177
　lesions from the, *149*
atrial septal structures
　deficiencies of, *180*
atrial septum, 175
　arrangement of the, 285
atrio-Hisian tracts, 138
atriotomy, 185
　left, 41
　opening the heart through an, 55
　right, 56, 58, 60, 64, 98, *131*, *133*, 176, 181, 184, 185, *187*, 195, 196, 222
　right-sided left, 62
　standard, *124*
atrioventricular bundle, 135, 170
atrioventricular canal, 22, 34
　formation and septation of, 18, 22
atrioventricular canal, expansion of, *372*

atrioventricular conduction axis, 34, 133, *136*, *139*, *232*, 308
　branching component of, *135*
　location of, *139*
　path of, *309*
atrioventricular conduction tissue, 316
　in hearts with isomerism, *477*
atrioventricular connections, *141*, 169, *317*, *350*, *470*
　absence of, 312
　absence of the right, 399
　discordant, 347
　ventricular mass and, 164
atrioventricular cushions, 19
atrioventricular endocardial cushions, 22
atrioventricular groove, 13
atrioventricular junctions, 14, 20–22, 83, *158*, *165*, 202
　dilation of the, 235
　features associated with, 169
　fibrous, 126, 334
atrioventricular muscular strands, 139
atrioventricular node, 34, 36, 51
atrioventricular orifice, danger area of, *308*
atrioventricular septal defect, 249, 250
atrioventricular septal defects, *166*, *191*, 191, *195*, 200
　four-chamber cut and, *207*
　haemodynamic shunting and, 202
　left ventricular outflow tract in, 210
　septal defects, 176
　variant, *197*
　various forms of, 196, *199*
　with atrioventricular junction, 204, *209*
atrioventricular septal malalignment, *230*
atrioventricular septum, 175
atrioventricular valvar atresia, 300
atrioventricular valve
　anomalous attachment of, 249
　components of the, 89
atrioventricular valves, 77, 88–89, 234

Index

atrioventricular-arterial
  junctions, 321
atrium
  left, 63
  right, 145, 315, 351
  small right, 415
azygos venous system, 470
  azygos vein, 6, 9, 73, 132, 410, 412, 419
azygous vein
  dilated, 411

Bachmann's bundle, 50
biventricular atrioventricular
  connections, 471, See also
  atrioventricular
  connections
Blalock-Hanlon septostomy, 323
brachiocephalic artery, 72
brachiocephalic trunk, 6
bundle branch
  right, 138
bundle branch, left, 136, 137
bundles of Kent, 139

cardiac catheters, 65
cardiac cavities, 1
cardiac chambers, 55, 283, 465, 467
  anatomy of, 41, 48
cardiac conduction system
  development of, 34–37
cardiac impulse
  conduction system and, 34
cardiac lymphatics, 131–132
cardiac malformations, 46, 465
cardiac rhythm
  problem of, 138–144
cardiac subsystems, valves and, 108
cardiac valves, 81
cardiomyocytes, 34, 50
cardiovascular malformations
  of the aortic arch, 430
Carnegie stage 10, 12
Carnegie stage 11, 11, 12
Carnegie stage 12, 13, 13, 24
  pharyngeal arches, 437
Carnegie stage 13, 14, 18, 20, 24
  cavities of developing heart at, 19
  embryo at, 19
  human embryo at, 20
  left ventricle and the, 22
Carnegie stage 14, 15, 24, 27, 438
  atrioventricular canal at, 20
  human embryo at, 28
  the cranial button and, 28
Carnegie stage 15, 30, 34, 439
  human embryo at, 36
Carnegie stage 16
  human embryo at, 21
  pharyngeal arches at, 439
Carnegie stage 17, 23
  dissected heart at, 21
  embryo at, 34
Carnegie stage 18
  extrapericardial arterial
    pathways at, 35

Carnegie stage 19, 34
  human embryo at, 36
Carnegie stage 20, 32, 440
  arterial pathways, 35
Carnegie stage 21, 15, 18
  pulmonary root, 32
Carnegie stage 23, 33, 38
  echocardiographic projection
    at, 33
Carnegie stages 15 and 16, 28
Carnegie stages 18–19
  developing human heart at, 22
Carnegie stages 19, 24
caval vein, 3
cavotricuspid isthmus, 148
cleft, true, 238
coarctation lesion, 428
complete median sternotomy, 1
computed tomogram, 168
concordant and discordant
  connections, 159
concordant atrioventricular
  discordant ventriculo-arterial
  connections with, 322
concordant atrioventricular and
  discordant ventriculo-
  arterial connections, 321
concordant atrioventricular
  connections, 321
concordant ventriculo-arterial
  connections, 315
conduction system, 133
congenital atresia, 459
congenital cardiac
  malformations
  describing, 153
congenital heart disease
  arrhythmia surgery for, 148–149
congenital malformations, 9
congenital pulmonary valvar
  stenosis
  treatment of, 254
congenital pulmonary venous, 419
congenital segmental stenosis, 418
coronary arterial circulation, 121
coronary arteries, 335, 336, 386
  anomalies of the, 456
  anomalous epicardial course, 459
  anomalous origin of, 456–459
  communications between the, 459
  epicardial, 459
  morphology of the, 333, 339
coronary arteries, the, 113–126
coronary artery
  anomalous origin of the left, 457
  congenital atresia of the left, 459
  left, 457
  origin of the right, 459
  silk ligature and the left, 456
coronary circulation, 109–111, 113

coronary arteries, 113–126
coronary veins, 127–129
  development of, 38, 39
coronary files, 83
coronary sinus, 109, 130, 195, See
  left atrium communication
  with, 190
  unroofing of the, 186, 190
coronary veins, the, 127–129
Cox maze III/IV procedures, 148
cryoablation lesions, 150

deficient atrioventricular
  septation, 264
dextrocardia, 465
dextroposition, 465
dextrorotation, 465
direct surgical correction, 316
discordant atrioventricular and
  ventriculo-arterial
  connections, 322
discordant atrioventricular
  connections, 467
discordant ventriculo-arterial
  connections, 310, 321
  Fontan procedure and, 315
distal outflow cushions, 22
diverticulum of Kommerell, 442, 445
  dual compressing fibrous
    remnants of, 445
dominant right ventricle, 312
dorsal mesenchymal protrusion, 13
double inlet and double outlet
  right ventricle, 310
double inlet atrioventricular
  connection, 300
double inlet left ventricle, 163, 302, 404
double inlet right ventricle, 311
double inlet to the dominant
  ventricle, 319
double inlet ventricle, 309
double inlet, to a dominant right
  ventricle, 301
double outlet right ventricle/
  ventricles, 170, 172, 322, 367, 368
  abnormal ventriculo-arterial
    connection to, 261
  ductal anomalies and, 448
  with subpulmonary defect, 235
double outlet the right ventricle/
  ventricles, 359
double outlet ventricle, 353–368
doubly committed and juxta-
  arterial, 332
doubly committed subarterial
  ventricular septal defects.
  See also ventricular septal
  defects
ductal anomalies, 448–451
dysplastic valves, 238, 239

Ebstein's malformation, 140, 145, 236, 236, 239, 316, 318, 344, 349

surgical treatment for, 238
Ebsteins' malformation, 238
echocardiographic plane, 222
Eisenmenger's syndrome, 411
electrocardiogram
  adult type of, 34
embryonic period, end of, 38
endocardial primordiums, 11
endothelial cardiac tube, 11
endothelial-to-mesenchymal
  transformation, 22
epigastrium, 466
Eustachian ridge, 54
Eustachian valve, 315
exteriorisation, of the heart, 465, 467
extrapericardial arterial
  pathways, 33, 35

fasciculo-ventricular
  connections, 138
fetal development, 38–39
fibromuscular tunnel, 248
fibrous raphe, 435
fibrous shelf, 348
fibrous tissue tag, 348
fibrous triangle, 83
fishmouth arrangement, 29
fixed stenosis, 247
fixed subaortic obstruction, 248
Fontan procedure, 299, 309, 312, 315
  conversion procedure, 149
  failed Fontan circulations, 148
  Fontan circulation, 132, 133, 146, 235, 283, 285, 300, 301, 316, 347
  modified, 316
  surgical palliation and, 312
free-standing septoparietal
  trabeculations, 263

Gerbode defect, 60
Gerbode defects, 191, 220, See
  also atrioventricular septal
  defects
  direct, 194
German Working Group, 87
Glenn procedure, 307
great arteries, the, 2, 170, 361
  access to, 4
  adventitial coverings of, 41
  double outlet connections and, 169
  posterior surface of, 41
  transposition of, 321
gross fibroelastosis, 284
gross lymphangiectasia, 286
gross pulmonary valvar
  insufficiency, 270

heart tube
  cardiomyocytes, 34
  linear, 11
  looping of, 11
heart, the
  abnormal positioning of, 465, 466

479

Index

heart, the (cont.)
  abnormal segmental
    connections and, 283
  after a pericardial incision, 42
  an infant, 460
  atrial arrangement, 154–158
  base of, 350
  Carnegie stage 13, 25
  chamber planes in, 176
  conduction axis reconstructed, 137
  displacement of, 451
  dissected, 21
  double outlet right ventricle, 353–368
  essential anatomy, 299
  exteriorisation of, 465, 467
  fibrous skeleton of the, 55–60
  four-chamber echocardiographic view, 177, 229, 313
  hypoplasia of the left, 316
  intracardiac malformations of, 172
  left morphology, 476
  left side of the reconstructed, 473
  location of, 1
  mirror-image organs arrangement and, 422
  myocardial bridging and, 128, 461
  outlet of the right ventricle, 263
  position of, 171–172
  right-sided, 409, 466–467
  right-sided atrium, 476
  segments of, 153
  septal structures in, 175
  surgery and the lymphatic drainage, 131–132
  surgical approaches to the, 1–9
  the position and support of the valves in, 80–88
  unroofing of the coronary sinus, 188
  valvar anatomy of, 77
  valvar complexes of, 77, 80
  vascular pedicle of the, 71
  with isomeric atrial appendages, 468–471
  with transposition, 339
hepatic venous connections, abnormal, 407
hepatocardiac channels, 13
His, Wilhelm, 13
hole, closing clinically significant, 215
Holmes heart, 400
Horner's syndrome, 9
human development, 11
hypertrophy, 263
  right-sided, 467
hypoplastic left heart syndrome, 164, 283, 286, 290, 293, 294, 297, 299, 313, 316, 318, 416
  aortic stenosis and, 291

atrioventricular connection and, 284
intact atrial septum and, 295
mitral valve and, 285
pulmonary truck and, 297
right atrium and, 294
inferior caval vein, 470
  abnormalities of, 408–411
inferior cavo-tricuspid isthmus, 146
inferior sinus venosus defect, 184
infero-caudal margin, 262
infero-caudal rim, 262
infero-septal recess, 102
infundibular morphology, 170
interatrial communications, 177, 190, 426
  superior sinus venosus, 407
  surgical treatment of, 188
interatrial shunting, 177
intercostal muscles, 5
intercostal neurovascular bundle, 5
intercostal space
  fourth, 4
  second left, 73
  sixth, 4, 7
intermediate sinus venosus defect, 186
interventional catheterization, 451
interventricular communication, 262, 365
interventricular membranous septum, 262
intracardiac anatomy of tetralogy, 264
intracardiac malformations, 470
intrapericardial arterial trunks, 27, 33
isolated pulmonary stenosis, 253
isolated ventricular inversion, 399, 400
isomeric atrial appendages
  problems with, 468–471
isomeric left atrial appendages, 405
isthmus, 148, 288
  aortic, 5, 34, 286
  atresia of the, 431
  constriction of aortic, 428
  inferior cavo-tricuspid, 145
  of the transverse arch, 284
  septal, 145

juxta-arterial, 228
juxta-arterial interventricular communication, 374
Juxta-arterial ventricular septal defect, 216, 223, 228, 229, 262, 267, 326, 343–346, 361–364, 374, 377, 380, 430

Koch's triangle, 195

Lancisi, muscle of, 94
laryngeal nerve, 6, 7

latissimus dorsi, preservation of, 5
left appendages, 154, 165, 408
  isomeric, 470
  isomerism of the, 156
  morphologically, 44, 476
left atrium. See also right atrium
  morphologically, 60–61
left coronary artery, circumflex branch of the, 124
left isomerism, 157, 158, 406, 411, 465, 470
  arterial trunks and, 400
left superior caval vein, 408
left ventricle/ventricles, 457
  morphologically, 68, 71
left-sided incomplete left ventricle, 311
Leiden convention, 115
lesions, 283, 299
  anatomic, 264
  cryoablation lesions, 150
  in transposition, 325
  pathological, 234
  subpulmonary obstruction and, 347
  tetralogy of Fallot and, 264
levoatrial cardinal vein, 286, 411–412, 418
linear tube. See heart tube
lower sternum, 466
lung/lungs
  cobble-stoning of, 286
  hypoplastic left heart and right, 295
  posterior retraction of the, 5
lymphangiectasia, gross, 286
lymphatic drainage system, 131

Mahaim connections, 143
malalignment ventricular septal defect, 327
malposition, 393
Marshall, ligament of, 73
Marshall, vein of, 15
maze procedure, 146
medial papillary muscle, 219, 221
mediastinum, 1
  entering the, 41
  middle, 5
  pericardial sac in the, 3
  vessels and nerves within, 2
membranous septum, area anterior to, 144
mesenchymal cap, 13
mesocardiums, 11
middle mediastinum, 5
mirror-imaged atrial arrangement, 323
mitral atresia, 283, 313, 316, 318, 411
mitral valve, 90–93, 92, 239, 240
  aortic leaflet of the, 83
  imperforate, 319
  mural leaflet of the, 90
  papillary muscles of the, 93
  parachute arrangement of the, 242

morphogenesis, 11
morphological method, 153–154
mural leaflet, 92
muscle of Lancisi, 94
muscular defect, 221, 223
muscular hypertrophy, 254
muscular inlet defect, 327
muscular outlet septum, 363
muscular rims, 224, 327, 382
  deficiency of the, 218
  superior, 223
muscular ventricular septum, 20, 221
  misalignment of, 230
Mustard procedure, 323–325
myocardial fishmouth, 29
myocardial-arterial junctions, 61, 65, 68, 70, 71, 77, 78, 79, 86, 98, 100, 101, 148, 242, 280
  anatomic, 147
  circular anatomic, 65
myocardium, 11

neonatal development, 38–39
nodoventricular connections, 138
nodule of Arantius, 95
Norwood sequence, 285
Norwood sequence of procedures, 285

ostium primum defect, 195, 242, 377
outflow tract, 31
outflow tract tachycardias
  substrates for, 147, 148
outlet septum, 354
outlet ventricular septal defects, muscular, 332
oval fossa, 50, 53
  defect within the, 184
  defects within the, 177, 184

pacemaker electrodes, 65
paired dorsal aortas, 11
parachute deformity, 238, 239
paraspecific pathways, 138
partial defects, 203
pathological lesions, 234
pathways
  left-sided, 139
  right-sided accessory, 139
pericardial cavity
  arrangement of, 41
pericardial recess, 41
pericardial reflection, 72
pericardium, 41
perimembranous defects, 219, 222, 326, 327, 343
perimembranous ventricular septal defect, 346
persistent truncus arteriosus, 377
pharyngeal arch arteries, 25
pharyngeal arches, 24, 25, 395, 437, 437, 438, 439
  fourth, 27
pharyngeal mesenchyme, 13, 26
  growth of, 13

phrenic nerves, 3–4, *4*, 5, 6
  left, 73
pleural space, 5
polysplenia, 468
postero-caudal deviation, *332*
Postero-inferiorly, 73
primary atrial foramen, 34
primary ring, 34
prolapse, 89, 92, 221, 238
  leaflet of the aortic valve, 223
  mitral valve leaflets, 85
  of a leaflet, 89
  of the leaflets, 225, 252, *257*
proximal septal defect, aortic arch and, 430
pulmonary arterial anomalies, 448–451
pulmonary arterial sling, *451*
pulmonary arteries, 73, *75*, 264, *281*, *307*–308, 315
pulmonary artery/arteries
  anomalous origin of the right, *449*
  conduit from the morphologically right ventricle to the, 347
  conduit to from left ventricle, 309
  development of, 27
  intrapericardial, 169, *369–371*
  left, *448*, *450*
  left from the right pulmonary artery, *450*
  right, 448, *449*
pulmonary atresia, 255, 264, *317*, 347, 369
  with ventricular septal defect, 264
pulmonary collateral arteries, 266
pulmonary hypertension, 448
pulmonary hypertensive vascular disease, 449
pulmonary pathways, *449*
  formation and septation of, 24, 33
pulmonary root
  opening of, *147*
pulmonary stenosis, 344, 470
pulmonary trunk, 71, *259*, 321, *See also* pulmonary arteries
  and left pulmonary artery, 451
  dilation of, *279*
  hypoplastic left heart syndrome and, *297*
pulmonary trunk, atretic, *371*
pulmonary valvar insufficiency, 270
pulmonary valvar leaflets, 83, 119
  absence of, 271
pulmonary valve, the, 69, 81, 105–107, 147, *258*, 343, 357, 364
  dysplasia of the leaflets of the, *258*
pulmonary veins, 418, *420*
  congenital segmental stenosis, *418*
pulmonary venous atrium, 323
pulmonary venous connection

totally anomalous, *420*
pulmonary venous connections, 418–426
pulmonary venous tributaries, 38

Rastelli or Nikaidoh operations, 332
restrictive subaortic infundibulum, *435*
restrictive ventricular septal defect, *431*, *436*
retro-esophageal right subclavian artery, 433
right appendages
  intracardiac malformations, 470
  isomerism of the, 156, 470
  morphologically, 154
right atrioventricular connection, absence of, *314*
right atrium, 46, *60*. See opening of, 53
right superior caval vein, *407*, *414*
  with brachiocephalic vein, *409*
right ventricle/ventricles, 60, *See also* left ventricle
  apical component of the, 65
  morphologically, 61, *68*
Ross procedure, 107

second heart field, 11
secundum defects, 177, *184*
Senning procedure, 323–325
septal defects, 175, *180*
  perimembranous, 333
septal deficiency, 60
septomarginal trabeculation, 67, 95, 222, 224, 261, 262, 325, 361
septoparietal trabeculations, 67, *67*, *172*, 177, *180*, 226, 262, 268
  deviated septum and, 261
  free-standing, 263
  malaligned muscular outlet septum and the, *353*
  muscular outlet septum and the, *261*
serratus anterior, preservation of, 5
shelf
  fibrous, *348*
  subvalvar fibrous, 247
Shone's syndrome, 239
sinus impulse, 34
sinus node, 34, *308*
sinus venosus defects, 177, *181–188*, 426
sinutubular junction, *72*, 241
solitary zone of apposition, 244
spina vestibuli, 13
splenic morphology, 470
splenic syndromes, 470
stenosis
  isolated pulmonary, 253
  treatment of congenital pulmonary valvar, 254
sternotomy, *466*
  complete median, 1

median, 3, *42*, 188
subaortic defect, 353
subaortic obstruction, 249
subaortic outflow tract, *251*
subclavian arteries
  left, 6, *9*
subclavian sympathetic loop, 9
subpulmonary infundibular stenosis, 364
subpulmonary infundibulum, 243, *333*, *335*
  free-standing, 224
  myocardium of the, 33
subpulmonary infundibulum, removal of, *107*, *113*
subvalvar fibrous shelf, 247
subvalvar obstruction
  dynamic, 250
subvalvar stenosis, 246
superior caval vein, 181
  abnormalities of the right, 407–408
  cannulation of the, 323
  connected to the left atrium, *414*
  left, *189*
  persistence of the left, 411
superior intercostal vein, 6
  left, *8*
superior sinus venosus defect, *185*, *187*
supero-inferior ventricles, 467, *470*
supradiaphragmatic drainage, 419
supravalvar aortic stenosis, 252
supravalvar stenosis
  true, 254
supraventricular crest, *66*, 123
  formation of, *179*
supraventricular tachycardias
  substrates for, 144, *147*
surgical correction, direct, 316
sutureless repair, 418
swiss cheese septum, 221
systemic venous connection, 411, *415*
  totally anomalous, *415*
systemic venous drainage, 470
systemic venous sinus, 11
systemic venous tributaries, 13

Taussig-Bing malformation, *362*, *435*
tendon of Todaro, 51, 133, *See* tertiary interventricular communication, 217
tetralogy of Fallot, 148, *171*, 235, *261*, 261, *270*, *276*, *353*, 353–359, 368, 372, 407
  and an atrioventricular septal defect, *272*
  ductal anomalies and, 448
  Eisenmenger's syndrome and, 411
  lesions and, 264, 270
  morphology of, 364
  normal outflow tract and, 261

outflow tracks in heart with, *171*
overriding aortic valve and, 263
statistics and, 446
with pulmonary atresia, 255, *274*
tetralogy, intracardiac anatomy of, 264, *See also* tetralogy of Fallot
Thebesian valve, *131*
thoracic artery, 3
thoracic duct, 6, *430*
  location of, *132*
thoracotomy
  anterior right or left, 9
  lateral, 3
  muscle sparing, 5
  right, 6
  standard lateral, 4
thymus gland, *2*, *3*, 5, 72
  in an infant, *3*
trachea, *442*
transposition, 148, 321, *322*, 339, 393
  congenitally corrected, 321, 334, *339*, *344*, *351*
  muscular defect, *328*
  perimembranous defect with, *326*
  position of the aorta in, *334*
  specimen of, *324*
  stranding and overriding tricuspid valve, *329*
  ventricular septal defects and, *326*
  with perimembranous defect, *328*
  with ventricular septal defect, *330*
  without any other anomaly, 343
triangle of Koch, 51, *57*, 138, 140–143, 175, *177*, 191, 218, 219, 231, *238*, 238, 307, 325, 334, 426
  ablation at base of, 144
  atrial boundary of the, 85, *87*
  atrial septum and, 193
  atrioventricular conduction axis and, 133, *309*
  boundaries of, 56
  conduction axis and, 108, *109*
  conduction tissues within the, *134*
  landmarks of, *176*
  location of, *56*
triatrial hearts, 154
tricuspid atresia, 148, 312, *315*
  absence of the right atrioventricular connection and, 399
  causes of, 316
  classical, *307*, *315*
  Ebstein's malformation and, 238
  left-sided atresia and, 316
  morphologically right atrium and, 312

Index

tricuspid valve, 93–95
  parachute malformation of the, 239
  straddling and overriding, 234
  straddling of the, 235
trisinuate root, 242
truncal relationships. *See also* valvar relationships
tubular aorta, *458*
tubular hypoplasia, 285
Turner syndrome, 245
twisted atrioventricular connections, *467*, *470*

umbilical venous tributaries, 14
univentricular atrioventricular connections, 158, *161*, *163*, 299, 312
  hearts with, 169
univentricular hearts, 148, 160, 299
upper sternum, *467*

vagus nerves, 3, 5–9, 73, 451–453
valvar anatomy
  importance of, 77
valvar aortic stenosis, 242
valvar complexes, 77, *80*
valvar morphology, 161–163
valvar orifice, 234
valvar relationships, 170
valvar stenosis, 344
valves
  atrioventricular, 88–89
  atrioventricular and arterial, 80–88
  mitral valve, 90–93
  tricuspid valve, 93–95
Van Praagh, Richard, 153, 159, 383
vascular rings, 437, *447*
vein of Marshall, 15
venous plexuses, 11
venous tributaries,
  reconstruction of, *16*
ventral aortas, 11
ventricle/ventricles
  formation of the, 22–23
  incomplete right, *404*
  left, *404*
  left-sided, *351*
  left-sided morphologically right, *403*
  morphologically left, *393*
  septal surface of the right, *180*
ventricular conduction tissues, 307
ventricular cone, *46*, 285
ventricular infundibulum
  right, 83
ventricular loop, 11, 18
  formation of, 24
ventricular mass, 169
ventricular myocardium, 34
ventricular outflow tract, 27, 170, 263, 355, 372, 395
  dissection of the, *179*
  dissection the right of the, *66*
  left, 22, 23, 60, 83, 102–105, *104*, 108, 196, 246, 327
  left ventricular entrance and, 356
  narrowing of the, 210
  narrowing of the left, 206
  obstructions in, 325, 344
  obstructions in the left, 250
  obstructions in the right, 240, *See also* tetralogy of Fallot
  opening the heart through the, 379
  right, 71, 327, *379*
  rotation of, 332
  stenosis of the right, 252
  with transposition, *331*
ventricular pre-excitation, 138–144
ventricular relationships, 167–169
ventricular repair, 235
ventricular septal defect, 252, 305, 326
  malalignment, *327*
  restrictive, *431*, *436*
ventricular septal defects, 226, *330*
  anatomy of, 264
ventricular septum, 175, 176, 249
  musculature of the, *224*
ventricular tachycardias
  curing, 147
ventricular topology, 470
  basic patterns of, 165
ventriculo-arterial connections, *163*, *168*, 169, 226, 392, 453
  concordant, 169, 235, *330*, 399, *403*
  discordant, 169
ventriculo-arterial junctions, 77, 169, 170, 263, 321, 369
ventriculo-infundibular fold, 107, 111, 170, 246, 247, 248, 261, 262, 263, 327, 361–365
  fusing with the septomarginal trabeculation, 222, 224, 262
  fusion with septal band, 325
  left-side, 110
  medial margin of, 143
  underside of, 95
  with the supraventricular crest, 123, *179*, 261
ventriculo-pulmonary arterial junction
  rights, *279*
visceral heterotaxy, 407

Wolff–Parkinson–White syndrome, 138, 139

xiphoid process, 1